P9-DTS-182

Handbook of
Implicit
Cognition
and
Addiction

Handbook of
Implicit
Cognition
and
Addiction

EDITORS

REINOUT W. WIERS
University of Maastricht, The Netherlands

ALAN W. STACY
University of Southern California

SAGE Publications
Thousand Oaks ▪ London ▪ New Delhi

Copyright © 2006 by Sage Publications, Inc.

All rights reserved. No part of this book may be reproduced or utilized in any form or by any means, electronic or mechanical, including photocopying, recording, or by any information storage and retrieval system, without permission in writing from the publisher.

For information:

Sage Publications, Inc.
2455 Teller Road
Thousand Oaks, California 91320
E-mail: order@sagepub.com

Sage Publications Ltd.
1 Oliver's Yard
55 City Road
London EC1Y 1SP
United Kingdom

Sage Publications India Pvt. Ltd.
B-42, Panchsheel Enclave
Post Box 4109
New Delhi 110 017 India

Printed in the United States of America on acid-free paper

Library of Congress Cataloging-in-Publication Data

Handbook of implicit cognition and addiction / edited by Reinout W. Wiers, Alan W. Stacy.
    p. cm.
Includes bibliographical references and index.
ISBN 1-4129-0974-0 (cloth)
    1. Substance abuse—Handbooks, manuals, etc. 2. Compulsive behavior—Handbooks, manuals, etc. 3. Cognition—Handbooks, manuals, etc. I. Wiers, Reinout Willem Henry Jon, 1966- II. Stacy, Alan W.
RC564.H3583 2006
362.2′5—dc22

2005015545

05   06   07   08   09   10   9   8   7   6   5   4   3   2   1

Acquiring Editor:	Jim Brace-Thompson
Editorial Assistant:	Karen Ehrmann
Production Editor:	Sanford Robinson
Copy Editor:	Taryn L. Bigelow
Typesetter:	C&M Digitals (P) Ltd.
Indexer:	Jeanne Busemeyer
Cover Designer:	Janet Foulger

Library
University of Texas
at San Antonio

Contents

CHAPTER 1

Implicit Cognition and Addiction: An Introduction

Reinout W. Wiers and Alan W. Stacy

IMPLICIT COGNITION

Until recently, most research on cognitive processes and drug abuse has focused on theories and methods of explicit cognition. When explicit cognition is assessed, people are asked directly to introspect about the causes of their behavior, usually through traditional questionnaires. It may be questioned, however, to what extent such methods reflect fundamental aspects of human cognition and motivation. Therefore, basic cognition researchers have turned to indirect methods to assess implicit cognitions, defined as "introspectively unidentified (or inaccurately identified) traces of past experience that mediate feeling, thought, or action" (Greenwald & Banaji, 1995; see De Houwer, Chapter 2, for issues regarding the definition of implicit cognition). In this book, we use the term "implicit" to refer to indirect measures as well as to implicit, automatic processes that are likely assessed by these measures (cf. De Houwer, Chapter 2). Assessing implicit cognitions has several potential benefits:

1. Implicit measures may assess cognitive processes that are unavailable to introspection.

2. These approaches are less sensitive to self-justification and social desirability.

3. Implicit and explicit cognitions explain unique variance or different aspects of behavior.

4. Implicit cognition approaches provide a new important bridge between diverse disciplines as well as human and animal research on addiction.

In this handbook, research from a variety of relevant disciplines is brought together for the first time, including major cognitive and biological approaches to addiction, basic research on implicit cognition and dual-process models, and implications of these new views for prevention and treatment are discussed. This is done by experts working in the addictions or in allied fields such as experimental psychopathology, health psychology, cognitive science, and neuroscience. As editors, we are very happy that many experts doing work in different areas of research (often not directly related to addiction) agreed to contribute to this book. The authors include an approximately equal representation of scholars from North

America and Europe, where most of the research on implicit cognition and addiction has been conducted.

In many of the chapters, one of the systems that steers addictive behaviors is an associative system. The importance of associations or connections, broadly defined, can be traced from Aristotle, the British empiricists, and William James to contemporary work on connectionist and associative memory models of memory, modern learning theories, implicit social cognition, and neuroscience. A focus on connections among elements (e.g., concepts, affects, groups of neurons, etc.) is a different way of viewing the basis of cognition than is a focus on the elements themselves or stored facts/if-then rules about those elements (see Deutsch & Strack and McEvoy & Nelson, Chapters 4 and 5, respectively). A simple way to think about connections is that a memory or cognition does not occur in isolation. It is usually triggered (activated or engaged) by something else, either in perception or memory. This "something else" must be connected to the memory or cognition to act as a trigger, and a trigger (e.g., seeing a bottle of wine) may have a hierarchy of strength of connections with other phenomena (e.g., negative affect, positive affect, arousal, nonaffective concepts, images, etc.). Indeed, there is also evidence that associations may automatically trigger actions in the absence of conscious recollection or intentional retrieval (see Palfai, Chapter 26). Automatic activation could occur through a number of different architectures, which have different ways of modeling connections and the operation of activation (e.g., Hintzman, 1990; Smith & DeCoster, 1998). Some of these architectures can readily model higher-order cognitions such as schemas (Hintzman, 1986) or emergent properties of cognition (Bechtel & Abrahamsen, 2002), revealing that patterns of interconnection and activation across multiple units constitute more than "simple associationism."

Associations, whether measured with reaction time (RT) tests, word association, attentional bias, or other tests outlined in this book or inferred from biological measures have different implications than the storage of facts or rules. Connections involving implicit systems or processes may often have the following characteristics: They take time to establish or strengthen; once established, they operate autonomously when engaged, not requiring the intervention of other systems; they are relatively resistant to change (although they are sensitive to context effects; see Deutsch & Strack, Chapter 4; Krank & Wall, Chapter 19); and they originate from both cultural and personal experiences, including experiences involving reinforcement and affect (see McEvoy & Nelson, Chapter 5; Stacy et al., Chapter 6).

Finally, many authors have come to the conclusion that there must be a second system, or set of systems, that is rule-based and has limited capacity and that this second system also has some influence on behavior (e.g., Bechara et al., Chapter 15; Deutsch & Strack, Chapter 4; Evans & Coventry, Chapter 3; Wiers et al., Chapter 22; Yin & Knowlton, Chapter 12). An important issue, also for interventions in this domain, concerns the interplay between these systems. From this perspective, there are different ways to change addictive behaviors. First, one may attempt to change something in the automatic system. Modern learning psychology has indicated that extinction of once-established associations may be difficult if not impossible (see Hermans & Van Gucht, Chapter 32; Wiers et al., 2004). There may, however, be viable alternatives, such as increasing aversive associations (which has an old tradition; see Wiers et al., Chapter 22), strengthening associations between triggers of addictive behaviors with alternative behaviors (e.g., Palfai, Chapter 26; Prestwich et al., Chapter 29), or "attentional retraining" procedures (see de Jong et al., Chapter 27; Fadardi et al., Chapter 9).

Second, there may be ways to use the second rule-based system in changing behavior. Mere inhibition of impulses from the associative system may be counterproductive (see Palfai, Chapter 26), but this system may be used to establish alternative associations (e.g., Palfai, Chapter 26) or to counter the influence of the associations on behavior (e.g., Marlatt & Ostafin, Chapter 33).

ADDICTION

Before turning to a brief introduction of the sections in this book, the second part of the title of the book may need some clarification. Why did we use the term "addiction" and not "substance dependence," as current psychiatric classification schemas would want us to categorize the disorders central in this book? The first reason is that we did not want to restrict ourselves to addictive behaviors that involve substances, because interesting work is done with respect to other addictions, such as gambling (see Evans & Coventry, Chapter 3; Zack & Poulos, Chapter 24). Second, some of the applications in the book refer to prevention of addictions; also from that perspective the general term addiction seemed most appropriate. Third, in many current conceptualizations of addiction (unlike current psychiatric classification schemes) appetitive motivations are important (Robinson & Berridge, 2003; Stewart et al., 1984; Wise and Bozarth, 1987). The related concept of "incentive sensitization" (Robinson & Berridge, 1993, 2003), based on work in animal models, has stirred enthusiasm in recent theorizing about implicit cognitive processes involved in addiction. Sensitization refers to the hypersensitization of mesolimbic circuits to drug effects and drug-associated stimuli. Robinson and Berridge (1993, 2003) proposed that psychologically this leads to the excessive attribution of incentive salience to drug-related representations, causing

pathological "wanting." Implicit "wanting" is "similar to implicit memory and to unconscious perception (e.g., blindsight), which can occur and influence behavior without conscious awareness" (Robinson & Berridge, 2003, p. 36). Implicit "wanting" need not lead to subjective wanting, and can influence behavior without it (see also Berridge & Robinson, Chapter 31). The incentive-sensitization theory has been linked to a variety of implicit cognitive mechanisms in addiction, including the most dominant ones: attentional bias and implicit drug associations (e.g., Chapters 10, 11, 17, 21, 22, 24, and 27). In addition, important transfer effects have been noted in animals (e.g., cross-sensitization, see Chapter 31) and recently similar findings have been reported in humans between different drugs (Ostafin & Palfai, Chapter 25) and between drugs and gambling (Zack & Poulos, Chapter 24), underscoring the use of "addiction" rather than substance dependence (note that the concepts of incentive motivation and sensitization are not represented in current psychiatric classification schemes). The link between neurobiological work on sensitization and implicit cognition in human addictions emphasizes the potential bridging function of implicit cognition in addiction, where so far human and animal work have been relatively isolated.

GENERAL OUTLINE
OF THE BOOK

The book consists of seven sections.

Section I focuses on general theoretical issues regarding implicit and explicit cognition in general and in relation to addiction. In Chapter 2, De Houwer argues that implicit measures are measurement outcomes that have certain functional properties that should be critically evaluated, as has been done for the related concept of automaticity. He concludes that to the extent that implicit measures reflect the automatic impact of attitudes and cognitions, they could provide a unique insight into the effects of automatic processing on real-life behavior. As noted above, many researchers have turned to the use of implicit measures from a dual-process perspective. The general idea is that human behavior is steered by two relatively independent systems, one of which can be characterized as fast, automatic, and associative, whereas the other is relatively slow, effortful, and controlled (Deutsch & Strack, Chapter 4; Evans & Coventry, Chapter 3; Strack & Deutsch, 2004). Emphasizing the relative independence of the processes, Evans (2003) paraphrased them as "two minds in one head." From this perspective, the use of implicit measures may provide a unique window to tap into the fast, automatic, and associative processes that partly steer behavior (especially under circumstances when effortful control processes are difficult to engage; cf. Fillmore & Vogel-Sprott, Chapter 20). The chapters by Evans and Coventry (Chapter 3) and Deutsch and Strack (Chapter 4) have been inspired by research in the areas of cognitive and social psychology. Both chapters present general functional dual-process models and apply them to addiction. Both models are functional in the sense that they do not directly link the proposed systems to underlying neurobiological mechanisms (cf. Chapters 12 and 15 in Section III for neurobiologically based multiple-process models). Another area of research in which the implicit-explicit distinction has been prominent is memory research. McEvoy and Nelson (Chapter 5) review different techniques for studying implicit memory: the methods of savings and of indirect test instructions, and the process dissociation procedure (see also Chapter 20). They then describe their model of cued recall that incorporates both implicit and explicit memory processes (PIER2, which is described in Chapter 5; Nelson et al., 1998), and illustrate it with examples relevant to addictive behaviors.

Section II focuses on assessment paradigms and their theoretical basis. In the first chapter in this section, Stacy et al. (Chapter 6) discuss basic memory research on word association and illustrate how several well-supported cognitive models (such as PIER2) can use these assessments of association to help explain and understand addictive behaviors. In Chapter 7, Houben et al. describe a different assessment approach: reaction time tests of associations that have generated much recent enthusiasm about implicit measures. They describe several of the major reaction time tests, including different recent versions of the Implicit Association Test (IAT), the Extrinsic Affective Simon Task (EAST), and several semantic and affective priming tests, with applications to addiction. In Chapter 8, Goldman et al. group many different assessment paradigms under the umbrella of their general expectancy theory, contending that expectancies can be assessed with either direct or indirect methods. In this approach, "expectancies" are seen as reflections of different processing systems that are shaped by evolution to anticipate the future. In Chapter 9, Fadardi et al. discuss individualized versus general measures of implicit cognition. This issue is relevant for whatever assessment tool is used, because the assessment may show utility only when the stimuli are tailored to the individual. The final two chapters of Section II both focus on measures of attentional bias. Bruce and Jones (Chapter 10) review methods used to assess and understand attentional bias in addiction, with a focus on the use of the emotional or drug-related Stroop paradigm. The emerging picture over different tests is that there might be a continuity of attentional bias along the consumption continuum from light to heavy use to problematic use (but see Chapter 21). Field et al. (Chapter 11) review models that assume that attentional biases occur at early stages of stimulus processing, and that attentional biases are associated with subjective craving and the tendency to approach drug-related cues and discuss relevant empirical findings. These include studies that have used visual-probe tasks and eye movement monitoring techniques to investigate the component processes of biases in visual orienting to drug-related stimuli (attracting vs. maintaining attention). It is argued that attentional biases in addictive and appetitive behaviors are qualitatively different from those in anxiety. Despite their differences, each of the strategies outlined in these chapters converge on assessing fundamental cognitive and attentional biases and these biases are likely to channel behavior down certain routes, in either harmful or beneficial directions.

Section III focuses on brain mechanisms underlying addiction. In Chapter 12, Yin and Knowlton outline different types of learning and their different neural substrates (circuits rather than structures) and the different roles these systems play in addictive behaviors. In Chapter 13, Franken et al. review findings in humans with recent functional imaging techniques, concerning the neural correlates (neuroanatomy and neurotransmitters) of general psychological processes that play a role in addiction: reward, craving, attention, memory, and decision making. In Chapter 14, Mucha et al. discuss other physiological measures that can be used in humans to assess drug-related motivation in an indirect way, with an emphasis on the startle-response measures. A common theme is that indices of brain functioning in addiction in humans (e.g., psychophysiological measures, functional imaging techniques) can be viewed as another indirect way to assess motivation underlying addiction. There has been, however, a paucity of studies directly comparing indirect brain measures and indirect cognitive measures. In Chapter 15, Bechara et al. propose their neurologically inspired dual-process model to explain addictive behaviors. They present results that indicate that at least three different (nonexclusive) processes

can be involved in addictions: strong automatic appetitive associations, two different problems in the reflective system, and problems related to decision making and to impulse control. These different neurological problems may characterize subgroups of individuals prone to addictions. In the last chapter of Section III, Curtin et al. (Chapter 16) present a model of implicit and explicit motivational processes in drug use, integrating basic neuroscience research on cognitive control and research on bottom-up motivational processes. It is argued that both positive (approach) and negative reinforcement (withdrawal) motivation can be triggered automatically, and that craving is a function of cognitive control systems reacting to automatically activated tendencies to use drugs (cf. Tiffany, 1990). The model further states that other situations that recruit cognitive control will result in craving, such as response conflict and novel or unfavorable outcomes. This chapter provides a bridge to the next section.

Section IV presents work on the interplay between implicit and explicit cognitive processes, emotion and motivation, and context effects in addictive behaviors. In Chapter 17, Cox et al. present their motivational theory of current concerns. Current concerns influence behavior by keeping an individual oriented toward cues and actions that advance the attainment of the goal. The underlying process is thought to be unconscious, but goals usually become conscious. Applied to addictive behaviors, performing addictive behaviors to regulate one's emotions can become an automatized goal, resulting in an attentional bias. This model has important implications for treatment: It is important to set alternative goals (e.g., through motivational techniques) and the attentional bias may be unlearned (e.g., through attentional retraining). Regarding the association between emotions and drug use, Birch et al. (Chapter 18) conclude that there is little evidence for simple relationships. Models that take into account moderators like individual differences in drug-use motives, however, better explain the data. Motivational theories generally distinguish between two broad classes of motivation for drug use: positive and negative reinforcement (e.g., Cooper et al., 1995; Curtin et al., Chapter 16), and the scarce evidence is consistent with the idea that in individuals who have strong enhancement motives, positive emotions activate both implicit and explicit motivations to use alcohol or drugs. For negative reinforcement (drinking to relieve tension or negative affect), however, results are less consistent: A negative mood has been found to activate explicit but not implicit coping motives (Birch et al., Chapter 18; cf. Wiers et al., Chapter 22). Context has been known for some time to affect cognition, memory, and drug-use behaviors. Krank and Wall (Chapter 19) review and integrate this literature. Although "context" is usually thought of in physical terms, an emotion can also function as a context for drug use, and recent evidence suggests that context also plays an important role in assessment, both for more implicit (e.g., Mitchell et al., 2003) and more explicit assessment methods (e.g., Schwartz, 1999). In Chapter 20, Fillmore and Vogel-Sprott review the effects of alcohol and other drugs on the relative contributions of automatic versus controlled processes using the process dissociation approach. It is argued that the ability of drugs to promote a reliance on automatic influences could explain a broad range of behavioral effects observed in the drugged state, and provide new insights into factors that contribute to drug abuse.

Section V is organized by addictive behavior. In Chapter 21, Waters and Sayette systematically review the literature on automatic affective and motivational processes in smoking. They conclude that there are robust differences regarding an attentional bias for smoking-related stimuli in smokers, not found in nonsmokers, but that there appears to be no strong relation with heaviness of smoking or abstinence (cf. Chapter 10). In Chapter 22, Wiers et al. review the work on implicit cognition in relation to alcohol use and abuse, using the three broad categories of alcohol-related cognitions that have emerged from research using explicit measures: positive and negative reinforcement and negative expectancies. Most research has focused on positive reinforcement, revealing ample evidence for automatic appetitive reactions in heavy and problem drinkers (attentional bias, automatic arousal or approach associations). In addition, there is more scattered evidence for the existence of automatic negative associations. It is argued that implicit negative reinforcement expectancies may be difficult to assess because in contrast to positive and negative associations, they involve two different associations. Ames et al. (Chapter 23) review literature on implicit cognitions in drugs of abuse with an emphasis on substances other than alcohol and cigarettes. For a variety of substances, implicit memory association measures and reaction time measures have been found to successfully predict addictive behaviors and to predict a different portion of the variance in behavior than explicit measures. Ames and her colleagues also point at the importance of implementing these measures in intervention research. As indicated earlier, the other two chapters of this section review recent work on implicit cognition and gambling (Zack & Poulos, Chapter 24) and cross-drug effects (Ostafin & Palfai, Chapter 25).

Section VI focuses on implications of the implicit cognition approach for interventions (prevention and treatment) in addiction (readers interested in this topic should note that many chapters outside this section also make useful suggestions for interventions). In the first chapter of this section, Palfai (Chapter 26) discusses self-regulation in addictive behaviors. Usually self-regulation is seen as the product of conscious, controlled processing, which serves to counter impulsive tendencies to use drugs (cf. Chapters 3, 4, 15). Recent research in social cognition indicates, however, that automatic processes play an important role in self-regulation (in line with the automatic pursuit of goals proposed in Chapter 17). From this perspective, new strategies for interventions can be derived to harness implicit processes in support of alternative goals and behaviors. De Jong et al. (Chapter 27) review work in other areas of psychopathology (anxiety and eating disorders) on the role of implicit cognition in the etiology and maintenance of problem behaviors. Given promising results in these other areas, they suggest the possibility of attentional retraining in addiction interventions, a topic currently investigated in several labs. In Chapter 28, Krank and Goldstein focus on how implicit cognition can be used in understanding the etiology and prevention of addictive behaviors in adolescence. Importantly, they indicate that implicit cognition measures can be used to prospectively predict changes in drug-use behavior (alcohol and marijuana), including early transitional stages. They also review suggestions on countering the influence of implicit drug associations and the influence of alcohol advertising (e.g., inoculation training). In the final chapter of this section, Prestwich et al. (Chapter 29) review the recent literature on implementation intentions, an example of a specific form of planning (in if-then format) that has been found to successfully influence a variety of health behaviors in an automatic way. The application of this and other strategies in this section to addictive behavior provides an exciting new opportunity to improve intervention effects.

Section VII contains invited commentaries by outside experts not working directly on implicit cognition and addiction (except for one coauthor, Ostafin). Commentaries are provided by Sher, a leader in research on the

origins of addictive behaviors in humans (Chapter 30); by Berridge and Robinson, two of the leading researchers on neurobiological processes in addiction (Chapter 31); by Hermans and Van Gucht, experts on learning theory and psychopathology (Chapter 32); and by Marlatt (with Ostafin, Chapter 33), a leader in relapse prevention, who discusses clinical applications of implicit cognition. In the final chapter (34) we give our concluding comments, which address some common themes, directions for the future, and challenges.

FINAL NOTE

We hope that this volume will stimulate further research on implicit cognition and addiction. All chapters have been reviewed by the editors and at least two other peer reviewers, usually authors from other (related) chapters and in some cases outside experts. We believe this procedure has increased the quality of the chapters and stimulated their integration. As the contents of this volume illustrate, implicit cognition is a rapidly growing direction in addiction research. This is not surprising, given the current interest in implicit cognition in general and the fact that addictive behaviors strike many as "irrational" behaviors par excellence. We hope this book will help to further integrate research from different independent fields that are all relevant for a better understanding of the etiology, maintenance, and prevention or treatment of addictive behaviors. We hope that this book will both stimulate further research and theorizing in this area and provide the groundwork for new approaches in the prevention and treatment of addictive behaviors. Finally, we thank all authors for their contributions and reviews, and acknowledge the outstanding editorial assistance of James Pike, Brian Houska, and Deborah Jelinek. We also acknowledge support from grants from the National Science Foundation of The

Netherlands (N.W.O.) VIDI grant 452.03.005 and from the National Institute on Drug Abuse (DA 16094) for research by the editors and by several of the chapter authors.

REFERENCES

Bechtel, W., & Abrahamsen, A. (2002). *Connectionism and the mind: Parallel processing, dynamics, and evolution in networks* (2nd ed.). Malden, MA: Blackwell.

Cooper, M. L., Frone, M. R., Russell, M., & Mudar, P. (1995). Drinking to regulate positive and negative emotions: A motivational model of alcohol use. *Journal of Personality and Social Psychology, 69,* 990–1005.

Evans, J. St. B. T. (2003). In two minds: Dual-process accounts of reasoning. *Trends in Cognitive Science, 7*(10), 454–459.

Greenwald, A. G., & Banaji, M. R. (1995). Implicit social cognition: Attitudes, self-esteem, and stereotypes. *Psychological Review, 102*(1), 4–27.

Hintzman, D. L. (1986). "Schema abstraction" in a multiple-trace memory model. *Psychological Review, 93*(4), 411–428.

Hintzman, D. L. (1990). Human learning and memory: Connections and dissociations. *Annual Review of Psychology, 41,* 109–139.

Mitchell, J. P., Nosek, B. A., & Banaji, M. R. (2003). Contextual variations in implicit evaluation. *Journal of Experimental Psychology, 132,* 455–469.

Nelson, D. L., McKinney, V. M., Gee, N. R., & Janczura, G. A. (1998). Interpreting the influence of implicitly activated memories on recall and recognition. *Psychological Review, 105,* 299–324.

Robinson, T. E., & Berridge, K. C. (1993). The neural basis of drug craving: An incentive-sensitization theory of addiction. *Brain Research Reviews, 18,* 247–291.

Robinson, T. E., & Berridge, K. C. (2003). Addiction. *Annual Review of Psychology, 54,* 25–53.

Schwartz, N. (1999). Self-reports. How questions shape the answers. *American Psychologist, 54,* 93–105.

Smith, E. R., & DeCoster, J. (1998). Knowledge acquisition, accessibility, and use in person perception and stereotyping: Simulation with a recurrent connectionist network. *Journal of Personality and Social Psychology, 74*(1), 21–35.

Stewart, J., de Wit, H., & Eikelboom, R. (1984). The role of unconditioned and conditioned drug effects in the self-administration of opiates and stimulants. *Psychological Review, 91,* 251–268.

Strack, F., & Deutsch, R. (2004). Reflective and impulsive determinants of social behavior. *Personality and Social Psychology Review, 3,* 220–247.

Tiffany, S.T. (1990). A cognitive model of drug urges and drug-use behavior: Role of automatic and nonautomatic processes. *Psychological Review, 97,* 147–168.

Wiers, R. W., de Jong, P. J., Havermans, R., & Jelicic, M. (2004). How to change implicit drug-related cognitions in prevention: A transdisciplinary integration of findings from experimental psychopathology, social cognition, memory and learning psychology. *Substance Use & Misuse, 39,* 1625–1684.

Wise, R., & Bozarth, M. (1987). A psychomotor stimulant theory of addiction. *Psychological Review, 94,* 469–492.

Section I

DEFINITIONS, GENERAL THEORETICAL ISSUES, AND FUNCTIONAL DUAL-PROCESS MODELS

CHAPTER 2

What Are Implicit Measures and Why Are We Using Them?

JAN DE HOUWER

Abstract: I argue that implicit measures are measurement outcomes that have certain functional properties. The expression "indirect measure," however, refers to an objective property of the measurement procedure, being that the researcher does not assess the attitude on the basis of a self-assessment by the participant but on the basis of another behavior. With regard to the question of why one should use implicit measures, research suggests that they do not allow one to register stable structures in memory. It is also doubtful that they provide an index of implicit attitudes. But to the extent that implicit measures reflect the automatic impact of attitudes and cognitions, they could provide a unique insight into the effects of automatic processing on real-life behavior.

INTRODUCTION

For many years, psychologists have tried to measure attitudes and other cognitions in an attempt to understand, control, or predict human behavior. Most often, they have done so using questionnaires. More recently, there has been a growing interest in a new type of measures, often denoted "implicit" or "indirect" measures. Examples of such measures are the affective priming task (e.g., Fazio et al., 1995), the Implicit Association Test (IAT; e.g., Greenwald et al., 1998), the Extrinsic Affective Simon Task (EAST; e.g., De Houwer, 2003; De Houwer & Eelen, 1998), and the word association task (e.g., Stacy, 1997; see Fazio & Olson, 2003, for a review). Implicit measures such as these are now widely used in social psychology (e.g., Greenwald et al., 1998), clinical psychology (e.g., Teachman et al., 2001), personality psychology (e.g., Asendorpf et al., 2002), marketing (e.g., Brunel et al., in press), and health psychology (e.g., Stacy, 1997; Wiers et al.,

AUTHOR'S NOTE: Preparation of this chapter was supported by Grant G.0356.03 of the Fund for Scientific Research (Flanders, Belgium). The chapter is based on a talk that I presented at the first special interest meeting on the use of indirect measures of attitudes and associations in clinical and health psychology, August 2003, Diksmuide, Belgium. I would like to thank Agnes Moors, Roland Deutsch, Alan Stacy, and Reinout Wiers for their helpful suggestions on an earlier draft.

2002). Despite their immense popularity, it is often not clear what terms such as "implicit measure," "implicit attitude," or "implicit cognition" refer to. In this chapter, I examine what it might mean to say that a measure is implicit or indirect and look at the possible benefits of using these measures. Although my analysis applies to all available implicit and indirect measures, I will focus primarily on reaction time measures such as the IAT and affective priming task simply because these are currently the most popular ones.

WHAT ARE "IMPLICIT" AND "INDIRECT" MEASURES?

What Are "Implicit Measures"?

Many researchers use the expression "implicit measures" and "indirect measures" to refer to a class of measures that are supposed to be in some way different from more traditional questionnaire measures. But what is unique about these measures? What does it mean to say that a measure is implicit or indirect? To answer this question, it is important to realize that the term "measure" can be used in different ways. It can either be used to refer to the outcome of a measurement procedure (e.g., a particular score on a questionnaire or a particular pattern of performance such as an IAT or priming effect) or to the objective measurement procedure itself (e.g., the questionnaire itself as consisting of certain instructions and certain questions or the exact instructions and stimuli that are presented during a reaction time task). A measurement procedure can be called a measure in the sense that it can in principle be used to obtain an outcome that provides an index of a construct or entity. For example, putting someone on a scale is a measure of weight in the sense that it is a procedure one can follow to obtain an estimate of someone's weight. The number provided by the

scale is the outcome of the measurement procedure. This outcome can be called a measure of weight in that it is an estimate of the actual weight of the person. For an outcome to reflect a construct or entity (such as an attitude or weight), it must somehow be (partially) produced or determined by the construct or entity. In other words, there are some underlying processes through which the construct or entity produces or determines the outcome of the measurement procedure (e.g., the processes by which the weight of the person is translated into a value on the scale).

Let us now turn to the definitions of implicit measures that can be found in recent psychological literature. Researchers have argued that, contrary to traditional (explicit) measures, implicit measures provide an index of a certain attitude or cognition even though participants (1) are not aware of the fact that the attitude or cognition is being measured (e.g., Brunel et al., in press), (2) do not have conscious access to the attitude or cognition (e.g., Asendorpf et al., 2002), or (3) have no control over the measurement outcome (e.g., Fazio & Olson, 2003). What is clear from these definitions is that they do not refer to objective properties of the measurement procedure itself. A procedure is merely a set of guidelines about what one should do as a researcher. Rather, the definitions of "implicit measure" that can be found in the literature refer to the conditions under which the outcome of the procedure functions as an index of the to-be-measured attitude or cognition. In line with the available definitions, one can therefore say that the term "implicit measure" refers to certain functional properties of measurement outcomes: The outcome functions as an index of an attitude or cognition despite the fact that participants are unaware of the impact of the attitude or cognition on the outcome, are not aware of the attitude or outcome, or have no control over the outcome. Because a measurement outcome can only function as a measure by the grace of certain underlying processes (see above), the functional properties of a measurement outcome therefore actually refer to the conditions under which the underlying processes operate.

This analysis leads to four important conclusions. First, the term "implicit measure" refers to the functional properties of measurement outcomes (e.g., an IAT *effect* defined as the difference between the compatible and incompatible test block) rather than to the measurement procedure (e.g., a particular IAT task as involving certain stimuli, responses, and instructions). From now on, when I use the term "implicit measure," I thus refer to a measurement outcome rather than a measurement procedure. Second, because the term "implicit measure" can refer to several functional properties, it is necessary to specify which properties one has in mind. For instance, rather than claiming that a measure *is* implicit, one could say that a measure is implicit *in the sense that* participants are not aware of what the measurement outcome reflects. Third, to conclude that a measure is actually implicit in a certain sense, one has to verify empirically whether it possesses the specified functional properties. That is, it is necessary not only to examine whether the measure does provide a reliable index of the to be-measured attitude or cognition (that it is reliable and valid) but also whether specified conditions are met. For instance, before a measure can be called implicit in the sense of unaware, it needs to be verified empirically as to whether participants are indeed unaware of the fact that the outcome reflects a certain attitude or whether they are unaware of the attitude itself. Whether a measure is reliable and valid always needs to be checked (if it is not, the measurement outcome is not a measure in the true sense of the word). But if one makes the additional claim that a measure is implicit, one also needs to specify and examine its functional properties. Fourth, the various functional properties that have been assigned to implicit measures do not necessarily co-occur. For instance, if one can demonstrate that participants have little control over the outcome of a measurement procedure, this does not imply that the participants are unaware of the attitude or cognition that is being measured. Therefore, each functional property has to be examined for each measure separately. This is also why one always needs to specify in which sense a measure is implicit. If, for instance, a measure cannot be controlled by the participant but the participant is typically aware of the attitude or cognition that is being measured, one should describe this measure as a measure that is implicit in the sense of uncontrollable (but not in the sense of unaware).

I am thus arguing that a conditional approach of the term "implicit measure" is warranted. This approach is in many ways similar to a conditional approach of the concept "automaticity." Researchers such as Logan (1985) and Bargh (1992) correctly pointed out that the term "automaticity" can refer to several functional properties that often do not co-occur. Therefore, to say that a process is automatic, one needs to specify the properties that the process possesses (e.g., unconscious, involuntary, effortless, goal-independent, *and/or* controllable) and conduct extensive research to check for each automaticity property separately whether it applies to that process. A similar approach is needed if one wants to continue to use the term "implicit measure" in a meaningful manner. A conditional approach to the concept "implicit measure" would also avoid unproductive debates about whether a measurement outcome is "truly" implicit. Just like there are probably few processes that have all the properties of an automatic process, there are probably few measures that are implicit in all possible senses of the word. Therefore, findings that show that a measurement outcome does not have a particular property of implicit measures do not allow one to conclude that it is not "truly" implicit. A more productive approach is to examine in what sense the measure is implicit.

Because both "implicit" and "automatic" refer to functional properties, one could also use a conditional approach to examine whether and in what sense implicit measures are automatic measures. In fact, several of the functional properties that are attributed to implicit measures are actually properties that are also attributed to automatic processes. For instance, both implicit and automatic processes can be characterized as uncontrollable (participants cannot control the outcome of the process) or unconscious (either in the sense that participants are unaware of the fact that an effect was due to a particular process or that participants do not have conscious access to the process that produced the effect). It might even be useful to replace the term "implicit measure" with "automatic measure" because much more is known about the functional properties that the term "automatic" can refer to (e.g., Bargh, 1992; Logan, 1985; Moors & De Houwer, in press). Also, whereas "implicit" is most often used to refer to the property "unconscious," the term "automatic" is traditionally used to refer to a much wider range of functional properties. Replacing the term "implicit measure" with the term "automatic measure" might thus broaden the scope of research on the functional properties of these measures.

In sum, one can define an implicit measure as a measurement outcome that reflects a certain attitude or cognition in an automatic manner, where "automatic" needs to be specified in terms of the presence of one or more functional features. Although one can have a debate about which properties are central to the concept of automaticity (see Moors & De Houwer, 2004), the fact remains that one cannot use the term

"implicit measure" in a meaningful manner without (1) making explicit the functional properties of the measurement outcome that one is referring to, and (2) providing empirical evidence that supports these functional properties. Although such a conditional approach to the concept "implicit measure" or "automatic measure" is thus necessary and would avoid a lot of confusion, it is rarely adopted. In the next section, I briefly summarize some of the research that has examined the functional properties of so-called implicit measures that are used in current research.

Evidence for the Implicit or Automatic Nature of Implicit Measurement Outcomes

Are existing implicit measures implicit in the sense that participants are unaware of the fact that the measurement outcome measures something?

Surprisingly, whether participants are indeed unaware of the fact that implicit measures measure something is almost never examined. One study that did probe this suggests that, at least in some cases, participants do know what is measured. Monteith et al. (2001) interviewed participants about their experiences with a race IAT. During the race IAT, positive words (e.g., happy), negative words (e.g., disgusting), first names typical of white Americans (e.g., John), and first names typical of black Americans (e.g., Jamel) were presented one by one on the screen. Participants responded to each stimulus by pressing one of two keys on the basis of the category to which the stimulus belonged (i.e., positive, negative, white, black). As is typically found in race IAT studies, participants were slower when they pressed one key for positive words and black names and the other key for negative words and white names (incompatible task) than when they pressed one key for positive words and white names and the other key for negative words and black names (compatible task). Such a result is taken as evidence for the hypothesis that (white) American people have a more negative attitude toward black people than toward white people. What is interesting for the present purpose is that 64 percent of the participants noticed that they were faster in the compatible task than in the incompatible task. Of the participants who noticed that they were faster in the compatible task, 37 percent attributed this slower performance to the fact that they apparently had a more negative attitude toward black people than toward white people. This result strongly suggests that a substantial number of the participants are aware of what a race IAT measures.

Studies by Duscherer et al. (2002) suggest that participants are often also aware of affective Simon effects and the origins of such effects. They used a standard affective Simon task during which positive and negative nouns (e.g., FLOWER, CANCER) and adjectives (e.g., HAPPY, DISGUSTING) were presented one by one on a computer screen. Half of the participants were instructed to say "GOOD" whenever an adjective was presented and "BAD" whenever a noun appeared, irrespective of the (good or bad) meaning of the noun or adjective. The response assignments were reversed for the other participants (i.e., say "GOOD" to nouns and "BAD" to adjectives). Reaction times were slower when the meaning of the correct response was incompatible with the meaning of the presented word (e.g., say "GOOD" to DISGUSTING because it is an adjective; incongruent trial) than when the meaning of the correct response and the presented word matched (e.g., say "BAD" to CANCER because it is a noun; congruent trial). But when asked to guess what the purpose of the experiments was, almost 80 percent of the participants mentioned that the purpose was to see whether the match between the valence of the word and the response influenced the speed of responding. Importantly, participants who realized this also showed a bigger Simon effect (i.e., more delay and errors on incongruent trials). This suggests that the outcome of certain measurement procedures might in part depend on whether participants have an insight into the measure.

In sum, one cannot simply assume that existing implicit measures such as IAT and Simon effects are implicit in the sense that they reflect attitudes and cognitions even though participants are not aware that the outcome reflects these attitudes or cognitions. Instead, this property needs to be verified empirically before any claim can be made about it. Although initial studies suggest that participants are often aware of the purpose of popular implicit measures such as the IAT, it is likely that some measures are implicit in this sense. For instance, research has shown that affective priming effects can be found even when the primes are presented subliminally (e.g., Klauer et al., 2003). That is, when a target (e.g., HAPPY) is preceded by a subliminally presented prime stimulus that has the same valence as the target (e.g., FLOWER), participants need less time to respond to the target than when the target is preceded by a subliminally presented prime with a different valence (e.g., CANCER). One could use this procedure to measure attitudes. For example, in order to examine whether someone has a positive or negative attitude toward smoking, one could present a smoking-related prime word in a subliminal manner and examine whether responses are faster when this word is followed by positive targets (in which case one can infer a positive attitude toward smoking) or when the word is followed by negative targets (in which case one can infer a negative attitude toward smoking). If such a measure works, it is likely that participants are unaware of what the task measures simply because they are unaware of the priming stimuli (i.e., the smoking-related words). It remains to be seen, however, whether such an implicit measure produces reliable and valid results (see Banse, 2001, for data with regard to the limited reliability of subliminal affective priming measures).

Are implicit measures implicit in the sense that participants are unaware of the attitude or cognition that is measured?

Rather than being unaware of the fact that the measure is measuring something, participants might be unaware of the attitude or cognition that is being measured. Do existing implicit measures (i.e., measurement outcomes) provide an index of such unconscious attitudes or cognitions? As Fazio and Olson (2003) pointed out, this is almost never checked. Moreover, often participants do realize that they possess the attitude or cognition that is being measured. For instance, flower-insect IAT studies revealed that participants are faster when they need to press one key for flower names (e.g., TULIP) and positive words (e.g., HAPPY) and the other key for insect names (e.g., COCKROACH) and negative words (e.g., DISGUSTING) than in a task where the response assignments are reversed (i.e., press one key for flower names and negative words and the other key for insect names and positive words). This result is in line with the idea that most people have a more positive attitude toward flowers than toward insects. But in all likelihood, the participants were aware of the fact that they liked flowers more than insects. It thus seems safe to conclude that implicit measures such as the IAT can register attitudes and cognitions that are available to consciousness. Therefore, one cannot simply interpret an implicit measure such as the IAT effect as reflecting the strength of an unconscious attitude or cognition (also see Fazio & Olson, 2003).

This does not imply that implicit measures can never register attitudes or cognitions that participants are unaware of. For instance, Olson and Fazio (2001) used an evaluative conditioning procedure to induce a positive or negative attitude toward certain Pokemon characters. That is, they unobtrusively paired one Pokemon with negative stimuli (e.g., the picture of a dead cow) and another Pokemon with positive stimuli (e.g., the picture of a puppy). Afterward, participants indicated that they liked the first Pokemon less than the second one even though they were unaware of the fact that one Pokemon was previously paired with positive stimuli and the other with negative stimuli. These implicitly learned attitudes were also detected using an IAT and a subliminal affective priming procedure. One can thus conclude that measures such as the IAT and subliminal affective priming can detect attitudes that participants have learned unconsciously. But it remains the case that these measures can also be influenced by attitudes that participants have learned in a conscious, controlled manner. Moreover, one might argue that participants in the Olson and Fazio study were aware of their attitudes in the sense that they could consciously report which Pokemon they liked best. Their attitude was "implicit" only in the sense that they were not aware of the reasons for their attitudes and could thus not provide an accurate justification for their attitudes. I will discuss the issue of whether and in what sense attitudes can be unconscious or implicit in the second part of this chapter. For now, it is sufficient to realize that, although implicit measures might sometimes register unaware attitudes and cognitions, one can certainly not assume that the outcome of implicit measures provides a direct and exclusive index of such unaware cognitions.

Are implicit measures implicit in the sense that participants cannot strategically control the outcome of the measure?

One of the most popular reasons for using so-called implicit measures is that they are supposed to be less susceptible to deception and social desirability. This argument is based mainly on the assumption that participants cannot strategically control (the impact of the attitude or cognition on) the outcome of the measurement procedure. But what does the evidence tell us?

There are some studies in which participants were asked to fake a certain attitude on the IAT. Kim (2003) instructed participants to perform a race IAT in such a way that it would not provide evidence for a racial bias against black people. These instructions had no impact on IAT scores. Lowery et al. (2001), however, did find less evidence for racial prejudice as measured by the IAT when participants were asked to be as unprejudiced as possible. They also found that Caucasian (but not Asian) participants showed less prejudice on the IAT when the experimenter was black than when he or she was white. Banse et al. (2001) found that heterosexual participants were unable to fake a positive attitude toward homosexuality on the IAT. Asendorpf et al. (2002) and Egloff and Schmulke (2002) failed to find a significant effect of faking instructions on the outcome of IAT measures of shyness or anxiety. Steffens (2004), however, noted that in the studies of Banse et al., Asendorpf et al., and Egloff and Schmulke, there was a nonsignificant trend toward an effect of faking instructions (Cohen's *d* effect size of between .13 and .39, *M* = .23). Steffens argued that participants might be better able to fake a certain attitude on the IAT when they already had some experience with the IAT. To test this prediction, all participants completed the same IAT twice and were given faking instructions before completing the second IAT. Steffens observed a small effect of faking instructions on an IAT designed to measure conscientiousness and a large effect on an IAT designed to measure introversion and extroversion. In the latter case, participants who were instructed to fake extroversion on average had an IAT score that suggested that they were extroverted (i.e.,

faster when self and extroversion items were assigned to the same key) whereas participants who were instructed to fake introversion had an IAT score that classified them as introverted (i.e., faster when self and introversion items were assigned to the same key). Although these findings suggest that participants can control the outcome of at least some IATs, it should be noted that the impact of faking instructions on the IAT was smaller than the impact of such instructions on the outcome of questionnaires. One can thus still argue that IAT effects are less susceptible to faking than (some) traditional questionnaire measures. Moreover, in the study of Steffens (2004), there still was a significant correlation between the scores of individuals on the first administration of the IAT (at a time when they were not asked to fake) and their scores on the second IAT (when they were asked to fake). This suggests that participants are unable to completely hide their "true" attitudes and associations when asked to fake.

A closer inspection of the data of Steffens (2004) suggests that participants can fake a certain attitude or association on the IAT by intentionally slowing down their reaction times (or increasing the number of errors) during certain phases of the IAT. There is, however, also a more subtle manner in which participants can strategically influence the outcome of an IAT and other implicit measures. Research has shown that implicit measurement outcomes are very context-dependent (see Blair, 2002, for a review). For instance, Mitchell et al. (2003, Experiment 1) presented names of liked black athletes, disliked white politicians, positive words, and negative words. When participants were asked to respond to the names on the basis of occupation (athlete or politician) and to words on the basis of valence, the IAT revealed a more positive attitude toward black athletes than toward white politicians. When the race of the names was relevant (black or white), however, a more positive attitude toward white politicians was found. Likewise, Dasgupta and Greenwald (2001) found smaller race IAT effects (i.e., less prejudice against black people as measured by the IAT) when participants saw names of admired black Americans and disliked white Americans before completing the race IAT. This suggests that participants can influence the outcome of an IAT by intentionally retrieving certain information or paying attention to certain features. For instance, when participants complete an extroversion-introversion IAT and are asked to fake being extroverted, they might retrieve memories of events in which they behaved in an extroverted manner (Steffens, 2004). They might even imagine events that have never occurred.

As far as we know, little or no research has been done about the ability of participants to strategically control other implicit measurement outcomes such as affective priming and affective Simon effects. But given that participants can in principle temporarily change their attitudes and cognitions by intentionally retrieving or constructing certain information, one would expect that most implicit measurement outcomes will be sensitive to faking. One possible exception is the subliminal affective priming task. Because participants are unaware of the subliminally presented primes, they do not know what attitudes are measured. It is therefore unlikely that they know which attitude they need to fake (unless they can infer from the test context what the crucial attitude is).

Are implicit measures implicit in the sense of unintentional, goal-independent, and efficient?

Above I noted that the concept "implicit" refers to functional properties that are also associated with the concept "automatic." The latter concept, however, also includes other functional properties that are typically not linked to the concept "implicit." The most important of these properties are unintentional, goal-independent, and efficient

(e.g., Bargh, 1992; Moors & De Houwer, 2004). An implicit measurement outcome can be described as unintentional if it reflects the to-be-measured attitude or cognition even though participants do not have the intention to reveal their attitude or cognition (in that measure) or if the participants do not have the intention to retrieve information about the attitude or cognition. It can be described as goal-independent if the implicit measurement outcome reflects the attitude or cognition regardless of the processing goal that the participant has. Finally, it would be efficient when the attitude or cognition is reflected in the implicit measure even when the participant is engaged in other demanding tasks (see Moors & De Houwer, 2004).

For most of the implicit measures that have been proposed in recent years, it has not been examined whether they possess these automaticity properties. Probably this is due to the fact that "implicit" is most often interpreted as "unconscious." There is, however, some evidence concerning whether affective priming effects provide an automatic measure of attitudes (see Klauer & Musch, 2003, for a review). First, the unintentional nature of affective priming is supported by the observation that affective priming effects are found even when participants are told that the primes are not important and should be ignored (e.g., Hermans et al., 1994). This renders it unlikely (but not impossible) that priming effects are due to the fact that participants intentionally process the valence of the primes or use information about prime valence as a basis for responding to the targets. Another argument is that priming effects are typically found when the asynchrony between the onset of the prime and the onset of the target (i.e., SOA) is so short that participants do not have the time to intentionally process and strategically use the valence of the prime (e.g., Hermans et al., 2001). A final argument is that such effects also arise when the primes are presented subliminally (e.g., Klauer et al., 2003). One could indeed argue that participants cannot intentionally process the valence of the primes or use this to influence their performance if they are not aware of the presence of the primes.

Second, affective priming effects can be found even when participants do not need to evaluate the targets (e.g., when they are instructed to read the target words; see De Houwer & Randell, 2004, for an overview of the evidence). This suggests that affective priming effects reflect the valence of the primes even when participants do not have the conscious goal to process the valence of stimuli in the environment.

Third, the data of Hermans et al. (2000) suggest that the magnitude of affective priming effects is not reduced by the presence of a difficult secondary task. This supports the hypothesis that affective priming effects are based on relatively efficient processes.

Conclusion: Are implicit measures implicit?

It should be clear that there is no simple answer to this question. The brief (and certainly not complete) review of the available evidence shows that many measures that are typically described as implicit do not have all of the functional properties that can be subsumed under the term "implicit." Having said this, whether a measure has a certain property is probably not an all or none issue. For instance, although research shows that a substantial portion of the participants are aware of what a racial IAT measures, it is possible that a racial IAT effect can be found also in participants who are not aware of what the IAT measures (e.g., Monteith et al., 2001). Likewise, existing research shows that participants can control IAT effects under certain conditions, but also suggests that they have less control over IAT effects than over their scores in traditional questionnaire measures. Hence, one could say that IAT effects are implicit in that they can reflect attitudes or cognitions also in people who are

unaware of what the IAT effect measures and in the sense that participants have relatively little control over these effects. There is also research that supports the idea that most implicit measures rely on a mixture of automatic and nonautomatic processes. For example, IAT effects are known to depend on the exact labels that are used during the task or on how the presented stimuli are interpreted by the participants (e.g., De Houwer, 2001; Mitchell et al., 2003). Likewise, affective priming effects depend on how the participants classify the primes (e.g., Olson & Fazio, 2003). But regardless of whether functional properties are absolute or relative, the fact remains that they need to be clearly specified and examined empirically.

With regard to the latter point, it needs to be pointed out that in some cases, claims about the functional properties of a measurement outcome can be based on logical arguments with regard to the measurement procedure rather than on empirical evidence. For instance, it seems unlikely that participants can consciously control the outcome of an affective priming measure if the primes are presented subliminally. Nevertheless, in most cases, functional properties of measurement outcomes are not determined fully by the procedure but do need to be verified empirically. This review shows that many issues still need to be investigated. Such research is desperately needed, not only to arrive at a certain level of conceptual clarity, but also to get a better understanding of the measures that researchers are using.

What Are Indirect Measures?

Until now, I have used the term "measure" to refer to the outcome of a measurement procedure. But as I pointed out earlier, "measure" can also refer to the measurement procedure itself. It makes little sense to say that a measurement procedure is implicit. There is nothing unconscious, uncontrollable, or automatic about a procedure. A procedure is merely a set of objective guidelines that can only be characterized on the basis of the nature of these guidelines.

When regarded as procedures, what most so-called implicit measures have in common is that participants are not asked to self-assess the extent to which they hold a certain attitude or cognition. Instead, the attitude or cognition is assessed indirectly by examining its effect on other behavior. As such, most implicit measurement procedures can be characterized as indirect measures. In contrast, many traditional procedures for measuring attitudes or cognitions are direct. That is, participants are asked to respond to a question about the attitude or cognition of interest. For instance, to directly measure how much someone likes Belgian Trappist beer, one could ask the person to rate on a seven-point scale how much he or she likes Trappist beer. Whether a measure is direct or indirect is an objective property of the measure: If the measure involves asking participants to express the attitudes or thoughts that are measured, it is a direct measure. If the attitude or cognition is inferred from behavior other than a self-assessment of the participant, it is an indirect measure. There is no need to do research about this. The direct or indirect nature of the measure is determined simply by looking at its objective properties.

Note that the outcome of an indirect measurement procedure does not necessarily have the functional properties of implicit measures (e.g., unconscious, uncontrollable, automatic). Whether it does, needs to be determined on the basis of research. Also note that indirect measures can be based on self-report. In virtually all studies on the name-letter effect (e.g., Koole et al., 2001), for instance, participants are asked to express their liking of each letter of the alphabet on a Likert-type rating scale. Results typically show that people tend to

like letters that are part of their name better than other letters. The size of this effect can be regarded as an index of self-esteem. Although participants are asked to give self-reports, these self-reports are not about the attitude that one wants to measure. That is, participants are asked to express how much they like the letters and not how much they like themselves. The name-letter procedure is thus a direct measure of attitudes toward letters but an indirect measure of self-esteem. In fact, many of the measurement procedures that are currently used to obtain implicit measures of attitudes are based on verbal reports of one kind or the other (e.g., free association, word-stem completion, stereotypic explanatory bias; see Fazio & Olson, 2003, for a review). As noted by Vargas (2004), such indirect measures have a long history in psychology.

From this perspective, many traditional questionnaires can be also regarded as indirect measures. The well-known Minnesota Multiphasic Personality Inventory (MMPI), for instance, is a questionnaire that was designed to measure various personality traits (e.g., Butcher et al., 2003). It does not do so by asking participants to answer questions about the extent to which they believe that they possess a certain personality trait, but by asking them whether statements about feelings and behaviors apply to them. For instance, people who endorse the item "I have a good appetite" will receive a lower score on the depression scale. As such, the MMPI can be regarded as an indirect measure of personality. Some might argue that the results of questionnaires such as the MMPI are unlikely to be implicit because participants have control over their answers or might realize that certain traits are being measured. But as I have argued above, the implicit nature of the results of an indirect measure (be it a questionnaire or a reaction time task) needs to be determined on the basis of research. It is not because an indirect measure depends on the verbal answer of participants to certain questions that it by definition does not provide an implicit measure. Therefore, if one wants to claim that a certain questionnaire (or any other measure for that matter) does or does not provide an implicit measure, one has to clearly state the functional properties and the evidence on which this statement is based.

Just like indirect measures do not by definition provide implicit measures, direct measures do not by definition provide explicit measures. For instance, one can ask participants to express their liking of a certain object as quickly as possible and/or while performing a demanding secondary task. In such cases, participants might have little control over the expressed attitude (e.g., Wilson et al., 2000). But again, one should always verify what the functional properties of the measurement outcome are before claiming that it is an implicit measure.

From the above, it should be clear that indirect measures are not a separate class of measures next to the class of implicit measures. The qualification "direct/indirect" refers to the measurement procedure whereas the qualification "implicit/explicit" refers to the functional properties of the outcome of the measurement procedure. Each indirect measure produces an outcome for which it needs to be determined whether it can be characterized as implicit.

WHAT ARE THE POTENTIAL BENEFITS OF USING IMPLICIT MEASURES?

In this second part of the chapter, I will discuss why researchers would want to use implicit measures. Why do they want to have a measure that participants do not recognize as such, that registers attitudes and cognitions even when participants are not aware that they have them, or that participants

cannot control? I will evaluate the shortcomings and merits of three possible answers to this question: Implicit measures might provide a way to measure (1) stable attitudes and cognitions, (2) implicit attitudes and cognitions, or (3) automatically activated attitudes and cognitions. This section is thus about the constructs that implicit measures might reveal rather than the conditions under which the implicit measures reveal a certain construct (i.e., its functional properties). Note that the three constructs that I will address do not entirely overlap. For instance, stable attitudes and automatically activated attitudes are not necessarily implicit in the sense of unconscious. Likewise, stable attitudes are not necessarily activated automatically.

Can Implicit Measures Measure "True," Stable Attitudes or Cognitions?

Psychologists have for a long time assumed that attitudes and other associations in memory are stable structures that underlie behavior in a variety of situations (e.g., Allport, 1935; Beck, 1976). A perfect measure of attitudes and cognitions would directly tap into these underlying stable structures without being influenced by other factors. It is well-known, however, that traditional questionnaire measures can provide biased estimates. For instance, a participant can intentionally try to deceive the researchers, the measurement outcome can be affected by social desirability, and the outcome can depend heavily on properties of the context (e.g., how questions are formulated or who asks the questions; see Blair, 2002, p. 256). Implicit measures promised to provide a less biased estimate of attitudes and cognitions. The hope was that they would be less affected by deception and social desirability and would reflect stable structures. In part, this promise is fulfilled. Above, I have discussed data that suggest that compared to traditional measures, implicit measures such as the IAT are indeed less affected by intentional efforts to deceive. Moreover, there is some evidence that the correlation between implicit measures and traditional self-report measures increases if the impact of self-presentation on explicit measures is reduced (see Fazio & Olson, 2003). On the other hand, IAT effects (and most likely also other implicit measures) can at least sometimes and to a certain extent be faked. Even more important, implicit measures seem to be highly malleable. That is, they depend heavily on a variety of extraneous factors such as self-image enhancement, the social context in which the measure is taken, mental imagery, recently presented information, and focus of attention (see Blair, 2002, for a review). One can thus conclude that implicit measures are not miracle measures that provide an unbiased view of the "true," stable attitudes and cognitions that are assumed to underlie behavior.

Based on these and other findings, more and more researchers are questioning whether this quest for the "true" attitude or cognition makes sense (e.g., Blair, 2002; Mitchell et al., 2003). It is, for instance, likely that attitudes are in principle context-dependent because the context determines how an attitude object is represented or construed. For instance, smokers might have both a negative and a positive attitude toward smoking. Which attitude is activated will depend on which aspect of the concept "smoking" is activated. When the sociable character of smoking is highlighted by the context (e.g., a party), someone might hold a favorable attitude toward smoking. When the health implications of smoking are activated by the context (e.g., when confronted with an advertisement against smoking), the same person might evaluate smoking as negative. Another view is that attitudes and other associations in memory are not stable structures but temporary constructions that are formed in response to a particular situation. This would imply that the manner in which attitudes change across different contexts could itself provide an important source for predicting behavior.

Can Implicit Measures Measure Implicit Attitudes or Cognitions?

It is sometimes suggested that implicit measures are capable of measuring so-called implicit attitudes or implicit cognitions. But as is the case with the expression "implicit measures," it is often unclear what researchers mean when they use the term "implicit attitude" or "implicit cognition." Two papers are often cited in this context: Wilson et al. (2000) and Greenwald and Banaji (1995). It is important to note that in neither of these articles, implicit attitudes or cognitions are defined as unconscious attitudes or cognitions. Wilson et al. (2000, p. 119), for instance, "suspect that cases . . . in which people have no awareness of their implicit attitudes, are relatively rare." As I pointed out above, it is also rarely checked whether participants are aware of the attitudes that the implicit measure is supposed to register. Moreover, one cannot simply interpret an implicit measure as a measure of an attitude or cognition that participants are not aware of because participants are often aware of the attitude or cognition that is reflected in the implicit measure. One can thus conclude that implicit measures most often do not measure "implicit attitudes" or "implicit cognitions" in the sense of unconscious attitudes or cognitions.

The most frequently cited definition of "implicit attitude" is the one formulated by Greenwald and Banaji (1995, p. 8). They define an implicit attitude as "introspectively unidentified (or inaccurately identified) traces of past experience that mediate favorable or unfavorable feeling, thought, or action toward social objects." Note that implicit attitudes are thus not viewed as a separate structure or entity, but as an unconscious *effect* of the attitude or past experiences on current feeling, thought, or action. In other words, Greenwald and Banaji use the term "implicit attitude" as shorthand for the unconscious operation or effect of an attitude.

The views of Greenwald and Banaji (1995) are closely related to the MODE model of Fazio (1990; see below), except that Greenwald and Banaji put the emphasis on the unconscious operation of attitudes whereas Fazio emphasizes the automatic operation of attitudes. The term "automatic" can entail not only the functional property unconscious, but also other properties such as unintentional, fast, efficient, and/or goal-independent. There are possible downsides to focusing exclusively on the property unconscious. First, as is clear from the literature on implicit memory and implicit learning, there are serious difficulties with assessing whether participants are aware of something (e.g., Shanks & St. John, 1994). Second, the definition of Greenwald and Banaji raises questions about whether so-called implicit measures are privileged indicators of implicit attitudes. As we have seen above, there is evidence that participants can be aware that a certain attitude is measured by an implicit measure and can be aware of the attitude that is measured. In other words, neither the attitude, nor the effect of the attitude on implicit measures such as the IAT is necessarily "introspectively undefined." One could thus argue that these measures do not register implicit attitudes. Maybe the measures do register implicit attitudes in the sense that participants are not aware of the past experiences that led to the attitude that they are aware of and that they know is being measured. But if this is a sufficient criterion to state that a measure reflects an implicit attitude, then the outcome of direct measurement procedures can also be said to reflect implicit attitudes. People can indeed express their feelings toward an attitude object by using a rating scale even when the traces of past experience that mediate this favorable or

unfavorable feeling are introspectively undefined. For instance, I am able to say in a controlled manner that I like brussels sprouts even though I have no insight into the experiences that led to this positive evaluation. In fact, most preferences cannot be justified in this manner (e.g., Zajonc, 1980). Does this mean that direct measurement procedures are as suitable for measuring implicit attitudes as indirect measurement procedures? One might argue that implicit measures such as IAT effects are more suitable for measuring implicit attitudes because participants are not aware of the processes by which the attitude or past experiences produces a certain IAT effect. Although this might be true, one could say that participants also do not have full insight in how they translate a particular attitude or feeling into a particular score on a rating scale. In sum, although Greenwald and Banaji should be applauded for providing a definition of the concept "implicit attitude," their definition is problematic in some respects.

Wilson et al. (2000, p. 104) define implicit attitudes as "evaluations that (a) have an unknown origin (i.e., people are unaware of the basis of their evaluation); (b) are activated automatically; and (c) influence implicit responses, namely uncontrollable responses and ones that people do not view as an expression of their attitude and thus do not attempt to control." They assume that implicit attitudes can coexist with and differ from explicit attitudes. One person could thus simultaneously hold a positive implicit attitude toward a certain object, but a negative explicit attitude toward the same object. The implicit attitudes are viewed as attitudes that were once explicit but were replaced by a new explicit attitude. The past attitudes are, however, not overwritten but remain latent and operate automatically like habits.

Although the dual-attitude model of Wilson et al. (2000) has the merit of attempting to clarify the relation between different kinds of attitudes and the relation between attitudes and behavior, there are some potential problems with it. First, as I have argued above, the definition of implicit attitudes as attitudes that have an unknown origin (i.e., participants are unaware of the past experiences that led to the attitude) is problematic. Second, the characterization of implicit attitudes as habits that are overlearned seems incompatible with the observation that newly learned attitudes can be activated automatically and can be detected with implicit measures. For instance, De Houwer et al. (1998) showed that so-called Turkish words (in fact, they were nonwords) produce affective priming effects even when the meaning of these words was learned immediately before the start of the priming phase. Likewise, Gregg et al. (in press) found that nonsense labels will function as positive or negative concepts in an IAT after merely asking participants to suppose that one label is the name of a group of aggressive people whereas the other label is the name of a group of victims. It is difficult to imagine that such new attitudes were overlearned or habit-like. One could argue, however, that implicit measures will reflect newly learned attitudes only if they are not in conflict with older attitudes that have previously been (over)learned. There is indeed some evidence that IAT effects reflect older attitudes. For instance, Rudman (2004) found that smokers' (negative) implicit attitudes toward smoking were correlated with early (negative) experiences rather than recent experiences. Research on evaluative conditioning, however, suggests that previously learned attitudes can be changed by providing new experiences, even when participants are not aware of what caused their initial attitudes or the subsequent change in attitudes (e.g., Baeyens et al., 1989). Characterizing implicit attitudes as habit-like also suggests that they are rigid and context-independent. Studies show, however, that the attitudes that are

measured by implicit measures are instead highly malleable and context-dependent (e.g., Blair, 2002). The dual-process model therefore does not seem to give an adequate characterization of the types of attitudes that are measured by current implicit measures.

Can Implicit Measures Measure Automatically Activated Attitudes and Cognitions?

Fazio and Olson (2003, p. 301) argued that the MODE model of Fazio (1990) provides a useful framework for understanding the possible benefits of implicit measures. The MODE model "proposes that attitudes can exert influence through relatively spontaneous or more deliberative processes. The former involve judgments of, or behavior toward, an object being influenced by one's construal of the object in the immediate situation—perceptions that themselves can be affected by individuals' attitudes having been automatically activated upon encountering the attitude object. In contrast, deliberative processing involves a more effortful, cost-benefit analysis of the utility of a particular behavior." Importantly, deliberative processing will take place only when participants have the opportunity and are motivated to engage in such processing.

Most often, people do not analyze their attitudes toward stimuli in a conscious and deliberate manner. Rather, their behavior is guided by a spontaneous, automatic affective appraisal of the environment (e.g., Zajonc, 1980). Whereas traditional questionnaires typically measure consciously constructed and expressed attitudes, implicit measures could index the spontaneous, automatic evaluation of stimuli. Hence, implicit measures could be particularly suited to predict spontaneous, uncontrolled behavior. Fazio and Olson (2003) review evidence that indeed suggests that implicit measures are particularly helpful in predicting behavior that is intrinsically difficult to control or behavior in situations where people are not motivated or do not have the opportunity to control the impact of automatically activated attitudes on behavior.

The proposal of Fazio and Olson (2003) has many merits. First, rather than relying on the concept "implicit," it focuses on the distinction between automatic and deliberative processing. As I argued earlier, the concept "automatic" is more clearly defined than the concept "implicit"; it can be linked to a variety of testable functional properties, and it does not have the limitation of referring only to a state of awareness. Second, the proposal fits well with the characterization of implicit measures as measurement outcomes that can have certain functional properties that are typical of automatic processes. Implicit measures are measures that at least in some respects reflect the automatic influence of attitudes and cognitions on behavior. From the perspective of the MODE model, implicit measures are thus laboratory equivalents of the automatic influence of attitudes and cognitions on real-life behavior. Hence, implicit measures can provide a unique perspective on real-life behavior. This argument is closely related to the idea of transfer-appropriate processing (e.g., Roediger, 1990). That is, the closer the overlap between the processes that determine the measurement outcome and those that determine the actual behavior that one wants to predict, the more that the measurement outcome will be able to predict the behavior (also see Vargas, 2004). In fact, one could say that both the measurement outcome and the real-life behavior have certain functional properties (i.e., the processes through which an attitude or cognition influences the outcome or behavior operate under certain conditions). One could thus argue that the predictive value of the measurement outcome depends on the extent to which its functional properties overlap with the functional properties of the real-life behavior that one wants to explain. For instance, real-life, attitude-driven behavior that occurs when people do not have the conscious goal to evaluate stimuli in the environment might be related most to measurement outcomes that occur in the absence of a conscious evaluation goal.

CONCLUSION

Ultimately, the merits of implicit measures will be judged on the basis of whether and to what extent they provide unique insights into human behavior. On the one hand, the predictive power of implicit measures will depend on psychometric properties such as test-retest reliability and validity (i.e., whether they in fact register the attitudes and cognitions that one wants to measure). The fact that reliability and validity are essential for all possible measures is well-known and beyond dispute. The aim of this chapter was, however, to communicate that it is also important to consider the functional properties of the measure, especially in the case of so-called implicit measures. That is, if one claims that a measure reflects an attitude or cognition under a certain set of conditions, one does not only need to verify whether it indeed provides a reliable index of the to-be-measured attitude or cognition (i.e., that it is reliable and valid) but also to make clear which conditions one refers to and to verify whether these conditions are actually met. Not only is this necessary to reduce conceptual problems (e.g., what does it mean to say that a measure is implicit or explicit), based on the MODE model one could argue that it can also help optimize the predictive power of (implicit) measures. I therefore hope that my attempt to clarify what implicit measures are and why we should use them will facilitate future research with and about these measures.

REFERENCES

Allport, G. W. (1935). Attitudes. In C. Murchison (Ed.), *Handbook of social psychology* (pp. 133–175). Worcester, MA: Clark University Press.

Asendorpf, J. B., Banse, R., Mücke, D. (2002). Double dissociation between implicit and explicit personality self-concept: The case of shy behavior. *Journal of Personality and Social Psychology, 83,* 380–393.

Baeyens, F., Eelen, P., van den Bergh, O., & Crombez, G. (1989). Acquired affective-evaluative value: Conservative but not unchangeable. *Behaviour Research and Therapy, 27,* 279–287.

Banse, R. (2001). Affective priming with liked and disliked person: Prime visibility determines congruency and incongruency effects. *Cognition & Emotion, 15,* 501–520.

Banse, R., Seise, J., & Zerbes, N. (2001). Implicit attitudes toward homosexuality: Reliability, validity, and controllability of the IAT. *Zeitschrift für Experimentelle Psychologie, 48,*145–160.

Bargh, J. A. (1992). The ecology of automaticity. Toward establishing the conditions needed to produce automatic processing effects. *American Journal of Psychology, 105,* 181–199.

Beck, A. T. (1976). *Cognitive therapy and the emotional disorders.* New York: Meridian.

Blair, I. V. (2002). The malleability of automatic stereotypes and prejudice. *Personality and Social Psychology Review, 6,* 242–261.

Brunel, F. F., Tietje, B.C., & Greenwald, A.G. (in press). Is the Implicit Association Test a valid and valuable measure of implicit consumer social cognition? *Journal of Consumer Psychology.*

Butcher, J., Derksen, J., Sloore, H., & Sirigatti, S. (2003). Objective personality assessment of people in diverse cultures: European adaptations of the MMPI-2. *Behaviour Research and Therapy, 41,* 819–840.

Dasgupta, N., & Greenwald, A. G. (2001). On the malleability of automatic attitudes: Combatting automatic prejudice with images of admired and disliked individuals. *Journal of Personality and Social Psychology, 81,* 800–814.

De Houwer, J. (2001). A structural and process analysis of the Implicit Association Test. *Journal of Experimental Social Psychology, 37,* 443–451.

De Houwer, J. (2003). The extrinsic affective Simon task. *Experimental Psychology, 50,* 77–85.

De Houwer, J., & Eelen, P. (1998). An affective variant of the Simon paradigm. *Cognition & Emotion, 12,* 45–61.

De Houwer, J., Hermans, D., & Eelen, P. (1998). Affective and identity priming with episodically associated stimuli. *Cognition & Emotion, 12,* 145–169.

De Houwer, J., & Randell, T. (2004). Robust affective priming effects in a conditional pronunciation task: Evidence for the semantic representation of evaluative information. *Cognition & Emotion, 18,* 251–264.

Duscherer, K., Holender, D., & Molenaar, E. (2002). The Affective Simon Effect: How automatic, how specific? Unpublished manuscript.

Egloff, B., & Schmukle, S. C. (2002). Predictive validity of an implicit association test for assessing anxiety. *Journal of Personality and Social Psychology, 83,* 1441–1455.

Fazio, R. H. (1990). Multiple processes by which attitudes guide behavior: The MODE model as an integrative framework. In M. P. Zanna (Ed.), *Advances in experimental social psychology* (Vol. 23, pp. 75–109). San Francisco, CA: Academic Press.

Fazio, R. H., Jackson, J. R., Dunton, B. C., & Williams, C. J. (1995). Variability in automatic activation as an unobtrusive measure of racial attitudes: A bona fide pipeline? *Journal of Personality and Social Psychology, 69,* 1013–1027.

Fazio, R. H., & Olson, M. A. (2003). Implicit measures in social cognition research: Their meaning and use. *Annual Review of Psychology, 54,* 297–327.

Greenwald, A. G., & Banaji, M. R. (1995). Implicit social cognition: Attitudes, self-esteem, and stereotypes. *Psychological Review, 102,* 4–27.

Greenwald, A. G., McGhee, D. E., & Schwartz, J. L. K. (1998). Measuring individual differences in implicit cognition: The Implicit Association Test. *Journal of Personality and Social Psychology, 74,* 1464–1480.

Gregg, A. P., Banaji, M. R., & Seibt, B. (in press). Easier made than undone: The asymmetric malleability of automatic preferences. *Psychological Bulletin.*

Hermans, D., Crombez, G., & Eelen, P. (2000). Automatic attitude activation and efficiency: The fourth horseman of automaticity. *Psychologica Belgica, 40,* 3–22.

Hermans, D., De Houwer, J., & Eelen, P. (1994). The affective priming effect: Automatic activation of evaluative information in memory. *Cognition & Emotion, 8,* 515–533.

Hermans, D., De Houwer, J., & Eelen, P. (2001). A time course analysis of the affective priming effect. *Cognition & Emotion, 15,* 143–165.

Kim, D. Y. (2003). Voluntary controllability of the Implicit Association Test (IAT). *Social Psychology Quarterly, 66,* 83–96.

Klauer, K. C., Mierke, J., & Musch, J. (2003). The positivity proportion effect: A list context effect in masked affective priming. *Memory & Cognition, 31,* 953–967.

Klauer, K. C., & Musch, J. (2003). Affective priming: Findings and theories. In J. Musch & K. C. Klauer (Eds.), *The psychology of evaluation: Affective processes in cognition and emotion.* Mahwah, NJ: Lawrence Erlbaum.

Koole, S. L., Dijksterhuis, A., & van Knippenberg, A. (2001). What's in a name?: Implicit self-esteem and the automatic self. *Journal of Personality and Social Psychology, 80,* 669–685.

Logan, G. D. (1985). Skill and automaticity: Relations, implications, and future directions. *Canadian Journal of Psychology, 39,* 367–386.

Lowery, B. S., Hardin, C. D., & Sinclair, S. (2001). Social influence effects on automatic racial prejudice. *Journal of Personality and Social Psychology, 81,* 842–855.

Mitchell, J. P., Nosek, B. A., & Banaji, M. R. (2003). Contextual variations in implicit evaluation. *Journal of Experimental Psychology: General, 132,* 455–469.

Monteith, M. J., Voils, C. I., & Ashburn-Nardo, L. (2001). Taking a look underground: Detecting, interpreting, and reacting to implicit racial bias. *Social Cognition, 19,* 395–417.

Moors, A., & De Houwer, J. (in press). Automaticity. *Journal of Personality and Social Psychology.*

Olson, M. A., & Fazio, R. H. (2001). Implicit attitude formation through classical conditioning. *Psychological Science, 12,* 413–417.

Olson, M. A., & Fazio, R. H. (2003). Relations between implicit measures of prejudice: What are we measuring? *Psychological Science, 14,* 636–639.

Roediger, H. L. (1990). Implicit memory: Retention without remembering. *American Psychologist, 45,* 1043–1056.

Rudman, L. A. (2004). Sources of implicit attitudes. *Current Directions in Psychological Science, 13,* 79–82.

Shanks, D. R., & St. John, M. F. (1994). Characteristics of dissociable human learning systems. *Behavioral and Brain Sciences, 17,* 367–395.

Stacy, A. W. (1997). Memory activation and expectancy as prospective predictors of alcohol and marijuana use. *Journal of Abnormal Psychology, 106,* 61–73.

Steffens, M. (2004). Is the Implicit Association Test immune to faking? *Experimental Psychology, 51,* 165–179.

Teachman, B. A., Gregg, A. P., & Woody, S. R. (2001). Implicit associations of fear-relevant stimuli among individuals with snake and spider fears. *Journal of Abnormal Psychology, 110,* 226–235.

Vargas, P. T. (2004). On the relationship between implicit attitudes and behavior: Some lessons from the past, and directions for the future. In G. Haddock & G. R. Maio (Eds.), *Contemporary perspectives on the psychology of attitudes.* New York: Psychology Press.

Wiers, R. W., van Woerden, N., Smulders, F. T. Y., & de Jong, P. J. (2002). Implicit and explicit alcohol-related cognitions in heavy and light drinkers. *Journal of Abnormal Psychology, 111,* 648–658.

Wilson, T. D., Lindsey, S., & Schooler, T. Y. (2000). A model of dual attitudes. *Psychological Review, 107,* 101–126.

Zajonc, R. B. (1980). Feeling and thinking. Preferences need no inferences. *American Psychologist, 35,* 151–175.

CHAPTER 3

A Dual-Process Approach to Behavioral Addiction: The Case of Gambling

Jonathan St. B. T. Evans and Kenny Coventry

Abstract: In this chapter, we explore the relevance of the dual-process theory of thinking and reasoning (Evans, 2003) to the understanding of behavioral addictions, with particular reference to gambling behavior. It is clear that such addictions may reflect a process of implicit learning resulting in compulsive and apparently irrational behavior that may conflict with the individual's consciously expressed beliefs and desires. Our purpose here is to examine the detailed theoretical proposals of cognitive researchers about the nature of the underlying cognitive systems to provide a stronger understanding of how such dissociation and conflict may come about. We illustrate the relevance of this theoretical system to behavioral addiction by critical review and discussion of studies of the psychology of gambling.

In this chapter, we explore the relevance of the dual-process theory of thinking and reasoning (Evans, 2003) to the understanding of behavioral addictions, with particular reference to gambling behavior. Our purpose here is to examine the detailed theoretical proposals of cognitive researchers about the nature of the underlying cognitive systems to provide a stronger understanding of how such dissociation and conflict may come about. In the first part of the chapter, we will discuss the dual-process theory as it has been developed in the study of thinking, reasoning, and judgment. We consider the nature of the two systems of thinking and the evidence for their distinctive nature. In

the second part of the chapter, we will demonstrate the relevance of this theoretical system to behavioral addiction by examining studies of the psychology of gambling.

THE DUAL-PROCESS THEORY OF THINKING

The notion of dual systems of thinking entered psychology with the writings of Sigmund Freud, who distinguished between *primary process* and *secondary process*. Primary process thinking was motivated by wish-fulfillment and was seen as undirected and associative in structure whereas secondary process thinking was seen as rational, goal-directed problem solving. Although this Freudian perspective has limited overlap with contemporary dual-process theories, it is historically important for introducing the idea of unconscious thinking that may conflict with conscious processes and also for the proposal of the notion of *rationalization*. When behavior is caused by unconscious processes, he argued, the conscious mind may produce an explanation of that behavior in terms of conscious goals and desires. As we shall see, the notion of rationalization or confabulation (Stanovich, 2004) is an important feature in contemporary accounts.

It is useful to distinguish between dual-process and dual-system theories of thinking. The weaker, dual-process theories specify that there are two distinct processes of thinking that compete for control of our behavior. Examples are the heuristic-analytic theory of reasoning (Evans, 1989) and the distinction between associative and rule-based reasoning proposed by Sloman (1996). Stronger, dual-system theories ascribe the origin of these dual processes to biologically distinct cognitive systems with sharply differing evolutionary histories (Evans, 2003; Evans & Over, 1996; Reber, 1993; Stanovich, 1999, 2004). In our view, there is much evidence to support the stronger form of the theory but it clearly carries with it a good deal more theoretical assumptions than those required simply to distinguish the presence of two different kinds of thought. For this reason, some authors interested in the dual-process distinction stop short of endorsing the full-blown dual-systems account.

Dual-system theorists have attributed a number of differing characteristics to the thought processes arising from the two systems, to which we will give the neutral labels System 1 and System 2 (Stanovich, 1999). A number of these are summarized in Table 3.1. In general, System 1 is seen as rapid, parallel, computationally powerful, and associative or pragmatic in nature. This system is supposed to be ancient in its evolutionary origin and to share a number of its features—in particular a general learning algorithm—with the cognitive systems of higher animals. Its operation is unconscious with only final products reaching conscious awareness. System 2 is by contrast slow and sequential, making demands on central working memory resources, and hence is correlated with IQ. It is thought to be recently evolved and unique to anatomically modern humans. It is associated with abstract thought and domain general problem solving and may be described as conscious and volitional.

Before considering the nature of the processes in greater detail, we will illustrate the kind of evidence that has led researchers in the thinking and reasoning tradition to postulate a dual-processing mechanism. The archetypal phenomenon is that of belief bias in deductive reasoning.

The Belief Bias Effect

Suppose we ask you to evaluate a logical argument. You are told that you must assume the premises are true and decide, on this basis, whether the conclusion necessarily follows. For example, consider the following syllogisms:

> *1. No addictive things are inexpensive*
> *Some cigarettes are inexpensive*
> *Therefore, some addictive things are not cigarettes*
>
> *2. No police dogs are vicious*
> *Some highly trained dogs are vicious*
> *Therefore, some police dogs are not highly trained*

In the study of Evans et al. (1983), syllogisms like Example 1 were endorsed as valid

Table 3.1 Characteristics Typically Attributed to the Two Systems of Thinking in Strong Dual-Process Theories (see Evans, 2003)

System 1	System 2
Unconscious	Conscious
Evolved early	Evolved late
Shared with animals	Uniquely human
Nonverbal	Verbal
Rapid, parallel	Slow, sequential
High capacity	Low capacity
Domain specific	Logical, abstract
Pragmatic	Hypothetical
Independent of working memory and IQ	Related to working memory capacity and IQ

by 75 percent of participants, whereas those like Example 2 were endorsed as valid by only 10 percent. The astonishing thing about this is that the two syllogisms have precisely the same logical form: No A are B, Some C are B, therefore, Some A are not C. The argument is, in fact, invalid: The conclusion does not necessarily follow. The difference between 1 and 2 is that the conclusion of 1 is believable and that of 2 is unbelievable. A similar, but weaker, belief bias effect is shown for valid syllogisms. In the same study, participants endorsed 89 percent of valid arguments as valid when they had believable conclusions but only 56 percent when they had unbelievable conclusions. These findings have proved very reliable in the subsequent literature (see, for example, Klauer et al., 2000).

The participants in these experiments are adults of above-average intelligence (undergraduate students) who, despite being given clear deductive reasoning instructions, are unable to resist the influence of their prior knowledge and belief. Such content effects are commonly observed in deductive reasoning tasks (Evans, 2002) and the tendency to

contextualize all problems in the light of prior knowledge has been described as a "fundamental computational bias" by Stanovich (1999). Note, however, that in the study of Evans et al. (1983)—and later replications—there was a substantial effect of logic as well as belief on responding. Participants endorse far more valid than invalid arguments overall; but they also endorse far more believable than unbelievable conclusions overall. Evans et al. (1983) entitled their article "On the Conflict Between Logic and Belief in Syllogistic Reasoning." On the basis of protocol analyses, they argued for a *within-participant* conflict between a tendency to respond on the basis of logic or belief, with one process "winning" on some responses and the other process winning for others in the same individual participant.

If there are dual systems of the kind described in Table 3.1, we can well imagine that System 1 would prime the belief-based response, but that in response to the deductive reasoning instructions System 2 might try to inhibit this response and respond on the basis of logical reasoning. Are there really two minds in one brain competing to control our behavior in such a fashion? Recently, several different forms of evidence have been adduced to support precisely this kind of dual-process account. First, Stanovich and West (1997) have shown that participants of high intelligence are better able to resist pragmatic influences of prior belief when reasoning (supporting the view that general intelligence is associated with System 2 but not System 1 thinking). Second, when additional instructional emphasis is given to logical necessity, belief bias is significantly reduced, although not eliminated (Evans et al., 1994), and conversely when deductive reasoning instructions are relaxed, the influence of prior belief on reasoning becomes significantly more marked (e.g., Stevenson & Over, 1995). A third—and very striking form of evidence—comes from neural-imaging studies of reasoning. Goel and Dolan (2003) showed that when syllogisms are presented that put logic and belief in conflict (valid-unbelievable or invalid-believable) then the brain areas that were recruited were differentiated according to the response made. When a logically correct response was given, activity was recorded in the right prefrontal cortex but when belief-based responding was observed, the ventral-medial prefrontal cortex was recruited (see also Bechara et al., Chapter 15). These are areas that memory researchers have associated with executive control and semantic memory, respectively.

Recently, researchers have paid attention to the proposal that System 1 thinking is rapid and System 2 thinking is slow. A recent study of belief bias reported by Evans and Curtis-Holmes (in press) compared syllogistic evaluation under both free time and rapid response conditions (in the latter participants were allowed 5 seconds to read the premises and a further 5 seconds to make a response; under free time conditions, participants normally take at least 20 seconds per syllogism). The results of this study are shown in Figure 3.1.

As predicted, measures of belief bias were significantly increased and rates of logically correct responding reduced when the rapid response task was employed. Note that the effect is restricted to the belief-logic conflict problems. Providing extra reasoning time confers no benefit when the belief-based response is the same as the logically correct response.

Evidence for dual-process theory is provided by a much wider range of studies than those of belief bias or even of deductive reasoning (for reviews see Almor & Sloman, 1996; Kahneman & Frederick, 2002; Stanovich, 1999). As stated earlier, however, the belief bias effect is archetypical. As a range of experimental evidence suggests, belief-based System 1 processes appear to compete with analytic reasoning processes of System 2 within the same participants for control of their responding. It is almost like a horse race, in which the handicapper (experimenter) can shift the odds by various manipulations. For example, strong deductive reasoning instructions assist System 2 whereas time restrictions shift the odds in favor of System 1. To our knowledge, however, all reported studies of the belief bias effect show significant influences of both logic and belief to although the balance between them can be altered.

System 1 Thinking and Cognitive Biases

System 1 thinking is often referred to as *heuristic* processing. Heuristic thinking is rapid but uncertain in its outcomes and may be responsible for intelligent search of complex problem spaces (Newell & Simon, 1972) but also for cognitive biases (Gilovich et al., 2002). The term "heuristic" is not ideal, as it can be used in the sense of a consciously adopted strategy that would place it in System 2. The use of the term in the heuristic-analytic theory (Evans, 1989), however, clearly equates heuristic processing with System 1 processing. In this account, it was argued that

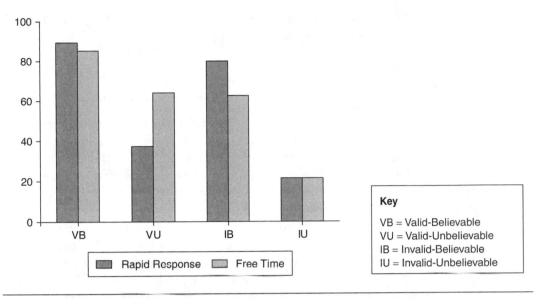

Figure 3.1   Rates of endorsement of syllogisms in the study of Evans and Curtis-Holmes (2004)

heuristic processes shape what is represented as relevant in reasoning and decision problems both by selectively representing presented information and by rapid retrieval of associated knowledge from long-term memory. Such processes may also be described by the term "pragmatic." Evans (1989) suggested that although subsequent analytic processing might intervene, the selective representations thus formed could be the cause of cognitive biases. Quite simply, people may attend to logically irrelevant information or overlook logically relevant features as a result. Recently, Kahneman and Frederick (2002) also make it clear that the famous heuristics and biases research program into the study of judgment under uncertainty (Gilovich et al., 2002; Kahneman et al., 1982) is consistent with a dual-process account in which heuristics arise from System 1 and can be overridden by analytic reasoning in System 2.

Any discussion of dual systems leads naturally into a debate about the nature of human rationality (Evans & Over, 1996; Stanovich & West, 2000). Why would we

(1) evolve or (2) learn to do things in a way that causes errors and biases? One line of argument is to question the external validity of psychological experiments and the appropriateness of the normative systems that psychologists use to judge right and wrong answers (Cohen, 1981). For example, in commenting on the belief bias effect, Evans and Over (1996) observe that in real life it is rational to reason from *all relevant belief*. Consider the two components of standard deductive reasoning instructions used in psychological experiments. First, one is required to assume the premises are true and to ignore any implicitly associated knowledge and belief. When would it be rational in everyday reasoning to ignore what you already know? Second, one is required to draw *necessary* conclusions by identifying what must be true, if the premises are true. The wealth of evidence suggests, however, that people prefer to draw pragmatically plausible conclusions that are held with a degree of belief and may be withdrawn in the light of further evidence (Evans & Over, in press; Oaksford & Chater, 2001).

Hence, it can be argued that heuristic processing frequently is adaptive in everyday life. Stanovich (1999, 2004), however, has made much of the fact that normatively correct solutions are often found by participants of very high intelligence. This suggests to him that abstract, analytic reasoning is often required for what he terms instrumental rationality in the modern technological world. He argues that System 1 thinking is an old system that evolved in an environment very different from the current world, a fact overlooked by many evolutionary psychologists who try to argue that all evolved thinking is necessarily adaptive (Stanovich, 2004; Stanovich & West, 2003). Thus, heuristic thinking will often lead to biases, unless moderated by intervention from the analytic system.

Behavioral addictions, such as problem gambling, must clearly be learned. The reason that such behaviors may seem maladaptive, as we shall explore in the second part of this chapter, is that they reflect on the nature of the general learning algorithm in System 1. This does not lead to explicit representations, reflective thought, or abstract, domain general reasoning. All of these require the facilities of the new brain in System 2. The old learning mechanism of System 1 responds, for example, to frequency information in the environment but does not encode theoretical understanding of probability. The knowledge it acquires is encapsulated in the domain in which it was learned. For example, people who acquire good statistical intuitions about sample size from experience (as opposed to theoretical study) are unable to transfer these concepts to a domain outside the one in which it was learned (Nisbett et al., 1983). It is also clear from the research on belief bias reviewed above that System 1 responding can be quite compulsive, often competing very effectively with System 2 even when an effort at analytic reasoning is being made. There is, however, a further complicating factor—the confabulatory

nature of System 2 thinking, to which we now turn.

System 2 Thinking and Its Interaction With System 1

The reader might object to the portrayal of dual systems above on the grounds that as people we do not feel as though we are perpetually in two minds, resolving conflict in our reasoning and decision making. Generally speaking, we feel "in control" and are able to provide a reasoned explanation for the choices we make. Our intuitions in this regard comply with folk psychology, otherwise known as belief-desire psychology, which is essentially a System 2 view of thinking favored by some philosophers and psychologists as well as by ordinary people (Haselager, 1997). In common with other dual-process theorists (see Stanovich, 2004, pp. 52–61), we believe that folk psychology makes a grave error in overlooking the influence of autonomous System 1 thinking on our behavior and by failing to understand the confabulatory nature of System 2. Our perception of unitary and controlling consciousness is essentially an illusion.

Nisbett and Wilson (1977), in their famous paper on "Telling More Than We Can Know," reviewed a wide range of evidence in cognitive and social psychology showing that (1) people are often unaware of the factors that caused their behavior and (2) they are nevertheless always willing to give a rational-sounding account of their actions. Nisbett and Wilson argued that people do not have access to the processes underlying their behavior but apply a priori causal theories when asked to introspect. In other words, people theorize about their own behavior when asked to explain it even though they are supposedly producing an introspective report on their mental processes.

We are not, of course, suggesting that analytic processes in System 2 simply serve to rationalize our own behavior. We know (see above) that analytic thinking is essential for hypothetical thinking about possibilities and for abstract, domain-general reasoning (Evans & Over, 1996; Stanovich, 2004). The essential fact remains, however, that the duality that is demonstrably present in our cognitive architecture is not reflected in our consciousness any more than it is in "common sense" folk psychology. In this respect, at least, Freud had it right. One function of the conscious mind is to rationalize unconsciously controlled behavior and retain an illusion of unity and control.

The implications of all this for compulsive and addictive behaviors are straightforward. Not only is System 2 not "in control" of such behavior but it also will be inclined to generate highly misleading verbal accounts. Thus, a smoker may rationalize her addiction by claiming that smoking helps her relax and concentrate and aids her work performance rather than attributing such "benefits" to the absence of withdrawal effects if she abstains. Depending upon education, she may also recruit System 2 resources to discredit medical or statistical evidence that she sees as exaggerating the risks. A heavy drinker may utilize the analytic system to explain that he chooses to drink because he is a sociable person and never gets out of control, thus effectively denying that he is an alcoholic in need of help and so on. We illustrate this process by examples drawn from the gambling literature in the second part of this chapter.

DUAL PROCESSES IN GAMBLING BEHAVIOR

Around 80 percent of the population in the Western world gamble (Walker, 1992). The forms on which they gamble vary considerably on a range of dimensions, including the degree of excitement involved, the time between decision points and outcomes, and the size and frequency of winning outcomes.

Although it has been noted that it is dangerous to treat gambling as a homogeneous activity (e.g., Coventry & Brown, 1993), most of these gambling forms involve chance completely, or a minimal degree of skill at best. This poses a problem for any notion of rationality relating to System 2 thinking. If one equates rationality with an understanding of normative decision theory where utility and monetary value are equated, then one should not gamble in the first place on chance games where the house set the odds so as to ensure a mean expected loss for the gambler. For example, roulette wheels include one or two zeros resulting in no payout for other bets that would otherwise have fair odds, say even money for red or black. Furthermore, not only do people gamble on games where there is no real hope of winning in the first place, but they also gamble very badly on games where there is the possibility of winning in the long term. Hence, in blackjack where one can win at somewhere between .5 and 2 percent (by card counting), players use strategies that deviate markedly from optimality (Keren & Wagenaar, 1985).

In the remainder of this chapter, we consider what Wagenaar (1988) has called "the gambling paradox," namely, why the majority of the population gambles in the face of systematic losses. We also, however, have a second goal. As Coventry (2002) has noted, most people do not gamble to the extent that their behavior becomes problematic. So what differentiates the so-called "pathological," "problem," or "addicted" gamblers from those who gamble less frequently, or stop before their gambling becomes a problem? We take each of these questions in turn.

Explaining Gambling Behavior

As Wagenaar (1988) argued, one possible explanation for gambling behavior is that participants misapply the heuristics that ordinarily serve them well, in situations where general principles do not apply. From a dual-systems theory perspective, the (older evolutionary) System 1 operates by means of utilizing patterns in past information to make future decisions via a general implicit learning mechanism. Real-world environments are "noisy," that is, they include random variation around patterns. Research has shown that people can learn to predict complex patterns in the environment when substantially noisy feedback is provided. Unless the patterns are very simple, however, the learning occurs implicitly (in System 1) without corresponding acquisition of explicit (System 2) knowledge (for example, see Evans et al., 2003).

The problem is that unlike natural environments, gambling games (e.g., roulette) are usually designed not simply to be noisy, but such that there is *no* sequential dependency between outcomes to be learned. Hence, an ancient System 1 learning mechanism that evolved to deal with noise in natural environments may inappropriately "learn" patterns where there are none to be found. What makes matters worse is that any resulting behavioral tendencies will then tend to be rationalized by System 2, as we shall see later. In line with our hypothesis, it has been proposed by Ladouceur and colleagues (e.g., Ladouceur et al., 1997) that the failure to understand the principle of the independence of successive events provides the crucial misunderstanding that underpins the explanation of gambling behavior at all levels.

The idea that gamblers use past information to make future decisions is consistent with so-called *evidential* theories. For example, Cohen (1979) argues that, as all relevant evidence required for the application of probability theory is not available to us, what needs to be done is to calculate the extent to which all relevant facts are specified in the information given. Thus, evidential models predict that bets are placed on the basis of the player's confidence that their prediction in the next outcome will come to fruition.

As Coventry (2002) has shown, in the gambling domain there is much evidence that direct exposure to gambling increases risk-taking behavior for both low-frequency and high-frequency gamblers (e.g., Ladouceur et al., 1987). This can be explained in terms of an increase in confidence over time as more information is available with which to construct a (implicit) theory for prediction. Peterson and Pitz (1988) provide similar evidence. They asked subjects to estimate the number of games won by a National League Baseball Team during a 163-game season. It was found that subjects' confidence in their answers was found to increase positively with the amount of salient evidence available. Similarly, Philips and Amrhein (1989) found in a game of computer blackjack that bet size increased as players had more time to place their bets. There is, therefore, much evidence that confidence in prediction increases as a function of the amount of evidence that is available and the amount of time that is available to evaluate that evidence.

There is also evidence that participants are happy to accept a cost to obtain information about past outcomes. Using a simple coin-tossing prediction paradigm ("heads" or "tails," with a different coin tossed on each trial), Ladouceur et al. (1997) let undergraduate students gamble with their participant payment fees in the hope that they would leave the laboratory with more money. The outcome of each coin toss was covered after it was initially shown, and participants were told that they had the option of paying a proportion of their subject payment fees in exchange for uncovering past outcomes. After debriefing the participants, Ladouceur et al. found surprisingly that the majority of participants did indeed pay to reveal past outcomes as they thought that this would help them make more accurate future predictions, despite being told in advance that the outcome of the coin-tossing task was not rigged.

There are many other demonstrations of the use of past outcomes on chance tasks.

Descending
WWWWWLWWWWLLLWWWWLLWLLWWLLLWLLLLW

Ascending
WLLLLLWLLLWWLLWLLWWWWLLLWWWWLWWWW

Random
WLWLLWLWLWWLLWLLWLWWWLWLWLLWLW

Figure 3.2   Sequences of wins and losses used by Langer and Roth (1975)

For example, Langer and Roth (1975) manipulated the sequence of wins and losses that subjects experienced on a coin-tossing task. Using three conditions, wins and losses were rigged so that all subjects experienced 15 wins and 15 losses over 30 trials (thus winning a chance number of times), but some participants won either mainly at the beginning (the descending condition), mainly at the end (the ascending condition), or evenly throughout the trials (see Figure 3.2 for the sequences used).

Langer and Roth (1975) found that those in the descending condition rated themselves as more skillful, remembered more wins, and thought that over future trials they would be more successful than those in either of the other two conditions. There was also an effect of an actor-observer manipulation such that those participating thought that they would do better than those observing but not participating directly. Finally, subjects believed that practice and distraction would influence performance on the task, again, mostly in the descending condition. Such a profile of behavior is what Langer and Roth term "the illusion of control," and has been shown for gamblers gambling across a range of gambling forms (e.g., Coventry & Norman, 1998; Reid, 1986; Wolfgang et al., 1984).

So, changing the availability of past outcomes, the pattern of those outcomes, and the sequence of wins and losses on a gambling task all affect the perception of the probability of future wins on such tasks. People generally are overconfident regarding future predictions given past information, and they use this past information erroneously during tasks. Indeed, it is well established that randomness is a concept people have great difficulty with, and additionally the view of this concept in the scientific community is also subject to variation (see Falk & Konold, 1997, for a discussion). As Coventry (2002) has argued, the gambler is in a sense rational to continue if System 1 produces a belief that there is a higher probability of winning than the probability of the task would warrant and this is not overridden by System 2 reasoning about the statistical structure of the game. But this still leaves the puzzle of why gamblers *continue* to gamble regularly (though not necessarily at problematic levels) given that they often lose?

There are a number of observations to make relevant to this point. First, if one observes a roulette table for any length of time, one of the first things one notices is that most gamblers place bets on many numbers at a time, spreading chips all over the roulette table for a single spin of the wheel. One of the consequences of this is that the gambler does win frequently, although the odds of the game have not changed and the mean expected outcome is just the same. As Wagenaar (1988) has noted, however, memory for events often errs in favor of remembering positive experiences, and forgetting the negative experiences. In other words, the feeling and memory of winning may be enough to allow the gambler to misperceive the likelihood of winning again in the future.

Second, there is much evidence accumulating that gamblers hold many erroneous beliefs about gambling. For example, Gaboury and Ladouceur (1989), Griffiths (1994), and Walker (1992) all provide evidence of erroneous perceptions across a variety of gambling forms using verbal protocols from gamblers, or the "think-aloud" method, as it has been referred to in this literature. In most cases, gamblers are trained to speak as they process during a task. Estimates of the percentages of erroneous beliefs reported by gamblers using this method range in this literature from 14 percent for regular gamblers and 2.5 percent for nonregular gamblers on slot machines to 87 percent for a group of roulette players. Such erroneous perceptions include the beliefs that in chance games (e.g., roulette) practice improves performance, that people can be on a hot winning streak, that distraction can adversely affect performance, and so on. Furthermore, it has been noted that some of these beliefs even transcend the immediate features of the game at hand. For example, Scolarios and Brown (1988; cited in Brown, 1993) catalog the presence of more bizarre and exotic cognitive distortions (than those cataloged by Wagenaar, 1988) from collected anecdotes of recovering self-diagnosed compulsive gamblers. For example, one gambler reported that gambling decisions were based on whether or not, on his way to the betting office, he won walking races with unsuspecting members of the public to secretly selected targets such as telephone boxes or lampposts. Brown (1993) argues that the heuristics and biases outlined by Kahneman et al. (1982), therefore, only represent the middle ground of a spectrum of cognitive distortions ranging from the bizarre through the erroneous to the almost rational.

In the gambling literature on discussions of these erroneous beliefs about gambling, it has often been assumed that such beliefs are causal (see, for example, Ladouceur & Walker, 1996). Dual-process theory, however, offers a more parsimonious account of where these beliefs come from as discussed in our earlier section on the interaction of Systems 1 and 2. As Coventry and Norman (1998) have argued, such erroneous perceptions may be post hoc rationalizations for one's gambling behavior, rather than causal explanations of it. In other words, gambling behavior is

actually controlled by System 1, as argued above, but System 2 kicks in afterward to confabulate beliefs compatible with gambling behavior. The false beliefs are actually a *consequence* not a cause of the gambling behavior. This account still leaves us with an unsolved problem, however. If all gamblers are like this, then why do only a small percentage of them lose control to the point where their gambling becomes addictive?

Loss of Control of Gambling Behavior and Gambling Addiction

There are a number of relatively recent findings in the literature that, when put together, provide clues to how addiction to gambling may occur. To begin with, gambling is associated with large increases in objective and subjective arousal, across a range of gambling forms (e.g., Anderson & Brown, 1984; Coventry & Hudson, 2001; Coventry & Norman, 1997; Griffiths, 1993). For example, Coventry and Norman (1997) found heart rate increases of up to 38 beats per minute over baseline during horse race betting in the off-course betting office. Furthermore, as Coventry and Norman (1998) have noted, gambling is also a task where participants are not conscious. Gamblers report losing track of time during gambling, standing outside themselves while gambling, feeling excited when gambling, and there is a lack of awareness of events outside the immediate task environment (see Diskin & Hodgins, 1999, 2001; Jacobs, 1988). Such dissociative experiences have been documented across a range of phenomena such as alcohol abuse and binge eating (Baumeister, 1991). The hallmarks for such states is that they involve both an attentional and an emotional component where people in such states exhibit a narrowing of attention with a particular focus on the experience at hand, and a related positive mood state that allows them to block out other life events of an unpleasant nature. Such experiences are common in the general population (Kihlstrom et al., 1994), but dissociative experiences of a pathological nature are much less common. It has been shown, however, that dissociative experiences during gambling are much more common in high-frequency gamblers than low-frequency gamblers (Kuley & Jacobs, 1988).

There is now evidence that there are complex interrelationships between degree of loss of control of gambling behavior, the extent of erroneous perceptions during gambling, and dissociation and arousal during gambling. Coulombe et al. (1992) found a significant positive correlation between the number of erroneous verbalizations and arousal as measured by heart rate in a group of video poker players consisting of both regular players and occasional players. The regular players also produced significantly more erroneous verbalizations than the occasional players, suggesting that post hoc (System 2) rationalizations are more common among high-frequency gamblers than low-frequency gamblers. Furthermore, it has been shown that there are correlations between erroneous perceptions during gambling, dissociation, and loss of control (Coventry et al., in preparation). One way of interpreting this pattern of intercorrelations is that gamblers vary in the need to be unconscious, and that gambling serves the function of escape from one's everyday environment when gamblers are unconscious during play. Therefore, the extent to which post hoc rationalizations are required through the activity of System 2 varies as a function of the need to escape from one's environment. The unconsciousness associated with the gambling experience in terms of cost-benefit analyses overrides the costs associated with loss of money and the consequences that follow from this. So if this is the case, how can one help addicted gamblers?

Implications for Treatment of Problem Gambling

There is emerging evidence, as we suggested previously, that it is possible to train System 2 to affect the extent to which System 1 dominates during a task. Ladouceur and colleagues (e.g., Ladouceur & Walker, 1996; Sylvain et al., 1997) have developed cognitive therapy for problem gamblers that addresses the erroneous perceptions that appear to underlie the clients' gambling behavior. In particular, the therapy targets the clients' lack of understanding of independence of events during gambling tasks. There is evidence that such an approach to therapy is successful, and indeed is more successful than other therapeutic techniques. For example, Sylvain et al. (1997) reported success rates using the cognitive correction of erroneous perceptions that were maintained at both 6- and 12-month follow-ups. Particularly striking during this therapeutic technique are the effects of recording verbalizations of addicted gamblers while they are gambling, and then playing the verbalizations back to the gamblers at a later point. Ladouceur (personal communication) observes that gamblers find it hard to believe how irrational the verbalizations they have produced during play actually are, and training gamblers about the real odds during a task and exposing how bizarre their decisions actually are during a task seems to be able to lead to a systemic decrease in their gambling behavior. Again, from a dual-process theory perspective, what this therapeutic technique appears to be doing is to train System 2 to interfere in the pervasive workings of System 1 thinking; it therefore reveals to gamblers exactly how irrational their previous behavior is from a System 2 perspective.

CONCLUSIONS

We have reviewed the dual-process approach to thinking and reasoning, and have shown that in gambling settings such a theory may have considerable value as a means of understanding both general gambling behavior and the behavior of a minority of gamblers who go on to develop addictive levels of play. It seems likely that gambling behavior may develop due to application of System 1 learning mechanisms that evolved to cope with noisy but nonetheless patterned environments. When applied within the artificial world of gambling forms that provide no predictability between successive events, this leads to false learning of relationships that are not actually present. Once established, the gambling behavior may then be maintained by cognitive biases such as the availability of successful and unsuccessful betting outcomes.

At the System 2 level, it is possible for people with appropriate education to understand the formal structure of gambling games and the inevitable expected losses involved. Doubtless many individuals do refrain from gambling for this reason. System 2, however, also has a strong confabulatory role in which biases resulting from System 1 processes may be rationalized, maintaining the illusion of conscious control. Hence, the commonly reported false theories of chance and probability people hold are more likely, in our opinion, to be the consequence rather than the cause of their gambling behavior. In effect, they are post hoc rationalizations constructed in System 2. The evidence suggests that this confabulation is particularly marked in persistent and problem gamblers. Preliminary outcome studies, however, provide support for the notion that System 2 can be trained to interrupt System 1 processes during play, and that such an approach has much utility.

REFERENCES

Almor, A., & Sloman, S. A. (1996). Is deontic reasoning special? *Psychological Review, 103*, 374–378.

Anderson, G., & Brown, R. I. F. (1984). Real and laboratory gambling, sensation seeking and arousal. *Journal of Psychology, 75*, 401–441.

Baumeister, R. F. (1991). *Escaping the self: Alcoholism, spirituality, masochism and other flights from the burden of selfhood*. New York: Guilford.

Brown, R. I. F. (1993). El papel de la activacion, distorsiones cognitivas y busqueda de sensaciones en las addicciones al juego. *Psicologia Conductual, 1*(3), 375–388.

Cohen, L. J. (1979). On the psychology of prediction: Whose is the fallacy? *Cognition, 7*, 385–407.

Cohen, L. J. (1981). Can human irrationality be experimentally demonstrated? *Behavioral and Brain Sciences, 4*, 317–370.

Coulombe, A., Ladouceur, R., Desharnais, R., & Jobin, J. (1992). Erroneous perceptions and arousal among regular and occasional video poker players. *Journal of Gambling Studies, 8*, 235–244.

Coventry, K. R. (2002). Rationality and decision making: The case of gambling and the development of gambling addiction. In J. J. Marotta, J. A. Cornelius, & W. R. Eadington (Eds.), *The downside: Problem and pathological gambling*. Reno: University of Nevada Press.

Coventry, K. R., & Brown, R. I. F. (1993). Sensation seeking, gambling and gambling addictions. *Addiction, 88*(4), 541–554.

Coventry, K. R., & Hudson, J. (2001). Gender differences, physiological arousal and the role of winning in fruit machine gamblers. *Addiction, 96,* 871–879.

Coventry, K. R., Laurie, A. D., & Dennis, I. (in preparation). *Gambling, dissociation and erroneous perceptions: Toward a model of loss of control of gambling behaviour.*

Coventry, K. R., & Norman, A. C. (1997). Arousal, sensation seeking and frequency of gambling in off-course horse racing bettors. *British Journal of Psychology, 88,* 671–681.

Coventry, K. R., & Norman, A. C. (1998). Arousal, erroneous verbalisations and the illusion of control during a computer-generated gambling task. *British Journal of Psychology, 89,* 629–645.

Diskin, K. M., & Hodgins, D. C. (1999). Narrowing of attention and dissociation in pathological video lottery gamblers. *Journal of Gambling Studies, 15*(1), 17–28.

Diskin, K. M., & Hodgins, D. C. (2001). Narrowed focus and dissociative experiences in a community sample of experienced video lottery gamblers. *Canadian Journal of Behavioral Science, 33*(1), 58–64.

Evans, J. St. B. T. (1989). *Bias in human reasoning: Causes and consequences.* Brighton, UK: Lawrence Erlbaum.

Evans, J. St. B. T. (2002). Logic and human reasoning: An assessment of the deduction paradigm. *Psychological Bulletin, 128,* 978–996.

Evans, J. St. B. T. (2003). In two minds: Dual process accounts of reasoning. *Trends in Cognitive Sciences, 7,* 454–459.

Evans, J. St. B. T., Allen, J. L., Newstead, S. E., & Pollard, P. (1994). Debiasing by instruction: the case of belief bias. *European Journal of Cognitive Psychology, 6,* 263–285.

Evans, J. St. B. T., Barston, J. L., & Pollard, P. (1983). On the conflict between logic and belief in syllogistic reasoning. *Memory & Cognition, 11,* 295–306.

Evans, J. St. B. T., Clibbens, J., Cattani, A., Harris, A., & Dennis, I. (2003). Explicit and implicit processes in multi-cue judgment. *Memory & Cognition, 31,* 608–618.

Evans, J. St. B. T., & Curtis-Holmes, J. (in press). Rapid responding increases belief bias: Evidence for the dual process theory of reasoning. *Thinking & Reasoning.*

Evans, J. St. B. T., & Over, D. E. (1996). *Rationality and reasoning.* Hove, UK: Psychology Press.

Evans, J. St. B. T., & Over, D. E. (In press). *If.* Oxford, UK: Oxford University Press.

Falk, R., & Konold, C. (1997). Making sense of randomness: Implicit encoding as a basis for judgment. *Psychological Review, 104,* 301–318.

Gaboury, A., & Ladouceur, R. (1989). Erroneous perceptions and gambling. *Journal of Social Behavior and Personality, 4,* 411–420.

Gilovich, T., Griffin, D., & Kahneman, D. (2002). *Heuristics and biases: The psychology of intuitive judgement.* Cambridge, UK: Cambridge University Press.

Goel, V., & Dolan, R. J. (2003). Explaining modulation of reasoning by belief. *Cognition, 87,* B11–B22.

Griffiths, M. D. (1993). Tolerance in gambling: An objective measure using the psychophysiological analysis of male fruit machine gamblers. *Addictive Behaviors, 18,* 365–372.

Griffiths, M. D. (1994). The role of cognitive bias and skill in fruit machine playing. *British Journal of Psychology, 85,* 351–369.

Haselager, W. F. G. (1997). *Cognitive science and folk psychology.* London: Sage.

Jacobs, D. F. (1988). Evidence for a common dissociative-like reaction among addicts. *Journal of Gambling Behavior, 4,* 27–37.

Kahneman, D., & Frederick, S. (2002). Representativeness revisited: Attribute substitution in intuitive judgement. In T. Gilovich, D. Griffin, & D. Kahneman (Eds.), *Heuristics and biases: The psychology of intuitive judgement* (pp. 49–81). Cambridge, UK: Cambridge University Press.

Kahneman, D., Slovic, P., & Tversky, A. (1982). *Judgment under uncertainty: Heuristics and biases*. Cambridge, UK: Cambridge University Press.

Keren, G., & Wagenaar, W. A. (1985). On the psychology of playing blackjack: Normative and descriptive considerations with implications for decision theory. *Journal of Experimental Psychology: General, 114*, 133–158.

Kihlstrom, J. F., Glisky, M. L., & Anguilo, M. J. (1994). Dissociative tendencies and dissociative disorders. *Journal of Abnormal Psychology, 103*, 117–124.

Klauer, K. C., Musch, J., & Naumer, B. (2000). On belief bias in syllogistic reasoning. *Psychological Review, 107*, 852–884.

Kuley, N. B., & Jacobs, D. F. (1988). The relationship between dissociative-like experiences and sensation seeking among social and problem gamblers. *Journal of Gambling Behavior, 4*(3), 197–207.

Ladouceur, R., Mayrand, M., & Tourigny, Y. (1987). Risk-taking behaviour in gamblers and non-gamblers during prolonged exposure. *Journal of Gambling Behaviour, 3*(2), 115–122.

Ladouceur, R., Paquet, C., Lachance, N., & Dubé, D. (1997). Study of a basic error in the perception of chance. *International Journal of Psychology, 31*(2), 93–99.

Ladouceur, R., & Walker, M. (1996). A cognitive perspective on gambling. In P. M. Salkovskis (Ed.), *Trends in cognitive and behavioural therapies*. New York: John Wiley.

Langer, E. J., & Roth, J. (1975). Heads I win, tails it's chance: The illusion of control as a function of the sequence of outcomes in a purely chance task. *Journal of Personality and Social Psychology, 32*(6), 951–955.

Newell, A., & Simon, H. A. (1972). *Human problem solving*. Englewood Cliffs, NJ: Prentice Hall.

Nisbett, R. E., Krantz, D. H., Jepson, D. H., & Kunda, Z. (1983). The use of statistical heuristics in everyday inductive reasoning. *Psychological Review, 90*, 339–363.

Nisbett, R. E., & Wilson, T. D. (1977). Telling more than we can know: Verbal reports on mental processes. *Psychological Review, 84*, 231–295.

Oaksford, M., & Chater, N. (2001). The probabilistic approach to human reasoning. *Trends in Cognitive Sciences, 5*, 349–357.

Peterson, D. K., & Pitz, G. F. (1988). Confidence, uncertainty, and the use of information. *Journal of Experimental Psychology: Learning, Memory and Cognition, 14*, 85–92.

Philips, J. G., & Amrhein, P. A. (1989). Factors influencing wagers in simulated blackjack. *Journal of Gambling Behavior, 5*, 99–111.

Reber, A. S. (1993). *Implicit learning and tacit knowledge*. Oxford, UK: Oxford University Press.

Reid, R. L. (1986). The psychology of the near miss. *Journal of Gambling Behavior, 2*, 32–39.

Sloman, S. A. (1996). The empirical case for two systems of reasoning. *Psychological Bulletin, 119*, 3–22.

Stanovich, K. E. (1999). *Who is rational? Studies of individual differences in reasoning*. Mahwah, NJ: Lawrence Erlbaum.

Stanovich, K. E. (2004). *The robot's rebellion: Finding meaning in the age of Darwin*. Chicago: University of Chicago Press.

Stanovich, K. E., & West, R. F. (1997). Reasoning independently of prior belief and individual differences in actively open-minded thinking. *Journal of Educational Psychology, 89,* 342–357.

Stanovich, K. E., & West, R. F. (2000). Individual differences in reasoning: Implications for the rationality debate. *Behavioral and Brain Sciences, 23,* 645–726.

Stanovich, K. E., & West, R. F. (2003). Evolutionary versus instrumental goals: How evolutionary psychology misconceives human rationality. In D. E. Over (Ed.), *Evolution and the psychology of thinking* (pp. 171–230). Hove, UK: Psychology Press.

Stevenson, R. J., & Over, D. E. (1995). Deduction from uncertain premises. *The Quarterly Journal of Experimental Psychology, 48A,* 613–643.

Sylvain, C., Ladouceur, R., & Boisvert, B. (1997). Cognitive and behavioural treatment of pathological gambling: A controlled study. *Journal of Consulting and Clinical Psychology, 65*(5), 727–732.

Wagenaar, W. A. (1988). *Paradoxes of gambling behaviour.* Hillsdale, NJ: Lawrence Erlbaum.

Walker, M. B. (1992). *The psychology of gambling.* Elmsford, NY: Pergamon.

Wolfgang, A. K., Zenker, S. I., & Viscusi, T. (1984). Control motivation and the illusion of control in betting on dice. *The Journal of Psychology, 116,* 67–72.

CHAPTER 4

Reflective and Impulsive Determinants of Addictive Behavior

ROLAND DEUTSCH AND FRITZ STRACK

Abstract: The way people judge and interact with their social environment does not only reflect what they believe or want. Cumulating evidence demonstrates that evaluative and stereotypic associations can shape social judgments and behavior in an automatic fashion that is sometimes opposed to a person's goals and beliefs. In the present chapter, we describe a comprehensive theory that explains social cognition and behavior as the joint function of a rule-based reflective system and an association-based impulsive system. In a second step, we apply our Reflective-Impulsive Model to selected phenomena in the realm of addictive cognition and behavior. We conclude that addictive behavior may in part be facilitated by the same mechanisms that underlie automatic social cognition and behavior.

INTRODUCTION

Probably the most intuitively compelling explanation of human behavior is that people do what they believe is good for them. Known as the Rational Model, this global explanation of behavior has been widely accepted in psychology (e.g., Ajzen, 1991; Bandura, 1977), economics, and the political sciences (e.g., Becker, 1976). Often, however, people seem to act in ways that contradict the rational model. They panic in objectively harmless situations, they behave aggressively although it only escalates the conflict, or they consume food or drugs to a self-destructive degree. Why does such behavior occur? One widespread explanation posits a lack of knowledge on the part of the actor as a cause. For instance, people may consume drugs because they mistakenly believe the benefits of consumption outweigh the costs (Becker & Murphy, 1988).

There are, however, instances of negative behavior that occur against all better

AUTHOR'S NOTE: Preparation of this chapter was partially supported by grants from the German Science Foundation (DFG) to Roland Deutsch (De 1150/1-1) and Fritz Strack (Str 264/19-1). We thank Antoine Bechara, Bertram Gawronski, Jan De Houwer, Regina Krieglmeyer, Alan Stacy, Reinout Wiers, and one anonymous reviewer for their helpful comments on an earlier version of this chapter.

knowledge (Berridge, 2003). Addicted persons are often very aware of the harmful long-term effects, but they continue their detrimental behavior (Robinson & Berridge, 2003). Pain or frustration may cause people to hurt other people or damage objects, even though they know that this is unfair or useless (Berkowitz et al., 1981). For a long time, such truly irrational behaviors were rationalized or ostracized from general psychology (Strack & Deutsch, 2004). More recently, these behaviors have gained considerable attention in social cognition research. Particularly, research has established that representations in memory such as stereotypes and attitudes can automatically shape cognition and behavior (for a review, see Greenwald et al., 2002), independent of what people know, believe, and endorse. Dissociations between automatic and controlled responses have stimulated the advent of dual-system models of social cognition and behavior (e.g., Lieberman et al., 2002; Smith & DeCoster, 2000; Strack & Deutsch, 2004). The core tenet of such models is that social behavior is determined by the joint operation of two systems that are characterized by qualitatively different representations and transformations of social information. The two systems may work synergistically or antagonistically, and, under specified conditions, they may promote seemingly irrational cognition and behavior.

Dual-system models may serve as a framework for understanding not only implicit/explicit phenomena in social cognition, but also addictive behavior and its cognitive predecessors (cf. Stacy, 1997; Tiffany, 1990). We will elaborate this idea by using our recently developed Reflective-Impulsive Model (RIM; Strack & Deutsch, 2004) as an example, because it integrates various findings from motivational science into the dual-system idea. Moreover, it is closely related to a neurological model of reflective and impulsive processes that has been outlined in this volume (Bechara et al., Chapter 15). Many psychological functions described in our general model of social cognition and behavior can be linked to the neural mechanisms of Bechara et al.'s model. There are, however, a few divergences, one of the most important being that our impulsive system describes a general memory system that also includes nonevaluative processes irrelevant to reinforcement, whereas the impulsive system as spelled out in Bechara et al.'s model specifically captures affective information-processing. In what follows, we will briefly describe the RIM (for a complete description, see Strack & Deutsch, 2004) and then discuss its potential implications for addiction research.

TWO SYSTEMS FOR SOCIAL BEHAVIOR

According to the RIM, social behavior is a common outcome of a Reflective System (RS) and an Impulsive System (IS), each operating according to different representations and computations, which jointly activate a *final common pathway to behavior* (Norman & Shallice, 1986).

Representation and Processing

The two systems represent the world as well as inner states of the organism in different ways. The IS consists of an associative network, in which activation automatically spreads between connected contents. It serves the function of long-term storage, where associative weights between contents change slowly and gradually. Frequently co-occurring representations of perceptual features, valence, and behavioral programs form associative clusters (see McClelland et al., 1995; Smith & DeCoster, 2000). Whole clusters or their parts can vary in accessibility according to the recency and frequency of their activation (Higgins, 1996). These clusters represent concepts in a concrete manner, because they include fragmentary reenactments of perceptions or behaviors related to the concept (cf. Barsalou, 1999; McClelland et al., 1995).

In contrast, operations of the RS are based on symbolic representations, which are momentary *re-representations* of concrete, modal concepts in the RS (cf. O'Reilly & Norman, 2002). Distinct symbols can be combined flexibly by abstract relations (e.g., *is a*, *is not*, etc.), which is the prerequisite for generating propositional representations containing truth-values. While this ensures great flexibility, the RS operates slowly, depends on intentions, and is easily disrupted by other processes. Because it also functions as a short-term memory store, representations must be construed constantly and fade without rehearsal. The long-term store of the RIM is associative in nature and resides in the IS, which may influence cognition and behavior autonomously, and from which information can be retrieved and converted into a symbolic, propositional format by the RS.

"Implicit social cognition" is often characterized as being unconscious, whereas "explicit social cognition" is assumed to be conscious. There is, however, ample reason to doubt the usefulness of this distinction (De Houwer, Chapter 2). For instance, fast automatic processes not only occur unconsciously, but can be accompanied by subjective experiences of like or dislike (e.g., Epstein, 1991; Russell, 2003). Similarly, controlled processes are not always fully conscious, and are often not accessible by introspection (e.g., Hassin, 2005). Therefore, we assume that both impulsive and reflective processes can occur consciously or unconsciously.

Judgments Versus Associations

Although the IS stores information about the environment, it cannot generate judgments and decisions. Because judgments and decisions relate objects and attributes, they need to be constructed in the RS, based on what is stored in the IS (see later section on system interactions). In general, this leads to a high convergence of associations and judgments. Under some conditions, however, associations and judgments may diverge. One important case is culturally transmitted but socially refuted and unrealistic attitudes or stereotypes, as in sexism or racism (e.g., Gaertner & Dovidio, 1986). In this case, people may exclude associations from their judgments, using effortful correctional strategies (e.g., Devine, 1989; Fazio, 1990).

Stability and Change

Evaluative or stereotypic associations are often characterized as being very enduring (e.g., Wilson et al., 2000). This is supported, for example, by the finding that evaluative associations are sustained even under conditions of extinction (e.g., Baeyens et al., 1988). In line with these observations, the RIM assumes that associative weights in the IS change only slowly and gradually. Concepts, however, are not meant to be single nodes in a network. Instead, they are distributed associative clusters containing codes from different sensory modalities, as well as from affective and behavioral systems. Because each of these components can receive independent activation, the way the IS responds to a particular stimulus is flexible, in spite of the fact that associative weights change only slowly. In line with this reasoning, numerous studies demonstrate that automatic evaluations and activation of stereotypes are context-dependent to a considerable degree (for a review, see Blair, 2002).

Analytic Limitations

The characteristics of the RS and IS imply that fast or unintentional processes are limited in their analytic capability (cf. Greenwald, 1992). Particularly, the RIM predicts that every process that relies on propositional representations depends on reflection. For instance, impulsive responses were demonstrated to be incapable of decoding verbal negations, unless the meaning of the negation had been highly trained (as in *no way*), or a well-defined opposite concept was readily accessible (Deutsch et al., 2004; Mayo et al., 2004). Negating associations presumably does not change the association itself, but merely adds a "false tag" to the link, which later needs to be interpreted by the RS (Fiedler et al., 1996; Ross et al., 1975). Another example for analytic limitations of the IS refers to the representation of time, which also requires propositional representations (Roberts, 2002). For instance, thinking about giving a fancy dinner next month requires ascribing the temporal qualifier *next month* to the representation of the dinner. Within the IS, processing stops at activating concepts. For instance, thinking of either a past or a future dinner is predicted to have the same effect on the IS. Generally speaking, the RIM implies that impulsive processes are myopic and that it takes reflection to construe the past and the future. Although there are some associative mechanisms that may lead to future-oriented behavior (Roberts, 2002), they appear to be limited to very specific behaviors (such as hoarding in animals) or depend on extended learning.

System Interactions

If two systems are indeed responsible for social cognition and behavior, how do they interact? Many recent models assume that impulsive responses can be controlled or corrected by reflection, but the RIM predicts even further interactions.

Reflection Influences
Impulsive Processes

Because the RS has only a short-term memory, propositions have to be constantly construed and rehearsed during operation (McClelland et al., 1995; O'Reilly & Norman,

2002; Smith & DeCoster, 2000), thereby activating concepts in the IS and thus changing its automatic reactivity. This is supported by several studies in the realm of attitudes and stereotypes (Blair, 2002). For instance, deliberate mental imagery of counterstereotypes reduces automatic stereotypic responding (Blair et al., 2001). Likewise, deliberately allocating attention to stereotype-relevant or -irrelevant categories can augment or attenuate automatic stereotyping (e.g., Macrae et al., 1997). Whereas this indicates that reflective activation can occur easily, the suppression of memory content appears to be particularly troublesome, and may even cause rebound effects (Wegner, 1994). In a similar vein, suppressing stereotypes may make the very stereotype more accessible (e.g., Macrae et al., 1994). Activation in memory, attention allocation, and inhibition of motor responses are seen as core means by which the RS can control unwanted cognitive and behavioral tendencies of the IS (Bechara et al., Chapter 15).

Impulsive Processes
Influence Reflection

Because the RS uses content from the IS to generate knowledge, as well as factual, evaluative, and behavioral decisions, it can be strongly influenced by the accessibility of conceptual content. The impact of accessibility on reflective judgments and decision making has been demonstrated in a plethora of studies, identifying the recency and frequency of prior activation as major determinants (Higgins, 1996). A further influence of impulsive responses on reflection rests upon the assumption that feelings of different qualities may be propositionally categorized, contextually qualified, and enter into reflection (e.g., Schwarz & Clore, 1983). For instance, affective responses toward stimuli may be used as judgmental cues in reflective decision making (e.g., Bechara et al., 1997, Bechara et al., Chapter 15). Also, knowledge about the self may be inferred from one's own behavior or from impulsively activated behavioral schemata, as described by attribution and self-perception theory (Bem, 1967).

Routes to Behavior

The core mechanism that mediates between information processing and behavior is a final common pathway, consisting of *behavioral schemata*, which compete for execution and receive input from reflective and impulsive processes. The RS activates behavioral schemata through decision making, whereas the IS activates behavioral schemata as a result of spreading activation.

Behavioral Schemata

We conceive of behavioral schemata as associative clusters that emerge in the IS through the frequent execution of behavior. They connect frequently co-occurring motor representations with both their antecedent conditions and their consequences (Schmidt, 1975), thereby mapping three types of associations. First, behavior-outcome associations will emerge (Elsner & Hommel, 2001). At a later point in time, these associations can be used by reflection to generate knowledge about how to reach a desired outcome. Second, situation-behavior associations will emerge (Miles et al., 2003), representing habits. Finally, associations between situations and outcomes will emerge, which may later elicit conditioned motivation (Rescorla & Solomon, 1967). Being part of the IS, behavioral schemata are subject to spreading activation and differ in their activation potential. Thus, the activation will spread to the remaining elements of the cluster if one part of a behavioral schema is activated.

Reflective and Impulsive Activation

Behavioral schemata support different forms of behavioral control, depending on the source of activation. At a given point in time, reflective and impulsive sources can activate schemata, which then compete for execution (Norman & Shallice, 1986). Processes in the RS scrutinize the desirability and feasibility of actions (Ajzen, 1991; Bandura, 1977), and finally activate appropriate behavioral schemata. Activation from impulsive processes results from a spread of activation from perception to behavioral schemata. Additionally, motivational factors such as deprivation will modulate the reactivity of the IS to environmental stimuli and hence it's behavioral responsiveness. Research indicates that anticipating desired effects of a behavior is a dominant way of translating intentions into behavior (e.g., Elsner & Hommel, 2001). At the same time, merely perceiving an opportunity for action, possible consequences, or the behavior proper will activate the corresponding schema, making the respective behavior more likely to occur (cf. Chartrand & Bargh, 1999; Dijksterhuis & Bargh, 2001).

Differential Predictability

Because the RS and the IS operate according to different principles, the two systems cause unique variance of behavior. Hence, measures of reflective processes (e.g., behavioral intentions) will predict behavior under different circumstances than measures of impulsive processes. For instance, measures of evaluative and stereotypic associations predict behaviors that are usually not under conscious control, such as facial expressions, gestures, or automatic approach and avoidance behaviors, whereas evaluative judgments have a stronger relation to controlled behaviors (e.g., Dovidio et al., 1997; Neumann et al., 2004). Moreover, the differential predictive validity of measures of impulsive and reflective processes is moderated by variables such as the actors' motivation to avoid prejudiced responses or to engage in effortful thinking (e.g., Fazio et al., 1995). In many cases, however, both systems are assumed to act in a synchronized fashion because reflection is based on what is available in the IS. Also, reflection temporarily alters the accessibility of concepts and behavioral schemata, and thus makes compatible responses more likely.

Motivational Mechanisms

Deprivation

Being deprived of a basic need calls for a rapid reversal of the situation and thus for a specific disposition to act. According to the RIM, such a disposition is created by a mechanism of reward and incentive learning (Dickinson & Balleine, 2002). If a state of deprivation is ended, the satisfying behaviors, their situational conditions, and the hedonic consequences will be associated with the representation of this deprivation. If the same state of deprivation occurs again, the satisfying behavioral schemata, their situational conditions, as well as the anticipated satisfaction will be activated. This way, deprivation will establish a *behavioral preparedness* and a *perceptual readiness* for relevant information in the environment. In support of this assumption, the deprivation of basic needs such as hunger and thirst was demonstrated to lower perceptual thresholds for need-relevant stimuli (Aarts et al., 2001). In addition, the associative mechanism outlined above predicts that the valence of objects or behaviors varies depending on deprivation (Cabanac, 1971). Whereas the associative cluster representing a need-relevant object (i.e., a slice of pie) generally contains representations of satisfaction (e.g., positive taste, joy of eating), deprivation will particularly activate this part of the cluster. Hence, the concept will temporarily have a more positive meaning in a deprived than in a satiated state (Ferguson & Bargh, 2004; Seibt et al., 2004; Sherman et al., 2003).

Motivational Orientation

Although deprivations direct behavior in a very specific manner, the IS is also endowed with a global motivational orientation, preparing the organism to decrease (approach) or to increase (avoidance) the distance toward an object (Cacioppo et al., 1993; Lang, 1995). Motivational orientations can be induced by several conditions. Many studies indicate that perceiving positive or negative stimuli automatically prepares the organism to execute approach or avoidance behaviors (Chen & Bargh, 1999; Förster & Strack, 1996). Moreover, extensive evidence suggests that the link between valence and behavior is bidirectional: Performing approach or avoidance behavior also facilitates the processing of compatible information (Förster & Strack, 1997; Neumann & Strack, 2000). Additionally, research indicates that negative affect, particularly the emotion of fear, induces avoidance motivation, whereas positive affect reduces avoidance motivation (Lang, 1995). There may be, however, specific exceptions to the link as proposed above. Particularly, some researchers have argued that anger—a negative emotion toward an aversive event—is associated with approach motivation (Carver, 2004). Finally, merely perceiving oneself approaching an object instantly enhances approach motivation, whereas perceiving oneself avoiding an object further increases avoidance motivation (Neumann & Strack, 2000).

APPLICATION TO ADDICTION

What are the merits of applying the RIM to addictive behaviors? On a general level, it can help integrate and organize research from different areas. On a more specific level, it may help identify interactions between processes that were previously considered in isolation. Some of the processes studied in addiction research (Robinson & Berridge, 2003) clearly belong to the RS, such as the regulation of action (Bandura, 1977), "rational choice" (Becker & Murphy, 1988), and explicit expectancies of drug effects (Goldman et al., 1999). Other mechanisms, however, are tied more closely to associative learning, such as conditioned withdrawal and tolerance (Siegel, 1979), drug habits (Tiffany, 1990), or incentive sensitization (Robinson & Berridge, 2003). Given the evidence for each of those processes, it is likely that all of them contribute to addictive behavior to some degree. Although these mechanisms differ in their operational principles, they interact at various stages. Therefore, it seems desirable to integrate them into one cognitive architecture.

In addition to these general benefits, the RIM may also have more specific implications for research and theory on addictive behavior. According to the operational principles of the IS, chronic consumption of psychoactive substances will lead to changes in the associative structure, which will strongly influence further processing and behavior. First, the representation of the drug in the IS will change with extended consumption (Stacy, 1997). Second, behavioral schemata will develop that are specific to a substance and may link the typical conditions and consequences of consumption. Third, addictive drugs usually induce tolerance, paired with cycles of withdrawal and satiation (Robinson & Berridge, 2003), and stimulate brain systems that are also relevant for natural reward (Kelley & Berridge, 2002). Therefore, the mechanisms that regulate impulsive responding in the case of deprivation may also operate in addiction. This impulsive setup may then cause situational cues and reflection to interact and facilitate addictive behaviors. In what follows, we describe three examples of such possible influences.

The Valence of Drugs

Consuming drugs often has immediate positive outcomes, but may give rise to negative outcomes in the more distant future (e.g., Jones & McMahon, 1994), which leads the RIM to predict that drugs are evaluatively ambivalent. The most obvious type of ambivalence can be understood as a conflict between the IS and RS. Just as beliefs and associations concerning social groups may produce opposing behavioral outcomes (e.g., Dovidio et al., 1997; Fazio et al., 1995), beliefs about drugs and drug-associations can diverge and determine behavior in antagonistic ways (e.g., Wiers et al., 2002). At the same time, however, the RIM also predicts antagonisms within the IS. First, they may arise if a substance is regularly consumed to end a negative feeling state (e.g., pain). Then, the drug and the behavioral representations of its consumption will become associated not only with the positive consequences of its consumption, but also with aspects of the preceding negative state (for a review of evidence, see Wiers et al., Chapter 22). Hence, the associative cluster in the IS will consist of both positive and negative elements, which may become accessible under different conditions. Second, associations that are verbally transmitted as opposed to being based on private experience may diverge. For instance, the word *cigarette* may be associated with negative attributes because of verbally transmitted information about cigarettes. At the same time, visual, gustatory, and olfactory representations of the object *cigarette* may be associated with positive feelings. Thus, depending on which part of the associative cluster representing the drug is more accessible (e.g., because of contextual priming) or which particular association (e.g., verbal vs. perceptual) is tapped, different valences may be obtained from implicit measures. In fact, some research indicates that drugs may be associated with negative attributes (Swanson et al., 2001 Wiers et al., 2002), whereas other studies demonstrate positive impulsive responses (Geier et al., 2000).

Craving and Compulsion

The mechanisms spelled out in the RIM may help to understand how drug urges—which may be elicited by drug cues, deprivation, and reflective operations—can facilitate compulsive consumption. Because reflection is assumed to be based on what is accessible in the IS, extreme states of the IS can alter what and how people think and decide about drugs. For instance, deprivation will render the representations of immediate drug-effects more accessible in the IS and hence direct thoughts toward the positive consequences of consumption. Likewise, if consumption schemata receive activation through deprivation, attention and thoughts will be biased toward those situations in which drugs were usually consumed. At the same time, the activated schemata will need less additional activation to exceed the threshold of execution. In turn, if reflection is centered on consumption, the drug, and its effects, impulsive activation of these concepts and schemata is predicted to be further enhanced. This vicious circle may finally push consumption schemata above the threshold of execution.

Analytic Limitations

Preventive and therapeutic action sometimes relies on verbally transmitted abstract concepts. Such intervention, if it requires propositional processing, may cause paradoxical effects. Take for instance the case of negated appeals, such as *alcohol does not make you sexy*. Such appeals activate the negated concepts in the IS, but the negation will only be effective in the RS. Hence, what is stored in the IS may actually oppose the intended meaning. In the case of the sentence *alcohol does not make you sexy*, the concepts *alcohol* and *sexy* may become associated in the IS. Evidence for this assumption comes from Farrelly et al. (2002), who compared the effectiveness of antismoking campaigns that used negations (e.g., *Don't smoke*) versus affirmative expressions (e.g., *Tobacco kills*). Exposed to negations, young adults were even more open to the idea of smoking, whereas the affirmative campaign positively changed attitudes toward tobacco. Similarly, drug-related intentions containing negations (e.g., *I will not touch these cigarettes*) will enhance the activation of the negated concept in memory (Palfai et al., 1997), thereby pushing the IS toward consumption. In a related vein, associations between the drug and the effects of consumption are predicted to have a short time horizon. Particularly, rich representations of immediate drug effects (e.g., activation, pleasure, or drowsiness) will automatically become part of the associative cluster representing the drug. Less proximate drug effects (e.g., social and health problems), however, cannot be integrated into the cluster via automatic learning. Instead, such relations must be established by reflective processes, based on language and abstract symbols. As a consequence, even when the negative proximate effects become part of the cluster, they are more abstract. In sum, reflective expectancies of drug effects and stored associations may differ with respect to the time horizon they can capture, and thus may direct behavior in opposing directions (Goldman et al., 1999).

SUMMARY AND CONCLUSION

In the present chapter, we have described a dual-system model of social cognition and behavior that can account for many phenomena observed in social-cognition research. On the one hand, behavior may be caused by decisions based on outcome expectancies. Decisions are generated in the RS, based on symbolic representation. On the other hand, behavior may be caused by a spread of activation in a simple associative network, the IS, which stores concepts in a multimodal manner with strong links to behavioral codes. Importantly, the two systems interact at various stages of processing. Reflection is based on information retrieved from the associative network and thus alters the reactivity of this system. At the same time, the activation of representations in the IS determines the ease of use for reflective operations. Thus, although the two systems follow different principles, they influence each other to a significant degree. Also, the architecture of the IS is dynamic in that its reactivity depends not only on the strength of associations, but also on the activation of representations, which may be influenced not only by situational cues, but also by motivational and reflective sources. Therefore, automatic evaluation may vary considerably. Moreover, the present framework de-confounds consciousness and processing systems. Both impulsive and reflective processes can occur in a conscious or unconscious manner.

From the present analysis, we conclude that dual-system models are powerful theoretical tools for integrating a wide range of phenomena from social psychology and beyond. Broad theories like the RIM can help unify research in different fields and may facilitate the convergence of language and concepts. Research on addiction has already adopted the distinction between automatic and controlled processes, and has successfully employed implicit measures of evaluative and conceptual associations. It is possible that the application of a broad dual-system model may have comparable merits.

REFERENCES

Aarts, H., Dijksterhuis, A., & De Vries, P. (2001). On the psychology of drinking: Being thirsty and perceptually ready. *British Journal of Psychology, 92,* 631–642.

Ajzen, I. (1991). The theory of planned behavior. *Organizational Behavior and Human Decision Processes, 50,* 179–211.

Baeyens, F., Crombez, G., Van den Bergh, O., & Eelen, P. (1988). Once in contact always in contact: Evaluative conditioning is resistant to extinction. *Advances in Behavioral Research and Therapy, 10,* 179–199.

Bandura, A. (1977). *Social learning theory.* Englewood Cliffs, NJ: Prentice Hall.

Barsalou, L. (1999). Perceptual symbol systems. *Behavioral and Brain Sciences, 22,* 577–609.

Bechara, A., Damasio, H., Tranel, D., & Damasio, A. R. (1997). Deciding advantageously before knowing the advantageous strategy. *Science, 275,* 1293–1295.

Becker, G. (1976). *The economic approach to behavior.* Chicago: University of Chicago Press.

Becker, G. S., & Murphy, K. M. (1988). A theory of rational addiction. *Journal of Political Economy, 96,* 675–700.

Bem, D. J. (1967). An alternative interpretation of cognitive dissonance phenomena. *Psychological Review, 73,* 185–200.

Berkowitz, L., Cochran, S. T., & Embree, M. C. (1981). Physical pain and the goal of aversively stimulated aggression. *Journal of Personality and Social Psychology, 40,* 687–700.

Berridge, K. C. (2003). Irrational pursuits: Hyper-incentives from a visceral brain. In I. Brocas & J. Carrillo (Eds.), *The psychology of economic decisions* (Vol. 1, pp. 17–40). Oxford, UK: Oxford University Press.

Blair, I. V. (2002). The malleability of automatic stereotypes and prejudice. *Personality and Social Psychology Review, 6*, 242–261.

Blair, I. V., Ma, J. E., & Lenton, A. P. (2001). Imagining stereotypes away: The moderation of implicit stereotypes through mental imagery. *Journal of Personality and Social Psychology, 81*, 828–841.

Cabanac, M. (1971). Physiological role of pleasure. *Science*, 1103–1107.

Cacioppo, J. T., Priester, J. R., & Berntson, G. G. (1993). Rudimentary determinants of attitudes: II. Arm flexion and extension have differential effects on attitudes. *Journal of Personality and Social Psychology, 65*, 5–17.

Carver, C. S. (2004). Negative affects deriving from the behavioral approach system. *Emotion, 4*, 3–22.

Chartrand, T. L., & Bargh, J. A. (1999). The chameleon effect: The perception behavior link in social perception. *Journal of Personality and Social Psychology, 76*, 893–910.

Chen, M., & Bargh, J. A. (1999). Consequences of automatic evaluation: Immediate behavioral predispositions to approach or avoid the stimulus. *Personality and Social Psychology Bulletin, 25*, 215–224.

Deutsch, R., Gawronski, B., & Strack, F. (2004). *At the boundaries of automaticity: Negation as reflective operation.* Manuscript submitted for publication.

Devine, P. G. (1989). Stereotypes and prejudice: Their automatic and controlled components. *Journal of Personality and Social Psychology, 56*, 5–18.

Dickinson, A., & Balleine, B. (2002). The role of learning in the operation of motivational systems. In H. Pashler & R. Gallistel (Eds.), *Steven's handbook of experimental psychology* (pp. 497–533). New York: John Wiley.

Dijksterhuis, A., & Bargh, J. A. (2001). The perception-behavior expressway: Automatic effects of social perception on social behavior. In M. P. Zanna (Ed.), *Advances in experimental social psychology: Vol. 33* (pp. 1–40). San Diego, CA: Academic Press.

Dovidio, J. F., Kawakami, K., Johnson, C., Johnson, B., & Howard, A. (1997). On the nature of prejudice: Automatic and controlled processes. *Journal of Experimental Social Psychology, 33*, 510–540.

Elsner, B., & Hommel, B. (2001). Effect anticipation and action control. *Journal of Experimental Psychology: Human Perception and Performance, 27*, 229–240.

Epstein, S. (1991). Cognitive-experiential self-theory: An integrative theory of personality. In R. Curtis (Ed.), *The relational self: Theoretical convergences in psychoanalytical, social, and personality psychology* (pp. 111–137). New York: Guilford.

Farrelly, M. C., Healton, C. G., Davis, K. C., Messeri, P., Hersey, J. C., & Haviland, M. L. (2002). Getting to the truth: Evaluating national tobacco countermarketing campaigns. *American Journal of Public Health, 92*, 901–907.

Fazio, R. H. (1990). Multiple processes by which attitudes guide behavior: The MODE model as an integrative framework. In M. P Zanna (Ed.), *Advances in experimental social psychology: Vol. 23* (pp. 75–109). San Diego, CA: Academic Press.

Fazio, R. H., Jackson, J. R., Dunton, B. C., & Williams, C. J. (1995). Variability in automatic activation as an unobtrusive measure of racial attitudes: A bona fide pipeline? *Journal of Personality and Social Psychology, 69*, 1013–1027.

Ferguson, M. J., & Bargh, J. A. (2004). Liking is for doing: The effects of goal pursuit on automatic evaluation. *Journal of Personality and Social Psychology, 87,* 557–572.

Fiedler, K., Armbruster, T., Nickel, S., Walther, E., & Asbeck, J. (1996). Constructive memory and social judgment: Experiments in the self-verification of question contents. *Journal of Personality and Social Psychology, 71,* 861–873.

Förster, J., & Strack, F. (1996). The influence of overt head movements on memory for valenced words: A case of conceptual-motor compatibility. *Journal of Personality and Social Psychology, 71,* 421–430.

Förster, J., & Strack, F. (1997). Motor actions in retrieval of valenced information: A motor congruence effect. *Perceptual and Motor Skills, 85,* 1419–1427.

Gaertner, S. L., & Dovidio, J. F. (1986). The aversive form of racism. In J. F. Dovidio & S. L. Gaertner (Eds.), *Prejudice, discrimination, and racism* (pp. 61–89). Orlando, FL: Academic Press.

Geier, A., Mucha, R. F., & Pauli, P. (2000). Appetitive nature of drug cues confirmed with physiological measures in a model using pictures of smoking. *Psychopharmacology, 150,* 283–291.

Goldman, M. S., Del Boca, F. K., & Darkes, J. (1999). Alcohol expectancy theory: The application of cognitive neuroscience. In H. T. Blane & K. E. Leonard (Eds.), *Psychological theories of drinking and alcoholism* (2nd ed., pp. 203–216). New York: Guilford.

Greenwald, A. G. (1992). New Look 3: Reclaiming unconscious cognition. *American Psychologist, 47,* 766–779.

Greenwald, A. G., Banaji, M. R., Rudman, L. A., Farnham, S. D., Nosek, B. A., & Mellott, D. S. (2002). A unified theory of implicit attitudes, stereotypes, self-esteem, and self-concept. *Psychological Review, 109,* 3–25.

Hassin, R. R. (2005). Non conscious control and implicit working memory. In R. R. Hassin, J. S. Uleman, & J. A. Bargh (Eds.), *The new unconscious.* New York: Oxford University Press.

Higgins, E. T. (1996). Knowledge activation: Accessibility, applicability, and salience. In E. T. Higgins & A. W. Kruglanski (Eds.), *Social psychology: Handbook of basic principles* (pp. 133–168). New York: Guilford.

Jones, B. T., & McMahon, J. (1994). Negative and positive alcohol expectancies as predictors of abstinence after discharge from a residential treatment programme: A one- and three-month follow-up study in males. *Journal of Studies on Alcohol, 55,* 543–548.

Kelley, A. E., & Berridge, K. C. (2002). The neuroscience of natural rewards: Relevance to addictive drugs. *The Journal of Neuroscience, 22,* 3306–3311.

Lang, P. J. (1995). The emotion probe: Studies of motivation and attention. *American Psychologist, 50,* 372–385.

Lieberman, M. D., Gaunt, R., Gilbert, D. T., & Trope, Y. (2002). Reflection and reflexion: A social cognitive neuroscience approach to attributional inference. In M. P. Zanna (Ed.), *Advances in experimental social psychology* (Vol. 34, pp. 199–249). New York: Academic Press.

Macrae, C. N., Bodenhausen, G. V., Milne, A. B., & Jetten, J. (1994). Out of mind but back in sight: Stereotypes on the rebound. *Journal of Personality and Social Psychology, 67,* 808–817.

Macrae, C. N., Bodenhausen, G. V., Milne, A. B., Thorn, T. M. J., & Castelli, L. (1997). On the activation of social stereotypes: The moderating role of processing objectives. *Journal of Experimental Social Psychology, 33,* 471–489.

Mayo, R., Schul, Y., & Burnstein, E. (2004). "I am not guilty" vs. "I am innocent": Successful negation may depend on the schema used for its encoding. *Journal of Experimental Social Psychology, 40*, 433–449.

McClelland, J. L., McNaughton, B. L., & O'Reilly, R. C. (1995). Why there are complementary learning systems in the hippocampus and neocortex: Insights from the successes and failures of connectionist models of learning and memory. *Psychological Review, 102*, 419–457.

Miles, F. J., Everitt, B. J., & Dickinson, A. (2003). Oral cocaine seeking by rats: Action or habit? *Behavioral Neuroscience, 117*, 927–938.

Neumann, R., Hülsenbeck, K., & Seibt, B. (2004). Attitudes towards people with AIDS and avoidance behavior: Automatic and reflective bases of behavior. *Journal of Experimental Social Psychology, 40*, 543–550.

Neumann, R., & Strack, F. (2000). Approach and avoidance: The influence of proprioceptive and exteroceptive cues on encoding of affective information. *Journal of Personality and Social Psychology, 79*, 39–48.

Norman, D. A., & Shallice, T. (1986). Attention to action. Willed and automatic control of behavior. In R. J. Davidson, G. E. Schwartz, & D. Shapiro (Eds.), *Consciousness and self regulation: Advances in research* (pp. 1–18). New York: Plenum.

O'Reilly, R. C., & Norman, K. A. (2002). Hippocampal and neocortical contributions to memory: Advances in the complementary learning systems framework. *Trends in Cognitive Sciences, 6*, 505–510.

Palfai, T. P., Monti, P. M., Colby, S. M., & Rohsenow, D. J. (1997). Effects of suppressing the urge to drink on the accessibility of alcohol outcome expectancies. *Behavior Research and Therapy, 35*, 59–65.

Rescorla, R. A., & Solomon, R. L. (1967). Two-process learning theory. *Psychological Review, 73*, 151–182.

Roberts, W. A. (2002). Are animals stuck in time? *Psychological Bulletin, 128*, 473–489.

Robinson, T. E., & Berridge, K. C. (2003) Addiction. *Annual Review of Psychology, 54*, 25–53.

Ross, L., Lepper, M., & Hubbard, M. (1975). Perseverance in self-perception and social perception: Biased attributional processes in the debriefing paradigm. *Journal of Personality and Social Psychology, 32*, 880–892.

Russell, J. A. (2003). Core affect and the psychological construction of emotion. *Psychological Review, 110*, 145–172.

Schmidt, R. A. (1975). A schema theory of discrete motor skill learning. *Psychological Review, 82*, 225–260.

Schwarz, N., & Clore, G. L. (1983). Mood, misattribution, and judgments of well-being: Informative and directive functions of affective states. *Journal of Personality and Social Psychology, 45*, 513–523.

Seibt, B., Häfner, M., & Deutsch, R. (2004). *Prepared to eat: How immediate affective and motivational responses to food cues are influenced by food deprivation.* Manuscript submitted for publication.

Sherman, S. J., Rose, J. S., Koch, K., Presson, C. C., & Chassin, L. (2003). Implicit and explicit attitudes toward cigarette smoking: The effects of context and motivation. *Journal of Social and Clinical Psychology, 22*, 13–39.

Siegel, S. (1979). The role of conditioning in drug tolerance and addiction. In J. D. Keehn (Ed.), *Psychopathology in animals: Research and treatment implications* (pp. 143–168). New York: Academic Press.

Smith, E. R., & DeCoster, J. (2000). Dual process models in social and cognitive psychology: Conceptual integration and links to underlying memory systems. *Personality and Social Psychology Review, 4,* 108–131.

Stacy, A. W. (1997). Memory activation and expectancy as prospective predictors of alcohol and marihuana use. *Journal of Abnormal Psychology, 106,* 61–73.

Strack, F., & Deutsch, R. (2004). Reflective and impulsive determinants of social behavior. *Personality and Social Psychology Review, 3,* 220–247.

Swanson, J. E., Rudman, L. A., & Greenwald, A. G. (2001). Using the implicit association test to investigate attitude-behavior consistency for stigmatized behavior. *Cognition and Emotion, 15,* 207–230.

Tiffany, S. T. (1990). A cognitive model of drug urges and drug-use behavior: Role of automatic and nonautomatic processes. *Psychological Review, 97,* 147–168.

Wegner, D. M. (1994). Ironic processes of mental control. *Psychological Review, 101,* 34–52.

Wiers, R. W., van Woerden, N., Smulders, F. T. Y., & de Jong, P. (2002). Implicit and explicit alcohol-related cognitions in heavy and light drinkers. *Journal of Abnormal Psychology, 111,* 648–658.

Wilson, T. D., Lindsey, S., & Schooler, T. Y. (2000). A model of dual attitudes. *Psychological Review, 107,* 101–126.

CHAPTER 5

Measuring, Manipulating, and Modeling the Unconscious Influences of Prior Experience on Memory for Recent Experiences

CATHY L. McEVOY AND DOUGLAS L. NELSON

Abstract: Understanding an individual's current behavior demands that we consider the prior experiences of the person in the same or similar contexts. These prior experiences leave memory traces that can implicitly influence how new experiences are interpreted and remembered. In this chapter, we describe how researchers use implicit measures of memory to explore these influences. We include the method of savings, indirect test instructions, the process dissociation procedure, and the PIER2 model of cued recall that formalizes the influence of unconscious processes on the conscious retrieval of recently experienced events. We discuss how memories that may not be consciously processed can, nonetheless, cue maladaptive thoughts and behaviors such as substance abuse.

INTRODUCTION

One of the fascinating characteristics of human cognition is the complex interaction between what we previously experienced and how we currently think and behave. This relationship is obvious when we observe phobic reactions to innocuous stimuli, increased drug use in settings associated with previous abuse, or reluctance to develop new relationships following an unsuccessful marriage. Clearly, we do not behave in a vacuum divorced from our past history. Rather, it is our history that makes us unique, and in the absence of that history our behavior would be largely a function of the current environment.

Much of the memory research over the past century has either ignored the influence of

AUTHOR'S NOTE: This research was supported by grants AG13973 from the National Institute on Aging to C. L. McEvoy and MH16360 from the National Institute of Mental Health to D. L. Nelson. Correspondence should be addressed to Cathy L. McEvoy, School of Aging Studies, University of South Florida, 4202 Fowler Ave. MHC1348, Tampa, FL 33620. E-mail: cmcevoy@luna.cas.usf.edu prior experience or attempted to minimize it. Interestingly, the father of experimental memory research, Hermann Ebbinghaus, did not succumb to this urge. He recognized that the "vanished mental states" of previous experiences continue to exist in memory and exert an influence even though the specific memories "do not return to consciousness at all" (1885/1964, p. 2). Nevertheless, for most memory researchers past experience represents a noisome source of experimental error. For others, however, it represents a tantalizing window on how prior experiences unconsciously shape our encoding and retrieval of current experiences. In this chapter, we will describe how researchers have used implicit measures of memory to explore the influence of experience on current behavior. We first will describe three techniques for studying implicit memory—the method of savings, indirect test instructions, and the process dissociation procedure. Then we will discuss in-depth a model of cued recall that incorporates both implicit and explicit memory processes (PIER2, D. Nelson et al., 1998) that is an alternative to other methods of studying implicit memory. As shown below and in the chapter by Stacy et al. (Chapter 6), the model suggests cognitive processes that may underlie or at least co-occur with addictive behaviors.

IMPLICIT MEMORY

The Method of Savings

While researching the learning of new materials, Ebbinghaus (1885/1964) noted that some materials could be learned more quickly than others and that the rate of relearning was faster than the rate of original learning. He developed the method of "savings" as a measure of memory for information that had been learned at one time, but could no longer be recalled explicitly. Savings refers to the difference between the number of trials needed to attain a criterion level of memory performance during an initial learning experience compared with attaining the same level after some retention interval. The assumption is that, even though the material may not be explicitly recallable after the retention interval, if it can be relearned faster than it was originally learned (showing savings), then there must be "continuing existence" of a memory trace for the material.

Early research on amnesic patients who have severely impaired explicit memory demonstrated savings in a wide variety of tasks. Milner et al.'s (1964) patient showed savings in relearning perceptual-motor tasks, despite a lack of explicit awareness of having ever engaged in those tasks. Warrington and Weiskrantz (1968) presented patients with fragmented words or pictures and had them identify each stimulus. Progressively more detail was added until the patient could identify the stimulus. After a retention interval, savings was determined by having the patient perform the completion task again. As with skill learning, amnesic patients showed savings on fragment completion even though they did not remember doing the task before and could not recognize intact stimuli as having been previously experienced.

Other researchers have used savings to explore unconscious influences on memory in normal subjects. Kolers (1976) had students read texts printed in an inverted format. As much as a year later, they showed savings in rereading inverted text. T. Nelson (1978) used savings to demonstrate that small amounts of information remained in memory even when recognition was at chance level. The savings measure is particularly useful in studying memory over long periods of time, when explicit recall may be at floor but implicit memory is still viable. The method, however, is time-consuming, requiring relatively long retention intervals. As a consequence, much of the research on implicit memory has used testing instructions to contrast explicit and implicit uses of memory.

Indirect Testing Instructions

The majority of research on implicit uses of memory has employed indirect testing instructions. Subjects are exposed to stimuli under a cover story that does not mention testing memory of the items. After this exposure, trial subjects are asked to perform another task. This might involve completing word fragments, in which some of the letters are missing (W _ R L _) to make the first word that comes to mind, or generating associated words to presented cues. The subject sees a set of cues that are related to the exposed words, plus a set of control cues that are related to nonexposed words. The test instructions are worded to disguise the connection between the exposure trial and the test. The measure of implicit memory is the difference in target production for the exposed items versus the nonexposed control items, reflecting repetition priming from a recently established memory trace for the targets. Implicit memory usually is contrasted with explicit memory for the same stimuli. Explicit instructions ask the subject to respond with a related item that was included in the exposure trial. Thus, the exposure trial and the test cues are held constant, with the only difference being the directness of the test instructions.

Test instructions have been used to study implicit and explicit memory in college students, children, older adults, neurological patients, and so on, and to study memory for stimuli that subjects may hesitate to recall explicitly (obscenities, etc.). Research on implicit memory blossomed in the 1980s (see Graf & Masson, 1993, for an excellent review), demonstrating significant influences from automatic or unconscious memory that are evident even in the absence of intention to remember. The early impetus for this research was the finding of relatively spared implicit memory in amnesic patients with severely impaired explicit memory (e.g., Graf et al., 1984). The research with amnesic patients suggests that priming is more intact than is explicit memory, and that the amount of priming is influenced by the types of materials used and the relationships between the test cues and the targets. These results have been used to argue for different memory systems underlying explicit versus implicit memory as well as for unique systems for processing perceptual versus conceptual information (e.g., Tulving & Schacter, 1990). Other researchers (e.g., Roediger & Blaxton, 1987) have argued for a transfer-appropriate processing explanation of these dissociations. For the purposes of this chapter, what matters is not so much whether retrieval of different materials under different instructions is mediated by different processes, different systems, or both, but rather, what can we learn about the influence of previously acquired information on retrieval of recently presented information?

Research on normal subjects using manipulations of testing instructions has suggested that the magnitude of priming effects depends on a variety of factors. When a conceptual test is used, priming generally is affected by conceptual manipulations, such as levels of processing and elaboration (Hamann, 1990; Srinivas & Roediger, 1990; but see also Light et al., 2000; D. Nelson et al., 1992). Items processed with a more elaborate or semantic encoding tend to show larger priming effects than those processed with a more structural encoding orientation, such as naming vowels. Such manipulations also have substantial influence on explicit tests of memory, such as cued and free recall and recognition. Manipulations of physical characteristics of the stimulus, such as changes in modality between the exposure and test trials have much less influence when a conceptual test is used. In contrast, these manipulations have large effects on priming when a perceptual task is used (such as perceptual identification), whereas semantic manipulations have less influence.

Manipulations of test instructions have yielded a large and important body of research on the conscious and unconscious contributions to memory retrieval. Much of the literature has focused on the issue of what memory processes (or memory systems) underlie performance in each of the tasks. One issue that became apparent relatively early was whether the tasks used in these studies were "process pure." That is, when a subject performs a stem completion task under indirect testing instructions, does this involve only implicit memory, and when the stem completion task is performed under direct testing instructions does this involve only explicit memory? This question has at least two important implications.

First, to what extent is performance in an implicit memory task contaminated by explicit retrieval? Subjects may notice that when they complete one of the test stems with the first word that comes to mind, the word happens to be one from the previous task. They might then use explicit retrieval of previously exposed words to try to complete the stems, rather than reporting the first word that comes to mind. To what extent was performance produced by implicit processes, and to what extent was it produced by explicit retrieval? The contamination is critical when comparing groups or conditions in which explicit retrieval might be confounded. For example, aging has a large effect on explicit memory, but a much smaller effect on implicit memory (La Voie & Light, 1994; McEvoy et al., 1995). Do younger subjects show greater repetition priming because they are more likely to notice a connection between the test cues and items from the exposure task, and then use their superior explicit retrieval to produce more of the target items during the implicit test? If so, then the age difference in implicit memory may simply reflect contamination from explicit memory, which clearly shows large age differences. This concern is also relevant when studying groups that may vary in motivation to explicitly retrieve, such as drug abusers.

Researchers attempt to reduce or identify explicit contamination in implicit tasks by disguising the connection between the test cues and the exposure trial. These disguises include clever test instructions that divert attention away from the exposure episode, filled delays between exposure and test, and the inclusion of test cues for nonexposed items to lessen the likelihood of subjects noticing the connection. Finally, subjects may be asked after the test is completed whether they noticed anything special about the items on the test trial.

The second issue arising when indirect and direct tests are considered pure measures of implicit and explicit memory, respectively, is that these assumptions ignore any possible contribution to explicit recall from implicit memory processes. As mentioned earlier, many researchers studying explicit memory consider the influence of prior knowledge to be a source of uncontrolled noise, and they tend to ignore its influences. An ignored influence is still there, however, and such influence means that a direct test of memory does not provide a pure measure of explicit, conscious retrieval processes. If we assume that performance on explicit tests of memory include both conscious and unconscious memory processes, how do we separate out those influences? This is much more complex than the possible contamination of implicit performance by explicit recall. It is not possible, for example, to ask subjects whether they used unconscious retrieval to recall items from the exposure trial.

Two lines of research are relevant to how the unconscious influences of prior knowledge on explicit memory can be studied. Jacoby (1991) developed a method, referred to as the process dissociation procedure, which uses test instructions and mathematical decomposition of performance to separate the contributions of conscious and automatic processes to intentional recall. D. Nelson and his colleagues (D. Nelson et al., 1998) developed a formal model of cued recall (PIER2) in which manipulations of the structure of prior knowledge are used to assess its influence on recall. Each will be described below.

Process Dissociation Procedure

The process dissociation procedure was developed by Jacoby (1991) and colleagues as a more "process pure" measure of the contributions of consciously controlled and automatic processes in memory. The procedure is based on the assumption that the probability of correct recall in an explicit task is a function of both conscious recollective processes and automatic processes, and that these processes can be put in opposition to one another through test instruction manipulations. Subjects are presented with a study list of words then receive related test cues. Subjects receive inclusion test instructions for half of the cues and exclusion instructions for the other half. In the inclusion instruction, they are told to recall a studied word that fits the test cue. In the exclusion instruction they are told to use the test cue to produce a word that fits the cue that *was not* on the study list. In other words, if they thought of a studied word they were supposed to exclude it and produce a different, unstudied, word.

In the inclusion condition subjects might produce the studied target because they recollected it, with a probability of R, or because it was automatically brought to mind, with a probability of A. Thus, the probability of responding with a target in the inclusion condition equals $R + A (1 - R)$. In the exclusion condition, if subjects think of a

target and recollect that it was in the study list they will not give it as their response because the instructions tell them to exclude studied items. They will only give a studied word if it is automatically brought to mind and they *do not* recollect that it was from the list. Thus, the probability of responding with a target in the exclusion condition equals $A (1 - R)$. Because the target can be produced in the inclusion condition from either recollective or automatic processes, but can be produced in the exclusion condition only from automatic processes, the difference between these two conditions (Inclusion – Exclusion) provides an estimate of recollection (R), which can be used to solve the equation for A ($A =$ Exclusion $/ 1 - R$).

The process dissociation procedure has been used to separate the influences of automatic and conscious processes on memory. Of particular interest in this chapter are studies showing differential effects of a variable on recollection, compared with its effects on automatic processes. For example, manipulating level of processing (Toth et al., 1994), amnesia (Verfaellie & Treadwell, 1993), and normal aging (Jennings & Jacoby, 1993) appear to have larger effects on recollection than on familiarity processes, whereas perceptual fluency manipulations show the opposite pattern (LeCompte, 1995).

Although the process dissociation procedure has been criticized regarding some of its assumptions (e.g., Curran & Hintzman, 1997; Graf & Komatsu, 1994), it continues to be widely used to study the automatic and conscious components of memory (see Yonelinas, 2002, for a review). It should be used with care, particularly when the probability of producing targets in the exclusion condition is low, resulting in large differences in base rates between the inclusion and exclusion conditions. It also is important to make sure that subjects understand the exclusion instructions, which may be a problem with individuals whose cognitive abilities are impaired by drug abuse, dementia, and so on. Thus, we next present a model of cued recall, PIER2, in which the automatic influences of prior knowledge are assessed through manipulations of materials, rather than through manipulations of test instructions.

PIER2

Experiencing a known word is assumed to implicitly activate related words from past experiences (e.g., Deese, 1965). For example, reading the word BEER activates associated concepts, such as *drink, wine, drunk, glass, vodka, alcohol*, and so on. These implicitly activated concepts generally do not come to consciousness, but nevertheless they can, and do, have systematic influences on the encoding and retrieval of the target word (BEER). We have developed a model of cued recall and recognition that attempts to explain these influences. The model is PIER2 (Processing Implicit and Explicit Representations) and it was designed to understand the linkage between what is known about a word and the likelihood that the word will be remembered when presented in a new episodic context (D. Nelson et al., 1998). To understand the PIER2 model, and the data that have shaped this model, we first have to describe how we measure what is known about familiar words.

Free Association as a Measure of Word Knowledge

We use free association as a means of measuring what people know about familiar words. In the free-association task, subjects are presented with a list of familiar words and are asked to write down the first word that comes to mind after reading each word. Approximately 125 to 180 subjects independently respond to each stimulus word. We then collate the responses from all of the subjects, producing a set of the different responses given by 2 or more subjects, and

the proportion of the subjects that gave each response. For example, of the 180 subjects who responded to the stimulus word BEER, 31 (or .17) of them gave the response *drink*, whereas 2 (or .01) of them gave the response *vodka*. The proportion of subjects giving each response is used as a measure of the relative strength of that response as an associate of the stimulus word. Thus, *drink* is considered to be a stronger associate of BEER than is *vodka*, but both are considered to be stronger associates of BEER than would be a word that was not given by any of the subjects. This is not to say that a word that was never given by any of the subjects in the normative task is not necessarily an associate of the stimulus. We assume that the free-association process picks up the strongest associates of a word, but that many other words are more weakly associated with the stimulus (D. Nelson et al., 2000; D. Nelson et al., 2004). Despite their limitations, free-association data provide the most reliable estimate of the strength relationships between words that is available to researchers (D. Nelson et al., in press).

In the process of collecting association norms, we discovered that words varied in the number of associates that they produced. We refer to this characteristic as a word's set size, with small set size generally defind as 7 or fewer associates and large set size as greater than 15 associates. We also discovered that the associations between words is much more complex than the individual direct connection from word A to word B. For example, the word BEER produces the words *wine* and *drunk*; the word WINE produces the words *beer, drink, alcohol, drunk*, and so on; and the word DRUNK produces the words *beer, alcohol, wine, drink*, and so forth. Thus, the set of associates of the word BEER are themselves likely to produce each other in independent normings of their associations, making BEER a word whose associates are relatively densely interconnected. We refer to this characteristic of words as their connectivity. We also measure the probability that a word's associates produce the originating word, a quality we refer to as resonance. In the above example, both WINE and DRUNK produced *bee*r as an associate, resulting in resonant connections. As will be seen later, our memory research suggests that both connectivity and resonance influence the likelihood that a target word will be recalled or recognized.

The Cued Recall Memory Task and the Effects of Prior Knowledge

Much of our work on the role of prior knowledge on memory for recent episodes has used the extralist cued recall task, and we will limit our discussion to the findings from that task. In extralist cued recall, subjects are presented with a list of words, usually 24 of them, one word at a time, for 3 seconds per word. Under the usual study conditions, subjects are asked to read each word aloud and try to remember as many as possible. No information is given at that time as to how memory will be tested. After the last word is presented, subjects either engage in a filler task, if the test is to be delayed, or receive the test instructions if an immediate test is to be given. The test instructions tell the subjects that they will now see a new set of words, each of which is meaningfully related to one of the studied words. They are to read each test cue aloud then attempt to recall a word from the list that is related to it. This test is self-paced and subjects are encouraged to guess if they are not sure. The extralist cued recall task requires subjects to rely on preexisting knowledge to determine whether a word is meaningfully related to the test cue. It is designed to mimic the many ways we use our preexisting knowledge to answer questions and remember episodes in our daily life.

Effects of the Strength of the Relationship Between the Cue and the Target

In the extralist cuing task the test cue is the initiating step for the retrieval process. Not surprisingly, the a priori strength of the relationship between the cue and the target has a large influence on the likelihood of correct recall (D. Nelson & McEvoy, 1979; D. Nelson et al., 1998). Cues that have a strong forward relationship to their targets are more likely to support correct recall than cues with weak forward relationships. Other links between the cue and target also influence recall. As shown in Figure 5.1, a cue and target can have a direct forward link (from WINE to BEER), a direct backward link (from BEER to WINE), and indirect links. Indirect links include shared associates and mediating associates. Shared associates are words that are produced by the cue and by the target, such as *alcohol* and *drink*. Mediated connections occur when an associate of the cue, such as *bottle* or *champagne*, in turn produces the target as one of its associates.

All four of these types of connections have consistent effects on recall. The presence of a backward link from the target to the cue increases the likelihood that the cue will be effective in prompting recall (D. Nelson et al., 1998). Just as stronger forward connections from the cue to the target increase the probability of recall, so too do stronger backward connections. Indirect connections also affect recall. The presence of both shared associate and mediated connections increases the probability of correct recall, although these effects are not as large as those observed with direct connections (D. Nelson & Zhang, 2000). Overall, it is clear that a cue can provide multiple routes to a sought-after target, and that the likelihood of correct recall is an additive effect of the many available routes.

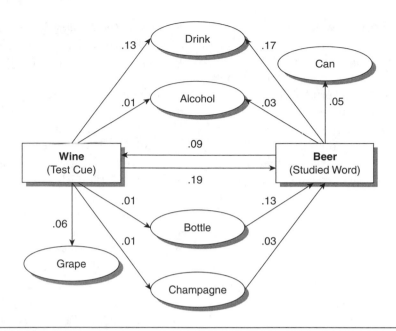

Figure 5.1   Preexisting links between the test cue WINE and the studied target word BEER

Effects of the Number of Associates of the Test Cue and the Target

In the above section, we described the different types of connections between a cue word and its target, and how each type of link has a positive impact on probability of recall. But what of those associates of the cue and of the target that do not link the two together, either directly or indirectly? Our early work showed that cues that had larger sets of associates were less effective than cues with smaller sets, and that targets with larger sets of associates were less likely to be recalled (D. Nelson & Friedrich, 1980; D. Nelson & McEvoy, 1979). We referred to these, respectively, as cue set size effects and target set size effects, and they appear to contradict the results described earlier—that the greater the number and strength of indirect connections from the cue to the target, the higher the probability of correct recall. The two sets of findings seem to suggest that

more associates are beneficial (the effects of shared and mediating associates), and that more associates are harmful (the effects of cue and target set size). How can these findings be reconciled?

Our earlier work on cue and target set size effects did not separate the influences of linking versus nonlinking associates. More recently, with the expansion of our norms to include independent normings for thousands of the responses in the sets, we are able to determine which associates are linking associates between a cue and target (such as *drink*, *alcohol*, *bottle*, and *champagne*) and which are nonlinking (such as *grape* and *can*). Set size effects appear to result from competition engendered by the nonlinking associates of the cue and target. When a test cue is presented during recall, accessing knowledge about that word should help recall if it connects to the target, but it should hinder recall if it misdirects retrieval processes away from, and hence competes with, the target. That is exactly what was observed when the strength of linking and nonlinking associates was manipulated (D. Nelson & McEvoy, 2002).

Effects of Connectivity and Resonance

Words do not stand alone as isolated entities. As was described earlier, our association norms suggest that some words have sets of associates that are densely interconnected, whereas other words may have the same number of associates but with far fewer interconnections among them. Do these differences in connectivity influence memory for the words? It seemed unlikely, as these associates are not consciously experienced and they do not necessarily link the cue with the target. Unlikely though it may have seemed, our research indicates that high connectivity words are more likely to be recalled and recognized than are low connectivity words (D. Nelson et al., 1998; D. Nelson et al., 2001). We also know that words with high levels of resonance (most of their associates produce the target as an associate) are more likely to be recalled than words with low levels of resonance (D. Nelson et al., 1998). The effects of connectivity and resonance are particularly interesting because they suggest that increasing activation anywhere within the target's associative set enhances its familiarity (D. Nelson et al., 2003).

Thus, the target word is the specific concept that was studied and must be retrieved during test, but the likelihood that it will be retrieved depends on the entire set of concepts linked to the target and the test cue. This finding has implications for understanding the cognitive processes that underlie substance abuse. Seemingly neutral stimuli may provoke drug use if those stimuli have unconsciously been associated with drugs in the past, and are now activated by cues that may have never themselves been associated with drugs.

The PIER2 Model: Encoding and Retrieval Assumptions

PIER2 is a model of cued recall and recognition that was designed to explain the influences of prior knowledge on memory for recently experienced familiar words (see D. Nelson & Zhang, 2000, for computational aspects of the model). The effects of cue-to-target connections, associative set size, connectivity, and resonance described above constitute the bulk of findings that PIER2 attempts to explain. This model provides a formal description of the implicit encoding processes that take place when a familiar word is experienced and the implicit retrieval processes that occur during extralist cued recall and recognition.

PIER2 assumes that when a person experiences and comprehends a familiar word, several processes are engaged that result in encoded representations for the word. An explicit representation is formed as the result of conscious processes directed toward the word. These processes may include noticing specifics about the context in which the word was experienced (an unusual type font, the fact that a BEER sure would taste good right about now, etc.). Explicit processes might also include orienting tasks or strategies that the subject uses in an attempt to remember the word. Explicit processes help tie the word to the encoding context and increase its accessibility as a response to a related test cue.

An implicit memory representation is also established during encoding as a result of unconscious activation processes. Comprehending the word activates related associates, producing a memory trace that reflects the number and strengths of the interconnections of these associates. The implicit activation process during encoding, and the representation resulting from it, reflects the cumulative activation accruing to a target from its associates. Figure 5.2 shows three associates of the word BEER that theoretically would be

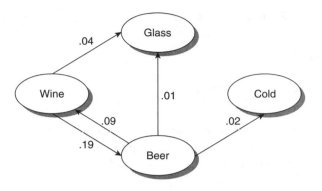

Figure 5.2   Associative strengths between BEER and its associates

activated. These are only a small portion of the associates related to BEER, but for simplicity of illustration we are limiting the figure to three associates. The values shown in the figure are taken from the association norms and are assumed to reflect relative strengths between the words. Thus, we assume that when BEER is experienced, *wine, glass,* and *cold* are activated with relative strengths of .09, .01, and .02, respectively. We also assume that the interconnecting and resonant links are activated in parallel with the forward links from the target word. Thus, the interconnecting link between *wine* and *glass* is activated with a strength of .04, and the resonant link from *wine* to BEER is activated with a strength of .19. PIER2 makes the assumption that activation from these sources add together with the target's initial activation level of 1.0 to produce a total activation strength (D. Nelson et al., 2003). With this simplified set of associates, the activation strength for the word BEER is 1.35. The total activation level of a target is increased by having more and stronger interconnections among its associates and more and stronger resonating links back to the target. This increased activation level makes the target more accessible during the memory test, and this is reflected in the connectivity and resonance effects observed in cued recall and recognition.

When memory is tested with extralist cued recall, subjects must use their prior knowledge about the cue to access the memory representation established during study. For example, the cue word WINE might be presented as a prompt for the target BEER, with the instruction to recall a recently presented word that is meaningfully related to the cue. For this cue to be effective, it must have some connection with the target in the individual's experiences prior to entering the lab. According to PIER2, the likelihood of retrieving the target is the product of a cue and target intersection process. This intersection process computes the ratio of links that bind the cue and target to the total links from the cue and from the target. Going back to Figure 5.1, the direct links from the cue WINE to the target BEER and from BEER to WINE, as well as the indirect links between the cue and target (e.g., the associates *drink, alcohol, bottle,* and *champagne*) are all connecting links that increase the likelihood that BEER will be recalled in response to the cue WINE. In contrast, the nonlinking associates of the cue (e.g., *grape*) and of the target (e.g., *can*) decrease the likelihood that BEER will be recalled in response to WINE. Typically, the great majority of the associates of both the cue and the target are nonlinking, or competitors. The intersection process uses activation strengths of the cue and its associates, as estimated from the association norms, and of the target and its associates, as estimated from the target activation calculations described above. These activation strengths enter into the numerator of the ratio if they are linking connections (forward, backward, shared associate, or mediating links). The denominator of this ratio includes activation strengths of all the associates activated by the cue or the target. Thus, the greater the strength of the linking connections compared with nonlinking connections, the larger the numerator relative to the denominator, and the greater the probability of retrieving the target in response to the test cue.

The cue-target intersection process explains why a target may be recalled with a very high probability in response to cue A, with a moderate probability in response to cue B, and almost never recalled in response to cue C. Cue A might be a word that shares a large proportion of associates with the target, or has one or more very strong shared or mediated associates, or has a strong forward or backward connection with the target. Any and all of these linking connections will increase the numerator of the cue-target intersection process. Interestingly, even a cue with no measurable forward direct connection to the target may still be effective if it has a strong backward connection from the target or has one or more relatively strong shared or mediated associates (D. Nelson et al., 1998). Cue B may be only moderately effective because the strength of its connecting links with the target is partially balanced out by the strength of its nonlinking associates. Finally, Cue C may not be effective in prompting recall because it has very few, or very weak linking connections to the target, or because it has one or more very strong nonlinking associates that compete with the target for retrieval. Thus, it is not possible to assign a "memorability score" to a word in isolation from the cue used to prompt its recall. Cued recall is a complex memory task

that uses one's prior knowledge to access a sought-after target in response to a provided cue. Prior knowledge about the cue and target are necessary for the cue to be effective, and connecting links help support recall. The contents of prior knowledge about the cue and target that do not link the two together, however, actually hinder recall. It is not what you know; it is whether your knowledge of connecting concepts is greater than your knowledge of competing concepts.

CONCLUSION

PIER2 was specifically designed to explain the effects of previous experiences on memory for current experiences. As Ebbinghaus (1885/1964) noted more than 100 years ago, the two cannot be divorced from one another. We do not remember in a vacuum, and any attempt to understand why we remember some things and not others must necessarily take into consideration our prior experiences with the events to be remembered and with the cues available to prompt our memory. Recent research on implicit memory using testing instructions and the process dissociation procedure have demonstrated that much of the work of remembering is unconscious. PIER2 provides a way of studying the unconscious influences on memory that are inevitable whenever we attempt to learn or remember something that has meaning. Unconscious activation of prior knowledge has a significant influence on recall in a laboratory setting, and it seems like a small leap to assume that the influence is even greater when we are remembering important events in the richness of our daily activities. Do we remember events exactly as they occurred, or as they are interpreted through the lens of our prior experiences with similar events? How do experiences such as drug abuse alter how an event is remembered? How can a therapist cue memory for events that have become associated with drug use, in an attempt to modify those associations? A fuller understanding of the unconscious influences on memory arising from prior experiences is essential to answering these questions and to understanding how retrieved memories shape the behaviors that lead to drug misuse and abuse.

REFERENCES

Curran, T., & Hintzman, D. L. (1997). Consequences and causes of correlations in process dissociation. *Journal of Experimental Psychology: Learning, Memory, and Cognition, 23,* 496–504.

Deese, J. (1965). *The structure of associations in language and thought.* Baltimore, MD: Johns Hopkins University Press.

Ebbinghaus, H. (1964). *Memory: A contribution to experimental psychology* (H. A. Ruger & C. E. Bussenius, Trans.). New York: Dover. (Original work published 1885)

Graf, P., & Komatsu, S. (1994). Process dissociation procedure: Handle with caution! *European Journal of Cognitive Psychology, 6,* 113–129.

Graf, P., & Masson, M. E. J. (Eds.). (1993). *Implicit memory: New directions in cognition, development, and neuropsychology.* Hillsdale, NJ: Lawrence Erlbaum.

Graf, P., Squire, L. R., & Mandler, G. (1984). The information that amnesic patients do not forget. *Journal of Experimental Psychology: Learning, Memory, and Cognition, 10,* 164–178.

Hamann, S. B. (1990). Level-of-processing effects in conceptually driven implicit tasks. *Journal of Experimental Psychology: Learning, Memory, and Cognition, 16,* 970–977.

Jacoby, L. L. (1991). A process dissociation framework: Separating automatic from intentional uses of memory. *Journal of Memory and Language, 30,* 513–541.

Jennings, J. M., & Jacoby, L. L. (1993). Automatic versus intentional uses of memory: Aging, attention, and control. *Psychology and Aging, 8,* 283–293.

Kolers, P. A. (1976). Reading a year later. *Journal of Experimental Psychology: Human Learning and Memory, 2,* 554–565.

La Voie, D. J., & Light, L. L. (1994). Adult age differences in repetition priming: A meta-analysis. *Psychology and Aging, 9,* 539–553.

LeCompte, D. C. (1995). Recollective experience in the revelation effect: Separating the contributions of recollection and familiarity. *Memory & Cognition, 23,* 324–334.

Light, L. L., Prull, M. W., & Kennison, R. F. (2000). Divided attention, aging, priming in exemplar generation and category verification. *Memory & Cognition, 28,* 856–872.

McEvoy, C. L., Holley, P. E., & Nelson, D. L. (1995). Age effects in cued recall: Sources from implicit and explicit memory. *Psychology and Aging, 10,* 314–324.

Milner, M., Corkin, S., & Teuber, H. L. (1964). Further analysis of the hippocampal amnesic syndrome: 14 year follow-up study of H.M. *Neuropsychologia, 6,* 215–234.

Nelson, D. L., Drydal, G. M., & Goodmon, L. B. (in press). What is pre-existing strength? Predicting free association probabilities, similarity ratings, and cued recall probabilities. *Psychonomic Bulletin & Review*.

Nelson, D. L., & Friedrich, M. A. (1980). Encoding and cuing sounds and senses. *Journal of Experimental Psychology: Human Learning and Memory, 6,* 717–731.

Nelson, D. L., & McEvoy, C. L. (1979). Encoding context and set size. *Journal of Experimental Psychology: Human Learning and Memory, 5,* 292–314.

Nelson, D. L., & McEvoy, C. L. (2002). How can the same type of prior knowledge both help and hinder recall? *Journal of Memory and Language, 46,* 652–663.

Nelson, D. L., McEvoy, C. L., & Dennis, S. (2000). What is free association and what does it measure? *Memory & Cognition, 28,* 887–899.

Nelson, D. L., McEvoy, C. L., & Pointer, L. (2003). Spreading activation or spooky action at a distance? *Journal of Experimental Psychology: Learning, Memory, and Cognition, 29,* 42–52.

Nelson, D. L., McEvoy, C. L., & Schreiber, T. A. (2004). The University of South Florida Free Association, rhyme, and word fragment norms. *Behavior Research Methods, Instruments, & Computers, 36,* 402–407.

Nelson, D. L., McKinney, V. M., Gee, N. R., & Janczura, G. A. (1998). Interpreting the influence of implicitly activated memories on recall and recognition. *Psychological Review, 105,* 299–324.

Nelson, D. L., Schreiber, T. A., & Holley, P. E. (1992). The retrieval of controlled and automatic aspects of meaning on direct and indirect tests. *Memory & Cognition, 20,* 671–684.

Nelson, D. L., & Zhang, N. (2000). The ties that binds what is known to the recall of what is new. *Psychonomic Bulletin & Review, 7,* 604–617.

Nelson, D. L., Zhang, N., & McKinney, V. M. (2001). The ties that bind what is known to the recognition of what is new. *Journal of Experimental Psychology: Learning, Memory, and Cognition, 27,* 1147–1159.

Nelson, T. O. (1978). Detecting small amounts of information in memory: Savings for nonrecognized items. *Journal of Experimental Psychology: Human Learning and Memory, 4,* 453–468.

Roediger, H. L., & Blaxton, T. A. (1987). Effects of varying modality, surface features, and retention interval on priming in word fragment completion. *Memory & Cognition, 15,* 379–388.

Srinivas, K., & Roediger, H. L., III (1990). Classifying implicit memory tests: Category association and anagram solution. *Journal of Memory and Language, 29,* 389–412.

Toth, J. P., Reingold, E. M., & Jacoby, L. L. (1994). Toward a redefinition of implicit memory process dissociations following elaborative processing and self-generation. *Journal of Experimental Psychology: Learning, Memory, and Cognition, 20,* 290–303.

Tulving, E., & Schacter, D. L. (1990). Priming and human memory. *Science, 247,* 301–306.

Verfaellie, M., & Treadwell, J. R. (1993). Status of recognition memory amnesia. *Neuropsychology, 7,* 5–13.

Warrington, E. K., & Weiskrantz, L. (1968). Amnesia: A disconnection syndrome? *Neuropsychologia, 20,* 233–248.

Yonelinas, A. P. (2002). The nature of recollection and familiarity: A review of 30 years of research. *Journal of Memory and Language, 46,* 441–517.

Section II

ASSESSMENT OF IMPLICIT COGNITION IN ADDICTION RESEARCH

Word Association Tests of Associative Memory and Implicit Processes: Theoretical and Assessment Issues

ALAN W. STACY, SUSAN L. AMES, AND JERRY L. GRENARD

Abstract: Word association is one of the most commonly used measures of association in cognitive science. These tests have been used to infer association parameters in normative studies, to derive cues and primes used in diverse paradigms (semantic priming, cued recall, illusory memory), to test implicit memory in experimental studies, and to suggest the operation of implicit processes in nonexperimental work. This chapter briefly outlines some of the historical routes and current controversies about association and summarizes basic cognitive research applying associative tests. The authors then describe benefits and limitations of the tests, as well as implications for theory and interventions on drug use.

This chapter briefly outlines some of the historical routes of word association and then summarizes several of the major streams of basic cognitive research revealing the value of these tests. We delineate several current controversies from this basic research and suggest why they are critical for understanding drug-related cognitions and behavior. We then address benefits, limitations, and further implications of the tests.

A BRIEF HISTORY OF WORD ASSOCIATION

The concept of association can be traced back to Aristotle and was not refined substantially until the effort of the British empiricists (Dawson, 2004). Some of Aristotle's primary concepts such as contiguity, similarity, and sequence effects anticipated a variety of associationist and connectionist models of the last

AUTHOR'S NOTE: This chapter was supported by a grant from the National Institute on Drug Abuse, DA16094.

century and today. In the 19th century, John Mill's philosophical work on association was a precursor of contemporary notions that associations can come together in new constellations that have emergent properties. William James (1913) elaborated on the importance of cognitive sequences, suggesting that one brain state leads to activity of another state that has been previously associated with the first. This idea and other concepts from James (e.g., pattern association) anticipated a number of subsequent developments in connectionist models (Dawson, 2004) that have been viewed as substantial elaborations or expansions of earlier associationism evolved to embrace emergent properties, distributed representations, nonlinear activation rules, and other innovations (Bechtel & Abrahamsen, 2002). As revealed below, association is still alive and well in contemporary cognitive research.

Word association has become one of the primary methods used to infer association in cognitive research, whether cast in terms of associative or connectionist models. The first research the authors found using this method was conducted by Francis Galton in 1879 (Crovitz, 1970). Although he is better known for his interest in evolution and heredity, he also studied the association of ideas in thought (Boring, 1950). Galton's results influenced the subsequent work of Jung (1910) as well as Wundt and Catell (Cattell & Bryant, 1889; Thorne & Henley, 2001).

Freud began developing his method of free association for psychoanalysis in 1892 and might have been influenced by Galton (Thorne & Henley, 2001), but the method does not normally use word association tests. Instead, the patient is expected to talk freely about a symptom or a dream (Freud, 1995). On the other hand, free association as it is used in studies of verbal behavior and cognition implies free word association, in which the participant is instructed to respond with

the first word or series of words that come to mind when presented with a word or phrase as a stimulus (Woodworth, 1921). In a controlled word association test, the participant is instructed to respond with words from a certain category (e.g., name animals that are mammals; Woodworth, 1921).

Word association was used later in the last century by both behaviorists (e.g., Cook & Skinner, 1939) and cognitive psychologists (e.g., Cramer, 1968; Deese, 1959a). Some of this research has had major influences on contemporary approaches. For example, Deese's (1959b) research has been substantially extended in recent studies on illusory memory, Underwood's (1965) concept of implicit associative response has influenced contemporary theories, and Noble's (1952) work on continuous association influenced later research on associative structures relevant to culture and drug use.

CONTEMPORARY COGNITIVE PARADIGMS REVEALING THE VALUE OF WORD ASSOCIATION

Although a few researchers have reported on the reliability of word association measures or norms (e.g., Preece, 1978; Stacy et al., 1993; Szalay et al., 1970), most cognitive research on this task provides evidence of predictive value rather than psychometric information. Findings from contemporary paradigms have revealed that word association norms predict cognitive responses that are often attributed to implicit or automatic processes. These findings may mirror at least some of the implicit processes that are engaged when behavior choices, such as drug use, are made. Many of these paradigms attempt to uncover processes that occur spontaneously, without the need for extensive deliberation, conscious recollection of events, or the conscious weighing of pros and cons.

Semantic Priming

In semantic priming, responses to a target stimulus (e.g., the word *cat*) are facilitated (i.e., speeded up compared to some baseline) if the target is preceded by a related prime word (e.g., *dog*). The most common procedure is lexical decision, where targets are either words or nonword letter strings (e.g., atcs) and primes are related words, unrelated or neutral words, or other variations (e.g., nonword letter strings). The participant's task is to indicate whether the target stimulus is a word or not, usually on two computer keys labeled yes or no. Another commonly used semantic priming paradigm is word naming (pronunciation), which is similar in presentation of prime/target pairs but requires naming the target word out loud rather than lexical (word/nonword) decision. In both lexical decision and naming, a common finding is that reaction times for decisions or naming are decreased if a target is preceded by a related prime compared to a neutral prime, although facilitation effects depend on the specific type of prime-target relation (Hutchison, 2003; Neely, 1991). Semantic priming has been used to infer a variety of automatic cognitive processes, most commonly spreading activation among nodes in memory (Collins & Loftus, 1975; Neely, 1991). There are several more recent theoretical explanations (e.g., Masson, 1995; Plaut & Booth, 2000).

Word association comes into play in semantic priming because the definition and pairing of prime-target pairs as "related" frequently has been based on word association norms. Indeed, word association norms have often yielded prime-target pairs that reveal priming effects in lexical decision and naming (for review, see Hutchison, 2003). Thus, word association seems to measure some sort of relationship that has relevance well beyond the word association task itself.

This picture, however, is complicated by a number of considerations involving the nature of the relationship uncovered in word association. This relationship may be primarily lexical (word based), semantic (e.g., categorical), conceptually based (but not categorical), or it may reflect some combination of levels. This is not a trivial issue, because the nature of the relationship assessed by both word association and semantic priming could place important limits on the utility of these tasks in research on behavior. For example, lexical associations may not have much utility beyond predicting word use, whereas conceptual or semantic relations likely imply a much broader range of relevance.

The Lexical View

Lexical associations represent co-occurrences in word use, in written or spoken language. One view is that semantic priming is not really semantic but instead involves associations only at the lexical level (Shelton & Martin, 1992). This position is based in part on findings showing that automatic semantic priming effects are often obtained when prime-target pairs are associated on the basis of word association norms, but are less consistently obtained when prime target pairs are related on the basis of certain semantic relations such as category coordinates (for review, see Hutchison, 2003) or similarity in the absence of association (e.g., Shelton & Martin, 1992). This common interpretation relies heavily on the critical assumption that word association measures only lexical associations. Indeed, much of this research assumes that if word association norms, but not semantic relations, predict facilitation in lexical decision, then lexical associations must govern semantic priming.

Conceptual Associations

In this section a concept is defined as something (e.g., a tree) that is represented in memory in, or accessible through, diverse modalities. A tree is not just the word itself (or its graphemic and phonemic linguistic representations). Memories about trees can be activated by the sight of a tree in the environment, by pictures, smells, touch, words, and related thoughts. Thus, a concept is not bound to a single perceptual modality. If words do indeed activate concepts, then it is plausible that word associations may reflect conceptual associations. Thus, tests of word association may index *concept* co-occurrence in everyday experience. For example, associations between *tree* and *leaf* may be detectable in word association not just because of co-occurrence in language, but also because of co-occurrence in a variety of visual experiences. A conceptual association has much more far-reaching implications for behavior than an association restricted to the lexical (word) system. For example, if semantic priming mimics activation of concepts in everyday encounters with a variety of cues differing in modality, then a semantic priming effect may provide a glimpse at concept activation processes relevant to behavior choices. Concept activation is relevant to behavior in a variety of approaches (e.g., Bargh et al., 1996), including those that address affect and behavior (Fazio, 2001).

Unfortunately, there is little evidence available to weigh the lexical association versus conceptual association views. One way to evaluate some of the necessary (but not completely sufficient) conditions of the conceptual association view is to examine associations across different modalities (e.g., words and pictures). Only a few relevant studies, however, have been conducted (Hines et al., 1986; Saffran et al., 2003).

A "Pure" Semantic View and Alternative Measurements

Semantic relationships are frequently defined in terms of similarity (shared features) or category relations, but an examination of published norms reveals a variety of other meaningful relations, such as functional, script, instrument, synonym, antonym, and other relationships (Hutchison, 2003). At least one class of theory relies heavily on a similarity-based semantic model (Masson, 1995; McRae & Boisvert, 1998). In this class of connectionist model, semantic priming is explained by the similarity between the prime and target, or more specifically, between the activation states engaged by the prime and target. A prime facilitates responses to a target to the extent that the two states match in their patterns of activation across elementary features (Masson, 1995). Despite earlier evidence from several studies showing that similarity did not produce semantic priming, MacRae and Boisvert demonstrated that similarity effects on automatic priming can be found in the absence of normative association (but see Wentura, 2000). This finding shows that association (whether lexical or conceptual) may not be the only route through which exposure to one stimulus facilitates responses to another. Affective priming is yet another route (Spruyt et al., 2004).

This work suggests that word association is not the only viable index of relation. Effects of similarity, however, are not as consistent as are effects of normative association (Hutchison, 2003; McRae & Boisvert, 1998). In addition, similarity judgments yield a *symmetric* association, whereas word association can detect *asymmetric* relations; asymmetric relations have important empirical and theoretical manifestations (Nelson et al., 1998; see also McEvoy & Nelson, Chapter 5). Nevertheless, similarity and other indexes of relationship are worthy of additional research because they do sometimes predict semantic priming in the absence of normative association and word association is certainly not immune from controversy (McRae & Boisvert, 1998; Ratcliff & McKoon, 1994).

Mixed Association and Semantic Models

In a recent comprehensive review, Hutchison (2003) concluded that both associative and semantic processes influence semantic priming responses. This conclusion can be accommodated by a "localist" perspective (spreading activation; Collins & Loftus, 1975) and by some distributed, connectionist models. For example, in Plaut and Booth's (2000) distributed memory model, associative effects are explained in terms of transition probabilities, in which the network learns transitions between patterns of activation through training in which one pattern follows another. In essence, the network represents habitual transitions, such that pattern A facilitates responding to pattern B to the extent that A transitioned to B in previous experience; this transition may constitute a predictive relationship akin to modern conceptions of a Pavlovian relation (Rescorla, 1988). Plaut and Booth's definition of a semantic effect is similar to other connectionist theories (Masson, 1995), whereby pattern A facilitates responding to B to the extent that the two patterns are similar in terms of shared features; that is, the network has fewer changes to make from pattern A to B. As outlined earlier, there are many additional definitions of semantic relations beyond similarity. Some of these definitions may be indistinguishable from Plaut and Booth's associative effect. For example, many functional or script relations likely involve transitions learned in the past. Plaut

and Booth provide one of the few contemporary approaches to semantic priming that seems to acknowledge that the associative process could operate at the concept level (cf. Nelson et al., 1998; Spruyt et al., 2004).

Clearly, word association is still quite relevant to semantic priming research. In fact, the exact source or level of the relationship uncovered in word association may be fundamental for inferences about the nature of semantic priming and its relevance to behavior. To the extent that semantic priming effects involve automatic activation processes, associations uncovered in word association norms foretell which words or concepts more readily activate (or transition to) other words or concepts. It is not a large leap to suggest that individual differences in these associations should predict concept activation at the individual level (Stacy et al., 1997) and behavior (Stacy, 1997; Szalay et al., 1993). The authors outline some evidence for this view in a subsequent section.

Conceptual Priming

This term is usually restricted to paradigms that incorporate distinct encoding (study) and test trials. The test trials include indirect tests of memory that have been classified as conceptually driven tasks. Implicit memory research classifies word association as a conceptual test of implicit memory (Toth, 2000; Vaidya et al., 1995; Zeelenberg et al., 1999). Studies investigating word association and conceptual priming, however, vary in the extent to which their procedures explicitly evaluate the assumptions of conceptually based, implicit processing.

Studies Using Amnesic Patients as Participants

Amnesic samples are relevant to inferences about implicit processing because the participants have deficits on direct tests of memory such as free recall. At least some assumptions about implicit versus explicit processes can be investigated because conscious recollection is impaired and clear dissociations between direct and indirect tests are revealed. Using this population, a variety of converging lines of evidence can sometimes be pieced together to make the case for a distinction in memory systems underlying different forms of memory (Ryan & Cohen, 2003).

Several studies have shown that word association can reveal memory priming in amnesic patients. Gardner and his colleagues (1973) found that amnesic Korsakoff patients revealed significant levels of priming in word association responses to categorical cues (an indirect test of exemplar generation) following a study trial in which exemplars were matched to categories. The amnesic patients revealed significantly less memory for exemplars on direct tests (free recall and cued recall), however, than did alcoholic control participants, revealing a decrement on tests referring back to the previous study episode. Exemplar generation using word association instructions in this study provides an example of the controlled association method (Cramer, 1968), in which the set of associative responses is restricted in the instructions in some fashion (e.g., category member, verb, noun, etc.). Studies of priming in free association among amnesic patients have shown similar findings of no impairment on the indirect test (word association) and decrements on direct tests (Levy et al., 2004; Schacter, 1985; Shimamura & Squire, 1984; Vaidya et al., 1995). Importantly, Vaidya et al.'s study demonstrated that priming in word association did not depend on perceptual match at study and test. A switch in modality from auditory during study to visual at test did not affect priming, suggesting a conceptual locus of the obtained priming effect.

Studies in Normal Samples

Several studies have focused on priming in word association using participants without memory impairments, providing information relevant to conceptual processes as well as to various associative memory parameters. For example, Zeelenberg and his colleagues (2003) manipulated the semantic context during an incidental study trial by presenting ambiguous target words within sentence contexts that were either congruent or incongruent with subsequent cue words presented during a word association test. In Experiment 2 from the same research series, a similar design was used but semantic context was varied more subtly by varying the sense of nonambiguous words. In both studies, sentence context affected priming. The authors concluded that "this finding is largely consistent with the view that priming in word association depends largely on conceptual processes" (Zeelenberg et al., 2003, p. 658). Other studies in normal samples also find significant priming effects in word association following incidental study trials, showing the predictive utility of several connection parameters that may underlie the effects (Nelson & Goodmon, 2002; Zeelenberg et al., 1999). The values of connection parameters (e.g., association strength, associative set size) are based on word association norms, further revealing the value of association tests.

Illusory Memory in Free Recall

Deese (1959b) first found that extralist (nonstudied) intrusions on free recall of word lists could be predicted from the responses made to a critical item on word association tasks. Roediger and McDermott (1995) subsequently replicated and extended Deese's work, fostering a surge of additional research on illusory memory using what is now called the Deese-Roediger-McDermott paradigm (DRM).

Several studies using the DRM are particularly informative with respect to word association. McEvoy et al. (1999) manipulated associative strength based on word association norms and found that stronger preexisting connections from presented list words to the critical lures (i.e., backward associative strength) produced more false recall than weaker preexisting connection strength. Additionally, and consistent with Deese (1959b), McEvoy et al. (1999) found that stronger connectivity among the words in word lists decreased the likelihood of illusory memories. In evaluating the contribution of seven processes likely to influence false recall of critical lures, Roediger et al. (2001) found backward associative strength to be the best predictor ($r = .73$) of false recall, consistent with Deese (1959b) and McEvoy et al. (1999). The number of list items accurately recalled was the second best predictor ($r = - .43$) of false recall. Hicks and Hancock (2002) manipulated backward associative strength and also found that word lists with greater associative strength to the critical item were more likely to produce false recall. They attributed their findings to the strong activation of the critical item by semantic associates at encoding and not to biases at retrieval. Reich et al. (2004) showed how the DRM could be usefully applied to alcohol-related cognitions, but they focused on recognition tests that are beyond the scope of this section.

Although the exact processes underlying illusory memories revealed from the DRM are still being studied, the research reviewed here provides evidence that activation from the presented words in the word lists seem to converge on, and prime, an associatively related, but nonpresented word (or concept). The effect of associative relationship is well predicted by word association norms.

Extralist Cued Recall

In extralist cued recall, participants are prompted with cue words during testing that were not provided during a previous study trial. The test instructions are direct, asking participants to recall words from a study list. Across numerous studies, several association parameters (cue-to-target association, set size, resonance, and connectivity) have been found to be good predictors of performance in this task (for reviews and definitions, see Nelson et al., 1998; Nelson et al., 2003; Nelson et al., 1992; McEvoy & Nelson, Chapter 5). Word association norms are used to derive the association parameters and have been found to be better predictors of extralist cued recall than have similarity ratings and word co-occurrence data (Nelson et al., in press).

Nelson and his colleagues (Nelson et al., 1998) have concluded that the effects of related associates on memory (and hence the association parameters) in extralist cued recall appear to emerge because of the implicit activation of those associates, akin to a priming effect. This view is based in part on Nelson et al.'s findings showing that associative set size effects occur regardless of the incidental or intentional nature of the study trial, regardless of whether test instructions refer to the study trial, and regardless of variations in instructions regarding guessing. Also, participants' ratings of set size do not correspond with associative set size as revealed in word association, suggesting that people's conscious cognitions about this process are independent from the apparently implicit process proposed by Nelson et al. On the basis of these and a number of related findings, Nelson and his colleagues assume the coexistence of independent implicit and explicit representations in memory, advanced in their theory of Processing Implicit and Explicit Representations, PIER1 and PIER2 (McEvoy & Nelson, Chapter 5; Nelson et al., 1998; Nelson et al., 1992). This theory also provides a viable explanation of findings in recognition (e.g., Nelson et al., 2003; Nelson et al., 1998), as well as results addressed earlier from conceptual priming in free association (Nelson & Goodmon, 2002) and illusory memory (McEvoy et al., 1999). In an analysis of associative parameters from over 29 controlled experimental studies, propositions from PIER2 fared better than did spreading activation (Nelson et al., 2003).

Summary of Basic Cognitive Research

Results from a variety of contemporary paradigms using word association norms, as well as earlier research, provide a remarkable empirical consensus of the utility of this simple test in basic cognitive research. It is a challenge to cognitive research to uncover an index of relation that is a better predictor of a wide variety of cognitive responses (cf. Nelson et al., 1998). Yet, there are a number of questions about the exact processes engaged in word association itself, as addressed in subsequent sections. The nature of these processes may be critical to addictive behaviors, contextual effects on these behaviors (Krank & Wall, Chapter 19), and interpretations of implicit processes.

APPLICATION AND PREDICTIVE UTILITY IN RESEARCH ON HEALTH BEHAVIOR

Examples of Assessment Strategies in Drug-Use Research

Variations of word association methods virtually identical to methods from basic cognitive research have been used in research on drug use and other health behaviors. Szalay and colleagues (e.g., Szalay et al., 1999) adapted the continued association methods of Noble (1952) to study the spontaneous distribution of continued free associations in drug users. With continued free associations, multiple (single-word) responses are obtained for the same cue, which is repeated in a column format (e.g., fun: ____; fun: ____; fun: ____). A variety of salient cues are offered as prompts. We have used an alternative, free-association method (Stacy, Ames, et al., 1996) that requires participants to write down the first word that comes to mind to single occurrences of each word in a list of different ambiguous cue words (e.g., fun: ____; draft: ____). Responses (e.g., "drunk") are binary coded (0 or 1) for consistency with the target behavior (e.g., alcohol use) and summed to form a scale used as a predictor of the behavior. We also have used controlled associations (Cramer, 1968), in which the potential set size of responses is restricted to a form of verb generation. With this task, participants are asked to write down the first behavior or action that comes to mind in response to one or several words (e.g., having fun: ____). There is preliminary evidence that priming in verb generation tasks is intact in amnesic patients (Seger et al., 1997) and measures an implicit, conceptual form of memory (Seger et al., 1999), but the support for free association is much broader. Pros and cons of free, controlled, and continuous association and measurement suggestions for applied work have been outlined previously (Stacy, Ames, & Leigh, 2004). Such indirect assessments, when not mentioning any particular behavior or encouraging recollection, seem likely to minimize self-perception processes and other executive or explicit-process effects on associative responses.

Summary of Drug-Abuse Findings

In previous research, we have argued that responses to word associations reflect associations in memory between cues, behaviors, and outcomes, and that these associations bias behavior decisions in a relatively spontaneous, possibly implicit manner (Ames & Stacy, 1998; Stacy, 1997). Szalay and his colleagues have advocated an essentially similar focus on the spontaneous effect of meaningful associations on drug use, as well as indirect assessment through word association (e.g., Szalay et al., 1999). Over a dozen studies provide evidence for the effectiveness of word association tasks as predictors of alcohol use, marijuana use, or HIV-risk behavior in diverse populations (for reviews, see Stacy, Ames, & Leigh, 2004; Szalay et al., 1999), and some of this research controls for potential confounders and moderators (e.g., ethnicity, gender, acculturation, sensation seeking, outcome expectancies) in the analysis (e.g., Palfai & Wood, 2001; Stacy, 1997). An updated review of much of this literature is provided by Ames et al. (Chapter 23). Overall, there is substantial empirical support for the utility of word association responses in predicting drug use.

Other Open-Ended Cognitive Tests Applicable to Health Behavior

Other open-ended tests applicable to health behavior share some similarities to word association. To our knowledge, however, most of these have not been used to predict responses in paradigms implicated in automatic or implicit processes (e.g., semantic priming, extralist cued recall). These other open-ended procedures include, for example, a variety of thought listing and think-aloud techniques used to infer chronic accessibility in social cognition (Bargh et al., 1986; Higgins et al., 1982), situation-specific cognitions that may inform therapeutic trials (Davison et al., 1997), and processes involved in coping (Cacioppo et al., 1997). A variation of this class of test asks participants to list how people feel when they engage in the behavior (Dunn & Goldman, 2000) or what outcomes of the behavior first come to mind (Stacy, Galaif, et al., 1996). Several other variations akin to word association

have proven to be empirically useful, as revealed by Goldman et al. (Chapter 8).

BENEFITS AND LIMITATIONS

Limits of Inference

Norms from word association predict apparently automatic or implicit processes in a variety of paradigms. Word association tests have been used successfully as indirect tests of conceptual priming, providing good evidence of functional properties that diverge from direct tests. Individual differences in word association responses predict behavior, consistent with some theories of implicit cognition. Although word association studies on drug use have relied on previously ascertained functional properties of these measures, no single study on drug use has itself fully examined properties that characterize implicit or automatic processes. Some guidelines are now available to improve future research in this area (De Houwer, Chapter 2).

One sense of implicit cognition, pervasive in research on implicit memory, focuses on responses in the absence of deliberate, conscious recollection of an event. Research reviewed earlier suggests that systematic word association responses *can* occur in the absence of these recollective processes though the findings do not imply that conscious, deliberate recollection never occurs. Another possibility is that although conscious recollection of an event is not engaged, processes other than an implicit association affect the response. One example of such a process is filtering (editing, censoring), which has been addressed only minimally in previous research (Stacy et al., 1997). If this threat increases Type I error, however, then it must involve a confounding relationship rather than random error. Some, but not all, potential confounders, such as personality (sensation seeking), habit, gender, acculturation, and outcome expectancies have been addressed in health-behavior research.

Conscious awareness of activated *content,* which characterizes word association responses, is different than deliberate or conscious recollection of the *source* of that content. Conscious awareness of content also does not imply that introspections about one's behavior affected that content. In a variety of findings from implicit memory research, including some research on word association (e.g., Vaidya et al., 1995), content can reach consciousness or awareness, the response can take some time, but the origins of the content are not known or identified by the participant. This presumed functional quality should be further investigated in drug-use research.

Relative Cognition

Word association is one of the few measures of cognition capable of assessing target cognitions in competition with a large number of alternatives. This is because the response format leads to self-generation of responses that could be almost anything—a potentially vast set size (Nelson et al., 1998) or "fan" (Anderson, 1983) of alternatives. The importance of *relative* cognition and alternatives is emphasized in areas as diverse as advertising (Stacy, Pearce, et al., 2004; Stewart, 1989), traditional social learning theory (Rotter, 1954), and motivational theory (Cox et al., Chapter 17; Palfai, Chapter 26). Further, a number of models of memory instantiate memory competition, whether conceived of as an automatic or explicit form of memory. Yet, if alternatives are examined at all, most other indirect tests and direct tests of health-related cognitions do not evaluate cognitive responses to more than one or several alternatives. Word association, on the other hand, allows the investigator to study associations involving the "target" behavior or content of focus in

comparison to *all* other possibilities, even though the alternatives are not explicitly mentioned. One might expect this to be a hopeless method, given that so many responses are possible. Nevertheless, the reviewed data support the view that something quite systematic is revealed in these tests.

Context and Larger Patterns of Association

Word association tests can be used to study context effects (Krank & Wall, Chapter 19). "Local" context effects, within the test itself, can be manipulated by varying the number and nature of cue words or by manipulating preceding items or the imagined context immediately before the requested associative response (Stacy et al., 1994; Stacy et al., 1997). Since everyday cognition is unlikely to be devoid of context, the study of local context effects in indirect tests of all types may improve the generalizability, and possibly predictive utility, of these tests. The manipulation of local context can also benefit the study of configural relations (Dosher & Rosedale, 1997). It is an empirical question whether local context, that is, context most likely to be processed in conjunction with the test item (e.g., an adjacent word), is more or less important than the global environmental context of the test, which may or may not be processed in a manner that affects test responses.

Another benefit of word association is that it can reveal a large pattern of connection across *many* concepts, and such larger patterns may be more important to behavior than one or several associations in isolation. A pattern of connection is particularly relevant to such theories as PIER2 (Nelson et al., 1998; McEvoy & Nelson, Chapter 5), Hopfield networks (e.g., Masson, 1995), and connectionist theories applied to social behavior (Smith & DeCoster, 1998). For example, results from studies on PIER2 show that parameters (such as resonance, connectivity, and set size) involving many associates of a target concept are important for activation of a target concept in memory, even when those associates are not presented during a study or test trial (Nelson et al., 2003; Nelson et al., 1998). It is conceivable that individual differences in connection patterns precede and predict experimentation with drugs and change further once drugs are tried. The study of patterns of association and activation across a fairly large number of elements is a different approach than the study of only several associations studied in isolation (e.g., only those that might represent expectancy for reinforcement).

Finally, associations, including larger patterns, revealed by word association tests are not applied in a theoretical vacuum. A number of theories are available to explain the development or learning of associations revealed by these tests, ranging from simple Hebbian learning rules applied to some connectionist networks (Masson, 1995) to multiple-trace explanations of associative memory (Hintzman, 1986). These approaches can be readily applied to associations involving affect or motivation as well as nonemotional concepts and have been useful in explaining drug use (Stacy, 1995).

Prevention and Treatment Interventions

Beginning with the work of Szalay and his colleagues, several investigators have provided guidelines for assessment of drug-use intervention effects through the study of word association (Stacy, Ames, & Leigh, 2004; Szalay et al., 1993; Szalay et al., 1999). The basic idea is that word association may reflect a change in associations, or creation of new associations, following an intervention. In some theories of implicit memory, such as dissociation and distinct representation models (for review, see Moscovitch, 2000), new

associations could affect behavior because they operate through implicit representations that do not require the participant to deliberately or consciously think back to previously learned information from a program—something people may not do very often. Implicitly activated cognitions would influence related behaviors, just as they influence related cognitions in models of implicit activation (Nelson et al., 1998); some assumptions from this view are consistent with theories arguing for biasing effects of memory activation on social behavior and judgment (e.g., Bargh et al., 1986; Fazio et al., 1986).

An alternative view, consistent with transfer appropriate processing (Morris et al., 1977; Roediger et al., 2002), focuses on the consistency of modes of processing across encoding and test trials. Much of value in what is learned in an intervention may not involve deliberate memorization processes but rather elaborations of new conjunctions of information. These elaborations may influence associations in memory, potentially one of the most active ingredients of the intervention (Stacy, Ames, & Knowlton, 2004). Tests of association, rather than tests of deliberate recollection or self-reflection, are likely more compatible with processes that strengthen associations. Further, tests of implicit conceptual memory, such as word association, may more closely reflect the type of spontaneous activation process engaged in everyday situations. If an intervention influences these tests, it might more readily transfer, influencing behavior in a relatively spontaneous manner. Word association may, in James's (1913, p. 257) terminology, capture "spontaneous trains of thought."

CONCLUSIONS

Word association tests clearly assess some type of association in memory relevant to a variety of cognitive responses and behaviors.

Associations derived from these assessments appear to operate at least relatively spontaneously on other cognitive responses. In a few paradigms using these tests, inferences of implicit processes are difficult to rule out. Many of the findings are indicative, though not conclusive, of a concept activation process. A number of theories of social cognition (Bargh et al., 1986; Fazio, 2001; Smith, 1996) and health behavior (chapters in this book) suggest that concept activation and its affective counterparts influence behavior. If associations uncovered in word association affect behavior, then their value is affirmed despite some current uncertainty about the exact nature of the association. Nevertheless, more research is needed to fully understand the properties of this test under different assessment conditions.

The degree of convergence from multiple lines of evidence regarding word association across divergent, independent paradigms is quite rare in cognitive research relevant to health behavior: these findings should not be ignored. Yet, potential confounders of word association also must be acknowledged. Overall, it is a challenge for cognitive research to provide evidence of a more generally useful, and less controvertible, test of association in cognition.

REFERENCES

Ames, S. L., & Stacy, A. W. (1998). Implicit cognition in the prediction of substance use among drug offenders. *Psychology of Addictive Behaviors, 12*(4), 272–281.

Anderson, J. R. (1983). *The architecture of cognition.* Cambridge, MA: Harvard University Press.

Bargh, J. A., Bond, R. N., Lombardi, W. J., & Tota, M. E. (1986). The additive nature of chronic and temporary sources of construct accessibility. *Journal of Personality and Social Psychology, 50*(5), 869–878.

Bargh, J. A., Chen, M., & Burrows, L. (1996). Automaticity of social behavior: Direct effects of trait construct and stereotype activation on action. *Journal of Personality and Social Psychology, 71*(2), 230–244.

Bechtel, W., & Abrahamsen, A. (2002). *Connectionism and the mind: Parallel processing, dynamics, and evolution in networks* (2nd ed.). Malden, MA: Blackwell.

Boring, E. G. (1950). *A history of experimental psychology* (2nd ed.). New York: Appleton-Century-Crofts.

Cacioppo, J. T., von Hippel, W., & Ernst, J. M. (1997). Mapping cognitive structures and processes through verbal content: The thought-listing technique. *Journal of Consulting and Clinical Psychology, 65*(6), 928–940.

Cattell, J. M., & Bryant, S. (1889). Mental association investigated by experiment. *Mind, 14,* 230–250.

Collins, A. M., & Loftus, E. F. (1975). A spreading-activation theory of semantic processing. *Psychological Review, 82*(6), 407–428.

Cook, S. W., & Skinner, B. F. (1939). Some factors influencing the distribution of associated words. *Psychological Record, 3,* 178–184.

Cramer, P. (1968). *Word association.* New York: Academic Press.

Crovitz, II. F. (1970). *Galton's walk: Methods for the analysis of thinking, intelligence, and creativity.* Oxford, UK: Harper & Row.

Davison, G. C., Vogel, R. S., & Coffman, S. G. (1997). Think-aloud approaches to cognitive assessment and the articulated thoughts in simulated situations paradigm. *Journal of Consulting and Clinical Psychology, 65*(6), 950–958.

Dawson, M. R. W. (2004). *Minds and machines: Connectionism and psychological modeling.* Malden, MA: Blackwell.

Deese, J. (1959a). Influence of inter-item associative strength upon immediate free recall. *Psychological Reports, 5,* 305–312.

Deese, J. (1959b). On the prediction of occurrence of particular verbal intrusions in immediate recall. *Journal of Experimental Psychology, 58,* 17–22.

Dosher, B. A., & Rosedale, G. S. (1997). Configural processing in memory retrieval: Multiple cues and ensemble representations. *Cognitive Psychology, 33*(3), 209–265.

Dunn, M. E., & Goldman, M. S. (2000). Drinking-related differences in expectancies of children assessed as first associates. *Alcoholism: Clinical and Experimental Research, 24*(11), 1639–1646.

Fazio, R. H. (2001). On the automatic activation of associated evaluations: An overview. *Cognition & Emotion, 15*(2), 115–141.

Fazio, R. H., Sanbonmatsu, D. M., Powell, M. C., & Kardes, F. R. (1986). On the automatic activation of attitudes. *Journal of Personality and Social Psychology, 50*(2), 229–238.

Freud, S. (1995). *The Freud reader.* New York: Norton.

Gardner, H., Boller, F., Moreines, J., & Butters, N. (1973). Retrieving information from Korsakoff patients: Effects of categorical cues and reference to the task. *Cortex, 9*(2), 165–175.

Hicks, J. L., & Hancock, T. W. (2002). Backward associative strength determines source attributions given to false memories. *Psychonomic Bulletin & Review, 9*(4), 807–815.

Higgins, E. T., King, G. A., & Mavin, G. H. (1982). Individual construct accessibility and subjective impressions and recall. *Journal of Personality and Social Psychology, 43*(1), 35–47.

Hines, D., Czerwinski, M., Sawyer, P. K., & Dwyer, M. (1986). Automatic semantic priming: Effect of category exemplar level and word association level. *Journal of Experimental Psychology: Human Perception and Performance, 12*(3), 370–379.

Hintzman, D. L. (1986). "Schema abstraction" in a multiple-trace memory model. *Psychological Review, 93*(4), 411–428.

Hutchison, K. A. (2003). Is semantic priming due to association strength or feature overlap? A microanalytic review. *Psychonomic Bulletin & Review, 10*(4), 785–813.

James, W. (1913). *Psychology.* New York: Henry Holt.

Jung, C. G. (1910). The association method. *American Journal of Psychology, 21*(2), 219–269.

Levy, D. A., Stark, C. E. L., & Squire, L. R. (2004). Intact conceptual priming in the absence of declarative memory. *Psychological Science, 15,* 680–686.

Masson, M. E. J. (1995). A distributed memory model of semantic priming. *Journal of Experimental Psychology: Learning, Memory, and Cognition, 21*(1), 3–23.

McEvoy, C. L., Nelson, D. L., & Komatsu, T. (1999). What is the connection between true and false memories? The differential roles of interitem associations in recall and recognition. *Journal of Experimental Psychology: Learning, Memory, and Cognition, 25*(5), 1177–1194.

McRae, K., & Boisvert, S. (1998). Automatic semantic similarity priming. *Journal of Experimental Psychology: Learning, Memory, and Cognition, 24*(3), 558–572.

Morris, C. D., Bransford, J. D., & Franks, J. J. (1977). Levels of processing versus transfer appropriate processing. *Journal of Verbal Learning and Verbal Behavior, 16*(5), 519–533.

Moscovitch, M. (2000). Theories of memory and consciousness. In E. Tulving & F. I. M. Craik (Eds.), *The Oxford handbook of memory* (pp. 609–625). London: Oxford University Press.

Neely, J. H. (1991). Semantic priming effects in visual word recognition: A selective review of current findings and theories. In D. Besner & G. W. Humphreys (Eds.), *Basic processes in reading: Visual word recognition* (pp. 264–336). Hillsdale, NJ: Lawrence Erlbaum.

Nelson, D. L., Drydal, G. M., & Goodmon, L. B. (in press). What is pre-existing strength? Predicting free association probabilities, similarity ratings, and cued recall probabilities. *Psychonomic Bulletin & Review.*

Nelson, D. L., & Goodmon, L. B. (2002). Experiencing a word can prime its accessibility and its associative connections to related words. *Memory & Cognition, 30*(3), 380–398.

Nelson, D. L., McEvoy, C. L., & Pointer, L. (2003). Spreading activation or spooky action at a distance? *Journal of Experimental Psychology: Learning, Memory, and Cognition, 29,* 42–52.

Nelson, D. L., McKinney, V. M., Gee, N. R., & Janczura, G. A. (1998). Interpreting the influence of implicitly activated memories on recall and recognition. *Psychological Review, 105,* 299–324.

Nelson, D. L., Schreiber, T. A., & McEvoy, C. L. (1992). Processing implicit and explicit representations. *Psychological Review, 99*(2), 322–348.

Noble, C. E. (1952). An analysis of meaning. *Psychological Review, 49,* 421–430.

Palfai, T. P., & Wood, M. D. (2001). Positive alcohol expectancies and drinking behavior: The influence of expectancy strength and memory accessibility. *Psychology of Addictive Behaviors, 15*(1), 60–67.

Plaut, D. C., & Booth, J. R. (2000). Individual and developmental differences in semantic priming: Empirical and computational support for a single-mechanism account of lexical processing. *Psychological Review, 107*(4), 786–823.

Preece, P. F. W. (1978). Three-year stability of certain word-association indices. *Psychological Reports, 42,* 25–26.

Ratcliff, R., & McKoon, G. (1994). Retrieving information from memory: Spreading-activation theories versus compound-cue theories. *Psychological Review, 101*(1), 177–184.

Reich, R. R., Goldman, M. S., & Noll, J. A. (2004). Using the false memory paradigm to test two key elements of alcohol expectancy theory. *Experimental & Clinical Psychopharmacology, 12*(2), 102–110.

Rescorla, R. A. (1988). Pavlovian conditioning. It's not what you think it is. *American Psychologist, 43*(3), 151–160.

Roediger, H. L., Gallo, D. A., & Geraci, L. (2002). Processing approaches to cognition: The impetus from the levels-of-processing framework. *Memory, 10*(5–6), 319–332.

Roediger, H. L., & McDermott, K. B. (1995). Creating false memories: Remembering words not presented in lists. *Journal of Experimental Psychology: Learning, Memory, and Cognition, 21*(4), 803–814.

Roediger, H. L., Watson, J. M., McDermott, K. B., & Gallo, D. A. (2001). Factors that determine false recall: A multiple regression analysis. *Psychonomic Bulletin & Review, 8*(3), 385–407.

Rotter, J. B. (1954). *Social learning and clinical psychology.* Oxford, UK: Prentice Hall.

Ryan, J. D., & Cohen, N. J. (2003). Evaluating the neuropsychological dissociation evidence for multiple memory systems. *Cognitive, Affective & Behavioral Neuroscience, 3*(3), 168–185.

Saffran, E. M., Coslett, H. B., & Keener, M. T. (2003). Differences in word associations to pictures and words. *Neuropsychologia, 41*(11), 1541–1546.

Schacter, D. L. (1985). Priming of old and new knowledge in amnesic patients and normal subjects. *Annals of the New York Academy of Sciences, 444,* 41–53.

Seger, C. A., Rabin, L. A., Desmond, J. E., & Gabrieli, J. D. E. (1999). Verb generation priming involves conceptual implicit memory. *Brain and Cognition, 41*(2), 150–177.

Seger, C. A., Rabin, L. A., Zarella, M., & Gabrieli, J. D. E. (1997). Preserved verb generation priming in global amnesia. *Neuropsychologia, 35*(8), 1069–1074.

Shelton, J. R., & Martin, R. C. (1992). How semantic is automatic semantic priming? *Journal of Experimental Psychology: Learning, Memory, and Cognition, 18*(6), 1191–1210.

Shimamura, A. P., & Squire, L. R. (1984). Paired-associate learning and priming effects in amnesia: A neuropsychological study. *Journal of Experimental Psychology: General, 113*(4), 556–570.

Smith, E. R. (1996). What do connectionism and social psychology offer each other? *Journal of Personality and Social Psychology, 70*(5), 893–912.

Smith, E. R., & DeCoster, J. (1998). Knowledge acquisition, accessibility, and use in person perception and stereotyping: Simulation with a recurrent connectionist network. *Journal of Personality and Social Psychology, 74*(1), 21–35.

Spruyt, A., Hermans, D., De Houwer, J., & Eelen, P. (2004). Automatic nonassociative semantic priming: Episodic affective priming of naming responses. *Acta Psychologica, 116*(1), 39–54.

Stacy, A. W. (1995). Memory association and ambiguous cues in models of alcohol and marijuana use. *Experimental & Clinical Psychopharmacology, 3*(2), 183–194.

Stacy, A. W. (1997). Memory activation and expectancy as prospective predictors of alcohol and marijuana use. *Journal of Abnormal Psychology, 106*(1), 61–73.

Stacy, A. W., Ames, S. L., & Knowlton, B. J. (2004). Neurologically plausible distinctions in cognition relevant to drug use etiology and prevention. *Substance Use & Misuse, 39,* 1571–1623.

Stacy, A. W., Ames, S. L., & Leigh, B. C. (2004). An implicit cognition assessment aproach to relapse, secondary prevention, and media effects. *Cognitive and Behavioral Practice, 11,* 139–149.

Stacy, A. W., Ames, S. L., Sussman, S., & Dent, C. W. (1996). Implicit cognition in adolescent drug use. *Psychology of Addictive Behaviors, 10*(3), 190–203.

Stacy, A. W., Galaif, E. R., Sussman, S., & Dent, C. W. (1996). Self-generated drug outcomes in high-risk adolescents. *Psychology of Addictive Behaviors, 10*(1), 18–27.

Stacy, A. W., Leigh, B. C., & Weingardt, K. R. (1993, November). *An individual-difference perspective applied to normative associative strength.* Paper presented at the annual meeting of the Psychonomic Society, Washington, DC.

Stacy, A. W., Leigh, B. C., & Weingardt, K. R. (1994). Memory accessibility and association of alcohol use and its positive outcomes. *Experimental & Clinical Psychopharmacology, 2*(3), 269–282.

Stacy, A. W., Leigh, B. C., & Weingardt, K. R. (1997). An individual-difference perspective applied to word association. *Personality and Social Psychology Bulletin, 23*(3), 229–237.

Stacy, A. W., Pearce, S. G., Zogg, J. B., Unger, J. B., & Dent, C. W. (2004). A nonverbal test of naturalistic memory for alcohol commercials. *Psychology & Marketing, 21*(4), 295–322.

Stewart, D. W. (1989). Measures, methods, and models in advertising research. *Journal of Advertising Research, 29*(3), 54–60.

Szalay, L. B., Carroll, J. F. X., & Tims, F. (1993). Rediscovering free associations for use in psychotherapy. *Psychotherapy: Theory, Research, Practice, Training, 30*(2), 344–356.

Szalay, L. B., Strohl, J. B., & Doherty, K. T. (1999). *Psychoenvironmental forces in substance abuse prevention.* Dordrecht, The Netherlands: Kluwer Academic.

Szalay, L. B., Windle, C., & Lysne, D. A. (1970). Attitude measurement by free verbal associations. *Journal of Social Psychology, 82*(1), 43–55.

Thorne, B. M., & Henley, T. B. (2001). *Connections in the history and systems of psychology* (2nd ed.). Boston: Houghton Mifflin.

Toth, J. P. (2000). Nonconscious forms of human memory. In E. Tulving & F. I. M. Craik (Eds.), *The Oxford handbook of memory* (pp. 245–261). London: Oxford University Press.

Underwood, B. J. (1965). False recognition produced by implicit verbal responses. *Journal of Experimental Psychology, 70*(1), 122–129.

Vaidya, C. J., Gabrieli, J. D. E., Keane, M. M., & Monti, L. A. (1995). Perceptual and conceptual memory processes in global amnesia. *Neuropsychology, 9*(4), 12.

Wentura, D. (2000). Dissociative affective and associative priming effects in the lexical decision task: Yes versus no responses to word targets reveal evaluative judgment tendencies. *Journal of Experimental Psychology: Learning, Memory, and Cognition, 26*(2), 456–469.

Woodworth, R. S. (1921). *Psychology: A study of mental life.* New York: Henry Holt.

Zeelenberg, R., Pecher, D., Shiffrin, R. M., & Raaijmakers, J. G. W. (2003). Semantic context effects and priming in word association. *Psychonomic Bulletin & Review, 10*(3), 653–660.

Zeelenberg, R., Shiffrin, R. M., & Raaijmakers, J. G. W. (1999). Priming in a free association task as a function of association directionality. *Memory & Cognition, 27*(6), 956–961.

CHAPTER 7

Reaction Time Measures of Substance-Related Associations

KATRIJN HOUBEN, REINOUT W. WIERS, AND ANNE ROEFS

Abstract: This chapter provides an overview of indirect RT measures of implicit associations, including the IAT, the EAST, and priming paradigms. Each indirect measure is described on a conceptual level and is illustrated with recent findings from addiction research. For each measure, a critical evaluation of its strengths and weaknesses is given including a discussion of its psychometric properties, the relativity of measured associations, its suitability for assessing ambivalence, and alternative accounts of effects by nonassociative processes. Recent modifications, such as the Single Target IAT, the GNAT, the Modified EAST and the Single Valence EAST that have been developed in response to some of the limitations of the measures described here are also discussed.

INTRODUCTION

Addiction research is currently exploring the value of implicit measures for assessing cognitions believed to be involved in the etiology and maintenance of addictive behaviors. Traditionally, addiction-related cognitions have been examined with self-report measures that ask respondents for introspection (see Wiers et al., Chapter 22). Self-report measures, however, have been criticized because of their susceptibility to self-presentation biases and the possibility that cognitive-motivational processes mediating addiction are not accessible through conscious introspection (e.g., Nisbett & Wilson, 1977; Stacy,

AUTHOR'S NOTE: First and second author are funded by a "VIDI" grant from the Dutch National Science Foundation (N.W.O.) awarded to the second author. The authors wish to thank Jan De Houwer, Martin Zack, Alan W. Stacy, and Tibor P. Palfai for helpful comments on the first draft of the manuscript. Correspondence concerning this chapter can be addressed to Katrijn Houben, Experimental Psychology; Uns 40; Maastricht University; PO BOX 616; 6200 MD Maastricht, The Netherlands. E-mail: K.Houben@psychology.unimaas.nl

1997). These two key problems of self-report measures have encouraged researchers to develop implicit measures that assess cognitions indirectly from behavior such as reaction time (RT).

Despite the increased use and popularity of implicit measures, the denotation of the term "implicit" remains confusing. Some have argued that the term refers to the measurement procedure (Fazio & Olson, 2003), whereas others believe that implicit measures have privileged access to automatically activated cognitions and tap different underlying processes than self-report measures (e.g., Cunningham et al., 2001; Stacy, 1997; Wilson et al., 2000). According to De Houwer (Chapter 2), these two views of implicit measures actually refer to different things, namely to the measurement procedure and the outcome of the measurement procedure, respectively. Following De Houwer, the terms "indirect" and "direct" are used here to denote measurement procedures, whereas the term "implicit" is used for cognitions assessed with indirect measures.

This chapter discusses the merits of a subset of indirect measures, namely indirect RT-based association measures. Several RT association measures, including the Implicit Association Test (IAT; Greenwald et al., 1998), the Extrinsic Affective Simon Task (EAST; De Houwer, 2003), and priming paradigms are described conceptually and illustrated with examples from addiction research. A critical review of strengths and weaknesses is given for each measure and recently developed modifications are discussed. For an extended overview of indirect measurement procedures see Wiers et al. (2004).

THE IMPLICIT ASSOCIATION TEST

The IAT (Greenwald et al., 1998) is a double categorization task that requires the classification of stimuli into four different categories

with two response keys. Typically, two categories represent the target concepts (e.g., alcohol vs. soft drinks) and two categories correspond to the poles of an attribute dimension (e.g., positive vs. negative). During the critical trials of the IAT, the target and attribute categories are assigned to two response keys in two different combinations. During one combination task, for example, participants have to classify both alcohol and negative words with one response key and soft drinks and positive words with the other. During the reversed combination task, alcohol and positive are assigned to the same key and soft drinks and negative to the other. Because performance will be better when concepts that are associated in memory are classified with the same response key (compatible), than when concepts sharing a response key are not or only weakly associated (incompatible), one of these combinations typically leads to faster and more accurate performance compared with the other. This performance difference is referred to as the IAT effect and is assumed to reflect the strength of implicit associations between the target and attribute categories (Greenwald et al., 1998).

Application to Addictive Behaviors

The IAT has already been used in numerous studies examining substance-related cognitions. For example, Swanson et al. (2001) and Huijding et al. (2005) compared smokers and nonsmokers' implicit smoking associations with valence. In both studies, both smokers and nonsmokers were found to have stronger negative implicit smoking associations compared with a number of different contrast categories such as sweets, exercise, and writing. Likewise, Field et al. (2004) used the IAT to examine cannabis users and nonusers' implicit cannabis associations compared with features of the natural environment. Nonusers showed stronger negative implicit cannabis associations compared to cannabis users. Wiers et al. (2002) measured heavy and light drinkers' implicit alcohol associations with the IAT in two dimensions: valence and arousal. Both heavy and light drinkers implicitly associated alcohol with negative valence compared with soft drinks, whereas only heavy drinkers demonstrated alcohol-arousal associations. These findings have been replicated in a sample of heavy drinkers (Wiers et al., 2005) and in a sample of patient drinkers (De Houwer et al., 2004). Palfai and Ostafin (2003a) recently modified the IAT by replacing the valence categories with approach and avoidance attributes. Results demonstrated that alcohol is associated with approach motivations (or action tendencies) in hazardous drinkers. Further, stronger alcohol-approach associations significantly correlated with urge to drink and arousal-reactivity in anticipation of alcohol consumption. Both the implicit arousal and the approach associations in heavy drinkers have been linked to the incentive-sensitization theory (Robinson & Berridge, 1993, 2003; see also Wiers et al., Chapter 22), which states that activation of a sensitized "wanting" system automatically increases attention, arousal, and approach responses, in the absence of "liking." Moreover, these findings underscore the usefulness of assessing substance-related associations in other dimensions than valence alone (e.g., arousal-sedation, approach-avoid), as has been demonstrated in other areas of psychopathology (e.g., Teachman et al., 2001; Teachman & Woody, 2003). Furthermore, the IAT can also be used with pictorial instead of verbal stimuli and has been shown to be robust against influence from such stimulus-related variations (Hofmann et al., 2004). To illustrate, Swanson et al. (2001) contrasted smoking pictures with nonsmoking pictures in an IAT and found both smokers and nonsmokers to have an implicit preference for nonsmoking pictures.

Strengths and Weaknesses

The IAT shows good internal consistency, in the region of .80. Stability over time is typically lower with an average test-retest value of .60 (e.g., Bosson et al., 2000; Cunningham et al., 2001; Greenwald & Nosek, 2001; around .70 for the alcohol IAT; Wiers et al., 2005). Promising results were also found regarding the convergent validity of the IAT (Cunningham et al., 2001; Greenwald & Nosek, 2001), though most studies have found correlations between indirect measures to be inconsistent, weak, and/or nonexistent (e.g., Bosson et al., 2000; Olson & Fazio, 2003). A large range of positive correlations between the IAT and direct measures have been found with a low but positive average of .24 (Hofmann et al., 2004).

The IAT, however, is not without limitations and recent research has uncovered problems that may compromise the interpretation of IAT effects. First, it is unclear which associations are assessed with the IAT. The IAT primarily measures associations between concepts at category level rather than at the level of individual exemplars (De Houwer, 2001, 2002). Exemplars can influence IAT effects by determining the target category context or supporting a category redefinition (Govan & Williams, 2004; Mitchell et al., 2003), but ultimately the categories determine IAT effects. This implies that category labels are important and that the IAT is vulnerable to influences of label associations (i.e., the "label effect"). In addition, IAT effects appear to be susceptible to contamination by culturally shared associative knowledge that is not necessarily personally endorsed (Karpinski & Hilton, 2001; Olson & Fazio, 2004).

Second, the IAT only provides a measure of the relative strength of implicit associations because the IAT requires two categories and two attribute categories (De Houwer, 2002). The bipolarity of the target dimension carries the implication that the IAT measures the strength of the association between one target concept and the attributes *relative to* the contrast target category. Therefore, conclusions about implicit associations of a single target category are unwarranted because the possibility always exists that the contrast category influenced IAT effects. Moreover, the bipolarity of the attribute categories prevents assessment of ambivalence, because it is impossible to find associations between a target category and both poles of the attribute dimension. This may be especially problematic for addictive behaviors, where ambivalence is typically quite strong (Conner & Sparks, 2002) and even at the core of some of its definitions (e.g., Orford, 2001).

Third, IAT effects are assumed to reflect the strength of implicit associations in memory (Greenwald et al., 1998) and, according to the analysis of De Houwer (2001), stimulus-response compatibility effects underlie IAT effects. Presumably, compatibility between the short-term associations of the response keys created by instructions and the intrinsic, long-term associations of the stimuli facilitates performance. Because IAT effects are based on the comparison of performance between two tasks, however, nonassociative processes can also influence IAT effects. Such an account of IAT effects is provided by Rothermund and Wentura (2001, 2004). They propose that salience or figure-ground asymmetries can cause IAT effects, independent of implicit associations. When one of the categories of an IAT dimension is more salient than the other, the most salient category will attract attention. This salient category becomes the so-called figure, whereas the other category constitutes the (back)ground. Subsequently, when both the target and attribute figure are mapped onto the same response, performance will be better compared with when one figure and one ground category are assigned to the same response. Similarly, the task-switching account (Mierke & Klauer, 2001, 2003) also

explains part of the IAT effects in terms of nonassociative processes: the IAT involves a switch between two different tasks (typically an easy and a difficult combination) and IAT effects are larger for people who have difficulties with task-switching, irrespective of their associations. This task-switching is thought to involve executive control processes and comes with a performance cost, causing slower and less accurate responding. This aspect of the IAT measurement procedure may be particularly worrying for comparisons of groups that differ in their task-switching abilities, such as young versus older or addicted versus nonaddicted participants.

Recent Developments

IAT Developments

Jajodia and Earleywine (2003) modified the IAT by eliminating attribute bipolarity to enable assessment of ambivalence toward alcohol. Attribute categories were presented in a unipolar format, by contrasting both positive and negative attributes with attribute categories made up of unrelated neutral words (e.g., basic, intermediate). Results showed implicit alcohol associations with both positive and negative valence relative to mammals, implying that implicit alcohol attitudes are in fact ambivalent. Furthermore, Houben and Wiers (2004) examined the extent to which the label effect, target and attribute bipolarity, and figure-ground asymmetries influence findings with alcohol IATs. In a first study, the influence of using the label "alcohol" versus the label "beer" was examined as well as the effect of using the contrast category "animals" instead of "soft drinks." Moreover, attribute bipolarity was eliminated by testing positive, negative, arousal, and sedation attributes relative to (different) neutral attribute categories. Results showed only minor effects of the labels and contrast categories and both alcohol and beer were very strongly associated with negative affect, strongly with positive affect and arousal, and moderately with sedation. These findings provide additional support for the existence of ambivalent implicit alcohol associations and underscore the need to assess implicit alcohol associations in a unipolar format with respect to the attributes. In a second study, participants performed visual search tasks (Rothermund & Wentura, 2004) to examine figure-ground asymmetries between categories that made up an IAT dimension in the first study. Results showed that the neutral categories were more salient than the positive, negative, and sedation categories, but showed no figure-ground asymmetries for the target dimensions or for the arousal-neutral dimension, suggesting that figure-ground effects cannot explain the IAT results of the first study.

According to Olson and Fazio (2004), some IAT properties might promote the use of extrapersonal (cultural) associations (cf. Karpinski & Hilton, 2001) by increasing the accessibility of normative information. Therefore, they introduced the personalized IAT (see also Fadardi et al., Chapter 9), which reduces this contamination by extrapersonal associations. First, it eliminates normative implications associated with the labels "positive" and "negative" through the use of the labels "I like" and "I dislike." Second, it uses attribute stimuli that are not normatively associated with valence but that have little evaluative consensus (large variability) while still being attitude-evoking (e.g., football, coffee). Finally, no error feedback is given to participants to avoid suggesting that there is a normative correct response. The personalized IAT was found to reveal less racial prejudice and was more strongly correlated with direct measures, suggesting a reduced influence of extrapersonal associations (Olson & Fazio, 2004). Nosek and Hansen (2004), in contrast, argue that the original and the personalized IAT both

capture unique attitude-relevant aspects, reflecting the multidimensionality of attitudes. In a series of studies, evidence for the multidimensionality of attitudes was found and results suggested that both IAT versions were capturing different aspects of these attitude constructs.

IAT Variants

Wigboldus et al. (2004) developed the Single Target IAT (ST-IAT), which is structurally similar to the IAT, with the difference that only one target category is used. Participants are instructed to classify both this target and one attribute category (e.g., alcohol and negative) with one response key and the other attribute category (e.g., positive) with the second response key. Unlike the IAT, the ST-IAT measures associations between only one target concept and the attributes without a second contrasting target category.

The GNAT (Go/No-Go Association Task; Nosek & Banaji, 2001) is another IAT variant designed to assess associations between a single target category and two poles of an attribute dimension. In this task, participants press one response key for targets and attributes (Go) and are instructed to ignore other stimuli (No-Go). The strength of associations is assessed by determining the extent to which stimuli belonging to the target category and one pole of the attribute dimension can be discriminated from distracter stimuli. As it is in the case of the ST-IAT, the target is first paired with one pole of the attribute dimension and subsequently with the other in two combination tasks. Differences in sensitivity between these two combinations reflect the association between the target and the attributes (Nosek & Banaji, 2001). One major advantage of the GNAT is that the task is very flexible with respect to the choice of the distracter set, allowing assessment of single associations with a target category (Nosek & Banaji, 2001). Dabbs et al. (2003)

used a portable version of the GNAT to assess smokers and nonsmokers' smoking attitudes. Preliminary results showed smokers to have a more favorable implicit attitude toward smoking compared with nonsmokers.

Both the ST-IAT and the GNAT are unipolar with respect to the target category and offer a way to assess associations with targets that do not have a natural opposing contrast, such as smoking. Both IAT variants, however, compare performance between two tasks, making nonassociative alternative accounts of effects possible. Also, since categories are labeled in both tasks, label effects may still influence results. Finally, attribute bipolarity remains a problem for both tasks when assessing associations that are possibly ambivalent.

THE EXTRINSIC AFFECTIVE SIMON TASK

The EAST (De Houwer, 2003) is a categorization task that allows measurement of single target associations within one task. In the EAST, attribute words (e.g., positive and negative) are typically classified by meaning with two response keys. Because of these task instructions, the response keys become extrinsically associated with the meaning of the attributes assigned to them, creating, for example, an extrinsically positive and an extrinsically negative response key. In contrast, target words (e.g., alcohol, soda) are classified with respect to an irrelevant stimulus property (e.g., color, shape) with the same two response keys. Participants, for example, may be instructed to respond with one key to positive words and to alcohol and soda stimuli that are presented in blue and to respond with the other key to negative words and to alcohol or soda targets that are presented in green. Subsequently, implicit associations between alcohol and valence are defined as the performance difference between giving an extrinsically positive response to a (blue) alcohol target and giving an extrinsically negative response to a (green) alcohol target.

Application to Addictive Behaviors

In a recent study, De Houwer et al. (2004) assessed implicit alcohol associations with an EAST in a sample of patients. Alcoholics were more accurate in responding to soft drink stimuli with an extrinsically positive response than with an extrinsically negative response, but showed no performance difference for alcohol stimuli. These results suggest that participants had a favorable attitude toward soft drinks and a neutral or ambivalent attitude toward alcohol. Wiers et al. (2003) assessed implicit alcohol associations with a valence-EAST and an arousal-EAST in drinking students and found that participants held implicit alcohol-arousal associations, replicating IAT findings (e.g., Wiers et al., 2002).

Strengths and Weaknesses

Until now, few studies have examined the reliability and validity of the EAST, although promising results have been obtained when assessing attitudes for which meaningful interindividual differences exist (De Houwer, 2003). Typically, EAST effect sizes are somewhat smaller than IAT effect sizes (De Houwer, 2003). Unlike the IAT, EAST effects are based on comparison of performance within one task, which makes nonassociative accounts of EAST effects (e.g., salience asymmetries, task-switching) less likely. Also, the EAST allows assessment of single associations between one target and the attributes, even when multiple target categories are used. Not only are target dimensions presented in a unipolar format, they are also presented without labels, making label effects less likely. The attribute dimension, however, is still presented in a bipolar format, making the EAST, like the IAT, unsuitable to assess ambivalent associations.

Recent Developments

Wiers et al. (2003) tested a Modified-EAST (M-EAST) for assessing multiple and ambivalent alcohol associations within one task. The M-EAST is structurally similar to the EAST, with the modification that target words now have to be classified by meaning and attributes by an irrelevant property. The M-EAST has the advantage that attribute dimensions are no longer bipolar. Because the targets are now bipolar again, however, only relative associations can be assessed. Using the M-EAST, Wiers et al. (2003) created an extrinsic alcohol and an extrinsic soft drink response key while positive, negative, arousal, and sedation attributes were presented in blue and green. Performance of heavy-drinking men was found to be better when making an extrinsically alcohol-related response compared to an extrinsically soft drink-related response to both arousal and sedation attributes. These results demonstrate implicit alcohol associations with both arousal and sedation. No reliable performance differences were found for positive and negative attributes.

De Liver et al. (2003) developed the Single Valence-EAST (SV-EAST) to enable the assessment of ambivalent attitudes. The SV-EAST is structurally similar to the EAST with attributes being classified by meaning and targets by an irrelevant property. Unlike the EAST, however, only one classification response is used (as in the GNAT). For example, attribute words require a response when they possess valence whereas attributes without valence have to be ignored. During one block, only positive and neutral attributes are presented or only negative and neutral attributes. Ambivalent (e.g., alcohol) and neutral targets are presented that require a classification response when presented in blue but have to be ignored when presented in green. The assumption is that responding to ambivalent targets will be superior compared with responding to neutral targets. The SV-EAST has the advantage that it presents both the target and attribute dimension in a unipolar format and without category labels.

PRIMING MEASURES

Sequential priming techniques are particularly useful for studying the associative structure of memory representations (Bargh & Chartrand, 2000). In semantic priming, associations are assessed between two different concepts and in affective priming, associations are assessed between a concept and its evaluation.

In *semantic* priming procedures, the presentation of a prime word or phrase, assumed to provide a semantic context, is followed by the presentation of a target word to which a response has to be generated. This response typically involves pronunciation of the target word (pronunciation task) or a word/non-word decision (lexical decision task). Targets can be semantically related or unrelated to the prime, and priming effects are demonstrated when response latencies or the percentage of errors for targets following unrelated primes are larger than for targets following a related prime (Bargh & Chartrand, 2000; Neely, 1991).

Affective or evaluative priming techniques involve the presentation of a prime that is evaluatively consistent or inconsistent with a subsequently presented target. The presentation of an attitude object as a prime is thought to activate any associated evaluations and hence facilitate the processing of and responding to evaluative consistent targets (Fazio, 2001; Klauer, 1998; Klauer & Musch, 2003). Most often, participants are asked to decide whether the target is "good" or "bad" (evaluative categorization task);

however, affective priming effects have also been found with the lexical decision task (e.g., Wentura, 2000) and the pronunciation task (under certain conditions; e.g., Hermans et al., 1994, 2001; Spruyt et al., 2002).

For both semantic and affective priming procedures, priming effects are indicated by an interaction between prime and target valence or meaning, showing faster performance when prime and target are congruent than when they are incongruent. Several accounts of priming effects have been proposed, including spreading activation (Fazio et al., 1986), response competition/facilitation (Klinger et al., 2000), affective-matching (Klauer, 1998; Klauer & Musch, 2003), and compound cue theory (Ratcliff & McKoon, 1988), but also more controlled processes like target expectancies (Neely, 1991).

Application to Addictive Behaviors

Using a semantic priming task, Hill and Paynter (1992) demonstrated faster responding to alcohol targets that were preceded by alcohol-related primes than to alcohol targets that were preceded by unrelated primes for alcohol-dependent drinkers. No such priming effect was found for the nondependent drinkers. Moreover, Weingardt et al. (1996) examined the association between alcohol and outcome states using a semantic priming task and were able to show that the presentation of positive outcomes of drinking alcohol facilitated the naming of subsequent alcohol-related words. Furthermore, results showed that more drinking experiences were accompanied by an increased priming effect. Zack and colleagues used semantic priming to assess associations between possible antecedents of drinking and alcohol. In line with this idea, Zack et al. (1999) showed that problem drinkers with high psychiatric distress displayed significant activation of alcohol concepts by negative affective primes. The opposite was also found in these problem drinkers: Negative concepts were primed by alcohol primes. Problem drinkers with low psychiatric distress showed inhibition in both these conditions. Zack et al. (2003) examined the association between alcohol and antecedent mood states and demonstrated faster pronunciation of alcohol targets following negative mood phrases in young drinkers with high- and low-anxiety sensitivity.

Palfai and Ostafin (2003b) used an affective priming task to examine the influence of alcohol consumption on the activation of alcohol outcome expectancies. Results indicated that, regardless of whether expectancy words were preceded by a neutral or an alcohol prime, participants responded faster to positive expectancies after consuming alcohol than after consuming a placebo beverage. Apparently, alcohol consumption increased the activation of positive expectancies but not associative memory links between alcohol and expectancies. Ostafin et al. (2003) modified the affective priming task by replacing positive and negative target words with targets related to approach and avoidance behavior. Results showed that alcohol-binge episodes and alcohol-related problems were correlated with weak associations between alcohol and avoidance tendencies, however, not with strong associations between alcohol and approach tendencies (see also Wiers et al., Chapter 22).

Strengths and Weaknesses

Priming has been proven to be useful, but effect sizes are typically small and reliability of individual differences is typically low (e.g., Bosson et al., 2000) to moderate (e.g., Cunningham et al., 2001). Priming measures are, however, only explained in terms of associative relationships and priming effects necessitate no comparison of different sets of words since the same stimulus words are used to make up both the congruent and the incongruent prime-target pairs. This avoids uncontrollable influences on priming effects such as effects of familiarity and salience (Klauer, 1998).

OTHER INDIRECT RT ASSOCIATION MEASURES

We will now briefly discuss two other measures that have been used in addiction research. A full review of these measures is unfeasible because of limited space and therefore, only the main task properties will be described for these measures and only some points of criticism will be given. First, the primed emotional Stroop task can be used to assess implicit associations by examining color-naming latencies for target words that are preceded by prime words. Participants are instructed to ignore the meaning of target words and only name the color of the words. Unlike in other indirect association measures, implicit associations are indicated in the primed emotional Stroop task by *slower* performance on trials where target words are preceded by a congruent prime. Both Kramer and Goldman (2003) and Stewart et al. (2002) have recently used the primed emotional Stroop to examine alcohol-related associations. In both studies, however, primes were presented for an unusually long period (2 seconds, stimulus onset asynchrony (SOA) = 5 seconds and 500 ms, SOA = 1300 ms, respectively) when compared with priming studies where priming effects have been found to dissipate at SOAs longer than 300 ms (e.g., Hermans et al., 2003). This makes the indirect nature of the test somewhat questionable.

Second, accessibility measures provide another way for measuring implicit associations. For example, participants can be instructed to respond to a series of expectancy words that are preceded by a prompt (e.g., "Alcohol makes me") by pressing one of two response keys (yes or no). The accessibility of expectancies is assessed by examining the time necessary to endorse expectancy items (e.g., Palfai, 2002; Palfai et al., 1997; Palfai et al., 2000). These accessibility measures are probably the closest to the direct self-report measures of all measures reviewed here, because they ask respondents to self-report on their cognitions while the accessibility of these cognitions is indirectly determined from response times.

DISCUSSION

Assessment of substance-related cognitions with indirect measures has provided new insights into the cognitions involved in addictive behaviors. There are at least two reasons for supplementing traditional direct self-report measures with indirect measures: self-presentation biases and limited cognitive accessibility. In this chapter, an overview was provided of indirect RT measures of implicit associations. When comparing these measures, it is obvious that the largest effects can be obtained with the IAT. Several problems have been attributed to this test, however, and IAT effects can be explained by both associative and nonassociative accounts. Therefore, IAT effects probably do not only reflect implicit associations in memory, but also reflect artifacts of the measurement procedure. In response to these problems, several other indirect association measures have been developed, such as the ST-IAT, the EAST, and the GNAT, which overcome some, but not all of the problems associated with the IAT measurement procedure. Priming procedures, on the other hand, appear to be less susceptible to nonassociative factors. Accounts of priming effects are primarily in terms of semantic or affective relationships between concepts and none explain priming effects in terms of artifacts of the measurement procedure. Typically, priming effects are also smaller than, for example, IAT effects, possibly because effects are not enlarged by nonassociative effects and reflect only the associations of interest.

One general limitation that applies to most indirect measures reviewed here is that these measures do not fully capture the directionality of implicit associations. Because targets typically both precede and follow attributes, an association between alcohol and an attribute can reflect both an association with an expected outcome (e.g., alcohol-positive: Drinking alcohol causes a positive mood) or with an antecedent (e.g., positive-alcohol: When in a positive mood, one should drink alcohol). This temporal sequence of associations is not addressed by current RT-based indirect measures. For example, it remains puzzling that people continue to use addictive substances while IAT research continues to find evidence that these substances are implicitly associated with negative valence. One possible explanation is that

associations with addictive substances are typically ambivalent and this conclusion seems to be supported by recent research. Alternatively, it is possible that negative stimuli act as a cue for using addictive substances while addictive substances activate positive expectancies (see Wiers et al., Chapter 22). This directionality issue as well as the meaning of implicit negative substance associations should be addressed by future research on implicit drug associations.

We hope this review of RT measures of implicit associations will stimulate further research on the processes underlying the effects of these measures. We trust this will lead to further improvements of indirect association measures that can be applied in addiction research as a supplement to direct self-report measures. Ultimately, such an approach could lead to a better understanding of automatic processes in addictive behaviors and their treatment.

REFERENCES

Bargh, J. A., & Chartrand, T. L. (2000). The mind in the middle: A practical guide to priming and automaticity research. In H. T. Reis (Ed.), *Handbook of research methods in social and personality psychology* (pp. 25–285). New York: Cambridge University Press.

Bosson, J. K., Swann, W. B., & Pennebaker, J. W. (2000). Stalking the perfect measure of implicit self-esteem: The blind men and the elephant revisited? *Journal of Personality and Social Psychology, 79,* 631–643.

Conner, M., & Sparks, P. (2002). Ambivalence and attitudes. *European Review of Social Psychology, 12,* 37–70.

Cunningham, W. A., Preacher, K. J., & Banaji, M. R. (2001). Implicit attitude measures: Consistency, stability, and convergent validity. *Psychological Science, 12,* 163–170.

Dabbs, J. M. J., Bassett, J. F., Brower, A. M., Cate, K. L., DeSantis, J. E., & Leander, N. P. (2003, May/June). *A portable version of the Go/No-Go Association Task (GNAT).* Poster session presented at the 15th annual convention of the American Psychological Society, Atlanta, GA.

De Houwer, J. (2001). A structural and process analysis of the implicit association test. *Journal of Experimental Social Psychology, 37,* 443–451.

De Houwer, J. (2002). The implicit association test as a tool for studying dysfunctional associations in psychopathology: Strengths and limitations. *Behavior Therapy and Experimental Psychiatry, 53,* 115–133.

De Houwer, J. (2003). The Extrinsic Affective Simon Task. *Experimental Psychology, 50,* 77–85.

De Houwer, J., Crombez, G., Koster, E. H. W., & De Beul, N. (2004). Implicit alcohol- related cognitions in clinical samples of heavy drinkers. *Journal of Behaviour Therapy and Experimental Psychiatry, 35,* 275–286.

de Liver, Y., Wigboldus, D., & van der Pligt, J. (2003). De structuur van ambivalente attitudes. In D. Wigboldus, M. Dechesne, E. Gordijn, & E. Kluwer (Eds.), *Jaarboek sociale psychologie* (pp. 217–226). Delft, The Netherlands: Eburon.

Fazio, R. H. (2001). On the automatic activation of associated evaluations: An overview. *Cognition & Emotion, 15,* 115–141.

Fazio, R. H., & Olson, M. A. (2003). Implicit measures in social cognition: Their meaning and use. *Annual Review of Psychology, 54,* 297–327.

Fazio, R. H., Sanbonmatsu, D. M., Powell, M. C., & Kardes, F. R. (1986). On the automatic activation of attitudes. *Journal of Personality and Social Psychology, 50,* 229–238.

Field, M., Mogg, K., & Bradley, B. P. (2004). Cognitive bias and drug craving in recreational cannabis users. *Drug and Alcohol Dependence, 74,* 105–111.

Govan, C. L., & Williams, K. D. (2004). Changing the affective valence of the stimulus items influences the IAT by re-defining the category labels. *Journal of Experimental Social Psychology, 40,* 357–365.

Greenwald, A. G., McGhee, D. E., & Schwartz, J. L. K. (1998). Measuring individual differences in implicit cognition: The implicit association test. *Journal of Personality and Social Psychology, 74,* 1464–1480.

Greenwald, A. G., & Nosek, B. A. (2001). Health of the implicit association test at age 3. *Zeitschrift für Experimentelle Psychologie, 48,* 85–93.

Hermans, D., De Houwer, J., & Eelen, P. (1994). The affective priming effect: Automatic activation of evaluative information in memory. *Cognition & Emotion, 8*(6), 515–533.

Hermans, D., De Houwer, J., & Eelen, P. (2001). A time course analysis of the affective priming effect. *Cognition & Emotion, 15*(2), 143–165.

Hermans, D., Spruyt, A., & Eelen, P. (2003). Automatic affective priming of recently acquired stimulus valence: Priming at SOA 300 but not at SOA 100. *Cognition & Emotion, 17,* 83–99.

Hill, A. B., & Paynter, S. (1992). Alcohol dependence and semantic priming of alcohol related words. *Personality and Individual Differences, 13,* 745–750.

Hofmann, W., Gawronski, B., Gschwendner, T., Le, H., & Schmitt, M. (2004). *A meta-analysis on the correlation between the implicit association test and explicit self-report measures.* Manuscript submitted for publication.

Houben, K., & Wiers, R. W. (2004). *Assessing implicit alcohol associations with the IAT: Fact or artifact?* Manuscript submitted for publication. Implicit alcohol associations: Influence of target category labels and contrast categories in a unipolar IAT [Abstract]. *Alcoholism: Clinical and Experimental Research, 28*(5-Suppl.), 102A.

Huijding, J., de Jong, P. J., Wiers, R. W., & Verkooijen, K. (2005). Implicit and explicit attitudes towards smoking in a smoking and a non-smoking setting. *Addictive Behaviors, 30,* 949–961.

Jajodia, A., & Earleywine, M. (2003). Measuring alcohol expectancies with the implicit association test. *Psychology of Addictive Behaviors, 17,* 126–133.

Karpinski, A., & Hilton, J. L. (2001). Attitudes and the implicit association test. *Journal of Personality and Social Psychology, 81,* 774–788.

Klauer, K. C. (1998). Affective priming. In W. Stroebe & M. Hewstone (Eds.), *European Review of Social Psychology* (Vol. 8, pp. 67–103). Chichester, UK: Wiley.

Klauer, K. C., & Musch, J. (2003). Affective priming: Findings and theories. In J. Musch & K. C. Klauer (Eds.), *The psychology of evaluation: Affective processes in cognition and emotion* (pp. 7–49). Mahwah, NJ: Lawrence Erlbaum.

Klinger, M. R., Burton, P. C., & Pitts, G. S. (2000). Mechanisms of unconscious priming: I. Response competition, not spreading activation. *Journal of Experimental Psychology, 26*(2), 441–455.

Kramer, D. A., & Goldman, M. S. (2003). Using a modified Stroop task to implicitly discern the cognitive organization of alcohol expectancies. *Journal of Abnormal Psychology, 112,* 171–175.

Mierke, J., & Klauer, K. C. (2001). Implicit association measurement with the IAT: Evidence for effects of executive control processes. *Zeitschrift für Experimentelle Psychologie, 48,* 107–122.

Mierke, J., & Klauer, K. C. (2003). Method-specific variance in the Implicit Association Test. *Journal of Personality and Social Psychology, 85,* 1180–1192.

Mitchell, J. P., Nosek, B. A., & Banaji, M. R. (2003). Contextual variations in implicit evaluation. *Journal of Experimental Psychology, 132,* 455–469.

Neely, J. H. (1991). Semantic priming effects in visual word recognition: A selective review of current findings and theories. In D. Besner & G. W. Humphreys (Eds.), *Basic processes in reading: Visual word recognition* (pp. 264–337). Hillsdale, NJ: Lawrence Erlbaum.

Nisbett, R. E., & Wilson, T. D. (1977). Telling more than we can know: Verbal reports on mental processes. *Psychological Review, 84,* 231–259.

Nosek, B. A., & Banaji, M. R. (2001). The Go/No-Go Association Task. *Social Cognition, 19,* 625–664.

Nosek, B. A., & Hansen, J. (2004). *The associations in our heads belong to us: Measuring the multifaceted attitude construct in implicit social cognition.* Unpublished manuscript.

Olson, M. A., & Fazio, R. H. (2003). Relations between implicit measures of prejudice: What are we measuring? *Psychological Science, 14,* 636–639.

Olson, M. A., & Fazio, R. H. (2004). Reducing the influence of extra-personal associations on the implicit association test: Personalizing the IAT. *Journal of Personality and Social Psychology, 86,* 653–667.

Orford, J. (2001). Addiction as excessive appetite. *Addiction, 96,* 15–31.

Ostafin, B. D., Palfai, T. P., & Wechsler, C. E. (2003). The accessibility of motivational tendencies toward alcohol: Approach, avoidance, and disinhibited drinking. *Experimental & Clinical Psychopharmacology, 11,* 294–301.

Palfai, T. P. (2002). Positive outcome expectancies and smoking behavior: The role of expectancy accessibility. *Cognitive Therapy and Research, 26,* 317–333.

Palfai, T. P., Monti, P. M., Colby, S. M., & Rohsenow, D. J. (1997). Effects of suppressing the urge to drink on the accessibility of alcohol outcome expectancies. *Behaviour Research and Therapy, 35,* 59–65.

Palfai, T. P., Monti, P. M., Ostafin, B., & Hutchison, K. (2000). Effects of nicotine deprivation on alcohol-related information processing and drinking behavior. *Journal of Abnormal Psychology, 109,* 96–105.

Palfai, T. P., & Ostafin, B. D. (2003a). Alcohol-related motivational tendencies in hazardous drinkers: Assessing implicit response tendencies using the modified-IAT. *Behaviour Research and Therapy, 41,* 1149–1162.

Palfai, T. P., & Ostafin, B. D. (2003b). The influence of alcohol on the activation of outcome expectancies: The role of evaluative expectancy activation in drinking behavior. *Journal of Studies on Alcohol, 64,* 111–119.

Ratcliff, R., & McKoon, G. (1988). A retrieval theory of priming in memory. *Psychological Review, 95,* 385–408.

Robinson, T. E., & Berridge, K. C. (1993). The neural basis of drug craving: An incentive-sensitization theory of addiction. *Brain Research Reviews, 18,* 247–291.

Robinson, T. E., & Berridge, K. C. (2003). Addiction. *Annual Review of Psychology, 54,* 25–53.

Rothermund, K., & Wentura, D. (2001). Figure-ground asymmetries in the Implicit Association Test (IAT). *Zeitschrift für Experimentelle Psychologie, 48,* 94–106.

Rothermund, K., & Wentura, D. (2004). Underlying processes in the Implicit Association Test: Dissociating salience from associations. *Journal of Experimental Psychology: General, 133,* 139–165.

Spruyt, A., Hermans, D., De Houwer, J., & Eelen, P. (2002). On the nature of the affective priming effect: Priming of naming responses. *Social Cognition, 20,* 227–256.

Stacy, A. W. (1997). Memory activation and expectancy as prospective predictors of alcohol and marijuana use. *Journal of Abnormal Psychology, 106,* 61–73.

Stewart, S. H., Hall, E., Wilkie, H., & Birch, C. (2002). Affective priming of alcohol schema in coping and enhancement motivated drinkers. *Cognitive Behaviour Therapy, 31,* 68–80.

Swanson, J. E., Rudman, L. A., & Greenwald, A. G. (2001). Using the implicit association test to investigate attitude-behaviour consistency for stigmatised behaviour. *Cognition & Emotion, 15,* 207–230.

Teachman, B. A., Gregg, A. P., & Woody, S. R. (2001). Implicit associations for fear-relevant stimuli among individuals with snake and spider fears. *Journal of Abnormal Psychology, 110,* 226–235.

Teachman, B. A., & Woody, S. R. (2003). Automatic processing in spider phobia: Implicit fear associations over the course of treatment. *Journal of Abnormal Psychology, 112,* 100–109.

Weingardt, K. R., Stacy, A. W., & Leigh, B. C. (1996). Automatic activation of alcohol concepts in response to positive outcomes of alcohol use. *Alcoholism: Clinical and Experimental Research, 20,* 25–30.

Wentura, D. (2000). Dissociative affective and associative priming effects in the lexical decision task: Yes versus no responses to word targets reveal evaluative judgment tendencies. *Journal of Experimental Psychology: Learning, Memory, and Cognition, 26,* 456–469.

Wiers, R., de Jong, P. J., Havermans, R., & Jelicic, M. (2004). How to change implicit drug-related cognitions in prevention: A transdisciplinary integration of findings from experimental psychopathology. *Substance Use & Misuse, 39,* 1625–1684.

Wiers, R. W., Ganushchack, A., Van de Ende, N., Smulders, F. T. Y., & de Jong, P. J. (2003, May/June). Comparing implicit alcohol associations across different RT-measures: The Implicit Association Test (IAT) versus varieties of the Extrinsic Affective Simon Task (EAST). Paper presented at the 15th annual convention of the American Psychological Association, Atlanta, GA.

Wiers, R. W., van de Luitgaarden, J., van den Wildenberg, E., & Smulders, F. T. Y. (2005). Challenging implicit and explicit alcohol-related cognitions in young heavy drinkers. *Addiction, 100,* 806–819.

Wiers, R. W., van Woerden, N., Smulders, F. T. Y., & de Jong, P. J. (2002). Implicit and explicit alcohol-related cognitions in heavy and light drinkers. *Journal of Abnormal Psychology, 111,* 648–658.

Wigboldus, D., van Knippenberg, A., Holland, R., den Hartog, G., & Belles, S. (2001). Het verschil tussen relatieve en absolute vergelijking bij het testen van impliciete associaties. In D. A. Stapel, M. Hagedoorn, & E. van Dijk (Eds.), *Jaarboek sociale psychologie deel 1* (pp. 337–345). Delft, The Netherlands: Eburon.

Wigboldus, D. H. J., Holland, R. W., & van Knippenberg, A. (2004). Single target implicit associations. Manuscript submitted for publication.

Wilson, T. D., Lindsey, S., & Schooler, T. Y. (2000). A model of dual attitudes. *Psychological Review, 107,* 101–126.

Zack, M., Poulos, C. X., Fragopoulos, F., & Macleod, C. M. (2003). Effects of negative and positive mood phrases on priming of alcohol words in young drinkers with high and low anxiety sensitivity. *Experimental & Clinical Psychopharmacology, 11,* 176–185.

Zack, M., Toneatto, T., & Macleod, C. M. (1999). Implicit activation of alcohol concepts by negative affective cues distinguishes between problem drinkers with high and low psychiatric distress. *Journal of Abnormal Psychology, 108,* 518–531.

CHAPTER 8

Expectancy as a Unifying Construct in Alcohol-Related Cognition

MARK S. GOLDMAN, RICHARD
R. REICH, AND JACK DARKES

Abstract: Explanations of goal-directed behavior increasingly have highlighted the role of anticipatory processes, especially anticipation of reward. Because many researchers in both neurobiological and psychological domains often use the term "expectancy" to refer to these processes, we review the expectancy construct as a device for unifying explanation at these different levels of analysis. Appreciation of this role is essential for advancing expectancy assessment. To this end, we show how expectancies can be assessed using implicit (indirect) tasks. These studies have indicated that the content and organization of implicitly measured expectancies differ as a function of an individual's exposure to alcohol information, customary drinking level, and context, and that expectancies can directly influence drinking.

H umans are not robots. Experts in the domain of alcohol use, abuse, and addiction agree that drinking is not inevitably impelled by biological processes, but involves decision making (see Schultz, 2004). That is, regardless of the

AUTHOR'S NOTE: We would like to acknowledge and express our deepest appreciation for the work of Bruce C. Rather, a fellow expectancy researcher and close friend whose unexpected and untimely death was keenly felt by all who knew him. We also thank a long list of colleagues, graduate students, and research assistants whose contribution has made this program of research possible.

Mark Goldman is also currently serving as the Associate Director of the National Institutes on Alcohol Abuse and Alcoholism (NIAAA).

Preparation of this chapter was supported by NIAAA Grants 2R01 AA008333 and R01 AA011925.

Correspondence concerning this chapter should be addressed to Mark S. Goldman, Department of Psychology, PCD 4118G, University of South Florida, 4202 E. Fowler Ave., Tampa, FL, 33620–8200. E-mail: goldman@cas.usf.edu factors that have been shown to influence drinking, at some point the drinker chooses to seek alcohol, and then to drink.

Understanding of this decision making has been complicated, however, by two other characteristics of alcohol-related decision making. First, often drinkers report a lack of intention to drink or to drink as much as was consumed. In extreme cases, such drinking is characterized as "out-of-control." Second, the outcomes of drinking sometimes are sufficiently negative that observers (and, once sober, the drinker themselves) cannot believe that rational decision making was involved.

The apparent inconsistency of making a choice absent of intent and reason has led the alcohol field to pose decision-making models that could accommodate all these elements. The earliest model from the psychodynamic era posited "unconscious" psychological processes. Translated into the alcohol-treatment field, this notion became "denial"; that is, the drinker ignored available evidence of the toll that her or his drinking was taking. In either form, it was accepted that decisions were made, but were driven by forces of which the drinker was unaware. When the behavioral view gained strength, the notion became one of conditioning or habit, removing the mentalistic portion of the explanation. Again, decisions were understood to be made, but were conditioned entirely on acquired experience. At present, following the "cognitive revolution," the reconfigured model involves the distinction between "explicit" processes, of which the person is aware, and "implicit" or automatic processes, which influence behavioral output in the absence of awareness. In each case, the intent was the same: to accommodate the need for a decision-making mechanism with the recognition that decision making, especially about alcohol use, did not seem always to be conscious and rational. This "hidden" process has begged for assessment by those wishing to achieve a thorough understanding of addiction.

Just as in other applications of a cognitive model to psychopathology research (Denny & Hunt, 1992; Mathews & MacLeod, 1994), alcohol and addictions researchers addressed the role of implicit cognitive processes by importing concepts and methods from general cognitive psychology (see Stacy, 1997). This approach has proven valid; a number of studies have now shown a relationship between implicit task performance and actual alcohol consumption patterns (see Kramer & Goldman, 2003; Palfai & Wood, 2001; Reich & Goldman, in press; Reich et al., 2004; Reich, Noll, & Goldman, 2005; Stacy, 1995, 1997; Stacy et al., 1994; Wall et al., 2001; Wall et al., 2000; Wiers et al., 2002; Zack et al., 1999). Central to these experimental investigations of implicit cognitive decision making about alcohol use is the capacity to probe, in the laboratory, specific memory contents without directing attention to them. It has long been a central tenet of experimental psychology that deliberate reporting might lead to biases (individuals might wish to minimize or maximize their drinking, present a rosy picture of their internal experience, etc.). To circumvent this concern, researchers have capitalized on the recognition that the presence of particular stimuli (called "primes") may automatically and without the awareness of the individual activate related concepts in memory (Nelson, McKinney, et al., 1998). Furthermore, because differences in the strength of relationships between memory concepts as they are stored in a given individual may reflect (in part) that person's previous experiences with those concepts (Nelson, McKinney, et al., 1998), priming stimuli may effectively probe individual differences. In alcohol research, primes have ranged from alcohol-related words (Carter et al., 1998; Reich & Goldman, in press; Reich, Noll, & Goldman, 2005; Roehrich & Goldman, 1995; Wiers et al., 2002), to behavioral outcomes (Palfai & Wood, 2001; Stacy, 1997), affective cues (Stein et al., 2000; Zack et al., 1999), and videotaped, simulated, and actual operational bars (Reich et al., 2004; Roehrich & Goldman, 1995; Wall et al., 2001; Wall et al., 2000). Outcomes (dependent measures) have also varied in these implicit memory studies, including variations of key press latency (Wall et al., 2001; Wiers et al., 2002; Zack et al., 1999), free-associate response frequency (Palfai & Wood, 2001; Reich & Goldman, in press; Stacy, 1995, 1997; Stacy et al., 1994), word recognition and recall (Reich et al., 2004; Reich, Noll, & Goldman, 2005), and alcohol consumption itself (Carter et al., 1998; Roehrich & Goldman, 1995; Stein et al., 2000).

These strategies for assessing implicit/indirect memory have opened a new window onto the causal pathway to alcohol use and risk for alcohol excess. The introduction of these strategies has also been accompanied, however, by a number of cautions and questions, some associated with the use of these methods in general, and some specific to the alcohol and addictions fields. For these reasons, we would suggest that such assessment should be understood as still "under development" in relation to clinical applications. To begin with, importing methods from general cognitive psychology to any applied field necessitates methodological adjustments. Cognitive psychologists most often wish to study general memory processes independent of the complications of preexisting individual differences. As a consequence, they "tune" their experimental methods to minimize the influence of these individual differences, which they view as error or "noise." One exception to this strategy involves the deliberate study of the effects variations in previous experience with particular stimuli have on later memory for those stimuli or related material. But even in such studies, cognitive researchers most often carefully control exposure to the antecedent stimulus material in the laboratory to reduce the influence of preexisting experience. In contrast, alcohol and addictions researchers (as in other applied fields) wish to highlight individual differences as the basis for differential use and abuse of alcohol. Hence, applications of cognitive methods need to be "retuned" in this new domain. Such retuning often requires a good deal of innovation before reliable results can be obtained.

The use of implicit memory tasks also introduces various conceptual issues that pertain to the meaning and import of implicit processes. In the present context, these issues can be highlighted with a question: Just what are we assessing with implicit methods? For example, is implicit memory an entirely separate domain of memory that holds unique information as some researchers believe (see Schacter & Tulving, 1994), or are implicit memory findings merely a function of method differences (as other researchers would aver; e.g., Fazio & Olson, 2003)? At a more general level, how does the material that is accessed by implicit techniques relate to the processes that guide overall behavior, how do implicit measures relate to explicit measures, how does a particular implicit measure relate to other implicit measures, and so on? Some of these questions will be addressed later.

EXPECTANCIES

We first turn, however, to the central question of this chapter: Why is a chapter on alcohol expectancies included in a book on implicit cognitive processing? In addressing this question, we will first offer a theoretical context for assessing expectancies, and then will show that expectancies can be measured implicitly (as well as explicitly). Our overarching purpose is to suggest that not only can expectancies be assessed implicitly, but also that an expectancy perspective has the capacity to serve as a nexus between cognition, emerging neuroscience, and the recent explosion of knowledge about the influence of genetic mechanisms in complex behavior. When considering this perspective, please keep in mind that it is not the word *expectancy* that is of critical importance, but instead the recognition that the cognitive/information-processing system is in its essence a system shaped by evolutionary pressures to anticipate the future. Further elaboration on this perspective can be found in Goldman (2002). We acknowledge at the outset that we have attempted a synthesis of many disparate areas of research, because we believe that a transdisciplinary model offers possibilities for advancements that can complement work in specific domains. We also acknowledge that because the expectancy concept has emerged in so many areas of research, and has reflected so many local concerns in these areas, that we emphasize common elements when attempting a transdisciplinary integration.

BASIC ASSOCIATIONISM

Implicit cognitive processing has most often been addressed within the context of associationism. That is, it is assumed that two stimuli, or a stimulus and a cognitive template for a motor response, become linked in some fashion as they are stored in memory, so that the presentation of one will have an increased likelihood of calling forth the other (or the response). Although in the modern history of psychology many specific theories have been proposed of how the two stimulus representations are "glued" together in memory, all essentially specify a process for systematically searching memory storage. If all stimuli that an organism encountered were stored haphazardly, memory would not be functional. The "filing system" of humans goes beyond simple search, however. Because in the neural system the same item might be accessed via a number of associational routes, many association theories are characterized as networks, with nodes and links (e.g., Collins & Loftus, 1975).

MERGING MOTIVATION AND COGNITION

Associationist theories can provide an effective framework for understanding how a memory system might be organized and searched for information. Effectively searching the vast array of information in the brain for situationally appropriate information is not a trivial task. A full explanation of how the behavior of an organism is directed requires, however, additional theoretical elements that encourage pure information to be translated into overt behavior. These additional elements typically are addressed as motivation, reward, incentive, reinforcement, and punishment. Hence, informational items that are accessed by associational search at some point themselves must be associated to information about reward and punishment (Schultz, 2004). It is this final, critical information that specifies what searches will be undertaken, and what actions (behaviors) will be carried out to consummate the reward (or the avoidance of aversive stimuli).

In higher organisms, one may distinguish (at least) two kinds of motivational pathways. In the first, basic needs are regulated by a physiological signal that indicates that the internal system has moved, or will soon move, outside an acceptable biological range (e.g., hunger, thirst, feeling too "hot" or too "cold," etc.). This signal then initiates an associational search for information about the behavioral steps that need to be taken to bring the system back into balance (some adjustments of course occur purely at the physiological level—i.e., homeostasis—without recourse to behavioral outputs). The second kind of pathway accommodates those rewards that go beyond the adjustment of basic biological parameters. In this second pathway, contextual stimuli signal (via a number of neural pathways) that a rewarding condition may be achieved. Information that in some way represents the behavioral steps that may lead to the reward is then accessed via an associational pathway. Because many rewarding circumstances are not of the variety that would call for activation of the first kind of pathway (they signal an advantage rather than a current biological necessity), organisms have neural systems that appear designed to signal the availability of reward; that is, they anticipate that reward is imminent (Berridge & Robinson, 1998). It must also be noted that these pathways are not independent; the second system may provide payoffs for behaving in a manner that anticipates (and wards off) strong activation of the first pathway. It is beyond the present scope to thoroughly examine motivational systems, but it is essential to note that motivation must be linked to cognition. Consider Holland and Gallagher (2004, p. 148): "Recently, conventional associative learning paradigms have been adapted to allow systematic study of expectancy and action in a range of species, including humans. . . . 'Expectancy' refers to the associative activation of such reinforcer representations by the events that predict them, before the delivery of the reinforcer itself."

In sum, to produce behavior, associational pathways must lead to the anticipation of reinforcement. These extended pathways can be characterized as (one kind of) expectancies. That is, expectancies may be understood to be complex associational pathways that link contextual signals of the availability of reinforcers to the internal representations of behaviors (i.e., scripts, templates) that have some probability of achieving these outcomes. The essence of the expectancy model is that context leads to the *anticipation* of reward, and to the emission of reward-related behaviors. In this way, expectancy serves as the theoretical amalgam

of cognition (association) and motivation/emotion.

It must be emphasized that anticipating reward (and aversive consequences) is critical to survival (see Goldman, 2002, pp. 738–739). An inexorable feature of existence is that time moves forward; no situation or context is static. Changes occur from moment to moment; biological and behavioral adjustments always made reactively and after the fact would place the organism at a competitive disadvantage. Hence, organisms use information about the past to make predictions (place "bets") about the future. In everyday language, the word we have come to use to denote this information about past experience is memory. But memory, although most often viewed as a device for looking backward in time, is more likely to have evolved as a capacity to anticipate the future. Widely diverse scientific authors have recognized this fundamental characteristic of the nervous system: For example, Dennett (1991, p. 177) referred to brains as "in essence, just anticipatory machines." And more recently, Holland and Gallagher noted (2004, p. 148), "The utility of learning and memory lies not in reminiscence about the past, but in allowing us to act in anticipation of future events."

How are these information patterns stored? Each of our senses registers information in a manner that is consistent with the actual physical input of an external stimulus. For example, the visual system registers patterns of light using sensors that are sensitive to these patterns (Frishman, 2001), the auditory system registers where on a vibrating membrane sound waves produce the most displacement (Moore, 2001), and so on. As a consequence, the storage of this information can come in the form of actual physical enhancement of the pathways that move sensory input through the nervous system. The processes that enhance the nervous tissue that registers external stimulus patterns tie expectancy directly to the biological substrate that supports learning and memory. It is beyond the scope of the present chapter to fully discuss these processes, but they include gene expression that creates proteins that serve as the structure for elaborated synaptic connections on neurons.

The paragraph above describes the means by which the nervous system converts information about the external world into relevant actions. It does not speak, however, to which inputs are deemed meaningful and therefore are stored in the form of nervous system templates or maps, nor does it speak to the choice of behavior sequences for motor activity. What does speak to these questions is the increasing literature on nervous system mechanisms for signaling biological significance. These mechanisms are the basis of motivation, and also are tied directly to cognition/information processing and the expectancy concept.

At the current time, neuroscientists identify a few key brain pathways for registering biological significance. In one of these pathways, dopaminergic pathways running from the striatum to the nucleus accumbens and on to the frontal lobes are thought to convert "an event or stimulus from a neutral 'cold' representation (mere information) into an attractive and 'wanted' incentive that can 'grab' attention" (i.e., incentive salience; Berridge & Robinson, 1998, p. 313). Referring to these same pathways, Kupfermann et al. (2000, p. 1010) note, "dopaminergic neurons encode expectations about external rewards." Recent work by Matsumoto and Tanaka (2004, p. 178) goes on to indicate that the prefrontal cortex (anterior cingulate cortex) links these signals of biologically important inputs with actions "based on goal expectation and memory of action—outcome contingency."

A second means of registering biological significance centers on the amygdaloid complex, which has been identified as important for the expression of emotion (Holland &

Gallagher, 2004; Iversen et al., 2000). Obviously, a neural system supporting the experience of pleasure and displeasure would be instrumental in encouraging certain behaviors and discouraging others. Once again, however, the close linkage between this source of emotional expression and systems that subserve information processing makes certain sensed patterns of information more salient, and therefore more likely to be stored and acted upon (Holland & Gallagher, 2004; Phelps, 2004). This linkage is further demonstrated by research showing connections between motivational areas such as the nucleus accumbens and amygdala, and information-processing areas such as the hippocampus and frontal cortex (Cardinal & Everitt, 2004; Phelps, 2004). Corticosteroids released by the HPA axis in response to threatening circumstances also influence hippocampal memory storage (Heinrichs & Koob, 2004). This linkage between neurally processed information and motivation/emotion is well captured by the expectancy concept, and researchers in this domain routinely do just that (Holland & Gallagher, 2004; Phelps, 2004).

EXPECTANCIES AND ALCOHOL USE, ABUSE, AND DEPENDENCE

By integrating the cognitive/information-processing system with neurally based memory storage and emotional/motivational influences, the expectancy concept becomes applicable to alcohol use, abuse, and dependence (as well as drug abuse, and other excessive behaviors such as gambling). The mechanisms by which alcohol use is reinforced, and may in some individuals become problematic, are not separate from the normal biopsychosocial processes that control all behavior. In the case of problematic alcohol use, these mechanisms are sometimes characterized as "hijacked" by alcohol use.

The expectancy processes described earlier place everyday stimuli that co-occur with the availability of alcohol into memory as expectancy templates. Alcohol itself works on the system for tagging stimuli as biologically significant (incentive salience), and on emotional/motivational systems, to make these memories more indelible and salient, and thereby more influential within the overall decision-making process that leads to (or avoids) alcohol use.

If all humans share this substrate for storing memories and using these memories to anticipate and prepare for future events, why are not all of us at risk for excessive alcohol use? One answer is that we all are at some level of risk given the right circumstances; environments can either encourage or discourage particular levels and patterns of use. The most important predictor of drinking-related problems is availability of alcohol (Gruenewald et al., 1993). After holding availability constant, differential use is largely a function of individual differences. Pointing out that individual differences in usage patterns are a function of other individual differences does not advance the cause of explaining alcohol risk, however. It is critical to appreciate that the basis for the individual difference characteristics that we routinely invoke, such as emotional reactivity, personality, and sensitivity to alcohol, are the very mechanisms discussed above as the basis for creating memories and making them more or less salient. For example, Katner et al. (1996) compared genetically bred alcohol-preferring (P) rats with Wistar rats, concluding that, "the mere expectation of ethanol availability enhances the efflux of DA (dopamine) in the Nac (nucleus accumbens) of the P, but not the Wistar rat, which may play a role in the initiation or maintenance of ethanol seeking behavior in the P line" (p. 669). McCarthy et al. (2000) evaluated the expectancies of humans who differed genetically in the alcohol dehydrogenase (ALDH2) allele and

reported that the mechanism by which the allelic variation may influence use is by lowering positive expectancies and reducing the expectancy-drinking relationship. In sum, it is the ongoing interplay between basic mechanisms of incentive salience, emotional reactivity, and alcohol reactivity, and those influences that come from the environment that create expectancies and determine subsequent usage patterns.

EXPECTANCIES AS IMPLICIT MEMORY

Tolman (1932) first used *expectancy* as an attempt to explain *animal* behavior. Since his time, expectancy has been applied to many behavioral arenas, often to address nondeliberative information processing. For example, expectancy has been used to explain animal reward and reinforcement (Kupfermann et al., 2000; Schultz, 2004; Schultz et al., 1997), classical and operant conditioning (Dragoi & Staddon, 1999; Kirsch et al., 2004), comparative judgment (Ritov, 2000), medicinal effects of drugs (Kirsch & Scoboria, 2001), brain electrophysiology (ERP; Donchin & Coles, 1988), and music appreciation (Krumhansl & Toivaine, 2000). Hence, expectancy has always included implicit, as well as explicit, information processing within its scope of usage.

More recently, however, implicit/indirect cognitive methods have enlarged our access to the causal pathways to alcohol use and risk for alcohol excess. We will not review the extensive literature that supports alcohol expectancies as assessed by questionnaires as reliable correlates and even mediators of alcohol use (see Goldman et al., 1999), but this body of literature provides a useful background against which assessment by implicit measures can be evaluated. Although questionnaires are usually regarded to be explicit measures, close consideration of how individuals respond to such measures foreshadows one of the critical questions regarding the distinction between explicit and implicit measures. People may respond to agree/disagree or Likert-type response formats with conscious deliberation, but it is not possible to say with any certainty what determines such response patterns (e.g., Weinberger et al., in press). They may deliberately recollect a specific experience (from "autobiographical memory") in responding, or they may simply "go with their subjective feeling or impression" to guide their choice. The fact that the latter strategy is somewhat difficult to distinguish from implicit processing underscores the inherent difficulty in parsing one type of processing from the other (see Roediger, 2003). A related point is that, although it is obvious that implicit processes need not be verbal in nature, much of the research in this domain uses verbal stimuli. Therefore, some of the empirical findings may not reflect the implicit/explicit distinction per se, but instead reflect the nature of the human language system. And even here, the distinction is fuzzy, because the general cognitive literature supports both perceptually based and conceptually based implicit processing for text read from a page or computer screen (Blaxton, 1989). Hence, the strict separation of memory into two discrete repositories, implicit and explicit, is likely an oversimplification (Roediger et al., 1999); the nervous system seems to support many separate memory processes. Leaving these issues aside, it is the ability to assess implicit expectancies offered by human language that is the basis for the new window on expectancy operation.

ALCOHOL EXPECTANCIES AND MEMORY

We began investigating memory processes in alcohol-expectancy operation (and concomitantly, implicit assessment of expectancies) by mapping expectancy associational space in accord with Estes's (1991, p. 12) suggestion that memory "traces can be viewed as vectors or lists, as nodes in a network, or as points in multidimensional space." To this end, we collected individual associations to the prompt, "Alcohol makes one . . ." and used multidimensional scaling (MDS) to place scaled responses to these items into a hypothetical memory network. In adults (Rather & Goldman, 1994; Rather et al., 1992) and children (both prior to, and subsequent to drinking experience; Dunn & Goldman, 1996, 1998), the resulting network was well described using two orthogonal dimensions, valence (positive-negative) and arousal (sedation-excitation). Hence, each associate could be located in space in terms of its coordinates on these two dimensions. Although the data collection methods used were primarily explicit, the participants were certainly unaware of the networks generated based on the relationships among all expectancy items. For this reason, the MDS plots of these networks served as models of implicit memory storage. In these models, words in proximity were viewed as more likely to activate together than words more distant. Ancillary analyses showed that heavier drinkers were more likely to associate positive and arousing outcomes with drinking, and seemed to have tighter relationships among these outcomes than did lighter drinkers. The increased likelihood of coactivation of a variety of positive and arousing outcomes would make heavier drinkers more likely to drink. Of particular interest, children in their preadolescent years showed a greater likelihood of activating negative expectancies, but gradually shifted into an increased likelihood of activating positive/arousing expectancies as they aged into adolescence, whether drinking had been initiated or not. That is, changes in the expectancy network seemed to anticipate, and ready them, for later drinking.

We recently confirmed these "maps" of the expectancy-association network using a direct method rather than the indirect approach represented by MDS. The method used was perhaps the most direct means of accessing implicit associations, free association (Nelson et al., 2000). The central advantage of this approach is that the strength of association between memory concepts can be quantified as the probability that given one word or concept (e.g., *salt)* another will be produced (e.g., *pepper).* These probabilities can be used to establish models of memory operation (e.g., Nelson et al., 2003).

We first obtained free associations from 1,465 children in the 2nd to 12th grades, and then from 4,585 college students. Children's free associations essentially replicated the previous work using the MDS approach, validating the earlier MDS maps (Dunn & Goldman, 2000). Obtaining free associates from a large number of students allowed us to accomplish a task that not only was informative in explaining the incentive matrix for drinking, but also was informative for future research in general cognitive psychology. Previous free-association research (Nelson et al., 2000) had been conducted in a manner that could establish general population norms. To this end, groups of 100 to 200 participants responded with their first associate to a limited list of prompts. By iterating this procedure many times to many prompts, norms were derived that would characterize the average response for all English language speakers (Nelson, McEvoy, et al., 1998). By using our large sample of responses to a single prompt, however, we were able to establish norms for subgroups of drinkers (i.e., individual differences in alcohol cognitions; Reich & Goldman, in press). As drinking level increased, our norms showed a steady shift from negative and sedating expectancies, toward arousing and positive expectancies. This finding provided direct confirmation that lighter and heavier drinkers activated different concepts in response to the prompt, and showed that humans differ in their associational network as a function of individual differences.

Portraying the structure of alcohol expectancy networks was the initial step in studying a multistep process in which context initiates cognitions that lead to motivated behavior. Next, we examined whether the process of activation within the memory networks observed using MDS and confirmed by free association could be demonstrated via the experimental manipulation of alcohol cues; that is, whether the expectancy network in fact activated as predicted in response to stimuli that might signal a drinking opportunity. To this end, tasks developed by cognitive psychologists to test memory activation following implicit primes were used. First, we conducted a study using the Stroop technique (Kramer & Goldman, 2003) in which, following an alcohol (e.g., *vodka)* or alcohol-neutral (e.g., *milk)* prime, expectancy target words were ink-named. Activation was indexed as the relative difference in latency to ink-name alcohol and neutral primed trials (as a consequence of interference; the greater the activation, the slower the ink-naming). The target alcohol-expectancy words were selected based on alcohol-expectancy memory network dimensions determined in the studies noted above (arousal and valence). In this experiment, expectancy activation differed as a function of prime (alcohol/nonalcohol), level of customary consumption, and location of the expectancies in a network defined by the valence/arousal dimensions. Following an alcohol cue, the heaviest drinkers had slower latencies to ink-name arousing expectancy words (greater activation) when compared with other target words, whereas lighter drinkers had greater activation (interference) to sedating expectancy words. Hence, context differentially activated particular expectancies as a function of individuals' experience with alcohol.

We also have used the false memory paradigm (Deese, 1959; Roediger & McDermott, 1995) to examine expectancy activation in the MDS-derived network. Participants studied several 12-word lists (e.g., *hot, chilly, frigid, wet*) that were each associated to one nonstudied word (e.g., *cold*). In previous studies of such words, about 80 percent of participants remembered studying the nonpresented word. We developed a study list of alcohol-expectancy words and intentionally excluded three high-frequency positive and arousing expectancy words (based on the observed network structure: *confident, happy,* and *silly*) that, according to our network maps, naturally should have been part of that list. Participants studied this list in either a simulated bar or an alcohol-neutral room. In this way, we evaluated how a rich alcohol context (a simulated bar) might activate those alcohol-expectancy elements of the identified network that intentionally were not presented. Further, participants were split into heavier, lighter, and nondrinkers to explore how context affected individuals with different patterns of typical consumption. After controlling for the tendency to falsely remember any type of word, it was found that heavier drinkers' false memory for the three nonpresented positive/arousing words was significantly higher in the bar context than in the neutral room, whereas false memory rates were the same in both contexts for the other two drinker groups. In other words, for heavier drinkers only, the alcohol context created sufficiently strong memory activation to make participants "remember" positive and arousing expectancies that were never presented. In addition to confirming the relationships of expectancies in the network to each other, these results showed the responsiveness of expectancy activation to context.

After representing the structure of the alcohol expectancy-memory network and showing that elements within that structure could be activated in a manner predicted by the associational structure via manipulation of context, the next step necessary to support the logic of expectancy operation was to show that cognitions activated by alcohol cues would translate into actual drinking. To this end, we used priming techniques and a disguised beer "taste test" in two studies to demonstrate increased alcohol consumption following the presentation of alcohol-consistent cues. In the first study (Roehrich & Goldman, 1995), participants who believed they were in a "memory" study viewed one of two video clips from network television comedies. The clips were similar in content, with the central difference being the contextual location of the show. One show took place in a bar (*Cheers;* alcohol prime), the other in an inn at a breakfast table (*Newhart;* alcohol-neutral prime). The participants also were primed with either alcohol-expectancy words or alcohol-neutral words. Following the manipulation, participants exposed to alcohol primes consumed more alcohol during what they believed was an entirely separate "taste test" study. In fact, a dose- response relationship was observed in which increased alcohol priming led to more alcohol consumed. The group exposed to both alcohol-consistent primes drank most, the group that had both alcohol-neutral primes drank least, and the other two groups with one alcohol-consistent prime and one alcohol-neutral prime fell in between. These results supported the inference of a causal relationship between expectancy activation and alcohol consumption.

Because the above study did not include measures of whether the primes had actually activated the memory networks theorized to drive drinking, a further study (Stein et al., 2000) used a similar design in which alcohol-consistent primes were presented to participants. For this study, however, participants completed a recognition task to determine whether the alcohol expectancy primes had been activated. Although all cues elicited measurable drinking, a dose-response relationship was found, in which the level of consumption increased as the level of alcohol cues presented increased. Additionally, greater priming (activation) effects occurred for heavier drinkers. Other studies using similar methodology also have shown increases in consumption following exposure to alcohol-expectancy-like cues (Carter et al., 1998; Palfai, 2001).

SUMMARY AND CONCLUSION

In summary, methods adopted from cognitive psychology have been used (1) to explore the associative nature of, and to "map," the alcohol expectancy memory network, (2) to demonstrate that alcohol cues produce activation of this network in accord with the empirically determined models of that network, and (3) to show that exposure to such cues and the resultant cognitive activation also result in increased consumption. Aspects of these results have been replicated in laboratories beyond our own. At the level of cognition and behavior, therefore, the expectancy concept of implicit decision making about alcohol use has a reasonable empirical base.

What is perhaps more important, however, is that the expectancy concept is solidly tied to the multilevel (transdisciplinary) explanation of human cognition and motivation described earlier in this chapter. This explanation emphasizes that our entire neurobehavioral organization is directed toward anticipation of upcoming events, and preparation for maximization of payoffs (and minimization of punishment) from those events. Although it remains quite possible to carry out very useful science at a single level of explanation, advances in molecular biology, genetics, neuroscience, and behavior have allowed for increasingly integrated explanatory models. At the very least, models at any single level of explanation should be sufficiently informed by developments at the other levels so as to minimize inconsistencies. Along with a number of other researchers, we have used the expectancy concept as one such approach, and it is our belief that opportunities for further advances will come from this kind of transdisciplinary thinking.

REFERENCES

Berridge, K. C., & Robinson, T. E. (1998). What is the role of dopamine in reward: Hedonic impact, reward learning, or incentive salience? *Brain Research and Brain Research Reviews, 28,* 309–369.

Blaxton, T. A. (1989). Investigating dissociations among memory measures: Support for a transfer appropriate processing framework. *Journal of Experimental Psychology: Learning Memory, and Cognition, 15,* 657–668.

Cardinal, R. N., & Everitt, B. J. (2004). Neural and psychological mechanisms underlying appetitive learning: Links to drug addiction. *Current Opinion in Neurobiology, 14,* 156–162.

Carter, J. A., McNair, L. D., Corbin, W. R., & Black, D. H. (1998). Effects of priming positive and negative outcomes on drinking responses. *Experimental & Clinical Psychopharmacology, 6*(4), 399–405.

Collins, A. M., & Loftus, E. F. (1975). A spreading activation theory of semantic processing. *Psychological Review, 57,* 1–14.

Cooper, M. L., Frone, M. R., Russell, M., & Mudar, P. (1995). Drinking to regulate positive and negative emotions: A motivational model of alcohol use. *Journal of Personality and Social Psychology, 69*(5), 990–1005.

Deese, J. (1959). On the prediction of occurrence of particular verbal intrusions in immediate recall. *Journal of Experimental Psychology, 58,* 17–22.

Dennett, D. C. (1991). *Consciousness explained.* New York: Little, Brown.

Denny, E. B., & Hunt, R. R. (1992). Affective valence and memory in depression: Dissociation of recall and fragment completion. *Journal of Abnormal Psychology, 101*(3), 575–580.

Donchin, E. & Coles, M. G. (1988). Is the P300 component a manifestation of context updating? *Behavioral and Brain Sciences, 11*(3), 357–427.

Dragoi, V., & Staddon, J. E. R. (1999). The dynamics of operant conditioning. *Psychological Review, 106*(1), 20–61.

Dunn, M. E., & Goldman, M. S. (1996). Empirical modeling of an alcohol expectancy network in elementary school children as a function of grade. *Experimental & Clinical Psychopharmacology, 4*(2), 209–217.

Dunn, M. E., & Goldman, M. S. (1998). Age and drinking-related differences in the memory organization of alcohol expectancies in 3rd-, 6th-, 9th-, and 12th-grade children. *Journal of Consulting and Clinical Psychology, 66*(3), 579–585.

Dunn, M. E., & Goldman, M. S. (2000). Validation of multidimensional scaling-based modeling of alcohol expectancies in memory: Age and drinking-related differences in expectancies of children assessed as first associates. *Alcoholism: Clinical and Experimental Research, 24*(11), 1639–1646.

Estes, W. K. (1991). Cognitive architectures from the standpoint of an experimental psychologist. *Annual Review of Psychology, 42,* 1–28.

Fazio, R. H., & Olson, M. A. (2003). Implicit measures in social cognition research: Their meaning and use. *Annual Review of Psychology, 54,* 297–327.

Frishman, L. J. (2001). Basic visual processes. In E. B. Goldstein (Ed.), *Blackwell handbook of perception.* Malden, MA: Blackwell.

Goldman, M. S. (2002). Expectancy and risk for alcoholism: The unfortunate exploitation of a fundamental characteristic of neurobehavioral adaptation. *Alcoholism: Clinical and Experimental Research, 26*(5), 737–746.

Goldman, M. S., Darkes, J., & Del Boca, F. K. (1999). Expectancy mediation of biopsychosocial risk for alcohol use and alcoholism. In I. Kirsch (Ed.), *How expectancies shape experience.* Washington, DC: American Psychological Association.

Gruenewald, P., Millar, A., & Treno, A. (1993). Alcohol availability and the ecology of drinking behavior. *Alcohol Health & Research World, 17*(1), 39–45.

Heinrichs, S. C., & Koob, G. F. (2004). Corticotropin-releasing factor in brain: A role of activation, arousal and affect regulation. *Journal of Pharmacology and Experimental Therapeutics, 311*(2), 427–440.

Holland, P. C., & Gallagher, M. (2004). Amygdala-frontal interactions and reward expectancy. *Current Opinion in Neurobiology, 14,* 148–155.

Iversen, S., Kupfermann, I., & Kandel, E. R. (2000). Emotional states and feelings. In E. R. Kandel, J. H. Schwartz, & T. M. Jessell (Eds.), *Principles of neural science.* New York: McGraw-Hill.

Katner, S. N., Kerr, T. M., & Weiss, F. (1996). Ethanol anticipation enhances dopamine efflux in the nucleus accumbens of alcohol-preferring (P) but not Wistar rats. *Behavioral Pharmacology, 8,* 669–674.

Kirsch, I., Lynn, S. J., Vigorito, M., & Miller, R. M. (2004). The role of cognition in classical and operant conditioning. *Journal of Clinical Psychology, 60*(4), 369–392.

Kirsch, I., & Scoboria, A. (2001). Apples, oranges, and placebos: Heterogeneity in a meta-analysis of placebo effects. *Advances in Mind-Body Medicine, 17*(4), 307–309.

Kramer, D. A., & Goldman, M. S. (2003). Using a modified Stroop task to implicitly discern the cognitive organization of alcohol expectancies. *Journal of Abnormal Psychology, 112*(1), 171–175.

Krumhansl, C. L., & Toivane, P. (2000). Melodic expectations: A link between perception and emotion. *Psychological Science Agenda, 13*, 8.

Kupfermann, I., Kandel, E. R., & Iversen, S. (2000). Motivational and addictive states. In E. R. Kandel, J. H. Schwartz, & T. M. Jessell (Eds.), *Principles of neural science*. New York: McGraw-Hill.

Mathews, A., & MacLeod, C. (1994). Cognitive approaches to emotion and emotional disorders. *Annual Review of Psychology, 45*, 25–50.

Matsumoto, K., & Tanaka, K. (2004). The role of the medial prefrontal cortex in achieving goals. *Current Opinion in Neurobiology, 14*, 178–185.

McCarthy, D. M., Wall, T. L., Brown, S. A., & Carr, L. G. (2000). Integrating biological and behavioral factors in alcohol use risk: The role of ALDH2 status and alcohol expectancies in a sample of Asian Americans. *Experimental & Clinical Psychopharmacology, 8*, 168–175.

Moore, B. C. J. (2001). Basic auditory processes. In E. B. Goldstein (Ed.), *Blackwell handbook of perception*. Malden, MA: Blackwell.

Nelson, D. L., McEvoy, C. L., & Dennis, S. (2000). What is free association and what does it measure? *Memory & Cognition, 28*(6), 887–899.

Nelson, D. L., McEvoy, C. L., & Pointer, L. (2003). Spreading activation or spooky action at a distance. *Journal of Experimental Psychology: Learning, Memory, and Cognition, 29*(1), 42–51.

Nelson, D. L., McEvoy, C. L., & Schreiber, T. A. (1998). The University of South Florida word association, rhyme, and word fragment norms. Retrieved January 5, 2005, from *http://www.usf.edu/Free Association*

Nelson, D. L., McKinney, V. M., Gee, N. R., & Janczura, G. A. (1998). Interpreting the influence of implicitly activated memories on recall and recognition. *Psychological Review, 105*(2), 299–324.

Palfai, T. P. (2001). Individual differences in temptation and responses to alcohol cues. *Journal of Studies on Alcohol, 62*(5), 657–666.

Palfai, T. P., & Wood, M. D. (2001). Positive alcohol expectancies and drinking behavior: The influence of expectancy strength and memory accessibility. *Psychology of Addictive Behaviors, 15*(1), 60–67.

Phelps, E. A. (2004). Human emotion and memory: Interactions of the amygdala and hippocampal complex. *Current Opinion in Neurobiology, 14*, 198–202.

Rather, B. C., & Goldman, M. S. (1994). Drinking-related differences in the memory organization of alcohol expectancies. *Experimental & Clinical Psychopharmacology, 2*(2), 167–183.

Rather, B. C., Goldman, M. S., Roehrich, L., & Brannick, M. (1992). Empirical modeling of an alcohol expectancy memory network using multidimensional scaling. *Journal of Abnormal Psychology, 101*(1), 174–183.

Reich, R. R., & Goldman, M. S. (in press). Exploring the alcohol expectancy memory network: The utility of free associates. *Psychology of Addictive Behaviors*.

Reich, R. R., Goldman, M. S., & Noll, J. A. (2004). Using the false memory paradigm to test two key elements of alcohol expectancy theory. *Experimental & Clinical Psychopharmacology, 12*(2), 102–110.

Reich, R. R., Noll, J. A., & Goldman, M. S. (2005). Cue patterns and alcohol expectancies: How slight differences in stimuli can measurably change cognition. *Experimental & Clinical Psychopharmacology, 13*(1), 65–71.

Ritov, I. (2000). The role of expectations in comparisons. *Psychological Review, 107,* 345–357.

Roediger, H. L. (2003). Reconsidering implicit memory. In J. S. Bowers & C. J. Marsolek (Eds.), *Rethinking implicit memory* (pp. 3–18). New York: Oxford University Press.

Roediger, H. L., Buckner, R. L., & McDermott, K. B. (1999). Components of processing. In J. K. Foster & M. Jelicic (Eds.), *Memory: systems, process, or function.* New York: Oxford University Press.

Roediger, H. L., & McDermott, K. B. (1995). Creating false memories—remembering words not presented in lists. *Journal of Experimental Psychology: Learning, Memory, and Cognition, 21*(4), 803–814.

Roehrich, L., & Goldman, M. S. (1995). Implicit priming of alcohol expectancy memory processes and subsequent drinking behavior. *Experimental & Clinical Psychopharmacology, 3*(4), 402–410.

Schacter, D. L., & Tulving, E. (1994). What are the memory systems of 1994? In D. L. Schacter & E. Tulving (Eds.), *Memory systems 1994* (pp. 1–38). Cambridge, MA: MIT Press.

Schultz, W. (2004). Neural coding of basic reward terms of animal learning theory, game theory, microeconomics and behavioural ecology. *Current Opinion in Neurobiology, 14,* 139–147.

Schultz, W., Dayan, P., & Montague, P. R. (1997). A neural substrate of prediction and reward. *Science, 275,* 1593–1599.

Stacy, A. W. (1995). Memory association and ambiguous cues in models of alcohol and marijuana use. *Experimental & Clinical Psychopharmacology, 3*(2), 183–194.

Stacy, A. W. (1997). Memory activation and expectancy as prospective predictors of alcohol and marijuana use. *Journal of Abnormal Psychology, 106*(1), 61–73.

Stacy, A. W., Leigh, B. C., & Weingardt, K. R. (1994). Memory accessibility and association of alcohol use and its positive outcomes. *Experimental & Clinical Psychopharmacology, 2*(3), 269–282.

Stein, K. D., Goldman, M. S., & Del Boca, F. K. (2000). The influence of alcohol expectancy priming and mood manipulation on subsequent alcohol consumption. *Journal of Abnormal Psychology, 109*(1), 106–115.

Tolman, E. C. (1932). *Purposive behavior in animals and man.* New York: Appleton-Century-Crofts.

Wall, A. M., Hinson, R. E., McKee, S.A., & Goldstein, A. (2001). Examining alcohol outcome expectancies in laboratory and naturalistic bar settings: A within-subject experimental analysis. *Psychology of Addictive Behaviors, 15*(3), 219–226.

Wall, A. M., McKee, S. A., & Hinson, R. E., (2000). Assessing variation in alcohol outcome expectancies across environmental context: An examination of the situational-specificity hypothesis. *Psychology of Addictive Behaviors, 14*(4), 367–375.

Weinberger, A. H., Darkes, J., Del Boca, F. K., Greenbaum, P. E., & Goldman, M. S. (in press). Items as context: The effect of item order on factor structure and predictive validity. *Basic and Applied Social Psychology*.

Wiers, R. W., van Woerden, N., Smulders, F. T. Y., & de Jong, P. J. (2002). Implicit and explicit alcohol-related cognitions in heavy and light drinkers. *Journal of Abnormal Psychology, 111*(4), 648–658.

Zack, M., Toneatto, T., & MacLeod, C. M. (1999). Implicit activation of alcohol concepts by negative affective cues distinguishes between problem drinkers with high and low psychiatric distress. *Journal of Abnormal Psychology, 108,* 518–531.

CHAPTER 9

Individualized Versus General Measures of Addiction-Related Implicit Cognitions

Javad S. Fadardi, W. Miles Cox, and Eric Klinger

Abstract: The chapter considers the use of individualized versus generalized stimuli to assess implicit cognitive processes in addictive behaviors. Most studies have used generalized stimuli that were not specifically selected for each participant. A major advantage of doing so is that compiling the stimuli is straightforward. A uniform set of addiction-related stimuli, however, might not apply to all participants, who vary in their addiction-related habits and preferences. A limited number of studies have used individualized stimuli, which were selected to represent each participant's current concerns. The individualized approach offers promise for better understanding people's individual motives for using addictive substances. It also has therapeutic implications for helping problematic users to control their use.

Work stimulated by the motivational theory of current concerns (e.g., Cox & Klinger, 2004; Klinger & Cox, 2004) provides a lens through which to examine the relative merits of individualized versus general methods for assessing addiction-related implicit cognition. The theory addresses needs, goals, and the associated cognitive processes involved in goal pursuits. In this view, people's lives are organized around their perceptions of the various incentives available to them. When a person makes a commitment to acquiring a positive incentive or getting rid of a negative incentive, a goal is formed. Each goal represents a psychological *need* in a person's motivational system. To be fulfilled, various needs compete with each another to enter an individual's consciousness. Whether or not a given need can win out in the competition depends on various factors. One factor is the *urgency* of satisfying a need—attaining a positive incentive or avoiding a negative incentive. Another factor is the degree to which an incentive is *valued*. Needs with higher emotional values have higher priority for entering consciousness than those with lower values (Baars, 1988; Dehaene & Changeux, 2000; Dehaene et al., 1998; Klinger, 1977).

The emotions associated with incentives can affect an individual's inner world and direct his or her motivational system toward goal attainments (e.g., the goal of drinking alcohol). Because of the resulting cognitive orientation, the person will become preoccupied with goal-related stimuli. In their preoccupation, individuals continually pay attention to, or can easily be distracted by, stimuli related to their goal-attainment priorities.

In studying people's reactions to goal-related stimuli, investigators have the option of choosing the stimuli individually for each participant or using generalized stimuli that are the same for all people who are pursing the same goal. The following sections first discuss the importance of implicit cognitions, with an emphasis on attention and attentional bias in alcohol abuse, and, drawing on both our experiences and those of researchers working within other paradigms, proceed with advantages and disadvantages of using individualized versus generalized stimuli in measuring alcohol-related implicit cognitions.

THE ROLE OF IMPLICIT COGNITION

The role of attention as the *shuttle* between an individual's cognitions and emotions is well-known (Wilson & Gottman, 1996). Any selective activity, including prioritizing competing incentives in an explicit or implicit way, is channeled through the gate of attention. Attention is an essential process for interacting successfully with the environment. Humans' immediate environment is saturated with a large number of stimuli, among which only a limited number can be consciously dealt with at a given time. The main functions of attention are to smooth the progress of a fast and accurate flow of perceptual judgments and actions and to maintain processing resources on *selected* stimulus inputs (MacLeod & MacDonald, 2000). In other words, the attentional system underlies the detection,

selection, and monitoring of stimuli that are vital to the individual's needs, incentives, and goals. The mechanism through which such a priority is formed is not a one-way relationship between cognitions and emotions; rather, the relationship is interactive (e.g., Schooler & Eich, 2000; Williams et al., 1997). Nevertheless, incentives and goals, along with attendant emotions, exercise an important orienting influence on the direction of attention and other cognitive processes.

Studies have shown that such an orientation occurs both overtly and covertly. The identifying feature of implicit cognitions is that experience can influence an individual's decision making in ways of which the person is not aware (Greenwald & Banaji, 1995). Thus, the cognition-steering functions of goal pursuits and emotions proceed to a large degree unconsciously and automatically.

In this chapter, we discuss some of the paradigms that have been used to study automaticity in cognition and action in addictive behaviors. We give particular attention to the use of individualized versus generalized stimuli to assess these implicit cognitive processes. Finally, we consider the therapeutic implications of implicit cognitions—particularly attentional bias for substance-related stimuli—in continuation of and relapsing to addictive behaviors.

AUTOMATICITY IN COGNITION AND ACTION

Many aspects of humans' everyday lives (thinking, feeling, and behaving) are automatic (Bargh, 1997; Klinger, 1971; Moskowitz et al., 2004). For example, what would a person do if a fire alarm suddenly sounded? Does the person need to sit down and think about what to do? When the alarm enters the attentional system, it acts as a trigger that evokes a chain of automatic cognitive-behavioral reactions.

The automatic relationship between environmental cues, the attentional system, and cognitive-behavioral reactions apply to many aspects of everyday life. As Jastrow (1906) pointed out, individuals are conscious only of what they need to be conscious of. In other words, many aspects of people's everyday life are automatic, especially the frequently performed behaviors (Bargh & Chartrand, 1999). An example is driving a car by an experienced driver. New behaviors, however, require attention to each component (e.g., when one starts learning how to drive a car). With practice, components intertwine with higher-order units that require progressively less attention, such that eventually they fall out of consciousness; thereafter, they act as automatic behavioral chains. Therefore, it is not surprising to see an experienced driver, sitting on the passenger seat of a friend's car, automatically moving his or her right foot as an unconscious attempt to stop the car when there is a hazardous situation. Many of us who have been driving in a right-hand driving system (e.g., in the United States) for many years cannot easily adjust to a left-hand driving system in other countries (e.g., in the United Kingdom); a mistake that some of us make is opening the driver-side door when we should sit on the passenger side.

According to Bargh (1997), automatic behaviors can be triggered at three levels of complexity: (1) automatic perception (i.e., the perception-behavior link), (2) automatic evaluation (i.e., approach-avoidance), and (3) automatic goal-oriented behavior and motivation (i.e., auto-motivation). Automatic processes play an important role in sustaining various types of human psychopathology (Williams et al., 1996). A spider phobic cannot resist an automatic urge to avoid a spider despite knowing that the reaction is not proportional to the situation. Likewise, automatic reactions to environmental cues (e.g., beer cans on the sidewalk) play an important role in continuation of and relapsing to addictive behaviors (Tiffany, 1990; Wiers, Stacy, et al., 2002; Wiers, van Woerden, et al., 2002).

One feature of automatic reactions is that they are organized to be at least partially independent of consciousness. Therefore, implicit measures are needed to uncover the hidden dimensions of cognitive processes (Greenwald & Banaji, 1995), which lead an individual or a group of people to make judgments and behave in certain ways (e.g., Ekehammar et al., 2003; Moskowitz et al., 2004).

IMPLICIT COGNITIONS AND ADDICTIVE BEHAVIORS

The frequent failure of substance abusers to control their abusive behavior has led researchers to conclude that substance use is uncontrollable (e.g., Tiffany, 1990). The automatic sequence leading to decisions to use the substance can begin with exposure to substance-related stimuli. The interaction of preestablished psychological concerns with associated stimuli causes attentional resources to be disproportionately allocated to incentive-related stimuli (Klinger, 1977, 1978), in this instance to substance-related stimuli, leaving little room for other stimuli that require controlled processing. The selective attention—the *attentional bias*—to substance-related stimuli will evoke a chain of neurodopaminergic, emotional, and cognitive responses (Franken, 2003; Robinson & Berridge, 2003). This will activate a well practiced cognitive-behavioral sequence that culminates in the act of using a substance.

Methods for Studying Substance-Related Attentional Bias

There are different paradigms to study psychopathology-related attentional bias. They include association tasks (e.g., Stacy, 1997), word-coding tasks (e.g., Craik & Lockhart, 1972), and abstract knowledge acquisition utilizing artificial grammar learning (e.g., Pothos & Cox, 2002), and others. Each has been used to study cognitive processes that affect addictive behaviors in covert ways. According to Williams et al. (1996), experimental studies of attentional bias fall within two broad categories. The first comprises experimental paradigms based on the *facilitation effect*. Facilitation is reflected by decrements in attentional and sensory thresholds for concern-related stimuli (i.e., those stimuli that are related to an individual's own current goals). For instance, people show lower auditory (e.g., Parkinson & Rachman, 1980) and visual (e.g., Powell & Hemsley, 1984) thresholds for concern-related stimuli than for stimuli not related to their concerns, and they more frequently attend to, recall, and think about concern-related than nonconcern-related stimuli (Klinger, 1978; Klinger et al., 1981). The second category comprises experimental paradigms based on *interference effects*. Interference reflects decrements in performance (e.g., longer response latencies) from automatic, selective attention to those stimuli or stimulus features that should be ignored during a task. The classic Stroop test (Stroop, 1935) is an example. Whether they assess primarily selective attention or downstream processing priority is subject to debate (De Houwer, 2003; Williams et al., 1996).

Within Williams et al.'s (1996) second category, modified versions of the classic Stroop test (Stroop, 1935), called *addiction Stroop tests*, are sensitive to attentional bias for addiction-related stimuli (Cox et al., 2005). These Stroop tests have been used to study alcohol abuse (e.g., Bauer & Cox, 1998; Stormark et al., 2000), smoking (e.g., Gross et al., 1993; Wertz & Sayette, 2001), heroin dependence (Franken et al., 2000), and compulsive gambling (McCusker & Gettings, 1997). The common finding of these studies, regardless of the methods employed or the target substance (e.g., alcohol, heroin, or tobacco), is that abusers show stronger implicit cognitions related to the abused substance than nonabusers.

Alcohol Stroop tests are discussed in detail by Bruce and Jones (Chapter 10). Although on the alcohol Stroop alcohol abusers usually show greater attentional bias for alcohol-related stimuli than nonabusers, attentional bias for alcohol is not limited to alcohol abusers. For example, Fadardi and Cox (2004) found that alcohol-attentional bias predicted the amount of alcohol that social drinkers habitually consumed. Stacy and colleagues (1996) found that adolescents' implicit responses to substance cues and their expected outcomes from using the substances were stronger predictors of their marijuana and alcohol use than were various demographic variables (e.g., gender, socioeconomic status, and ethnicity).

More recently, investigators have developed the Implicit Association Test (IAT; Greenwald et al., 1998), which requests concept-discrimination judgments by pressing a key with the left hand for one concept category and pressing a key with the right hand for the other concept category. Examples of concept categories might be face pictures of one candidate for election versus face pictures of the opposing candidate, or pleasant words versus unpleasant words. The procedure pits semantic stimulus features—a target feature and a distractor feature presented simultaneously (e.g., a face picture of Candidate A [right key press] and, on the same screen, an unpleasant word [left key press])—against each other (in contrast to concordant stimulus features) and assesses effects on reaction time. As in the Stroop, the discrimination that would have been reasonably automatic were there only one salient feature or two concordant features is temporarily de-automatized when different salient features of the same stimulus automatically dispose to opposite responses, creating conflict and response delay (e.g., De Houwer, 2003).

There have been at least three investigations that have used the Implicit Association Test (IAT) to study implicit responses to alcohol. All used a constant set of stimuli for all participants rather than individualized stimuli. All reported associations between alcohol IAT measures with various aspects of alcohol use.

The first of these investigations (Wiers, van Woerden, et al., 2002) found that "heavy drinkers . . . strongly associated alcohol with arousal on the arousal IAT (especially men) and scored higher on explicit arousal expectancies than light drinkers. . . . On the valence IAT, both light and heavy drinkers showed strong negative implicit associations with alcohol that contrasted with their positive explicit judgments (heavy drinkers were more positive). Implicit and explicit cognitions uniquely contributed to the prediction of 1-month prospective drinking" (p. 648).

Similarly, Jajodia and Earleywine (2003) found that undergraduates' implicit positive expectancies of alcohol outcomes, as assessed with the IAT, were associated with recollections of the quantity, frequency, and maximum amounts of alcohol consumed during the preceding month. The implicit measures accounted for significant variance in each of the three alcohol-use variables that was not accounted for by explicit questionnaire measures.

Finally, in a study with hazardous drinkers, Palfai and Ostafin (2003) found that the alcohol IAT measure "is associated with binge drinking episodes [during the previous 30 days], perceived difficulty controlling alcohol use, and appetitive responses to alcohol cues" (p. 1149). It thus appears that the alcohol IAT constitutes a valid measure of implicit evaluations of alcohol use, and that it provides incremental information beyond that obtainable with explicit measures.

Within a given paradigm for studying implicit cognitions in addictive behaviors, inconsistencies exist. For example, addiction Stroop studies have been conducted with a diverse range of formats (e.g., card vs. computerized), different intertrial intervals, durations of stimulus presentation, the variables that have been controlled, and the number and type of stimuli. Therefore, no two addiction Stroop studies are exactly the same. There are various characteristics of the stimuli that might influence the ability of an addiction Stroop to identify addiction-related attentional bias (Cox et al., 2004). These characteristics include linguistic features of the stimuli, their emotional valence (e.g., positive or negative), whether they are generic addiction-related words or brand names, and whether the stimuli are *general* addiction-related words or *individually* chosen for each participant. Although many of these features have been addressed (see Cox et al., 2005), the relative influence of general versus individualized stimuli on attentional bias remains unresolved.

There also have been no attempts to individualize IAT stimuli. The "personalized" IAT (Olson & Fazio, 2004) attempts to individualize responses but uses standard stimuli. It does this by changing the evaluation categories *pleasant* and *unpleasant* to *I like* and *I don't like* and by choosing stimulus words of average pleasantness but with large standard deviations of pleasantness ratings. Thus, participants can evaluate stimulus words without reference to normative pleasantness, but the words are nevertheless the same for all participants in a given condition. Olson and Fazio (2004) reported higher correlations with explicit self-descriptions using the personalized version of the IAT than using the standard version. The next section discusses generality versus specificity of the stimuli in studies using Stroop tests and association tasks.

Generality Versus Specificity of Stimuli in Stroop Studies

Most current studies using implicit methods to characterize the covert aspects of addictive behaviors use stimuli that are assumed to apply to the average alcohol or other substance abuser. In other words, the stimuli representing a substance usually are not personally selected for each participant. Findings suggest that measures of implicit cognition that use generalized stimuli can detect the cognitions that trigger the act of drinking alcohol or using a drug (Wiers, Stacy, et al., 2002; Wiers, van Woerden, et al., 2002). The ability to detect the bias with such stimuli varies, however, both from one paradigm to another and from one study to another.

There is at least one advantage of implicit paradigms that use generalized stimuli: Compiling the stimuli is rather straightforward. This is because (1) the experimenter is better able than with personalized stimuli to compile a comparable category of neutral words in terms of various linguistic dimensions, especially in the case of modified versions of the Stroop test; and (2) there is no need to change each set of emotionally salient and neutral words from one participant to another. Another advantage is related to interpretability of the findings, because all participants are treated the same.

On the other hand, one might argue against the use of general addiction-related stimuli in assessing implicit cognition. One might question how well a set of addiction-related stimuli can apply to all participants, who vary from each other in terms of their addiction-related habits and preferences. The question seems even more relevant in the case of alcohol consumption. That is, alcohol-related concepts that could be included in implicit-cognition tests (e.g., the alcohol Stroop) vary dramatically among individual drinkers. For example, people who drink have preferred alcoholic beverages, and sometimes they know little about other alcoholic beverages or brand names. Many drinkers describe one beverage as their favorite, but they might find other beverages disgusting. Even within the generalized paradigm, there is no evidence on the relative potency of generic words for alcohol (e.g., alcohol, booze, drink, wine, beer, spirit) versus names of specific alcoholic beverages (e.g., Beck's, Budweiser, Smirnoff Vodka, Champagne) in detecting social and abusers' attentional bias for alcohol. Again, one might question the extent to which attentional bias is accurately evaluated with a test that includes stimuli that are highly valued by some people but unknown or disliked by other people, when both kinds of people complete the same test.

Unfortunately, there is currently insufficient research investigating the question of generality versus specificity of stimuli in tests of implicit cognition. Studies are now described that have used personalized stimuli to measure implicit cognitions. Only one of these studies used the alcohol Stroop test.

To evaluate the extent to which attentional bias for alcohol and other personally relevant concerns can predict drinking behavior, Cox et al. (2000) used a modified version of the emotional Stroop test that included alcohol-related, neutral, and an additional category of stimuli that were related to participants' current concerns (see Klinger, 1975, 1977, 1996; Klinger & Cox, 2004). Participants' current concerns were related to their goals in various life areas, such as health, education, and finances. Participants reported themselves committed to pursuing goals related to these concerns. The concern-related stimuli were individually chosen for each participant. For example, "divorce" was a stimulus for a participant who was concerned about his impending divorce. The word "dog" was selected for one who had a goal of acquiring a dog. "Weights" was used to represent another participant's concern about weight-lifting and bodybuilding. In another experiment, Cox et al. (2002) used personalized concern-related stimuli. Unlike the prior study, the alcohol-related stimuli were also personalized. That is, the alcohol-related stimuli were selected to represent each participant's favorite alcoholic beverage. Both studies indicated that larger interference from alcohol-related than from other concern-related stimuli (i.e., giving greater priority to drinking than to pursuing other goals) was associated with poorer treatment outcomes. Nonetheless, the effect size of the alcohol-related interference in the Cox et al. (2002) study was not larger than that of other alcohol Stroop studies (Cox et al., 2005). Clearly, it is not possible to draw firm conclusions about the power of personalized versus general alcohol Stroop paradigms based on one study.

In another study, Riemann and McNally (1995) asked student participants to name the colors of words that varied according to whether they were emotionally neutral or were highly or only slightly related to each participants' positive or negative current concerns. Responses were quickest for neutral words and slowest for words highly related to concerns, regardless of whether the concerns were positive or negative. This relationship was unaffected by whether participants had gone through a mood induction for neutral, anxious, or happy moods. Thus, the concern-relatedness of individualized stimuli influences the way in which participants implicitly cognitively process them, regardless of the valence of the stimuli and of the participants' current mood.

Studying implicit cognition related to pain, Andersson and Haldrup (2003) used 5 personalized pain words for each participant from a list of 16 words that the researchers had compiled. Each participant selected the 5 best descriptors of their pain. Threat-related and neutral words were also used. The interference for the pain-related stimuli in this study was not stronger than that found in other studies using generalized stimuli. The researchers interpreted this finding as in accordance with other findings suggesting a generally poor support for attentional bias for pain-related stimuli.

In general, then, investigations that have used personalized stimuli in modified versions of the Stroop test have found that these stimuli influence participants' cognitive processing independently of the participant's affective status. In Stroop studies, however, the advantages of using personalized stimuli over generalized ones or vice versa await future research.

Generality Versus Specificity of Automatic Effects on Cognition in Other Paradigms

There are also implicit cognition studies that have used paradigms other than modified versions of the Stroop test. One was a modification of dichotic listening methods (Klinger, 1978). Student participants heard two simultaneous 15-minute narratives, one in each ear, both from the same literary work. These narratives were unobtrusively modified at 12 places in each original narrative by inserting words that would presumably be associated with one of the participant's current concerns into one narrative and synchronously words that alluded to what may be a concern for some other participant in the opposite narrative. Participants were instructed to use a toggle switch to signal at all times the channel to which they were listening. A few seconds after each of these modified passages (embedding sites), the tape stopped with a signal for participants to report their last thoughts and the last segments of the tape they could recall hearing. The results showed highly significant differences in attention, recall, and thought content between sites related to participants' own concerns versus sites related to others' concerns. The rates of recall and stimulus-related thought content for own-concern-related sites were double those of the other sites.

These results not only confirmed the power of concern-related stimuli to influence cognition but also demonstrated the specificity of the effects to participants' own concerns. As another control, participants heard narrative pairs that had been taped for other participants. No such effects occurred with those tapes. Finally, recalled material and thought content were compared with modified wording that participants had not yet heard, because they were situated in a later portion of the session tape. As expected, the effects here failed to occur. These controls indicate the specificity of the effects to stimuli that were related to individuals' current concerns.

What these data did not establish conclusively is the extent to which these effects were truly implicit and automatic. To explore this, Hoelscher et al. (1981) played intermittently to sleeping participants a series of words or brief phrases that were related to their own concerns or to others' concerns, a few seconds after which they were awakened for a dream report. Participants reported Rapid Eye Movement (REM) dreams matchable to immediately preceding cues that were related to their own concerns about three times as often as they reported dreams matchable to cues of others' concerns. Again, a control rating of dreams against cues not yet heard found much weaker resemblance, indicating that the concern-related cues were responsible for the effect. Another investigation indicated effects of stimuli administered before sleep onset on later REM dreams (Nikles et al., 1998).

Because effects on sleeping participants must surely be implicit, these results suggest that the effects of concern-related cues on cognitive processing are substantially automatic. Furthermore, the stimuli in these cases were individualized, chosen as related to either the particular participant's concerns or to other participants' concerns. The results may be taken as indicating that individualized stimuli produce a stronger effect than general stimuli.

This conclusion was further buttressed by data from a lexical decision task (Young, 1987). Young's participants were to decide as quickly as possible whether each occurrence of a letter string on a computer screen was an English word. Button-press answers provided reaction times. The left side of the screen was taken up with computer-related verbal "garbage" that participants were instructed to ignore (which they seem to have done) but which sometimes contained a word associated with one of a participant's current concerns. When the target string was indeed a word, reaction time of reporting this was significantly slower if the garbage contained a concern-related word. Thus, concern-related stimuli seem to impose an extra cognitive-processing load even when they are peripheral and participants are consciously ignoring them. This strongly supports both the automaticity of the effect and its specificity to individuals' concerns and their associated cues.

In summary, then, attention, recall, and thought content appear to be substantially governed by people's current concerns about their goal pursuits, of which addictive substances are an instance. Having one's cognitive processing skewed toward addictive substances presumably helps to maintain behavior patterns in pursuit and consummation of the addictive substance. Recall Cox et al.'s (2000, 2002) findings that the degree of substance-related cognitive interference predicted treatment outcome.

NEUROPHYSIOLOGICAL EVIDENCE

The common finding of studies of implicit cognition is that it is an observable phenomenon that influences the rest of the cognitive and behavioral system. All of the studies discussed thus far have used implicit techniques that are based on either facilitation or interference. The consequences of forming implicit cognitions, such as attentional bias, have also been studied from physiological and neurological viewpoints in several experiments.

Greeley et al. (1993) and Stormark et al. (2000) reported that alcohol abusers had stronger skin-conductance responses to alcohol-related stimuli than to neutral stimuli. These stimuli were individualized to the extent that they were created with alcohol abuse in mind but were not otherwise individualized. This finding is consistent with previous findings that words selected to pertain to the particular participants' current concerns, largely nonsubstance-related, also produced elevated skin-conductance responses (Nikula et al., 1993). In addition, Stormark et al. (1997) found decelerated cardiac variability in a sample of alcohol abusers after they had been exposed to alcohol-related cues. Decelerated heart rate indicates a tendency to accept a stimulus, whereas accelerated heart rate reflects tendencies to reject it (Friedman & Thayer, 1998; Porges, 1992). The results, therefore, suggest that the alcohol abusers were distracted by the alcohol-related stimuli, and that the stimuli had positive emotional valence for them.

There is evidence from Event-Related Potentials (ERP) studies that the brain reacts to emotional stimuli no later than the P300 range, which begins at about 300 ms after being exposed to emotional cues (Klinger, 1996). These findings suggest that the activity of brain loci in processing concern-related stimuli starts at a nonconscious level.

Recently, using a single-stimulus presentation paradigm, Ingjaldsson et al. (2003) reported that alcohol abusers (but not control participants) showed strong heart rate decelerations in response to a masked alcohol stimulus presented for 30 ms. These responses did not occur to emotional words that were unrelated to participants' drinking habits. Using a shorter subliminal presentation of 16 ms, however, Bradley et al. (2004) did not find attentional deployment to smoking-related pictures.

The results of these studies confirm the impact of emotionally salient stimuli (e.g., alcohol) on the activity of the neurophysiological system that is independent of the method of presentation. The results also suggest that commitment to a goal causes automatic recognition of the goal-related cues before conscious semantic analysis of the cues occurs. Thus, when goals are established, their influence begins so early in cognitive processing that they can direct all cognitive processing toward a person's goals. Psychological processes involved in goal pursuits determine an individual's inner world by automatizing goal-related perceptual and cognitive activities. This automaticity might occur through conditioning of structural features of goal-related cues to some form of concern-related brain responses. Perhaps commitment to a goal automatically *sensitizes* people to respond to structural configurations of concern-related stimuli, including words, with enhanced nonconscious processing.

It should be noted that all substance-use-related studies of this kind that provided neurophysiological evidence tailored their stimuli to participants only in distinguishing between substance-related and nonsubstance-related stimuli; they were not otherwise individualized to represent participants' current concerns. Whether or not different results are obtained with completely individualized stimuli awaits future research.

THERAPEUTIC IMPLICATIONS

This section discusses the therapeutic implications of the important role that attentional bias for addiction-related stimuli plays in continuation of and relapsing to addictive behaviors. As described earlier, there is evidence that recently detoxified substance abusers have greater attentional bias for substance-related stimuli than control participants, and persistence of the attentional bias predicts later relapse after successful quitting. Therefore, it seems reasonable to develop interventions aimed at correcting abusers' and recent quitters' attentional bias and processing priority for their substance of abuse. Such an intervention might enhance abusers' ability to control the intrusion of substance-related stimuli into their attentional focus. The intervention should aim to intensify the inhibitory mechanisms that are responsible for suppressing abusers' attentional bias for substance-related stimuli. The intervention might serve two goals: (1) to reduce the automatic nature of abusers' selective attention to substance-related stimuli in their environment, and (2) to reduce the time they need to divert their attention away from these stimuli once these have captured their attention. Preliminary results from Fadardi and Cox's ongoing study to evaluate an intervention called the Alcohol Attention Control Training Program (AACTP) suggest that these goals are viable.

REFERENCES

Andersson, G., & Haldrup, D. (2003). Personalized pain words and Stroop interference in chronic pain patients. *European Journal of Pain, 7*(5), 431–438.

Baars, B. J. (1988). *A cognitive theory of consciousness.* London: Cambridge University Press.

Bargh, J. A. (1997). The automaticity of everyday life. In R. S. Wyer (Ed.), *Advances in social psychology* (Vol. 10, pp. 1–49). Mahwah, NJ: Lawrence Erlbaum.

Bargh, J. A., & Chartrand, T. L. (1999). The unbearable automaticity of being. *American Psychologist, 54*(7), 462–479.

Bauer, D., & Cox, W. M. (1998). Alcohol-related words are distracting to both alcohol abusers and non-abusers in the Stroop colour-naming task. *Addiction, 93*(10), 1539–1542.

Bradley, B. P., Field, M., Mogg, K., & De Houwer, J. (2004). Attentional and evaluative biases for smoking cues in nicotine dependence: Component processes of biases in visual orienting. *Behavioural Pharmacology, 15,* 29–36.

Cox, W. M., Blount, J. P., & Rozak, A. M. (2000). Alcohol abusers' and nonabusers' distraction by alcohol and concern-related stimuli. *American Journal of Drug and Alcohol Abuse, 26*(3), 489–495.

Cox, W. M., Fadardi, J. S., & Pothos, E. M. (2005). *The alcohol-Stroop test: Theoretical considerations and procedural recommendations.* Unpublished manuscript.

Cox, W. M., Hogan, L. M., Kristian, M. R., & Race, J. H. (2002). Alcohol attentional bias as a predictor of alcohol abusers' treatment outcome. *Drug and Alcohol Dependence, 68*(3), 237–243.

Cox, W. M., & Klinger, E. (2004). A motivational model of alcohol use: Determinants of use and change. In W. M. Cox & E. Klinger (Eds.), *Handbook of motivational counseling: Concepts, approaches, and assessment* (pp. 121–138). Chichester, UK: Wiley.

Craik, F. I., & Lockhart, R. S. (1972). Levels of processing: A framework for memory research. *Journal of Verbal Learning and Verbal Behavior, 11*(6), 671–684.

Dehaene, S., & Changeux, J. P. (2000). Reward-dependent learning in neuronal networks for planning and decision making. *Progress in Brain Research, 126,* 217–229.

Dehaene, S., Kerszberg, M., & Changeux, J. P. (1998). A neuronal model of a global workspace in effortful cognitive tasks. *Proceedings of the National Academy of Sciences of the United States of America, 95*(24), 14529–14534.

De Houwer, J. (2003). A structural analysis of indirect measures of attitudes. In J. Musch & K. C. Klauer (Eds.), *The psychology of evaluation: Affective processes in cognition and emotion* (pp. 219–244). Mahwah, NJ: Lawrence Erlbaum.

Ekehammar, B., Akrami, N., & Araya, T. (2003). Gender differences in implicit prejudice. *Personality and Individual Differences, 34,* 1509–1523.

Fadardi, J. S., & Cox, W. M. (2004a). *Can university students' alcohol-attentional bias and motivational structure predict their alcohol consumption?* Manuscript submitted for publication.

Franken, I. H. (2003). Drug craving and addiction: Integrating psychological and neuropsychopharmacological approaches. *Progress in Neuro-Psychopharmacology & Biological Psychiatry, 27*(4), 563–579.

Franken, I. H., Kroon, L. Y., Wiers, R. W., & Jansen, A. (2000). Selective cognitive processing of drug cues in heroin dependence. *Journal of Psychopharmacology, 14*(4), 395–400.

Friedman, B. H., & Thayer, J. F. (1998). Autonomic balance revisited: Panic anxiety and heart rate variability. *Journal of Psychosomatic Research, 44*(1), 133–151.

Greeley, J. D., Swift, W., & Heather, N. (1993). To drink or not to drink? Assessing conflicting desires in dependent drinkers in treatment. *Drug and Alcohol Dependence, 32*(2), 169–179.

Greenwald, A. G., & Banaji, M. R. (1995). Implicit social cognition: Attitudes, self-esteem, and stereotypes. *Psychological Review, 102*(1), 4–27.

Greenwald, A. G., McGhee, D. E., & Schwartz, L. K. (1998). Measuring individual differences in implicit cognition: The Implicit Association Test. *Journal of Personality and Social Psychology, 74,* 1464–1480.

Gross, T. M., Jarvik, M. E., & Rosenblatt, M. R. (1993). Nicotine abstinence produces content-specific Stroop interference. *Psychopharmacology (Berlin), 110*(3), 333–336.

Hoelscher, T. J., Klinger, E., & Barta, S. G. (1981). Incorporation of concern- and nonconcern-related verbal stimuli into dream content. *Journal of Abnormal Psychology, 49,* 88–91.

Ingjaldsson, J. T., Thayer, J. F., & Laberg, J. C. (2003). Preattentive processing of alcohol stimuli. *Scandinavian Journal of Psychology, 44*(2), 161–165.

Jajodia, A., & Earleywine, M. (2003). Measuring alcohol expectancies with the implicit association test. *Psychology of Addictive Behaviors, 17,* 126–133.

Jastrow, J. (1906). *The subconscious.* New York: Houghton Mifflin.

Klinger, E. (1971). *Structure and functions of fantasy.* New York: John Wiley.

Klinger, E. (1975). Consequences of commitment to and disengagement from incentives. *Psychological Review, 82*(1), 1–25.

Klinger, E. (1977). *Meaning and void: Inner experience and the incentives in people's lives.* Minneapolis: University of Minnesota Press.

Klinger, E. (1978). Modes of normal conscious flow. In K. S. Pope & J. L. Singer (Eds.), *The stream of consciousness: Scientific investigations into the flow of human experience* (pp. 225–228). New York: Plenum.

Klinger, E. (1996). Emotional influences on cognitive processing, with implications for theories of both. In P. Gollwitzer & J. A. Bargh (Eds.), *The psychology of action: Linking cognition and motivation to behavior* (pp. 168–189). New York: Guilford.

Klinger, E., Barta, S. G., & Maxeiner, M. E. (1981). Current concerns: Assessing therapeutically relevant motivation. In P. C. Kendall & S. D. Hollon (Eds.), *Assessment strategies for cognitive behavioral interventions* (pp. 161–196). New York: Academic Press.

Klinger, E., & Cox, W. M. (2004). Motivation and the theory of current concerns. In W. M. Cox & E. Klinger (Eds.), *Handbook of motivational counseling: Concepts, approaches, and assessment* (pp. 3–27). Chichester, UK: Wiley.

MacLeod, C. M., & MacDonald, P. A. (2000). Interdimensional interference in the Stroop effect: Uncovering the cognitive and neural anatomy of attention. *Trends in Cognitive Sciences, 4*(10), 383–391.

McCusker, C. G., & Gettings, B. (1997). Automaticity of cognitive biases in addictive behaviours: Further evidence with gamblers. *British Journal of Clinical Psychology, 36*(Pt. 4), 543–554.

Moskowitz, G. B., Li, P., & Kirk, E. R. (2004). The implicit volition model: On the preconscious regulation of temporarily adopted goals. In M. P. Zanna (Ed.), *Advances in experimental social psychology* (Vol. 36, pp. 317–413). Amsterdam, The Netherlands: Elsevier Academic.

Nikles, C. D., II, Brecht, D. L., Klinger, E., & Bursell, A. L. (1998). The effects of current-concern- and nonconcern-related waking suggestions on nocturnal dream content. *Journal of Personality and Social Psychology, 75,* 242–255.

Nikula, R., Klinger, E., & Larson-Gutman, M. K. (1993). Current concerns and electrodermal reactivity: Responses to words and thoughts. *Journal of Personality, 61,* 63–84.

Olson, M. A., & Fazio, R. H. (2004). Reducing the influence of extrapersonal associations on the Implicit Association Test: Personalizing the IAT. *Journal of Personality and Social Psychology, 86,* 653–667.

Palfai, T. P., & Ostafin, B. D. (2003). Alcohol-related motivational tendencies in hazardous drinkers: Assessing implicit response tendencies using the modified-IAT. *Behaviour Research and Therapy, 41,* 1149–1162.

Parkinson, L., & Rachman, S. (1980). Are intrusive thoughts subject to habituation? *Behaviour Research and Therapy, 18*(5), 409–418.

Porges, S. W. (1992). Vagal tone: A physiologic marker of stress vulnerability. *Pediatrics, 90*(3, Pt. 2), 498–504.

Pothos, E. M., & Cox, W. M. (2002). Cognitive bias for alcohol-related information in inferential processes. *Drug and Alcohol Dependence, 66*(3), 235–241.

Powell, M., & Hemsley, D. R. (1984). Depression: A breakdown of perceptual defence? *British Journal of Psychiatry, 145,* 358–362.

Riemann, B. C., & McNally, R. J. (1995). Cognitive processing of personally relevant information. *Cognition & Emotion, 9*(4), 325–340.

Robinson, T. E., & Berridge, K. C. (2003). Addiction. *Annual Review of Psychology, 54*(1), 25–53.

Schooler, J. W., & Eich, E. E. (2000). Memory for emotional events. In E. Tulving & F. I. M. Craik (Eds.), *Oxford handbook of memory* (pp. 379–394). New York: Oxford University Press.

Stacy, A. W. (1997). Memory activation and expectancy as prospective predictors of alcohol and marijuana use. *Journal of Abnormal Psychology, 106*(1), 61–73.

Stacy, A. W., Ames, S. L., Sussman, S., & Dent, C. W. (1996). Implicit cognition in adolescent drug use. *Psychology of Addictive Behaviors, 10*(3), 190–203.

Stormark, K. M., Field, N. P., Hugdahl, K., & Horowitz, M. (1997). Selective processing of visual alcohol cues in abstinent alcoholics: An approach-avoidance conflict? *Addictive Behaviors, 22*(4) 509–514.

Stormark, K. M., Laberg, J. C., Nordby, H., & Hugdahl, K. (2000). Alcoholics' selective attention to alcohol stimuli: Automated processing? *Journal of Studies on Alcohol, 61*(1), 18–23.

Stroop, J. R. (1935). Studies of interference in serial verbal reaction. *Journal of Experimental Psychology, 18,* 643–662.

Tiffany, S. T. (1990). A cognitive model of drug urges and drug-use behavior: Role of automatic and nonautomatic processes. *Psychological Review, 97*(2), 147–168.

Wertz, J. M., & Sayette, M. A. (2001). Effects of smoking opportunity on attentional bias in smokers. *Psychology of Addictive Behaviors: Journal of the Society of Psychologists in Addictive Behaviors, 15*(3), 268–271.

Wiers, R. W., Stacy, A. W., Ames, S. L., Noll, J. A., Sayette, M. A., Zack, M., et al. (2002). Implicit and explicit alcohol-related cognitions. *Alcoholism, Clinical and Experimental Research, 26*(1), 129–137.

Wiers, R. W., van Woerden, N., Smulders, F. T. Y., & de Jong, P. J. (2002). Implicit and explicit alcohol-related cognitions in heavy and light drinkers. *Journal of Abnormal Psychology, 111,* 648 658.

Williams, J. M. G., Mathews, A., & MacLeod, C. (1996). The emotional Stroop task and psychopathology. *Psychological Bulletin, 120,* 3–24.

Williams, J. M. G., Watts, F. N., MacLeod, C. M., & Mathews, A. (1997). Attention to emotional stimuli: Causes and correlates. In *Cognitive psychology and emotional disorders* (pp. 72–105). New York: John Wiley.

Wilson, B. J., & Gottman, J. M. (1996). Attention—the shuttle between emotion and cognition: Risk, resiliency, and physiological bases. In E. M. Hetherington & E. A. Blechman (Eds.), *Stress, coping, and resiliency in children and families. Family research consortium: Advances in family research* (pp. 189–228). Hillsdale, NJ: Lawrence Erlbaum.

Young, J. (1987). *The role of selective attention in the attitude–behavior relationship.* Unpublished doctoral dissertation, University of Minnesota, Minneapolis.

CHAPTER 10

Methods, Measures, and Findings of Attentional Bias in Substance Use, Abuse, and Dependence

GILLIAN BRUCE AND BARRY T. JONES

Abstract: The selective processing (attentional bias) of concern-related stimuli is thought to retard concern resolution. This chapter focuses on alcohol-related concerns and reviews the methods used to explore attentional bias in this area. Research with the Stroop paradigm is reviewed first and then research with a wide range of other paradigms. Strong evidence consistent with a differential alcohol related attentional bias between excessive and social drinkers is reviewed. Emerging evidence consistent with a corresponding effect between heavier and lighter social drinkers is also reviewed and the possibility that there might be a continuity of attentional bias along the consumption continuum is raised.

INTRODUCTION

Evolution, driven by the pressures of natural selection, has delivered an information-processing system with components that take advantage of environmental redundancy to improve efficiency and survival. *Selective attention* is one such component. It allows us to ignore volumes of behaviorally irrelevant information and process the behaviorally relevant. *Attentional bias,* discussed in this chapter, is one manifestation of selective attention. Although the functional benefits of selective attention predominate, research into substance use, abuse, and dependence suggests that it might sometimes cause problems. In this

chapter, the substance in focus is alcohol and the different methods used to explore the association between alcohol consumption and selective attention are described.

An attentional bias is said to be present when a particular stimulus source has more impact on cognitive life and behavior than might otherwise be expected. The extent of the attentional bias is usually *inferred* by *measuring* the extent of its impact on behavior. Two dozen papers employing a half dozen paradigms report attentional bias research in alcohol use, abuse, and dependence, 75 percent of which use modifications of the classical Stroop paradigm (Stroop, 1935). This chapter, therefore, begins with the logic behind the classical Stroop effect. It then extends to the use of modified versions of the Stroop in alcohol research, and subsequently to other more recently conceived paradigms.

In the classical Stroop task, words depicting the names of colors are presented to individuals who are asked to name as quickly as possible the color in which the word is set, while ignoring the meaning of the word itself. For example, the word might be "red" set in the color black, for which the correct response would be to say "black" (not "red"). It has been most frequently found that when the two colors involved are incongruent (e.g., the word "red" is set in black), color-naming times are slower than when they are congruent (e.g., the word "red" is set in red)—the classical Stroop effect. The processing of the semantic stimulus property is thought to interfere with the processing of the perceptual stimulus property. Since the instructions are to ignore the semantic property and process the perceptual property, the occurrence of the Stroop effect suggests that the semantic property might be processed *involuntarily* (or automatically or unconsciously).

Although the explanation of the classical Stroop effect became a focus of basic research in perceptual and cognitive psychology (see MacLeod, 1991), the involuntary component has also attracted the attention of researchers in the clinical domain who have modified the classical Stroop paradigm. In such modifications, the task remains unchanged—to name the color in which the word was set—but the distracting semantic content of the words relate to the psychopathology under scrutiny rather than the names of the colors. The extent to which involuntary processing of the psychopathology-related semantic content interferes with the color-naming task is a measure of the extent of the psychopathology-related attentional bias.

STROOP PARADIGM

Alcohol Abuse, Problem Drinking, and Dependence—Early Work

The initial work on attentional bias and alcohol dependence (Johnsen et al., 1994; Stetter et al., 1995) found that male alcoholics from treatment programs had an attentional bias toward alcohol-related words as compared with neutral words, a difference that was absent in controls. The early work suggested the Stroop findings were robust because two very different ways of implementing the Stroop gave similar results. This methodological difference is explained below.

Stetter et al.'s (1995) work was set in a spreading activation framework with nodes representing alcohol and neutral concepts (Collins & Loftus, 1975)—alcohol nodes/concepts would be more readily activated in alcoholics because of their alcohol history, with a potential for consuming processing resource. In their two studies, they used two composite stimuli cards presented in a counterbalanced order—the card Stroop. One card held 25 alcohol words in columns and the other 25 neutral words. Each of the words was repeated four times in one of four colors. Participants named the color of each word while ignoring its content. The difference between the color-naming times for the alcohol and neutral cards provided the measure of alcohol-related attentional bias. Having found an alcohol attentional bias in individuals in treatment ($n = 40$) but not in social drinking controls, it was concluded that the alcohol Stroop might be better at identifying alcoholics than traditional assessment tools with self-rating scales because it avoids the problem of "denial" accompanying self-report.

Johnsen et al. (1994) used a different implementation of the Stroop paradigm, often called the automated Stroop. Single words were presented on a computer monitor and color-naming times were measured by a voice-activated switch. The design they adopted was similar to Stetter's et al. (1995). Unlike Stetter, however, Johnsen et al. set their study within Tiffany's (1990) theoretical framework for addiction. Within this framework, the development of automatic or unconscious processes representing alcohol-seeking behavior is regarded as key to explaining addiction and the relative ease with which it is maintained. Like Stetter, they found that alcoholics ($n = 13$) had slower response times to alcohol words than to neutral words, which was not found with controls. Johnsen et al. suggested—"it may help explain why alcoholics, when exposed to internal or external cues for drinking, may act on these cues, despite their prior intention not to do so."

A Note on Terminology

Attentional bias normally refers to the within-participant comparison of the behavior alcoholics show toward alcohol stimuli compared with neutral stimuli. When an attentional bias toward alcohol stimuli is found in alcoholics but not in controls (or a lesser attentional bias is found in controls), it is helpful to call this a *differential* attentional bias—its value becomes evident in the next study reviewed.

Alcohol Abuse, Problem Drinking, and Dependence—More Early Work

Bauer and Cox (1998) returned to the possibility that attentional bias research might help the "elucidation of the cognitive mechanisms responsible for the development and maintenance of alcohol problems and lead to improved diagnosis, treatment and the monitoring of treatment outcomes" (p. 1539). They identified previous research, however, as confounding alcohol-relatedness and emotional valence in the alcohol category of words used. Consequently, it was

impossible, they claimed, to conclude whether it was the alcohol-relatedness or the emotional valence of the words that was driving the effect. Accordingly, Bauer and Cox designed a study with two categories of positive and negative emotional words in addition to the two categories of neutral and alcohol words traditionally used. Words were chosen from a word pool in which items had previously been rated for emotional valence and through which the mean emotional valence could be controlled. Using these four categories (10 words per category) in an automated Stroop paradigm with alcohol abusers in treatment ($n = 20$), Bauer and Cox found an attentional bias toward alcohol words significantly more than for positive or negative emotional words. Consequently, they concluded that the bias was predominantly driven by the alcohol rather than emotional content. Not only did they find this bias in alcohol abusers in treatment, but in contrast to the differential bias found in earlier studies they also found it in the nonabusing controls—a nondifferential attentional bias.

In a subsequent study explicitly set within Tiffany's (1990) addiction framework, Stormark et al. (2000) also addressed the issue of the role of emotional valence in the modified Stroop task. Their design, similar to Bauer and Cox's (1998), incorporated negative emotional words as well as alcohol and neutral words—although they only used four different words per category. By contrast, they found that alcoholics ($n = 23$) showed a Stroop effect to the category of emotional words that was almost the same as to the alcohol-related words—suggesting that the alcohol attentional bias found in alcoholics might be driven by the stimuli's negative emotional valence. Also in contrast to Bauer and Cox, Stormark et al. did not find an alcohol-related attentional bias in controls—that is, they found a differential alcohol-related attentional bias.

Comparison between these two studies is difficult, however, because there were several differences in detail—some of which are instructive. First, Stormark et al. (2000) used only 4 words per category whereas Bauer and Cox used 10. It is difficult to imagine a set of 4 safely representing any category. Moreover, the words chosen by Bauer and Cox (1998) were from a prestudy emotional valence rating exercise that ensured that each word did, indeed, capture the properties that were intended. Stormark et al. did not take this precaution. Second, whereas Bauer and Cox used a vocal response through a voice key, Stormark et al. used manual responses to one of several buttons. Because there is evidence that a larger Stroop effect is generated when the responses are, or include, vocal responses, there remains the possibility that Stormark et al.'s procedure was not as sensitive as Bauer and Cox's for detecting Stroop effects in controls. Third, Stormark et al. presented trials blocked by category, whereas Bauer and Cox randomized presentations. Under some circumstances, randomized presentations might reduce the Stroop effect because of the carryover of possible "emotional content" from alcohol to neutral words that would not occur in blocking (Sharma et al., 2001). In this case, the failure of Bauer and Cox to find a differential attentional bias might reflect this lack of sensitivity. Finally, Bauer and Cox used hospital blue-collar staff as controls whereas Stormark et al. did not and they might have had elevated alcohol-related attentional biases through their regular exposure to and having developed concerns about alcohol issues. It remains unclear from this evidence whether the alcohol Stroop effect is driven by the emotional content of the stimuli as well as (or even instead of) the semantic content.

A Lone Treatment Follow-Up Project

The perspective on alcohol attentional bias was changed, somewhat, by addressing the other current concerns an alcoholic might have in addition to their concern about alcohol (Cox & Klinger, 1990). Cox et al. (2002) argued that alcoholics would have a better chance of attenuating whatever involuntary processing of alcohol concepts they might have developed if they had significant positive concerns that could be used to help distract them (or that therapy could take advantage of). If, on the other hand, they had additional significant negative concerns, then distraction and escape might be much less likely—or the additional negative concerns might even promote excessive consumption themselves. Within this context, Cox et al. grasped the nettle and became the first (and, still, the only) group to assess attentional biases surrounding treatment in relation to treatment tenure and outcome. Two groups were used: alcohol abusers ($n = 23$) admitted to a treatment program who had their attentional biases measured on treatment entry and approximately 4 weeks later on discharge; and a control group drawn from the staff of the treatment unit who were measured over a corresponding period. The alcohol abusers were also followed up 3 months after discharge to evaluate their drinking. An automated Stroop procedure was used with three different categories of stimuli (10 stimuli per category)—alcohol-related, concern-related, and neutral.

This study differed from all other Stroop studies in two ways. First, alcohol stimuli were "individualized" to reflect the beverage preferences of each participant. In a pre-experiment, each participant rated for preference 30 textual logos of different alcohol beverages, the top 10 of which were selected for individual presentation in the alcohol category. Second, the contents of the concern-related category were also individualized by asking each participant to name concerns of theirs within each of the following areas: home and household matters, employment and finances, health and medical matters, and partner, family, and relatives. "Words" composed of nontextual symbols from a computer keyboard, having no emotional content, made up the neutral category. A more extensive treatment of "individualizing" can be found in Fadardi et al. (Chapter 9).

Cox et al. (2002) found that alcohol abusers who did not complete the treatment program had significantly higher interference times for the concern-related category than those completing the treatment program and controls. As Cox and Klinger's (1990) motivational framework suggests, this result indicates that there might be more to attentional bias (surrounding treatment, at least) than only alcohol-related attentional bias. It was also found that those with an unsuccessful treatment outcome at the 3-month follow-up had shown a significant increase in attentional bias toward alcohol stimuli from admission to discharge testing. The control group and those alcohol abusers who had a successful treatment outcome at follow-up, on the other hand, showed no corresponding change. Interference times to the concern-related category remained unchanged throughout. This shows that, at least within a treatment and follow-up context, increases in alcohol attentional bias is associated with "relapse." Curiously, Cox et al.'s study remains the only published treatment follow-up that measures attentional biases, in spite of the constant speculation that knowledge of alcohol-related attentional bias should help us better understand excessive consumption and inform treatment dynamics. Additional projects in this area of health care are long overdue.

Recent Replications of the Stroop Effect in Abusers, Problem Drinkers, and Dependents

More recently, there have been three Stroop studies replicating the findings of differential attentional bias in alcoholics (Lusher et al., 2004; Ryan, 2002; and Sharma et al., 2001).

Sharma et al.'s (2001) theoretical approach was embedded in the wider role of cognitions in health-compromising behaviors in general. They used the automated Stroop paradigm with alcohol and neutral categories (25 items per category). They used counterbalanced, blocked presentation of the items of the two different categories but with multiple repetitions of the blocks to test whether attentional bias in Stroop studies might be caused by social drinkers habituating to alcohol stimuli quicker than problem drinkers, rather than by problem drinkers attending to these stimuli more. In addition, they used two control groups—lighter/infrequent and heavier/frequent social drinkers—recognizing that, in earlier studies, finding or not finding an attentional bias in control groups might have been due to the accidental inclusion of more heavier or more lighter social drinkers as controls. They found an attentional bias for alcohol stimuli for both problem drinkers and heavier social drinkers but not for lighter social drinkers (each group *n* = 20). In other words, a differential attentional bias was found between alcoholics and the lighter-drinking control group but a nondifferential attentional bias between the alcoholics and the heavier-drinking control group (replicating Bauer & Cox, 1998). Importantly, no habituation effects were detected across the multiple presentations of the different category blocks, suggesting that the differential attentional bias they found was not driven by alcoholics' slower habituation to alcohol stimuli than other drinkers but by their enhanced processing of alcohol-related stimuli.

Whereas Sharma et al. (2001) sought to explore differential attentional bias with problem drinkers in treatment and university students acting as controls, Ryan (2002) used problem drinkers in treatment ($n = 30$) and staff from an alcohol-treatment service to help control for the experience of encountering alcohol-related concepts as opposed to the experience of drinking alcohol at excessive levels (like Bauer & Cox, 1998). The card version rather than the automated Stroop was used with vocal responses—but with only five different words in each of the alcohol and neutral categories. Consistent with Bauer and Cox's finding, Ryan found an attentional bias but no differential attentional bias—that is, both the experimental and control groups showed an attentional bias toward alcohol words. Ryan also measured "affective state" but found no relationship between this measure and attentional bias.

Finally, Lusher et al. (2004) in a larger study than most ($N = 64$) compared alcohol abusers in treatment with controls attending for general practitioner appointments. The automated Stroop was used with eight alcohol and eight neutral words each presented in category blocks and requiring button-pressing responses. A differential alcohol-related attentional bias was found consistent with Sharma et al.'s (2001) replication but not with Ryan's (2002) or Bauer and Cox's (1998). In common with Ryan, Lusher et al. also measured "mood" but found no relationship between mood and attentional bias. Finally, in an additional analysis, Lusher et al. tested to see whether severity of alcohol problem impacted on the attentional bias displayed by their individuals in treatment. Using the number of years with an alcohol problem as the analogue for severity and a median split technique to generate two levels of severity, they found no difference in attentional bias between the two groups. On the basis of this finding and also on the basis of Sharma's failure to find a differential attentional bias between their higher-drinking control group and treatment group, Lusher et al. speculate that drinkers in general might develop such a bias—including, at least, those who are heavy users, misusers, abusers, and dependents, but presumably not those who use at a relatively light and infrequent level. Lusher et al. recruit Tiffany's (1990) framework for addiction to explain their findings but they also point to Robinson and Berridge's (1993) cognitive neuroscience theory of addiction—incentive sensitization. With prolonged exposure to alcohol, neural sensitization and associative learning make stimuli that were present during alcohol consumption "powerful incentives," which, Lusher et al. note (in common with observations from the earliest studies), might elicit craving and help maintain addiction even in the face of mounting problems.

Alcohol Use

Lusher et al. (2004) suggest there might be a discontinuity of alcohol-related attentional bias between light, infrequent drinkers and, as a homogenous group, the remainder of drinkers. But if this were the case, it would be inconsistent with the relationship found between other (implicit and explicit) alcohol cognitions and consumption. For example, wide-ranging evidence indicates that increasing levels of alcohol consumption outcome expectancies are associated with increasing levels of consumption (see Jones et al., 2001). In addition, both alcohol-consumption outcome associations (Gadon et al., 2004) and alcohol-cue reactions (Greeley et al., 1993) increase with increasing levels of consumption. Consequently, it might be expected that a similar continuity exists between other cognitive constructs such as attentional bias and consumption. Findings from a number of

Stroop studies with social drinkers support this view and are reviewed below.

Using an automated Stroop with button-pressing responses, Cox et al. (1999) were the first to find a differential attentional bias toward alcohol-related stimuli between undergraduate heavy and light social drinkers (*n* = 30 per group). This was, however, only under "potentiated" conditions of test—that is, only with the heavier drinkers, toward alcohol stimuli and, critically, in a room full of alcohol rather than neutral posters. Subsequently, Cox et al. (2003) carried out a similar study in which the "potentiation" came from a sham blind-taste evaluation given before the Stroop procedure using either alcohol or soft drinks. In the Stroop design, they used four categories of word—alcohol, soft drink, cleaning product, and xxxx. For each participant, three sets of interference times were computed by subtracting their mean color-naming times for each of the three categories from the corresponding value for the alcohol category. They found a positive association between consumption and attentional bias for participants who were in the top third for consumption, who took part in the alcohol drink not soft drink sham-tasting evaluation, and only for the attentional bias measure computed by subtracting the soft drink from the alcohol times. Thus, there is evidence of a differential attentional bias among heavier rather than lighter social drinkers but only under specific conditions of test.

Only the most recent report (Bruce & Jones, 2004) on attentional bias in social drinkers using the automated alcohol Stroop paradigm (but using pictorial not textual stimuli), does not adopt potentiating methods. Twenty photographs of alcohol scenes and objects compared with 20 neutral scenes and objects were presented randomly in a block and replicated four times. Responses were made through one of three color-coded buttons. Interference times were calculated by subtracting for each participant their mean response time to neutral stimuli from alcohol stimuli. It was found that heavier social drinkers showed more interference than lighter social drinkers (a differential attentional bias with a "large" effect size; Cohen, 1992). Moreover, for the first of the four blocks, but not for the remaining blocks, there was a significant positive correlation (*r* = .43) between interference times and usual self-reported consumption. This correlation is the first demonstration with a "straight" Stroop paradigm and social drinkers, of a continuity (i.e., a relationship) of attentional bias underpinning a portion of the consumption continuum as opposed to a comparison between two points (i.e., a difference).

Conclusions Based on Extant Stroop Data

First, individuals in alcohol-problem treatment appear to consistently exhibit an attentional bias toward alcohol words. Second, there remains an issue of whether it is the words' alcohol-relatedness or their emotional valence that is behind the attentional bias (or even frequency of encountering them). Third, whether individuals in treatment exhibit a differential attentional bias as opposed to an attentional bias depends on the choice of control group. Fourth, in spite of the speculation on the role that attentional bias might have in relation to excessive alcohol consumption, prospective or follow-up studies are noticeable by their absence and limited to a single study. Finally, some limited evidence suggests that there might be a differential attention bias between individuals at different points of the social drinking region of the consumption continuum not just between its extreme regions.

What cognitive or perceptual processes are described by the term attentional bias? Ryan (2002) suggests that there might be a two-part process. Part 1 might, indeed, be characterized by salient stimulus properties grabbing attention in a preconscious, automatized, and involuntary way and the extent to which this occurs might reflect an individual's level of involvement with alcohol. This drives the Stroop effect. Part 1 is "noticing," triggering part 2, which might simply be described as thinking about alcohol now that it has been inserted in current consciousness. For those with serious alcohol problems that interfere with their lives, thinking might be represented by "ruminations" and might even generate craving and alcohol-seeking. For heavier and frequent social drinkers, it might be represented by mild urges and desires and an increased likelihood of seeking alcohol, whereas for lighter and infrequent social drinkers it might quickly pass from consciousness as other components replace it. Within a framework such as this, part 1 probably drives Stroop behavior but part 2 might also have some impact, especially in excessive consumers of alcohol.

PARADIGMS OTHER THAN THE STROOP

The use of the modified Stroop paradigm to measure attentional bias in alcohol research has not been without its critics. Algom et al. (2004), De Houwer (2003), and Fox et al. (2001), for example, have shown that the logic behind the classical Stroop effect does not necessarily extend to the effects measured using the modified Stroop. Consequently, alcohol research using paradigms other than the Stroop is reviewed next—first, research with excessive drinkers as the focus and, second, focusing on social drinkers.

Alcohol Abuse, Problem Drinking, and Dependence

Only three such studies have been reported with paradigms other than the Stroop.

Posner Paradigm

In the Posner paradigm (Posner & Snyder, 1975), the target and distracter components of the stimulus array are dislocated whereas in the Stroop they are spatially coincident. Under these new conditions of test, it is easier to conceptualize "attention diversion" than under the latter conditions. Stormark et al. (1997) recognized that alcoholics who were currently in recovery were once ready to approach alcohol but were now trying to avoid it. They adapted the Posner paradigm to evaluate this approach-avoidance process. They compared the performance of hospitalized alcoholics ($n = 10$) with social drinkers from a university population. The participants' task was to detect when an asterisk-target appeared on a computer screen either to the left or the right of a fixation point and to respond through a single button as soon as it did. The target appearance was cued by a word that could either be a valid cue (it appeared on the same side of the fixation point as would the target) or an invalid cue (on the opposite side). The cue words were drawn from an alcohol category and a neutral category (words in the neutral category had been screened for neutral emotional valence in a prestudy). Of critical importance, the cue-target interval was either short (100 ms) or long (500 ms). Stormark et al. reasoned that only the automatic, unconscious, or involuntary process relating to attention-engagement (approach) would be able to operate during the 100 ms cue-target interval. They also reasoned that additional disengagement processes (avoidance) would be likely during the longer 500 ms interval. Accordingly, Stormark et al. predicted that alcoholics' response times for invalid trials to alcohol words would be slower than to neutral words when the cue-target interval was 100 ms but faster when the cue-target interval was 500 ms—no such difference, and change in differences, would be seen in controls. The results were consistent with their predictions. They supported the view that there was, indeed, an involuntary attentional bias toward alcohol-related stimuli in alcoholics that was less or absent in controls. Moreover, this involuntary bias was followed by (probably more voluntary) efforts to disengage from the alcohol-related stimuli through processes that were probably driven by the negative emotional valence of the stimuli.

Dual-Task Paradigm

Not only did Waters and Green (2003) dislocate the target and distracter components of the stimulus array like Stormark et al. (1997), they also gave participants the tasks of monitoring and responding to both the components—a dual-task paradigm. Abstinent alcoholics (*n* = 25) and controls from the general population fixated the center of a screen where one of the digits one through eight would appear for 5 seconds. They were to make an "odd-even" judgment and respond using a two-button box. Additional text would appear in the periphery during some of the trials and they were to make a lexical decision "out of the corner of their eye" responding through a different two-button box. Three blocked categories of words (and their non-lexical counterparts) were used—alcohol, semantically related, and semantically unrelated. Forty-eight trials were given per block, half with digits at the fixation point and half with the additional text appearing at unpredictable locations in the periphery, half of which were words and half nonwords.

Waters and Green (2003) found that alcohol abusers' odd-even reaction times to the digits presented centrally were slowed when the peripheral distracters were alcohol words but not when they were words from the other two categories—control participants did not show this pattern. Lexical decision times in the alcohol category were also slowed in alcohol abusers but not in other categories, which

was not seen in controls. This is not consistent with the usual "attentional bias" predictions because it would be expected that the times would be quicker not slower on this basis. If the alcohol-related words had a negative emotional valence, however, it would be consistent with alcohol abusers avoiding processing them. Finally, Waters and Green also asked participants to recall the words from each of the different categories once the experiment was finished and found that alcohol abusers recalled the alcohol-related items better than the items from the other categories. The fact that the controls showed the same pattern, however, is not consistent with Tiffany's (1990) framework, which suggests that more elaborative processing should occur in alcohol abusers as compared with controls, which should, in turn, cause alcohol abusers to recall more of these words than should controls. Waters and Green concluded that, since in the dual-task paradigm there is a spatial shift in attention underpinning the Stroop effect, there is more support for Robinson and Berridge's (1993) theory from their dual-task paradigm than from the Stroop (1935) because the incentive-sensitization theory implies a shift in attention between stimuli out there in the environment.

Flicker Paradigm for Inducing Change Blindness

Finally, Bruce et al. (2004) and Jones et al. (in press) have adopted a paradigm to more directly test attentional bias that does not rely on the target-distracter feature of the paradigms described above. In the flicker paradigm for inducing change blindness, two identical stimulus arrays are presented to viewers in rapid, continuous succession, in register and separated by a mask (Rensink, 2002). A permanent change is made to one of the displays and the task is to "spot the difference" as the two almost identical arrays are flicked back and forth. The change is surprisingly difficult to spot—that is, induced change blindness. Rensink and particularly Turatto et al. (2003) have shown that unless "attention is sent to an object" a change is not detected. Accordingly, Jones et al. (2002) and Jones et al. (2003) have argued that change detection latency directly measures alcohol attentional bias if the change is made to an alcohol object in a scene. Bruce et al. and Jones et al. (2006) presented such a flickered change to an alcohol object to one group of problem drinkers ($n = 18$) and to a neutral object to another such group ($n = 18$). They used controlled photographs of alcohol and neutral (household) objects set in a 3×6 landscape rectilinear matrix with 3×3 alcohol-related items on one side and 3×3 neutral items on the other. The change was made to the photograph at the center of the appropriate 3×3 matrix. In problem drinkers, they found that change detection latencies were shorter to the alcohol change than to the neutral change—there was no difference between the two corresponding social drinking control groups. This is consistent with problem drinkers (but not controls) sending attention to alcohol but not to neutral objects—a differential attentional bias. In addition, support for a continuity of attentional bias within problem drinkers was found—a negative correlation ($r = -.51$) in the 18 problem drinkers given the alcohol change to detect, between change detection latency and severity of problem (the number of times they had previously been treated).

The results of the foregoing studies reveal an alcohol-related attentional bias in individuals drinking at a level that brings them into contact with treatment and using a range of paradigms in which either the target and distracter items are spatially dislocated or in which attention is measured directly. These results add to and are generally consistent with the results from the Stroop (1935) paradigm reviewed earlier in this chapter.

Alcohol Use

Evidence for a differential attentional bias within social drinking is limited when Stroop studies are reviewed but evidence from elsewhere is more compelling and is reviewed below.

Dot-Probe Paradigm

MacLeod et al. (1986) developed the dot-probe paradigm to measure attentional bias in emotional disorders in an effort to dislocate the target and distracter components of the stimulus array, confounded in Stroop studies. It has been widely used since. Townshend and Duka (2001) have extended its use to social drinkers. They presented pairs of alcohol and neutral stimuli briefly on a monitor, immediately followed by a dot probe in register with one of the stimuli of the pair. The task was to press one of two buttons as soon as the dot probe appeared. The logic was that if attention was captured by the alcohol-related item of the alcohol-neutral pair, response times to the probe appearing in register with the alcohol item would be quicker that when it appeared in register with the neutral item. Picture items were used in half of the study and text items in the other. The picture categories comprised alcohol and stationery items. Their word categories comprised alcohol items, too, but were subdivided into craving-related words and words representing relief from alcohol withdrawal. Stationery words representing the pictures were also included. Attentional bias scores were calculated by subtracting the response times when the probe and alcohol stimuli were in register from those when they were not. With the pictures, it was found that heavier social drinkers had higher attentional bias scores than did light, occasional social drinkers—a differential attentional bias. There was no such bias with word stimuli.

Johnsen, B. H., Laberg, J. C., Cox, W. M., Vaksdal, A., & Hugdahl, K. (1994). Alcoholic subjects' attentional bias in the processing of alcohol-related words. *Psychology of Addictive Behaviors, 8,* 111–115.

Jones, B. C., Jones, B. T., Blundell, L., & Bruce, G. (2002). Social users of alcohol and cannabis who detect substance-related changes in a change blindness paradigm report higher levels of use than those detecting substance-neutral changes. *Psychopharmacology, 165,* 93–96.

Jones, B. T., Bruce, G., Livingstone, S. & Reed, E. (in press). Alchol-related attentional bias in problem drinkers with the flicker change blindness paradigm. *Psychology of Addictive Behaviors.*

Jones, B. T., Corbin, W., & Fromme, K. (2001). A review of expectancy theory and alcohol consumption. *Addiction, 96,* 55–70.

Jones, B. T., Jones, B. C., Smith, H., & Copely, N. (2003). A flicker paradigm for inducing change blindness reveals alcohol and cannabis information processing biases in social users. *Addiction, 98,* 235–244.

Lusher, J., Chandler, C., & Ball, D. (2004). Alcohol dependence and the alcohol Stroop paradigm: Evidence and issues. *Drug and Alcohol Dependence, 75,* 225–231.

MacLeod, C., Mathews, A., & Tata, P. (1986). Attentional bias in emotional disorders. *Journal Of Abnormal Psychology, 95,* 15–20.

MacLeod, C. M. (1991). Half a century of research on the Stroop effect: An integrative review. *Psychological Bulletin, 109,* 163–203.

Posner, M. I., & Snyder, C. R. (1975). Facilitation and inhibition in the processing of signals. In P. M. Rabbit (Ed.), *Attention and performance* (Vol. 5, pp. 669–682) New York: Academic Press.

Pothos, E. M., & Bailey, T. M. (2000). The role of similarity in artificial grammar learning. *Journal of Experimental Psychology: Learning, Memory, and Cognition, 26,* 847–862.

Pothos, E. M., & Cox, W. M. (2002). Cognitive bias for alcohol-related information in inferential processes. *Drug and Alcohol Dependence, 66,* 235–241.

Rensink, R. A. (2002). Change detection. *Annual Review of Psychology, 53,* 245–277.

Robinson, T., E., & Berridge, K. C. (1993). The neural basis of drug craving: An incentive-sensitization theory of addiction. *Brain Research Reviews, 18,* 247–291.

Ryan, F. (2002). Attentional bias and alcohol dependence: A controlled study using the modified Stroop paradigm. *Addictive Behaviors, 27,* 471–482.

Sharma, D., Albery, I. P., & Cook, C. (2001). Selective attentional bias to alcohol-related stimuli in problem drinkers and non-problem drinkers. *Addiction, 96,* 285–295.

Stetter, F., Ackermann, K., Bizer, A., Straube, E. R., & Mann, K. (1995). Effects of disease-related cues in alcoholic inpatients: Results of a controlled "alcohol Stroop" study. *Alcoholism: Clinical and Experimental Research, 19,* 593–599.

Stormark, K. M., Field, N. P., Hugdahl, K., & Horowitz, M. (1997). Selective processing of visual alcohol cues in abstinent alcoholics: An approach-avoidance conflict? *Addictive Behaviors, 22,* 509–519.

Stormark, K. M., Laberg, J. C., Nordby, H., & Hugdahl, K. (2000). Alcoholics' selective attention to alcohol stimuli: automated processing? *Journal of Studies on Alcohol, 61,* 18–23.

Flicker Paradigm for Inducing Change Blindness

In the first application of the flicker paradigm in the alcohol field, Jones et al. (2003) used the same design as reported recently by Bruce et al. (2004), and Jones et al. (in press) above. Jones et al. (2003), however, used heavy- and light-drinking participants (undergraduates) not problem drinkers; and the array of alcohol and neutral objects (office gear) was naturally arranged and photographed on a table top with the two categories grouped side by side rather than have the individual photographs of the objects set in a rectilinear matrix. Half the heavier social drinkers were given the alcohol change and half the neutral change and the lighter drinkers were treated in the same way (groups $n = 20$). Heavier social drinkers detected the alcohol change quicker than did the lighter social drinkers. A "reverse" attentional bias was seen with the neutral change, however. Jones et al. (2003) interpreted this reverse as indicating that the alcohol objects captured the attention of the heavier drinkers and for this reason it took them longer to detect the change to the neutral object than it would the lighter drinkers (a feature not seen in the data of Bruce et al.).

Jones et al. (2002), in a study parallel to Jones et al.'s (2003) above, measured attentional bias in heavier and lighter social drinkers in a novel version of the flicker paradigm in which two (not one) changes were given to be detected—an alcohol and a neutral change were simultaneously presented to *compete* for participants' attention. In the instructions, however, participants were told that "*a* change would be made and their task was to detect *it*." Jones et al. (2002) had argued that such a procedure might be a more sensitive way of detecting attentional biases than using a single change. Their prediction was that individuals who detected the alcohol-related change when both changes were available would have higher usual consumption measures than individuals detecting the neutral change under the same conditions of test. The data supported the prediction.

Artificial Grammar-Learning Paradigm

Pothos and Cox (2002) note that alcohol-related attentional bias has been traditionally measured using relatively low-level, noninferential processes. They adopt the novel position that it would be surprising if these low-level processes were the only level of cognitive process that became "biased" through experience. To test this at a higher level (i.e., the level of implicit inference), they adopted an artificial grammar-learning (AGL) paradigm. In AGL, individuals are exposed in a training phase to sequences of symbols that obey a set of rules—only certain symbols can follow others in a grammatical sequence. They are simply asked to look at the different sequences. In a testing phase, they are then shown new sequences that obey the rules (grammatical, G) or do not (nongrammatical, NG) and they are asked to classify them as G or NG. If individuals can identify G above chance, they are said to have inferred some of the rules—a feature of implicit learning representing higher cognitive processes of rule inference, associations, and similarity principles (Pothos & Bailey, 2000).

Using an AGL framework, Pothos and Cox (2002) constructed an alcohol and a neutral version of the same AGL task. In other words, the symbols of the sequences were different but the rules governing the grammatical order of the symbols were the same. In the neutral version, the symbols were different cities and 23 different sequences were instantiated as airline routes. In the alcohol-related version, the 23 symbols were different drinks served to guests at a party. Contexts were generated to ensure that participants attended to the different sequences. Each sequence was presented three times for 5 seconds on a computer screen. Half of the heavy drinkers were exposed to the alcohol-related AGL and half to the neutral AGL ($n = 38$); the light drinkers were treated in the same way ($n = 12$). Pothos and Cox found that heavy drinkers exposed to the neutral AGL performed above chance in classifying G sequences at test but that those exposed to the alcohol AGL did not. Light drinkers performed above chance on both the neutral and alcohol AGL. They explain that the heavy-drinkers' performance on the alcohol AGL test as being due to the heavier drinkers processing the semantic content of the symbols rather than their sequential dependencies, which would impair the implicit learning, impacting on high-level structures.

The foregoing shows that a range of quite different paradigms provides evidence of a differential attentional bias within social drinking and adds to the limited findings with the Stroop (1935). Together, they increase the possibility that there exists a continuity of attentional bias along the consumption continuum and the correlational analyses from Bruce et al. (2004) and Jones et al. (in press) suggest that it might extend along its whole length. If this were so, then it would be consistent with the continuity that has been found with other alcohol cognitions such as alcohol-consumption outcome expectancies and associations and alcohol-cue reactions.

CONCLUSIONS

The evidence both for an alcohol attentional bias and a differential alcohol attentional bias appears robust—and the choice of control governs and informs on this. Much is gained from the range of very different paradigms that demonstrate it. The evidence also appears to indicate that, rather than being represented by a discontinuity between individuals drinking at a level that has brought them in contact with treatment and the rest, it might be better represented as a graded continuity along the length of the consumption continuum.

This also raises the possibility that the bias might be represented by multiple components rather than by a single one. It is likely, for example, that the resolution to the issue of whether the bias is driven by the semantic content or the emotional/anxiety content of a stimulus is resolved by finding evidence for both. It is also likely that the relative magnitude of the components could systematically change from one end of the consumption continuum to another. Indeed, an important research direction would be to make—at a series of different positions on the consumption continuum—within-participant comparisons between alcohol attentional biases to "liked" and "wanted" (to use the terminology from incentive-sensitization theory) or to positively and negatively valued features of the alcohol domain. The two-change flicker paradigm—developed by Jones et al. (2002) from the traditional one-change version used throughout psychology—in which two potential drivers of attentional capture are made to simultaneously compete side by side, would be an appropriate methodology because it effectively requires the individual's attentional system to make an "implicit forced choice."

It is widely claimed that attentional bias is a risk factor for the maintenance of excessive drinking and relapse, mediated by craving. In view of such wide claims, it is surprising that prospective studies have not been run and that craving has not been measured (particularly since the link between craving and subsequent consumption or relapse is controversial). In relation to treatment, it is difficult to know whether attentional bias might be a useful measure of treatment progress (for example, before and after measures of cue-exposure training) or a feature to be measured and

discussed with a view to the development of skills designed to cope with its effect. It might also be a treatment target.

Finally, although alcohol studies have captured the attention of substance use, misuse, abuse, and dependence more than has any other drug, oth in this book review work with n ates, and cocaine and with the s paradigms.

Algom, D., Chajut, E., & Lev, S. (2004). A rational look at the emotional St phenomenon: A generic slowdown, not a Stroop effect. *Journal of Ex mental Psychology: General, 133,* 323–338.

Bauer, D., & Cox, W. M. (1998). Alcohol-related words are distracting to alcohol abusers and non-abusers in the Stroop color-naming task. *Add 93,* 1539–1542.

Bruce, G., & Jones, B. T. (2004). A pictorial Stroop paradigm reveals an a attentional bias in heavier as compared with lighter social drinkers. *Jo Psychopharmacology, 18,* 531–537.

Bruce, G., Livingstone, S., Reed, E., Frame, M., Boyd, A., & Jones, B. T September). *The first use of the flicker paradigm (for inducing chan ness) in measuring alcohol attentional bias with social and problem* Presentation at Addictions 2004, Brisbane, Queensland, Australia.

Cohen, J. (1992). A power primer. *Psychological Bulletin, 112,* 155–159

Collins, A., & Loftus, E. (1975). A spreading-activation theory of sem cessing. *Psychological Review, 82,* 407–428.

Cox, W. M., Brown, M. A., & Rowlands, L. J. (2003). The effects of exposure on non-dependent drinkers' attentional bias for alcol *Alcohol and Alcoholism, 38,* 45–49.

Cox, W. M., Hogan, L. M., Kristian, M. R., & Race, J. H. (2002). A tional bias as a predictor of alcohol abusers' treatment outcom *Alcohol Dependence, 68,* 237–243.

Cox, W. M., & Klinger, E. (1990). Incentive motivation, affective alcohol use: A model. In W. M. Cox (Ed.), *Why people drink: alcohol as a reinforcer* (pp. 291–314). New York: Gardner Pres

Cox, W. M., Yeates, G. N., & Regan, C. M. (1999). Effects of alcoh nitive processing in heavy and light drinkers. *Drug and Alcoh 55,* 85–89.

De Houwer, J. (2003). On the role of stimulus-response and s compatibility in the Stroop effect. *Memory & Cognition, 31,*

Fox, E., Russo, R., Bowles, R., & Dutton, K. (2001). Do threaten or hold visual attention in subclinical anxiety. *Journal Psychology: General, 130,* 681–700.

Gadon, L., Bruce, G., McConnochie, F., & Jones, B. T. (2004) consumption outcome associations in young and mature ad The route to drinking restraint? *Addictive Behaviors, 29,* 1

Greeley, J. D., Swift, W., Prescott, J., & Heather, N. (1993). R related cues in heavy and light drinkers. *Journal of Stud* 359–368.

Stroop, J. R. (1935). Studies of interference in verbal reactions. *Journal of Experimental Psychology: General, 18,* 643–622.

Tiffany, S. T. (1990). A cognitive model of drug urges and drug-use behavior: Role of automatic and nonautomatic processes. *Psychological Review, 97,* 147–168.

Townshend, J. M., & Duka, T. (2001). Attentional bias associated with alcohol cues: Differences between heavy and occasional social drinkers. *Psychopharmacology, 15,* 67–74.

Turatto, M., Bettella, S., Umilta, C., & Bridgeman, B. (2003). Perceptual conditions necessary to induce change blindness. *Visual Cognition, 10,* 233–255.

Waters, H., & Green, M. W. (2003). Demonstration of attentional bias, using a novel dual task paradigm, towards clinically salient material in recovering alcohol abuse patients? *Psychological Medicine, 33,* 491–498.

CHAPTER 11

Attention to Drug-Related Cues in Drug Abuse and Addiction: Component Processes

MATT FIELD, KARIN MOGG,
AND BRENDAN P. BRADLEY

Abstract: According to several theories of addiction, drug-related stimuli should capture and hold attention, and elicit approach behaviors, in drug users (e.g., Robinson & Berridge, 1993, 2003; Franken, 2003). Such models assume that attentional biases for drug-related cues are "automatic," that is, they occur at early stages of stimulus processing, and that attentional biases are associated with subjective craving and the tendency to approach drug-related cues. This article reviews these models and relevant empirical findings, including studies that have used visual probe tasks and eye movement monitoring techniques to investigate the component processes of biases in visual orienting to drug-related stimuli, and implicit tasks that assess behavioral approach tendencies for drug-related cues.

INTRODUCTION

Drug-associated environmental stimuli are thought to influence drug-seeking behavior. There are numerous demonstrations that exposure to drug-related cues causes physiological, subjective, and behavioral reactivity in addicts (see Carter & Tiffany, 1999, for a review). In particular, increases in subjective drug craving and behavioral indices of drug-seeking are observed after exposure to drug-related cues. As reviewed in Bruce and Jones (Chapter 10) and Waters and Sayette (Chapter 21), drug users also show biased cognitive

AUTHOR'S NOTE: Much of the research described in this article was supported by grants awarded by the Wellcome Trust to Brendan Bradley and Karin Mogg (reference number 57076) and by the University of Southampton to Brendan Bradley, Matt Field, and Karin Mogg. Karin Mogg holds a Wellcome Senior Research Fellowship in Basic Biomedical Science. Correspondence should be addressed either to Brendan Bradley and Karin Mogg at the School of Psychology, University of Southampton, Highfield, Southampton SO17 1BJ, UK, or to Matt Field, who is now at the School of Psychology, University of Liverpool, Eleanor Rathbone Building, Bedford Street South, Liverpool L69 7ZA, UK.

processing of drug cues, which become the focus of attention at the expense of competing stimuli. This chapter will explore the cognitive and attentional processes that are involved in attentional biases in addiction, and the relationships between attentional bias for drug cues, approach behaviors directed toward drug cues, and drug-craving. We will also contrast the biases in specific attentional processes that are seen in addiction with those that are seen in other appetitive motivational states such as hunger, and aversive emotional states such as those seen in anxiety disorders.

THEORETICAL BACKGROUND

Contemporary theories propose that addiction is associated with biases in the attentional processing of drug-related cues, and that this biased cognitive processing may index the processes that underlie compulsive drug-seeking behavior in addiction, and may even mediate that behavior. These theories make clear predictions about the cognitive mechanisms that underlie attentional biases, and about the variables that will be associated with them. Historically, theories of addiction have emphasized either the positive incentive (e.g., Stewart et al., 1984) or the negative reinforcing (e.g., Wikler, 1948) properties of drugs of abuse, with more recent theories stressing the importance of cognitive and, specifically, attentional, factors in addiction (e.g., Cox & Klinger, 2004; Ryan, 2002). Recent incarnations of each of these approaches have all argued for the presence of attentional biases in addiction, and these models will be briefly reviewed here.

Many addiction theorists argue that addiction is maintained by the positive incentive properties of drugs and drug-related cues. For example, Stewart et al. (1984) proposed that, through a classical conditioning process, drug-related cues become associated with the positive reinforcing properties of drugs and, as a

consequence, those cues acquire conditioned incentive properties, thereby drawing the individual toward the drug, resulting in drug-taking (see also Tomie, 1996). Subsequently, in the incentive-sensitization theory, Robinson and Berridge (1993, 2003) evoked similar incentive learning mechanisms to explain the development of addiction. They suggested that repeated administration of drugs of abuse causes a sensitization of dopamine release in the nucleus accumbens and related circuitry of the mesolimbic dopamine system. They implicate the nucleus accumbens in incentive learning processes, and they argue that, as dopamine release increases in magnitude each time drugs are taken, this leads to a progressive increase in the incentive value of drugs, such that pathological motivation for the drug develops. Due to repeated pairings of drug-induced dopamine release with environmental drug-related cues, presentation of drug-related cues eventually produces a conditioned increase in dopamine release. This conditioned dopamine release causes environmental cues that are associated with drug-taking to acquire conditioned incentive properties, or "incentive salience." In behavioral terms, this means that a drug-paired cue acts as a powerful conditioned incentive that *"grabs attention, becomes attractive and 'wanted,' and thus guides behavior to the incentive"* (Robinson & Berridge, 1993, p. 261; emphasis in the original).

Robinson and Berridge (1993, 2003) propose that there are individual differences in susceptibility to sensitization. Consequently, individuals vary in the extent to which the dopamine system is prone to increasing the incentive value of drugs, and transforming drug-associated stimuli into incentive stimuli that grab attention. Therefore, an attentional bias for drug-related cues may provide a cognitive index of vulnerability to dependence, as well as dependence severity. A further tenet of the theory is that an attentional bias for drug-related cues is mediated primarily by automatic processes, which operate in early aspects of stimulus processing and which do not depend on intentional, controlled strategies. According to Ryan (2002) and Franken (2003), attentional bias may play an important role as a mediating link between the perception of drug cues, and drug-seeking behaviors in response to those stimuli. Specifically, like Robinson and Berridge (1993), Franken (2003) argues that presentation of drug cues increases the release of dopamine in the nucleus accumbens and associated structures in the mesolimbic dopamine system. This results in *"motor preparation and a hyperattentive state towards drug-related stimuli that, ultimately, promotes further craving and relapse"* (Franken, 2003, p. 563; emphasis added).

Other theorists argue that addiction is maintained because drugs alleviate the negative mood states that occur during drug withdrawal. According to Baker and coworkers (Baker, Brandon, et al., 2004; Baker, Piper, et al., 2004), the strong links between negative affect and the motivation to smoke may occur because negative affect *"inflate[s] the incentive value of smoking cues"* (Baker, Brandon, et al., 2004, p. 483; emphasis added). Baker, Piper, et al.'s (2004) model predicts that, when negative affect increases (for example, as a consequence of drug withdrawal or environmental stressors), drug-related cues become more salient. Thus, this model implies that attentional biases for drug cues may be enhanced by high negative affect, given that attention seems more likely to be allocated preferentially to information that is highly salient for the individual.

Finally, other theorists take a cognitive processing approach to addictive behavior and in doing so arrive at different explanations for attentional biases in addiction. Cox and Klinger (2004) argue that an addict who wishes to discontinue drug use will have a greater chance of success if they are able to engage in, and become easily distracted by, nondrug-related activities and concerns,

rather than drug-related concerns. Therefore, the degree to which addicts get easily distracted by (or have an attentional bias for) stimuli that relate to drug use rather than stimuli that are related to other concerns, should be directly associated with the risk of relapse. If an individual could narrow the attentional focus exclusively toward positive concerns that were not drug-related, even when faced with drug-related cues, their chances of maintaining abstinence over the long term should be high. McCusker (2001) and Sayette et al. (2000) propose that attentional biases provide a cognitive measure of an individual's motivation to use drugs. In fact, all theories that emphasize attentional biases in addiction predict that attentional biases for drug-related cues will be related to indices of drug-use motivation, such as drug craving, and this prediction will be addressed in this chapter.

In summary, a number of theories of addiction predict the presence of an "attentional bias" for drug-related cues in addiction, and also that the attentional bias is "automatic"; that is, it occurs at an early stage of cognitive processing, possibly before the drug user is aware of the stimuli. A common theme in these theories is the suggestion that subjective drug craving and the ability of drug cues to elicit approach behaviors should be correlated with measures of attentional bias. In the past decade, a considerable body of evidence has accumulated that enables us to evaluate these predictions, and this literature will be evaluated in the next section.

ATTENTIONAL PROCESSES AND CORRELATES OF ATTENTIONAL BIAS IN ADDICTION AND DRUG USE

Attentional Processes

According to several theorists, attentional biases for drug-related cues operate automatically and at very early stages of cognitive processing, such that addicts may shift their attention to drug-related cues before those cues have crossed the threshold of conscious awareness. Various cognitive paradigms have been used to explore the "automatic" nature of attentional biases for drug cues, and the results from these studies will be discussed below in order to address this issue.

Several studies have used subliminal presentation paradigms to examine biased processing of drug cues that are presented below the threshold of conscious awareness. Franken, Kroon, and Wiers, et al. (2000) used a "subliminal Stroop" paradigm to examine attentional bias for briefly presented heroin-related words in groups of heroin addicts and nonaddict controls. In this task, target words (either heroin-related or control words) were presented very briefly (16 ms) in a colored font and were then replaced with a masking stimulus (a row of x's) in the same color. Participants were instructed to name the color of the stimuli, and color-naming latencies were compared for heroin-related and control words. Postexperimental awareness checks confirmed that participants were unaware that words had been presented before the colored x's; therefore, if heroin-related words caused color-naming interference, they must have done so in the absence of participants' conscious awareness of those words. However, neither addicts nor controls showed differential color-naming interference from heroin-related and matched control words, suggesting no attentional bias in either group. When the same words were presented supraliminally (i.e., above the threshold of conscious awareness), then the heroin addicts, but not the control participants, were significantly slower to color-name the heroin-related rather than the matched control words, which is consistent with an attentional bias for the heroin-related words. Munafo et al. (2003) reported related findings in smokers: Supraliminally presented smoking-related words produced greater color-naming interference in smokers, than in nonsmokers. However, when those words were briefly presented and masked (which restricted the level of awareness of the word stimuli), there was only a trend for color-naming interference from masked smoking-related words in smokers, but this did not reach significance. Mogg and Bradley (2002) also included a masked version of the modified Stroop task in a study of the effect of nicotine deprivation on cognitive biases in smokers and found no evidence of a preconscious bias for masked smoking-related cues.

Bradley et al. (2004) used a visual probe task to investigate biased attentional processing of subliminally presented smoking-related pictures. Pictures are more naturalistic drug-related stimuli than words, and as such they may be expected to grab attention at an earlier stage of cognitive processing than words. In the Bradley et al. (2004) study, pairs of smoking-related and matched control pictures were presented very briefly (16 ms), and then followed by a pattern mask for a further 64 ms. Immediately after stimulus offset, a small visual probe appeared in the location that had been occupied by one of the pictures, and participants were instructed to make a rapid manual response to the probes. Reaction time (RT) to the probes therefore provides an index of attentional deployment: faster RTs to probes that replaced masked smoking-related rather than masked control pictures would indicate an attentional bias for masked smoking-related pictures. However, hypotheses were not supported, as smokers had similar response latencies to probes replacing masked smoking-related and control pictures, which suggests the absence of an attentional bias for subliminally presented pictures. However, when the smoking-related and control pictures were presented for longer durations (200 or 2,000 ms), and were not replaced by pattern masks (i.e., supraliminal presentation conditions), then smokers, but not nonsmokers, showed an attentional bias for the smoking-related pictures.

Thus, research so far has revealed no conclusive evidence of a preconscious bias for drug-related cues. The absence of a processing bias for subliminally presented drug-related stimuli does not preclude the existence of an "automatic" attentional bias that operates in the early stages of cognitive processing. For example, attention may be directed rapidly and reflexively to certain types of stimuli without this bias necessarily operating outside of awareness. Furthermore, current theories of spatial attention emphasize that the attentional system is not unitary, with important distinctions made between the processes that influence the initial orienting versus maintenance of attention (Allport, 1989; LaBerge, 1995). Orienting of covert attention can occur relatively rapidly and automatically, and it functions to program shifts in overt attention, that is, eye movements (Jonides, 1981; Kowler, 1995). By contrast, the maintenance of attention may be more likely to be influenced by strategic cognitive processes, which in turn may be influenced by motivational variables (LaBerge, 1995). Although many paradigms that are currently in use to measure attentional biases in addiction (e.g., the modified Stroop) are not suitable for investigating these component processes of attentional biases, other paradigms can yield information about biases in the initial shift versus maintenance of attention to drug-related cues (see Bruce & Jones, Chapter 10, and Waters & Sayette, Chapter 21, for further details of procedures for measuring attentional bias).

In the visual probe task, it is possible to manipulate the stimulus onset asynchrony (SOA), that is, the duration of time for which drug-related pictures are presented (i.e., the interval between the onset of picture cues and the onset of the probe). If pictures are presented briefly (e.g., for 200 ms or less),

then any observed attentional biases are likely to represent biases in the *initial orienting* of attention. By contrast, with longer SOAs (e.g., 2,000 ms), the attentional bias index is likely to represent a bias in the *maintenance of attention*. Another distinction has been drawn between relatively fast, automatic shifts of attention (e.g., occurring within 50 to 200 ms of a novel stimulus appearing in the visual field) and deliberate, intentional shifts of attention, which tend to have a slower time course (e.g., Egeth & Yantis, 1997). Therefore, in the context of a visual probe task, if an attentional bias is found when the picture pairs are shown relatively briefly (e.g., 200 ms), this could suggest that rapid, automatic processes may be playing an important role in mediating the attentional bias.

Several studies have demonstrated that addicted individuals have attentional biases for drug-related words or pictures that are presented for as little as 100 or 200 ms, in visual probe- and attentional-cueing tasks (Franken, Kroon, & Hendriks, 2000; Stormark et al., 1997). In addition, Bradley et al. (2004) demonstrated that smokers showed an attentional bias for smoking-related pictures that was not significantly different when pictures were presented for 200 and 2,000 ms. However, in one study, heavy social drinkers did not show an attentional bias for pictorial alcohol-related stimuli presented for 200 ms (Field, Mogg, & Zetteler et al., 2004). The findings of attentional shifts to stimuli that are presented very briefly (e.g., 100 to 200 ms) seem consistent with the predictions made by Franken (2003) and Robinson and Berridge (1993, 2003) that attentional biases are "automatic." However, unlike in the anxiety disorders (discussed below), attentional biases in addiction do not seem to be so automatic in the sense that they are evident for stimuli that are presented below the threshold of conscious awareness. Models of addiction may need to be modified in order to incorporate the data that suggest that attentional biases for drug cues may be limited in the extent of their automaticity. The available evidence, although limited, suggests that attentional biases are not so automatic that drug-related cues are selectively attended to before the drug user is aware of those cues.

Other research implicates both the orienting and the maintenance of attention in attentional biases in addiction. Several studies have used the visual probe task to demonstrate attentional biases for drug-related cues presented for 500 ms in opiate users (Lubman et al., 2000), smokers (Bradley et al., 2003; Ehrman et al., 2002; Hogarth et al., 2003; Waters, Shiffman, Bradley, et al., 2003), cannabis users (Field et al., 2004a), and heavy social drinkers (Field, Mogg, Zetteler, et al., 2004). Similar biases have also been found with a longer SOA of 2,000 ms in smokers (e.g., Bradley et al., 2003; Field et al. (2004b); Field et al., 2005; Mogg et al., 2003, 2005) and social drinkers (Field, Mogg, Zetteler, et al., 2004). The latter exposure time is clearly long enough to permit repeated shifts of attention between drug-related and matched control stimuli, therefore these results are consistent with a bias to maintain attention on drug-related cues.

In addition, in numerous studies in our laboratory, we have monitored smokers' eye movements while they complete the visual probe task with smoking-related and matched control pictures. Eye movement measures have several advantages over other methods of measuring attentional biases—primarily that they provide directly observable and ecologically valid measures of visual orienting. In our studies, we have measured the *direction* of initial fixations when smoking-related and matched control pictures are presented simultaneously, which provides a measure of the initial *orienting* of attention, and the *duration* of fixations to smoking-related and control pictures, which provides a measure of the

maintenance of attention. Therefore, eye movement monitoring permits the measurement of the orienting *and* the maintenance of attention to drug-related stimuli within the same trial. Our research indicated that smokers tended to maintain their gaze for longer on smoking-related pictures than control pictures, whereas nonsmokers did not demonstrate this attentional bias (Mogg et al., 2003). Moreover, in smokers, biases in the maintenance of attention to drug-related cues were associated with subjective drug craving and with behavioral approach tendencies for drug-related cues (Field et al. (2004b); Field et al., 2005; Mogg et al., 2003, 2005), as discussed below.

Cue Approach

According to models of addiction, attentional biases for drug-related cues are only one manifestation of the elevated incentive value of drug-related cues in drug users, as subjective (drug craving) and behavioral (approach behaviors directed toward the drug-related stimuli) responses should also be observed. For example, according to Franken (2003), drug-related cues grab attention, which leads to increased drug-craving and a tendency to direct approach behaviors toward those cues. Several recent studies have investigated the ability of drug-related cues to elicit approach behaviors. Palfai and Ostafin (2003) reported that hazardous levels of alcohol consumption were associated with facilitated approach tendencies for alcohol-related words, and Ostafin et al. (2003) demonstrated that binge drinkers had impaired avoidance tendencies for alcohol-related words. In our laboratory, we have used a novel paradigm, termed the "stimulus response compatibility" (SRC) task, to assess the ability of smoking-related cues to elicit approach behaviors. This task was developed from previous research by De Houwer and colleagues into implicit measures of stimulus valence (e.g., De Houwer et al., 2001). In this task, participants are required to categorize smoking-related and matched control pictures by making symbolic approach or avoidance movements in response to the cues. In several studies using the SRC task (Bradley et al., 2004; Field et al., 2005; Mogg et al., 2003), we demonstrated that smokers were faster to categorize smoking-related pictures when the appropriate response was an approach, rather than an avoidance, movement, which suggests that smokers tend to approach, rather than avoid, smoking-related cues. However, this bias to approach smoking-related cues was either absent (Bradley et al., 2004), or attenuated (Mogg et al., 2003), in nonsmokers, compared to smokers. In the studies where we examined the relationships between indices of attentional bias (i.e., orienting vs. maintenance of gaze) and the bias to approach smoking-related cues, we found that in smokers the approach bias was positively correlated with the maintenance of gaze on smoking-related cues, but not with biased orienting of gaze to those cues (Mogg et al., 2003, 2005). These demonstrations of interrelationships between cue approach and the maintenance of attention on smoking-related cues are theoretically important, and they lend support to incentive models that suggest that attentional bias and cue approach should be interrelated.

Subjective Craving

Drug craving is almost universally regarded as an important subjective correlate of attentional bias for drug-related cues. For example, Franken (2003) proposed that high levels of craving should cause enhanced attentional processing of drug-related stimuli. As will be described below, there is some evidence that demonstrates that drug craving and attentional bias are associated (see also Franken, 2003, for a review of studies that demonstrate a relationship between drug craving and attentional bias).

In smokers, craving increases with increasing periods of nicotine deprivation (Schuh & Stitzer, 1995), and nicotine deprivation enhances attentional biases in smokers (Field et al., 2004b; Gross et al., 1993; Waters & Feyerabend, 2000). Moreover, several studies have demonstrated positive correlations between cigarette craving and various measures of attentional bias, independently of any experimental manipulation of nicotine deprivation (Mogg & Bradley, 2002; Mogg et al., 2003, 2005; Sayette & Hufford, 1994; Waters, Shiffman, & Bradley et al., 2003; Zack et al., 2001). Associations between craving and attentional bias have also been reported in alcoholics (Sayette et al., 1994), cocaine addicts (Rosse et al., 1993; Franken, Kroon, & Hendriks, 2000), and recreational users of cannabis and alcohol (Field et al., 2004a; Field, Mogg, Zetteler, et al., 2004). On the other hand, numerous investigations of attentional bias in addiction either did not measure subjective craving, or did not report correlations between craving and attentional bias measures, whereas other studies have reported that such correlations were not statistically significant (e.g., Ehrman et al., 2002). Nonetheless, the widely replicated association between craving and attentional bias for drug cues across different drug classes suggests that the association is reasonably robust, especially considering that studies differ widely in the tasks used to measure attentional bias, and in the self-report measures of craving that were used (e.g., single item visual analogue scales versus multifactorial questionnaires).

Studies that monitor eye movements to smoking-related cues in smokers suggest that craving may be selectively associated with biases in the maintenance, rather than the initial shift, of overt attention to drug-related cues. In our initial eye movement study

(Mogg et al., 2003), we found that, in smokers, subjective cigarette craving was correlated with biases in the maintenance of gaze on smoking-related pictures. This demonstration of an association between subjective cigarette craving and the maintenance of gaze was subsequently replicated (Mogg et al., 2005). In two further studies, we experimentally manipulated craving by imposing 12 hours of nicotine deprivation (Field et al., 2004b), or by administering a moderate dose of alcohol (Field et al., 2005). In both of these studies, the manipulations were effective, as subjective cigarette craving was elevated by nicotine deprivation and by alcohol. Importantly, in both of these studies, the manipulations were selectively associated with an increased bias in the maintenance of gaze on smoking-related pictures, but they were not associated with an increased bias in the orienting of gaze. Comparable associations were reported by Rosse et al. (1993), who demonstrated that the duration of visual scanning of a cocaine-related cue was positively correlated with subjective cocaine craving, in a sample of cocaine addicts. Therefore, recent evidence suggests that, in cigarette smokers, subjective craving is selectively associated with biased maintenance of attention on drug-related cues, but not with biases in the orienting of attention to those cues.

These demonstrations of a selective association between subjective drug craving and biased maintenance of attention to drug cues, are perhaps not surprising. Drug craving is a subjectively experienced motivational state, and the maintenance of attention is thought to be under the influence of strategic cognitive processes and motivational variables (LaBerge, 1995). However, the initial orienting of attention may occur more automatically and may be strongly influenced by simple stimulus features, such as brightness and color (Egeth & Yantis, 1997).

ATTENTIONAL BIASES FOR NONDRUG INCENTIVE STIMULI AND AVERSIVE STIMULI

This chapter has considered the cognitive processes and correlates of attentional biases in drug addiction. However, attentional biases for concern-relevant stimuli are not exclusively a feature of addiction: Attentional biases are also evident in emotional disorders such as anxiety, as well as for nonpathological motivational states such as hunger. This presents an interesting question: Why are different disorders and motivational states associated with similar cognitive biases? We suggest that closer examination and comparison of the component processes of biases in anxiety and appetitive motivational states (including addiction) reveal that these attentional biases may actually be quite different, and as such, they may be subserved by different underlying mechanisms.

There is evidence that when "normal" appetitive motivational states, such as hunger, are activated, they are associated with an attentional bias for motivationally relevant stimuli. Mogg et al. (1998) and Placanica et al. (2002) used visual probe tasks with food-related and matched control words to assess attentional bias. Both studies reported that hungry individuals demonstrated an enhanced attentional bias for the food-related words (i.e., faster reaction times to respond to probes that replaced food-related words than control words). Interestingly, Mogg et al. (1998) also investigated attentional bias for subliminally presented food-related words in a modified visual probe task in which the word stimuli were briefly presented and then masked before probes were presented. With this task, there was no evidence of a processing bias for the food-related words. Therefore, the limited available evidence suggests that appetitive motivational states such as hunger do not appear to be associated with preconscious processing of motivationally relevant cues (i.e., food cues), which has an interesting parallel with findings from the addiction literature (reviewed above), which have similarly suggested the absence of an attentional bias for subliminally presented drug-related stimuli (see de Jong et al., Chapter 27, for further discussion of motivational influences on cognition).

Cognitive models of anxiety (e.g., Mogg & Bradley, 1998), predict that anxious individuals will show a vigilance-avoidance pattern of attentional biases for highly threatening stimuli. That is, while anxious individuals may initially orient their attention toward threatening stimuli in the environment, this may be followed by a tendency to reduce the maintenance of attention on these stimuli, in order to reduce subjective discomfort. The evidence is broadly supportive of this view. Individuals with anxiety disorders show attentional biases for threatening stimuli that are presented below the threshold of conscious awareness in modified Stroop (e.g., Mogg et al., 1993) and visual probe paradigms (Mogg, et al., 1995). Individuals with anxiety disorders also show biased orienting of gaze (i.e., overt shifts of attention) to threatening rather than control stimuli (Mogg et al., 2000). Furthermore, Bradley et al. (2000) found that individual differences in social anxiety level were correlated with the bias to shift gaze to negative facial expressions rather than positive facial expressions.

However, some studies suggest that after initial orienting of attention to threatening stimuli, anxious individuals show subsequent attentional avoidance of those stimuli. For example, Hermans et al. (1999) found that individuals with spider phobia spent more time viewing pictures of spiders compared to pictures of flowers in the first 500 ms of stimulus presentation, but from 1 s to 3 s they demonstrated reduced maintenance of gaze on the spider pictures. By contrast, a nonfearful control group demonstrated increased maintenance of gaze on the spider pictures, relative to flower pictures, throughout the trial. Using a visual probe task, Mogg and Bradley (in press) found that, in comparison with nonfearful participants, individuals with high levels of spider-fear showed a greater attentional bias for briefly (200 ms) presented spider pictures, and that this bias in the high-fear group significantly reduced as the exposure duration increased, so that it was no longer evident when pictures were presented for 2,000 ms. Rohner (2002) monitored eye movements in response to pairs of emotional faces and found that, after initial orienting to angry faces (in the first 1 s of stimulus presentation), high-trait anxious individuals were more likely than low-anxious individuals to avert their gaze from angry faces (i.e., reduced maintenance of gaze on threat cues in anxious participants in the 2 s to 3 s interval after stimulus onset). In addition, Mogg, Bradley, Miles, et al. (in press) found that individuals with high levels of blood-injury fear showed an attentional bias toward high-threat cues presented for 500 ms in a visual probe task, but avoidance of them when presented for 1,500 ms, which is consistent with a vigilant-avoidant pattern of attentional bias for high-threat cues.

Therefore, when we compare patterns of attentional biases in addiction and in anxiety, several consistent differences are apparent. Addiction appears to be associated with biases in the maintenance of attention on drug-related stimuli (e.g., as reflected by eye movement studies of cigarette smokers, described earlier). However, biases in attention have not so far been found for drug-related stimuli that are presented below the threshold of awareness, and there is evidence that subjective drug craving is associated with biased maintenance of attention on drug-related stimuli. By contrast, research into attentional biases in anxiety suggests a vigilance-avoidance pattern of attentional bias for threat cues: Threatening stimuli are initially oriented to, even when presented below the threshold of conscious awareness, but intense fear-related stimuli are subsequently avoided, such that biases in the maintenance of attention tend to reflect reduced, rather than increased, maintenance of gaze on the stimuli of interest. In addition, individual differences in anxiety appear to be associated with the bias in initial orienting toward concern-related stimuli. These fundamental differences in the types of attentional biases that are associated with addictions and anxiety disorders may imply that these biases have dissociable neural bases. Clarification of the neural basis for attentional biases in different emotional and motivational states is a key target for future research.

TREATMENT IMPLICATIONS

So far, research into attentional biases has mainly focused on evaluating hypotheses that are derived from theories of addiction that predict the existence of these biases, and elucidating the underlying cognitive mechanisms. There has been little research as yet relating to treatment implications. However, this is a potentially important area for further development. For example, recent research suggests that an attentional bias for drug cues may be of clinical significance in predicting treatment outcome (Waters, Shiffman, Sayette, et al., 2003). Furthermore, according to Franken (2003), attentional biases for drug cues may be an important determinant of drug craving, cue approach, and drug-seeking behavior. Therefore, if drug users could be trained to allocate their attention away from drug-related cues, this may in turn reduce their craving and drug-seeking behavior. Such attentional training could be extended to "high-risk" situations, thereby reducing craving and the risk of relapse to drug-taking in these situations. According to Franken's model, such an approach may not prevent drug-related cues from attracting attentional resources in the first instance, but it may prevent this attentional bias from growing in strength and provoking further increases in drug craving.

CONCLUDING COMMENTS

In this chapter, we have discussed the component processes of attentional biases in addiction, and how these may be related to cue approach, and drug craving. Although this is a relatively new area of research, the evidence to date suggests that attentional biases in addiction do not appear to operate preconsciously, and that drug craving and cue approach may be primarily associated with biases in the maintenance of attention to drug-related cues. Consideration of the cognitive mechanisms that mediate attentional biases in addiction, normal appetitive motivational states, and emotional states and disorders, such as anxiety, suggests that appetitive and aversive motivational states may be associated with biases in different components of selective attention. This in turn suggests that there may be important distinctions between the underlying cognitive and neural bases for attentional biases in these different disorders.

REFERENCES

Allport, A. (1989). Visual attention. In M. I. Posner (Ed.), *Foundations of cognitive science* (pp. 631–682). Cambridge, MA: MIT Press.

Baker, T. B., Brandon, T. H., & Chassin, L. (2004). Motivational influences on cigarette smoking. *Annual Review of Psychology, 55,* 463–491.

Baker, T. B., Piper, M. E., McCarthy, D. E., Majeskie, M. R., & Fiore, M. C. (2004). Addiction motivation reformulated: An affective processing model of negative reinforcement. *Psychological Review, 111,* 33–51.

Bradley, B. P., Field, M., Mogg, K., & De Houwer, J. (2004). Attentional and evaluative biases for smoking cues in nicotine dependence: Component processes of biases in visual orienting. *Behavioural Pharmacology, 15,* 29–36.

Bradley, B. P., Mogg, K., & Millar, N. (2000). Covert and overt orienting of attention to emotional faces in anxiety. *Cognition & Emotion, 14,* 789–808.

Bradley, B. P., Mogg, K., Wright, T., & Field, M. (2003). Attentional bias in drug dependence: Vigilance for cigarette-related cues in smokers. *Psychology of Addictive Behaviours, 17,* 66–72.

Carter, B. L., & Tiffany, S. T. (1999). Meta-analysis of cue reactivity in addiction research. *Addiction, 94,* 327–340.

Cox, W. M., & Klinger, E. (2004). A motivational model of alcohol use: Determinants of use and change. In W. M. Cox & E. Klinger (Eds.), Handbook of motivational counseling: Concepts, approaches, and assessment (pp. 121–138). Chichester, UK: Wiley.

De Houwer, J., Crombez, G., Baeyens, F., & Hermans, D. (2001). On the generality of the affective Simon effect. *Cognition & Emotion, 15,* 189–206.

Egeth, H. E., & Yantis, S. (1997). Visual attention: Control, representation, and time course. *Annual Review of Psychology, 48,* 269–297.

Ehrman, R. N., Robbins, S. J., Bromwell, M. A., Lankford, M. E., Monterosso, J. R., & O'Brien, C. P. (2002). Comparing attentional bias to smoking cues in current smokers, former smokers, and non-smokers using a dot-probe task. *Drug and Alcohol Dependence, 67,* 185–191.

Field, M., Mogg, K., & Bradley, B. P. (2004a). Cognitive bias and drug craving in recreational cannabis users. *Drug and Alcohol Dependence, 74,* 105–111.

Field, M., Mogg, K., & Bradley, B. P. (2004b). Eye movements to smoking-related cues: Effects of nicotine deprivation. *Psychopharmacology, 173,* 116–123.

Field, M., Mogg, K., & Bradley, B. P. (2005). Alcohol increases cognitive biases for smoking cues in smokers. *Psychopharmacology, 180,* 63–72.

Field, M., Mogg, K., Zetteler, J., & Bradley, B. P. (2004). Attentional biases for alcohol cues in heavy and light social drinkers: The roles of initial orienting and maintained attention. *Psychopharmacology, 176,* 88–93.

Franken, I. H. A. (2003). Drug craving and addiction: Integrating psychological and neuropsychopharmacological approaches. *Progress in Neuro-Psychopharmacology & Biological Psychiatry, 27,* 563–579.

Franken, I. H. A., Kroon, L. Y., & Hendriks, V. M. (2000). Influence of individual differences in craving and obsessive cocaine thoughts on attentional processes in cocaine abuse patients. *Addictive Behaviors, 25,* 99–102.

Franken, I. H. A., Kroon, L. Y., Wiers, R. W., & Jansen, A. (2000). Selective cognitive processing of drug cues in heroin dependence. *Journal of Psychopharmacology, 14,* 395–400.

Gross, T. M., Jarvik, M. E., & Rosenblatt, M. R. (1993). Nicotine abstinence produces context-specific Stroop interference. *Psychopharmacology, 110,* 333–336.

Hermans, D., Vansteenwegen, D., & Eelen, P. (1999). Eye movement registration as a continuous index of attention deployment: Data from a group of spider anxious students. *Cognition & Emotion, 13,* 419–434.

Hogarth, L. C., Mogg, K., Bradley, B. P., Duka, T., & Dickinson, T. (2003). Attentional orienting towards smoking-related stimuli. *Behavioural Pharmacology, 14,* 153–160.

Jonides, J. (1981). Voluntary versus automatic control over the mind's eye movements. In J. Long & A. Baddeley (Eds.), *Attention and performance IX* (pp. 187–203). Hillsdale, NJ: Lawrence Erlbaum.

Kowler, E. (1995). Eye movements. In S. M. Kosslyn & D. M Osheron (Eds.), *Visual cognition* (pp. 215–265). Cambridge, MA: Harvard University Press.

LaBerge, D. (1995). *Attentional processing.* Cambridge, MA: Harvard University Press.

Lubman, D. I., Peters, L. A., Mogg, K., Bradley, B. P., & Deakin, J. F. W. (2000). Attentional bias for drug cues in opiate dependence. *Psychological Medicine, 30,* 169–175.

McCusker, C. G. (2001). Cognitive biases and addiction: An evolution in theory and method. *Addiction, 96,* 47–56.

Mogg, K., & Bradley, B. P. (1998). A cognitive-motivational analysis of anxiety. *Behaviour Research and Therapy, 36,* 809–848.

Mogg, K., & Bradley, B. P. (2002). Selective processing of smoking-related cues in smokers: Manipulation of deprivation level and comparison of three measures of processing bias. *Journal of Psychopharmacology, 16,* 385–392.

Mogg, K., & Bradley, B. P. (in press). Time course of attentional bias for fear-relevant stimuli in spider-fearful individuals. *Behaviour Research and Therapy.*

Mogg, K., Bradley, B. P., Field, M., & De Houwer, J. (2003). Eye movements to smoking-related pictures in smokers: Relationship between attentional biases and implicit and explicit measures of stimulus valence. *Addiction, 98,* 825–836.

Mogg, K., Bradley, B. P., Hyare, H., & Lee, S. (1998). Selective attention to food-related stimuli in hunger: Are attentional biases specific to emotional and psychopathological states, or are they also found in normal drive states? *Behavior Research and Therapy, 36,* 227–237.

Mogg, K., Bradley, B. P., Miles, F., & Dixon, R. (in press). Time course of attentional bias for threat scenes: Testing the vigilance-avoidance hypothesis. *Cognition & Emotion.*

Mogg, K., Bradley, B. P., & Williams, R. (1995). Attentional bias in anxiety and depression: The role of awareness. *British Journal of Clinical Psychology, 34,* 17–36.

Mogg, K., Bradley, B. P., Williams, R., & Mathews, A. (1993). Subliminal processing of emotional information in anxiety and depression. *Journal of Abnormal Psychology, 102,* 304–311.

Mogg, K., Field, M., & Bradley, B. P. (2005). Attentional and evaluative biases for smoking cues in smokers: An investigation of competing theoretical views of addiction. *Psychopharmacology, 180,* 333–341.

Mogg, K., Millar, N., & Bradley, B. P. (2000). Biases in eye movements to threatening facial expressions in generalized anxiety disorder and depressive disorder. *Journal of Abnormal Psychology, 109,* 695–704.

Munafo, M., Mogg, K., Roberts, S., Bradley, B. P., & Murphy, M. (2003). Attentional bias in cigarette smokers, ex-smokers and never-smokers on the modified Stroop task. *Journal of Psychopharmacology, 17,* 311–317.

Ostafin, B. D., Palfai, T. P., & Wechsler, C. E. (2003). The accessibility of motivational tendencies towards alcohol: Approach, avoidance, and disinhibited drinking. *Experimental & Clinical Psychopharmacology, 11,* 294–301.

Palfai, T. P., & Ostafin, B. D. (2003). Alcohol-related motivational tendencies in hazardous drinkers: Assessing implicit response tendencies using the modified-IAT. *Behaviour Research and Therapy, 41,* 1149–1162.

Placanica, J. L., Faunce, G. J., & Job, R. F. S. (2002). The effect of fasting on attentional biases for food and body shape/weight words in high and low eating disorder inventory scorers. *International Journal of Eating Disorders, 32,* 79–90.

Robinson, T. E., & Berridge, K. C., (1993). The neural basis of drug craving: An incentive-sensitisation theory of addiction. *Brain Research Reviews, 18,* 247–291.

Robinson, T. E., & Berridge, K. C. (2003). Addiction. *Annual Review of Psychology, 54,* 25–53.

Rohner, J. C. (2002). The time-course of visual threat processing: High trait anxious individuals eventually avert their gaze from angry faces. *Cognition & Emotion, 16,* 837–844.

Rosse, R. B., Miller, M. W., Hess, A. L., Alim, T. N., & Deutsch, S. I. (1993). Measures of visual scanning as a predictor of cocaine cravings and urges. *Biological Psychiatry, 33,* 554–556.

Ryan, F. (2002). Detected, selected, and sometimes neglected: Cognitive processing of cues in addiction. *Experimental & Clinical Psychopharmacology, 10,* 67–76.

Sayette, M. A., & Hufford, M. R. (1994). Effects of cue exposure and deprivation on cognitive resources in smokers. *Journal of Abnormal Psychology, 103,* 812–818.

Sayette, M. A., Monti, P. M., Rohsenow, D. J., Gulliver, S. B., Colby, S. M., Sirota, A. D., et al. (1994). The effects of cue exposure on reaction time in male alcoholics. *Journal of Studies on Alcohol, 55,* 629–633.

Sayette, M., Shiffman, S., Tiffany, S. T., Niaura, R. S., Martin, C. S., & Shadel, W. G. (2000). The measurement of drug craving. *Addiction, 95(Suppl. 2),* S189–S210.

Schuh, K. J., & Stitzer, M. L. (1995). Desire to smoke during spaced smoking intervals. *Psychopharmacology, 120,* 289–295.

Stewart, J., de Wit, H., & Eikelboom, R. (1984). The role of conditioned and unconditioned drug effects in the self-administration of opiates and stimulants. *Psychological Review, 91,* 251–268.

Stormark, K. M., Field, N. P., Hugdahl, K., & Horowitz, M. (1997). Selective processing of visual alcohol cues in abstinent alcoholics: An approach-avoidance conflict. *Addictive Behaviors, 22,* 509–519.

Tomie, A. (1996). Locating reward cue at response manipulandum (CAM) induces symptoms of drug abuse. *Neuroscience & Biobehavioral Reviews, 20,* 505–535.

Waters, A. J., & Feyerabend, C. (2000). Determinants and effects of attentional bias in smokers. *Psychology of Addictive Behaviors, 14,* 111–120.

Waters, A. J., Shiffman, S., Bradley, B. P., & Mogg, K. (2003). Attentional shifts to smoking cues in smokers. *Addiction, 98,* 1409–1417.

Waters, A. J., Shiffman, S., Sayette, M. A., Paty, J. A., Gwaltney, C. J., & Balabanis, M. H. (2003). Attentional bias predicts outcome in smoking cessation. *Health Psychology, 22,* 378–387.

Wikler, A. (1948). Recent progress in research on the neurophysiological basis of morphine addiction. *American Journal of Psychiatry, 105,* 329–338.

Zack, M., Belsito, L., Scher, R., Eissenberg, T., & Corrigall, W. A. (2001). Effects of abstinence and smoking on information processing in adolescent smokers. *Psychopharmacology, 153,* 249–257.

Section III

BRAIN MECHANISMS

CHAPTER 12

Addiction and Learning in the Brain

HENRY H. YIN AND BARBARA J. KNOWLTON

Abstract: Addiction can be viewed as a maladaptive form of learning. This chapter discusses the relevant types of learning implicated in addiction and their neural substrates. First, we describe the associative structures of various learning processes—abstract descriptions of the content of learning based on behavioral studies. We then attempt to link various types of adaptive behavior and their modification by distinct learning processes to specific neural substrates. In particular, we argue that parallel but interacting cortico-basal ganglia networks in the cerebrum provide the neural implementations of associative structures from learning theory, and that abnormal interactions between these networks could result in addictive behavior. Finally, we discuss the implications of such a conceptual framework for our understanding of addiction.

INTRODUCTION

Learning through experience is critical for producing adaptive behavior. Addiction, however, is a maladaptive manifestation of the brain's capacity to change as a result of experience. In this chapter, we discuss the different types of learning implicated in addiction and their neural substrates.

Addictive drugs can cause long-term changes in the same brain regions involved in learning reinforced by natural rewards such as food and sex. Although there is now much knowledge about how drugs alter the functioning of neurons at the cellular and molecular level (Berke & Hyman, 2000; Gerdeman et al., 2003), it remains unclear how such alterations lead to the behavioral phenomena that comprise addiction. A coherent conceptual framework can only emerge once we understand the global processes implicated in addiction at the level of behavior. What kinds of behavioral changes are induced by the taking of addictive drugs? How can they be classified? And what are the physiological mechanisms underlying these changes? As these questions suggest, the analysis of behavior is a crucial step in bridging findings from the neuroscience laboratory to the clinic.

Consider an organism that learns to perform actions for rewards. For example, a rat may learn to press a lever for food or cocaine. In this simple situation, three different types of learning can be discerned. First, the rat may learn the relationship between its action (A) and the outcome (O)

(A-O association). In other words, it may learn that pressing the lever leads to a certain reward. Second, the rat can also learn, at the same time, an association between the environmental stimuli (S) and the response (R) (S-R association). For example, an association may be formed between the cues in the testing chamber and the lever press, so that these cues can automatically elicit the response. In this case, the behavior is not produced because it leads to food, but rather "habitually." And finally, the testing chamber cues can be associated with the reward directly. This is designated as a Pavlovian stimulus-outcome, or S-O association. The environmental stimuli function as Pavlovian conditional stimuli predicting reward. In our example, the rat will produce preparatory responses when it is in the chamber where reward is expected, for example, salivation if the reward was food, or physiological changes that ready the body for cocaine.

These abstract descriptions of learning (A-O, S-R, and S-O), also called associative structures, are based on many decades of experimental work using Pavlovian and instrumental conditioning (Bolles, 1972). It is likely that all three processes take place as an individual gains experience with drugs. We will describe how these different types of learning can be experimentally dissociated in the laboratory and how they inform the study of addiction.

PREDICTION AND CONTROL: THE PAVLOVIAN/ INSTRUMENTAL DISTINCTION

In the study of learning, a critical distinction exists between Pavlovian conditioning and instrumental learning. Pavlovian conditioning is the paradigmatic type of stimulus-stimulus associative learning that takes advantage of the largely innate reflexes, or unconditional responses (URs), to biologically salient events such as reward or pain. Because these URs can easily be measured in the laboratory, Pavlov was able to use them to study the fundamental processes underlying associative learning in general. In appetitive Pavlovian conditioning, with which we are concerned, the association in question is that between a stimulus and a reward.

By contrast, in instrumental learning, not only does the animal encode the relationship between actions and their outcomes, it is also able to exert control over its own actions, thereby controlling the occurrence of the outcomes (Balleine & Dickinson, 1998). Thus, the instrumentally controlled action (A) is to be distinguished from all other responses, such as habits and reflexes. In Pavlovian learning, the conditional response elicited (CR) does not cause the outcome, but merely prepares for it. For instance, a dog learns that the sound of a bell predicts food and salivates to the bell, but this response merely prepares for the food consumption that is to follow. Because these Pavlovian responses are not instrumentally controlled by the action-outcome (A-O) contingency, they persist even when that contingency is reversed, that is, when food is taken away whenever the CR is generated (Hershberger, 1986; Holland, 1979). This manipulation, called omission, is a litmus test for assessing the "instrumentality" of a particular behavior. But it should be pointed out that in the natural world, the salivation response to predictors of food is usually followed by food, since there is no mischievous experimenter to reverse this relationship that has operated for millions of years on the evolution of the organism. Hence the innateness of these Pavlovian responses, which are phylogenetically "stamped in" by regularities in the natural world.

From Actions to Habits

Within the class of instrumental actions, a further distinction can be made between goal-directed actions controlled by the explicit expectancy of the outcome and stimulus-driven habits controlled by antecedent stimuli. This distinction between actions and habits has yet to be widely recognized, but it has far-reaching implications for the study of addiction.

Goal-directed actions are intentional, deliberate actions performed to achieve an outcome. In A-O learning, the action is mediated by the belief that it will lead to a specific outcome that is desired by the organism. As such, changes in outcome value as well as the causal efficacy of the action are expected to change performance (Dickinson & Balleine, 1993). If an outcome is no longer desired, or if the action fails to predict the previously experienced outcome, the action should decrease in frequency. For example, if the behavior of the drug user was controlled by an A-O relationship between drug seeking and the effects of the drug, he would stop seeking drugs after experiencing harmful consequences. To be considered goal-directed, then, performance must be sensitive to changes in outcome value as well as to changes in the A-O contingency (Dickinson & Balleine, 1993).

Behavioral assays have been developed to dissociate goal-directed actions from habits (Dickinson, 2000). For example, a rat may be trained to perform two actions, each yielding a distinct reward. After training, one of the rewards can be devalued by prefeeding that reward to satiety (Dickinson, 2000). This procedure is known as outcome devaluation. When tested without the delivery of reinforcers (to ensure that any change in behavior is due to existing knowledge), if the rat selectively reduces performance of the action earning the devalued reward relative to the other action, then its behavior is under the control of the A-O contingency. On the other hand, degradation, like omission, is a direct manipulation of the instrumental contingency. Just as devaluation reduces the value of the outcome, so degradation reduces the causal relationship between action and outcome by equating the rate of reward in the presence and in the absence of action. This manipulation is also expected to reduce performance if the behavior is goal-directed.

Unlike Pavlovian CRs, S-R habits involve arbitrary actions that are nonspecific, rather than preparatory responses linked to specific rewards (e.g., leg flexion rather than salivation). Like Pavlovian CRs, however, habits are not controlled by the expectancy of the outcome. They persist even if the outcome is no longer desirable. For example, a drug user who persists in seeking drugs despite having experienced harmful consequences shows behavior similar to the observed behavior of animals after habit formation.

According to current views on instrumental learning, habit formation takes place in parallel with A-O learning and, under certain conditions, can assume control over instrumental behavior. The amount of training appears to be an important variable in this regard. In a pioneering study, Adams found that overtraining produced responding impervious to outcome devaluation, whereas moderate training did not (Adams, 1982). This shift in the control of behavior after extensive training was interpreted as an instance of habit formation. It was also shown that this change in sensitivity to devaluation was not simply due to the number of responses performed, but rather to the number of rewarded responses—a finding in accord with the traditional idea that S-R associations are stamped in by subsequence reinforcement.

In addition, the schedule of reinforcement also determines variations in sensitivity to outcome devaluation. Two classes of such schedules are commonly used. In ratio schedules, each response is rewarded according to a fixed or variable probability; more responses earn more rewards. In interval schedules, the additional requirement of time is in place, so that only the first response after a scheduled time interval is rewarded, and all responses during that interval are futile. This is also a common feedback function: for example, checking one's e-mail many times a day will not lead to more messages than checking it once during the average interval between messages.

A well-controlled comparison of the schedules demonstrated that interval schedules produce habitual responding whereas ratio schedules do not (Dickinson et al., 1983). The difference in sensitivity to changes in outcome value must therefore be due to differences in the schedules used. As the correlation between behavior and reward is high in ratio schedules but low in interval schedules (Baum, 1973), the lack of exposure to the A-O contingency under interval schedules could result in poorer acquisition of the A-O association (Dickinson, 1989).

Although the underlying mechanisms remain unknown, this finding suggests that drug-taking is more likely to become habitual under an interval schedule of reinforcement. For example, if the reinforcing effects of a drug are similar during a period of time regardless of how frequently drug-seeking actions were initiated during that period, this situation could promote more habit formation than if each drug-seeking behavior led to a fixed amount of reinforcement. Differences in the ability to transfer actions into habits could possibly contribute to individual differences in the predisposition to become addicted to drugs.

MULTIPLE-SYSTEMS PERSPECTIVE

From the above outline of the associative structures of three different learning processes, S-O, A-O, and S-R (see Table 12.1), we may summarize the three functional systems as follows: Pavlovian responses are not modified by their consequences because they are relatively fixed responses to certain biologically salient stimuli and predictors of such stimuli. On the other hand, instrumental actions are modified by their consequences, via instrumental learning, but in two very different ways. Habit formation involves the strengthening of an S-R association by subsequent reward. By contrast, the A-O system involves the encoding of specific features of the outcome, including its value, which controls the performance of the action. Although these different processes can be dissociated, in many situations they tend to interact, and it is their interaction that sheds light on the problem of addiction.

Researchers have long suggested that different types of learning have different neural substrates. According to an influential proposal by Mishkin et al. (1984), the hippocampus is involved in cognitive learning (such as stimulus-stimulus associations), whereas the striatum is involved in S-R learning. Although not explicitly discussed by Mishkin, A-O associations would be an example of cognitive learning in that these associations can flexibly direct behavior. According to this view, the hippocampus plays a role in learning but is not the ultimate storage site of cognitive memories.

A set of studies using the cross maze (Restle, 1957) produced evidence in support of Mishkin et al.'s (1984) claim of a dissociation between learning systems (Packard & McGaugh, 1996). For example, rats were trained to start in the south arm of the maze and make a left turn to enter the west arm to find food. Whether the rats were learning the location of the food or simply a left-turn habit was tested by now starting the rat in the north arm. If the rat turns to the left, it will enter the east arm, whereas to reach the food (in the west arm) it will need to make a right turn—a different and non-habitual response. Using this task, Packard and McGaugh showed that, after moderate training, most rats used the place strategy when

Table 12.1 Different functional systems characterized by different learning processes

Associative structure	Definition	Behavioral criteria
Stimulus-outcome (S-O)	Pavlovian association between a neutral stimulus and its biologically salient outcome: a type of stimulus-stimulus association.	Insensitive to manipulation of A-O contingency, e.g., omission. Unconditional response (UR) to biologically salient stimulus (US).
Action-outcome (A-O)	Association between a self-generated action and its outcome: e.g., lever press → food. A type of declarative knowledge traditionally described as a "belief" in folk psychology. Only received adequate experimental analysis in the last two decades.	Sensitive to manipulation of A-O contingency. Sensitive to post-training change in outcome value (e.g., devaluation). Rapid acquisition, promoted by the use of two outcomes and feedback schedules with high A-O contingency such as ratio schedules.
Stimulus-response (S-R)	Association between a stimulus and a response, thought to be strengthened by a subsequent reward (law of effect). Also known as habits, and formerly believed to control all instrumental responses.	Reduced sensitivity to manipulation of A-O relation. Insensitive to post-training change in outcome value (e.g., devaluation). Gradual acquisition, promoted by extended training and by feedback schedules with reduced exposure to A-O contingency such as interval schedules.

tested, but after extensive training they switched to a response strategy. This finding is consistent with the idea that overtraining produces habitual responding. Moreover, with inactivation of the dorsal part of the striatum, the rats tended to use the place strategy despite overtraining, but inactivation of the hippocampus had the opposite effect—so that the response strategy was used more frequently even early in training (Packard & McGaugh, 1996). In other words, the seemingly same behavior (maze running) could be under different types of control (by different parts of the brain), and a behavioral assay could be used to identify the type of control in question.

A similar dissociation was also discovered in humans. Knowlton et al. (1996) examined the performance of Parkinson's patients on a weather prediction task, in which multiple stimuli (cues) are associated with one of two responses (sun or rain key), and feedback was given after each trial. Each stimulus is only probabilistically associated with the right outcome (akin to partial reinforcement). Patients with Parkinson's disease were impaired on this task, though they showed normal explicit memory for the test. Parkinson's disease results in the depletion of dopamine from the striatum due to cell death in the substantia nigra. As the dorsal part of the striatum has the highest concentration of dopamine receptors in the brain, it is probably where the lack of dopamine innervation found in Parkinson's disease would have the most striking effects, suggesting that dopamine input to the dorsal striatum in particular could be involved in S-R learning.

BEYOND HABIT LEARNING IN THE DORSAL STRIATUM

The dorsal striatum has long been known to be involved in instrumental responses (Divac et al., 1967; Konorski, 1967). These early studies, however, were performed without the benefit of the contemporary distinction between actions and habits in the analysis of instrumental conditioning. Because the dorsal striatum is a large and heterogeneous structure receiving input from the entire cerebral cortex, the question naturally arises as to whether, like the cortex itself, it is also functionally specialized.

Previous studies have established that the lateral region of the dorsal striatum differs from the medial region in connectivity, distribution of various receptors, and mechanisms of synaptic plasticity (Joel & Weiner, 2000; Partridge et al., 2000; West et al., 1990). This raises the possibility that the lateral and medial regions within the dorsal striatum can be functionally dissociated— that, for example, the dorsolateral striatum (DLS) is involved in S-R learning whereas the dorsomedial striatum (DMS) is involved in A-O learning.

Yin et al. (2004) took advantage of the established differences between ratio and interval feedback schedules to examine the neural substrates of A-O and S-R learning. They examined the effects of dorsolateral striatal lesions on S-R learning using interval schedules known to generate habitual learning insensitive to outcome devaluation. After training, the reward (sucrose solution) was then devalued in all rats by inducing a taste aversion to it. The key test came when these rats were returned to the chamber. Lever pressing of control rats was not reduced by devaluation, as expected. In contrast, though rats with pretraining lesions to the DLS could learn to press a lever for sucrose solution normally, they reduced responding after devaluation relative to the controls. These results suggest that, their habit system having been disrupted by the lesion, they learned the response as a goal-directed action.

To assess the role of the DMS in A-O learning, Yin et al. (in press) used a training procedure with two actions and two outcomes under variable ratio schedules. As shown in many behavioral studies, such a training schedule results in behavior that is clearly controlled by the expectancy of the outcome (Colwill & Rescorla, 1986). One area of the DMS, the posterior dorsomedial striatum (pDMS), which receives projections from both medial prefrontal cortical areas involved in planning as well as from limbic regions such as the basolateral amygdala, was shown to be a critical substrate for the acquisition and expression of goal-directed actions. Both pretraining and post-training lesions of the pDMS abolished sensitivity to devaluation and degradation, and reversible inactivation of this area selectively abolished sensitivity of performance to degradation and devaluation. The pDMS, then, appears to be a crucial neural substrate for the learning and expression of goal-directed actions.

In another study, it was shown that the pDMS is also involved in flexible responding based on place cues (Yin & Knowlton, 2004). After pretraining lesions, rats were trained to retrieve food from the west arm of the maze, starting from the south arm, by turning left at the choice point. Unlike the other groups, most of the rats in the pDMS group turned left, using the response strategy on both probe tests, and unable to use place cues to guide behavior flexibly. This conclusion is in accord with a growing body of work showing the role of the DMS in flexible responding (Devan & White, 1999; Gold, 2003). Note that the key manipulation in the place/response procedure, namely the probe test with the opposite starting point, is similar to a reversal in the A-O contingency. Previously, a particular turn would lead to the arm with food, but with the 180-degree rotation of the starting point, the same turn would lead to the previously unreinforced arm. Therefore, it is not surprising that lever-pressing controlled by the instrumental contingency shares common neural substrates with the use of the place strategy on the maze.

To summarize, lesions or inactivation of the pDMS disrupt the goal-directed neural circuit involved in A-O learning, under conditions that usually lead to the learning of flexible and instrumentally controlled behavior. Insensitivity to devaluation and degradation as well as the predominant use of the response strategy characterize habits in general. Together, these findings are in accord with previous studies suggesting a role of the associative striatum in working memory and outcome expectancy (Divac et al., 1978; Levy et al., 1997), and falsify the hypothesis that the dorsal striatum, as a whole, mediates S-R habit learning.

DIVIDING THE BRAIN

It should be clear from the above discussion that the traditional contrast between hippocampus-dependent learning and striatum-dependent learning (Mishkin et al., 1984) is inadequate. In fact, as recent studies have shown, even within the hippocampus, the dorsal and ventral regions can be functionally dissociated (Bannerman et al., 2004). At the level of behavior, there appears to be more heterogeneity *within rather than between* structures like the hippocampus and the striatum. We therefore need to reconsider the overall conceptual framework provided by the generally accepted account of multiple memory systems, an account largely based upon traditional anatomical entities dating back hundreds of years.

According to the most comprehensive model of brain organization available, projection neurons in the cerebrum can be divided into two large classes by the type of neurotransmitter they carry: The glutamate-containing cells are found in the cortex, whereas the GABA-containing cells are found in the nuclei. The nuclei (or basal ganglia) can be further divided into the striatum and the pallidum (Swanson, 2000). Each part—cortex, striatum, and pallidum—is a large and highly heterogeneous structure, and all cerebral structures can be reclassified as one of these three classes. Regardless of the controversial details in this model, its most prominent feature is the emphasis on the cortico-nuclei motif, the logic of which is the basis of the parallel loops model of the basal ganglia (Alexander & Crutcher, 1990). In other words, a *cortico-basal ganglia (cortico-BG) network is the fundamental motif of cerebral organization* (see Figure 12.1).

The cortical component is the major source of influence on the striatal component, which in turn controls the pallidal component, which is of course then capable of reentering the thalamocortical network as well as directly controlling brainstem motor control networks and other limbic structures implicated in arousal. Undoubtedly, each of these structures, by virtue of unique physiological properties, has unique "computational" properties, but at the level of behavior what matters is the integrated functioning of a distributed network comprising various elements. A cerebral circuit is a network consisting of different cortical, striatal, and pallidal components. The integration of various physiological processes within these components results in the output of the network, and only this output is behaviorally "meaningful" and detectable by behavioral assays.

The corticostriatal projections are organized by cortical regions so that, roughly, the limbic cortex projects to the limbic striatum (mainly the nucleus accumbens), the

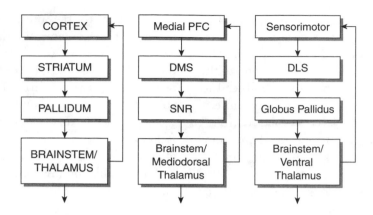

Figure 12.1 Schematic illustration of the cortico-basal ganglia motif. The cortico-basal ganglia motif is the basic functional unit of cerebral organization at the level of behavior. Two examples of this organization are given for the associative and sensorimotor networks. DMS (dorsomedial striatum), PFC (prefrontal cortex), SNR (substantia nigra pars reticulata), DLS (dorsolateral striatum). Note that there is considerable overlap between these networks, which is not emphasized in the illustrations.

association cortex projects to the dorsomedial, or associative, striatum, and the sensorimotor cortex projects to the dorsolateral or sensorimotor striatum (Reep et al., 2003). Likewise, the cerebrum can be divided into three major functional networks—limbic, associative, and sensorimotor (Figure 12.2). Each network has a labile set of components including cortical, striatal, and pallidal structures. Seen in this light, DLS and DMS, by virtue of their different patterns of connectivity, are to be classified as different components in different cortico-BG networks. The dorsal striatum is functionally specialized because the DLS and the DMS mediate different functions. But because they do so as critical components in larger cortico-BG circuits, the respective functions in question, for example, A-O learning and S-R learning, are widely distributed.

According to the present framework, neural activity within a given network during behavior tends to be similar. For example, if the dorsolateral prefrontal cortex exhibits certain properties when the animal is performing a task, the caudate nucleus (DMS),

the main striatal component of this network, is then expected to exhibit similar activity. Between networks, however, the neural correlates of behavioral variables are expected to show important differences, which should reflect the differences between the respective functions of these networks in behavior. Much evidence has already been accumulated in support of this general claim, and we will briefly review some of the relevant data.

LIMBIC NETWORK (S-O)

Further divisions within this network are not only possible but likely, but with the limited data available these are lumped together (Cardinal et al., 2002). In general, the limbic network is involved in assigning value to objects in the world and maintaining such value in memory.

The basolateral amygdala (BLA) complex appears to be a critical substrate for S-O learning, especially for associating a neutral stimulus with the incentive significance of the reward (Cardinal et al., 2002).

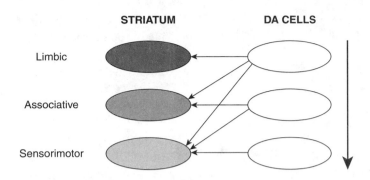

Figure 12.2 Schematic illustration of the hierarchical organization of the cortico-BG networks and a possibility for interaction between different networks. Interactions between levels could be implemented by the reciprocal connections between the striatum and the dopamine (DA) cells in the substantia nigra.

BLA-lesioned rats are also incapable of assigning incentive values to specific rewards: As they cannot tell whether one food is more valuable than another, their choice behavior is also impaired by this fundamental deficit (Balleine et al., 2003). Similarly, the orbitofrontal cortex is also critical in S-O learning. The activation of projections from the orbitofrontal cortex to the nucleus accumbens are closely tied to the expression of addictive behaviors (see Kalivas, 2004, for a review). Neural activity in the orbitofrontal cortex can represent the value of rewards, and can be modulated by the current motivational state (Rolls, 2000). This area appears to be involved in higher-order integration of the properties of rewards (as well as punishers), and could play an important role in how emotion directs instrumental behavior (Bechara, 2004). The BLA and the orbitofrontal cortex appear to be complementary structures involved in a similar function. It is not clear, however, which subcortical components participate in this network functionally, though they probably include structures such as the basal nucleus of the stria terminalis, the centromedial amygdala, as well as parts of the ventral striatum.

There is, in addition, considerable evidence suggesting that the "energizing" of instrumental behavior by a Pavlovian conditioned stimulus, a phenomenon known as Pavlovian-instrumental transfer, also depends on the limbic network. Although Pavlovian conditioning does not involve voluntary responses, the presence of a Pavlovian-conditioned stimulus can facilitate learned instrumental responses. This transfer of incentive from one motivation system to another appears to depend on the nucleus accumbens. Lesions of the accumbens do not impair Pavlovian S-O learning or instrumental A-O learning, but specifically abolish the energizing of instrumental learning by the Pavlovian CS (Corbit et al., 2001). While the Pavlovian S-O system itself is characterized by limited flexibility in its motor outputs (e.g., CRs lack instrumental control by the A-O contingency), it is able to exert control over the instrumental action system, and the ventral striatum appears to be a critical locus at which this process takes place. Interestingly, it has been shown that previous exposure to amphetamine enhances Pavlovian-incentive transfer (Wyvell & Berridge, 2001). Thus, experience with drugs may facilitate this interaction between the S-O system and instrumental behavior.

ASSOCIATIVE NETWORK (A-O)

The entire dorsal striatum, and its cortical connections, can be viewed as the substrate of instrumental actions. But within this larger system, a clear division can be established between the associative and sensorimotor networks, corresponding to the A-O and S-R systems, respectively.

As already discussed, the associative striatum (or DMS, akin to the caudate nucleus in primates) is important for A-O learning. This region is heavily connected with the prefrontal cortex, and considerable evidence shows that the prefrontal cortex is also involved in A-O learning (Balleine & Dickinson, 1998; Corbit & Balleine, 2003; Leon & Shadlen, 1999; Tsujimoto & Sawaguchi, 2002; Tsujimoto & Sawaguchi, 2004a, 2004b). Moreover, the associative striatum in primates (i.e., caudate nucleus) is involved in working memory (Levy et al., 1997; Lewis et al., 2004). Lesions of the head of the caudate, impair performance on spatial delayed response and delayed alternation tasks (Divac et al., 1967; Divac et al., 1978; Levy et al., 1997). Like the prefrontal cortex (Leon & Shadlen, 1999), caudate activity is also strongly modulated by anticipation of reward. Such anticipatory firing is only found when the monkey performs an action that yields a reward (Hassani et al., 2001). Studies of monkeys performing a saccade task have observed that neural activity in the caudate is modulated by reward expectancy (Hikosaka et al., 2000; Kawagoe et al., 1998). Thus, the associative network mediates transient retrospective memory of actions, and prospective memory, or expectancy, of actions and outcomes (Barraclough et al., 2004; Haruno et al., 2004; Konorski, 1967). This network is characterized by great representational flexibility (Leon & Shadlen, 1999; Wallis & Miller, 2003). The respective roles of the prefrontal cortex and the associative striatum in goal-directed actions, however, remain to be clarified.

SENSORIMOTOR NETWORK (S-R)

The sensorimotor network comprises the sensorimotor cortices and their targets in the basal ganglia, beginning with the dorsolateral striatum, which is the equivalent of the putamen in primates. The outputs of this circuit are directed at motor cortices generally, via reentry into the thalamocortical network, and at brain stem motor networks. In monkeys, putamen neurons displayed more movement-related activity than caudate neurons (Kanazawa et al., 1993; Kimura et al., 1993). The onset of the movement-related neurons was time-locked to the visual cue, and ended with the beginning of the movements (Kimura, 1990; Kimura et al., 1990; Kimura et al., 1992). There is now clear evidence that neurons in this region respond to the discriminative stimulus in cued movements, and in self-timed movements the neural activity increases more gradually, building up just before movement onset (Lee & Assad, 2003). This pattern is consistent with the idea that the circuit is involved in S-R habit learning. Studies of rats performing instrumental tasks have found similar results, as well as convincing evidence that cells in the sensorimotor striatum can undergo long-term and systematic changes under these conditions (Carelli et al., 1997; Jog et al., 1999). Such forms of long-term plasticity have been viewed as neural correlates of S-R learning, and though the physiological mechanisms underlying this type of learning remain unclear, dopamine has been implicated as the reinforcement signal strengthening the S-R association (Wickens et al., 2003).

INTERACTION BETWEEN SYSTEMS AND THE HIERARCHICAL ORGANIZATION OF ACTION

Although these circuits may operate somewhat independently, there are also ample opportunities for the circuits to interact (Joel & Weiner, 1994, 1997). For instance, it has long been known that the limbic striatum can exert control over the motor striatum via indirect connections with the midbrain (Nauta, 1989). Recent anatomical evidence suggests the intriguing possibility of serial propagation of information from the limbic level to the sensorimotor level (Joel & Weiner, 2000).

Thus, the networks reviewed above could be arranged hierarchically. The limbic level, for instance, could constitute the highest level of this hierarchy. The intermediate level would then consist of the associative cortico-BG circuit; the lowest level, the sensorimotor cortico-BG circuit. From this perspective, the DMS and the DLS participate in a hierarchically higher associative level and a hierarchically lower sensorimotor level. The propagation of signals from the limbic level to the sensorimotor level, then, would represent the translation of motivation into action (see Figure 12.1).

In support of this view, there is evidence that overtraining of a behavior shifts activity from the associative circuit to the sensorimotor circuit. Learning of new motor responses, for example, activated the caudate nucleus and the prefrontal cortex, whereas with well learned sequences, the site of activation shifts to the putamen and motor cortices. When well trained subjects were asked to pay attention, the prefrontal cortex as well as the caudate nucleus were activated again (Jueptner, Frith et al., 1997; Jueptner, Stephan, et al., 1997). Attention to action requires the involvement of higher levels, but once a task is well learned, only the sensorimotor level is needed for its performance. This may also be understood as a shift from controlled to automatic behavior. With habit formation, behavior shifts from a higher level of functional integration to a lower one—more specifically, from the associative cortico-BG network to the sensorimotor cortico-BG network.

IMPLICATIONS FOR THE TREATMENT OF ADDICTION

Having outlined the basic learning processes implicated in addiction, we now consider their clinical implications. As a result of exposure to substances that exploit the brain's natural machinery for learning, neural circuits reviewed above are altered, resulting in addiction. In light of what has been discussed so far, how should we characterize the behavior of the addict?

According to one hypothesis, abnormally enhanced habit formation in the dorsal striatum underlies addiction (Everitt & Wolf, 2002; Gerdeman et al., 2003). This account classifies addiction as a type of habit learning. Instead of habit learning generated by natural reinforcers under natural conditions, addiction is generated by artificial means, namely the chemical substances in drugs of abuse that target the same neural circuitry. Presumably, drugs of abuse are simply more powerful reinforcers of the S-R habit. This position is supported by the persistence of addiction despite harmful consequences and the tendency to relapse under stress or re-exposure to cues originally associated with the drug taking (Everitt & Wolf, 2002).

In a recent review, however, Robinson and Berridge (2003) argued that although S-R learning explains the automaticity of some aspects of addiction, it fails to explain the motivational compulsion of addiction. This argument raises an important issue: The organism cannot possibly show sensitivity to devaluation and degradation if it failed to learn the specific A-O contingency. But just because it fails such tests does not mean that the A-O contingency was not "encoded" in the first place. It could simply be a failure of the A-O contingency to control behavior performance. Addicts may of course be aware of the contingency between their actions and outcomes, even though such a contingency is not controlling their behavior.

There is already considerable evidence for the habitual control of drug-seeking behavior (Dickinson et al., 2002; Miles et al., 2003; Olmstead et al., 2000; Vanderschuren & Everitt, 2004). For example, unlike actions earning lemon-sucrose solution, actions earning a cocaine-sucrose solution were not affected by outcome devaluation (Miles et al., 2003). In addition, prolonged self-administration of cocaine also rendered drug-seeking insensitive to harmful consequences such as shock (Vanderschuren & Everitt, 2004).

There is also considerable evidence for the involvement of the dorsal striatum in drug-seeking behavior. In particular, studies have implicated dopamine in the potentiation of drug-seeking. Cocaine-seeking is associated with increased levels of extracellular dopamine in the dorsal striatum, but not in the ventral striatum (Ito et al., 2002) and posttrial infusions of dopamine receptor agonists into the dorsal striatum enhanced the acquisition of win-stay habit learning, a task that is insensitive to outcome devaluation (Packard & White, 1991; Sage & Knowlton, 2000). Drugs of abuse can therefore (perhaps via the dopamine system) affect the sensorimotor cortico-BG network in potentiating habitual behavior that is impervious to changes in outcome value.

Drugs of abuse certainly possess strong emotional salience to addicted users—a fact not captured by the S-R account of addiction. As already mentioned, however, one possible way for the different cortico-BG networks to interact is through spiraling connections between the striatum and the dopaminergic cells in the midbrain (see Figure 12.2). Dopaminergic cells projecting to the sensorimotor striatum also receive inputs from the limbic striatum, suggesting that the S-O system can exert direct control over the S-R system (Joel & Weiner, 2000). If we focus on the possible interactions between the functional systems delineated above, there is indeed the promise of reconciling the two dominant explanations of addiction: the idea that addiction is essentially enhanced habit learning, and the idea that addiction is due to abnormally heightened "incentive salience" assigned to stimuli associated with drug-taking (Robinson & Berridge, 2003). In light of the associative structures reviewed in this chapter, the former account attributes addiction to the S-R system (enhanced strength of the S-R association), whereas the latter account attributes addiction to the S-O system (enhanced association between environmental stimuli and incentive attributes of the drug itself). Both accounts are supported by empirical evidence, but the interactive and hierarchical organization of the cortico-BG networks, as reviewed above, suggests that these explanations are not mutually exclusive. Results from a recent behavioral study, indeed, has suggested that the ability for Pavlovian cues to enhance instrumental responding is significantly enhanced by the overtraining of that instrumental response. That is, the control of the S-O system over instrumental responding may be particularly strong for habits (Holland, 2004). The intriguing finding suggests that once responding has become habitual (S-R), it is more susceptible to being potentiated by the S-O system. This implies that habitual drug users may be particularly likely to seek out drugs in environments that have been associated with positive reinforcement. An interesting possibility is that this is due to links between the limbic and the sensorimotor networks via the midbrain dopaminergic cells.

CONCLUSION

To understand how addiction might occur, it is necessary to understand the various learning processes involved, how they modify behavior, and how they interact. In this chapter, we have described three functional systems, each with distinct behavioral characteristics and mechanisms of learning (S-O, A-O, and S-R). Recent work in neuroanatomy has suggested that this continuum of behavioral flexibility and capacity for modification by environmental feedback finds a corresponding continuum in the cortico-BG networks in the cerebrum (limbic, associative, and sensorimotor). According to the views presented here, addiction is not limited to a discrete aberration in a single learning process, but rather involves multiple learning processes in these networks, and moreover could affect the mechanisms of interaction between them.

Different symptoms of addiction can be classified according to their respective neural substrates. For example, relapse may be more likely to occur when the cues present have been associated with the effects of a drug. As the cues have acquired incentive value based on their Pavlovian association with the reinforcing effect of the drug, they can potentiate drug-seeking behavior. This is an instance of enhanced incentive salience of environmental stimuli due to S-O learning, mediated by the limbic cortico-BG network, and the incentive salience could be transferred to the associative and sensorimotor cortico-BG networks, perhaps via the dopaminergic cells in the midbrain. For example, the ritualistic behavior of addicts in a familiar drug-taking environment could be linked to the S-R habits.

The demarcation of learning processes, therefore, has important implications for treatment. Each aspect of addiction can be treated separately by targeting the different learning systems. Different types of addiction should also be treated differently by weighing the relative contribution of different cortico-BG networks. And since we have identified interactions between networks as being particularly important for addiction, it is also important to identify and alter potentially harmful interactions between these systems. Pharmacological interventions could then reduce these harmful interactions, while behavioral treatment may be helpful in shifting control of behavior away from habits. Naturally, such a project as outlined here has barely begun, and considerable research is needed to clarify addiction along these lines. We nevertheless believe that progress will be rapid so long as research on addiction is grounded in, and guided by, our understanding of the fundamental learning processes at the level of neural systems.

REFERENCES

Adams, C. D. (1982). Variations in the sensitivity of instrumental responding to reinforcer devaluation. *Quarterly Journal of Experimental Psychology, 33B*, 109–122.

Alexander, G. E., &, Crutcher, M. D. (1990). Functional architecture of basal ganglia circuits: Neural substrates of parallel processing. *Trends in Neurosciences, 13*, 266–271.

Balleine, B. W., & Dickinson, A. (1998). Goal-directed instrumental action: Contingency and incentive learning and their cortical substrates. *Neuropharmacology, 37*, 407–419.

Balleine, B. W., Killcross, A. S., & Dickinson, A. (2003). The effect of lesions of the basolateral amygdala on instrumental conditioning. *Journal of Neuroscience, 23*, 666–675.

Bannerman, D. M., Rawlins, J. N., McHugh, S. B., Deacon, R. M., Yee, B. K., Bast, T., et al. (2004). Regional dissociations within the hippocampus—memory and anxiety. *Neuroscience & Biobehavioral Reviews, 28,* 273–283.

Barraclough, D. J., Conroy, M. L., & Lee, D. (2004). Prefrontal cortex and decision making in a mixed-strategy game. *Nature Neuroscience, 7,* 404–410.

Baum, W. M. (1973). The correlation-based law of effect. *Journal of the Experimental Analysis of Behavior, 20,* 137–153.

Bechara, A. (2004). The role of emotion in decision-making: Evidence from neuropsychological patients with orbitofrontal damage. *Brain and Cognition, 55,* 30–40.

Berke, J. D., & Hyman, S. E. (2000). Addiction, dopamine, and the molecular mechanisms of memory. *Neuron, 25,* 515–532.

Bolles, R. (1972). Reinforcement, expectancy, and learning. *Psychological Review, 79,* 394–409.

Cardinal, R. N., Parkinson, J. A., Hall, J., & Everitt, B. J. (2002). Emotion and motivation: The role of the amygdala, ventral striatum, and prefrontal cortex. *Neuroscience & Biobehavioral Reviews, 26,* 321–352.

Carelli, R. M., Wolske, M., & West, M. O. (1997). Loss of lever press-related firing of rat striatal forelimb neurons after repeated sessions in a lever pressing task. *The Journal of Neuroscience, 17,* 1804–1814.

Colwill, R. M., & Rescorla, R. A. (1986). Associative structures in instrumental learning. In G. Bower (Ed.), *The psychology of learning and motivation* (pp. 55–104). New York: Academic Press.

Corbit, L. H., & Balleine, B. W. (2003). The role of prelimbic cortex in instrumental conditioning. *Behavioural Brain Research, 146,* 145–157.

Corbit, L. H., Muir, J. L., & Balleine, B. W. (2001). The role of the nucleus accumbens in instrumental conditioning: Evidence of a functional dissociation between accumbens core and shell. *Journal of Neuroscience, 21,* 3251–3260.

Devan, B. D., & White, N. M. (1999). Parallel information processing in the dorsal striatum: Relation to hippocampal function. *Journal of Neuroscience, 19,* 2789–2798.

Dickinson, A. (1989). Expectancy theory in animal conditioning. In S. B. Klein & R. R. Mowrer (Eds.), *Contemporary learning theories* (pp. 279–308). Hillsdale, NJ: Lawrence Erlbaum.

Dickinson, A., & Balleine, B. W. (1993). Actions and responses: The dual psychology of behaviour. In N. Eilan et al. (Eds.), *Spatial representation: Problems in philosophy and psychology* (pp. 277–293). Malden, MA: Blackwell.

Dickinson, A., Nicholas, D. J., & Adams, C.D. (1983). The effect of the instrumental training contingency on susceptibility to reinforcer devaluation. *Quarterly Journal of Experimental Psychology: Comparative & Physiological Psychology, 35,* 35–51.

Dickinson, A., Wood, N., & Smith, J. W. (2002). Alcohol seeking by rats: Action or habit? *Quarterly Journal of Experimental Psychology-B, 55,* 331–348.

Divac, I., Markowitsch, H. J., & Pritzel, M. (1978). Behavioral and anatomical consequences of small intrastriatal injections of kainic acid in the rat. *Brain Research, 151,* 523–532.

Divac, I., Rosvold, H. E., & Szwarcbart, M. K. (1967). Behavioral effects of selective ablation of the caudate nucleus. *Journal of Comparative Physiological Psychology, 63,* 184–190.

Everitt, B. J., & Wolf, M. E. (2002). Psychomotor stimulant addiction: A neural systems perspective. *Journal of Neuroscience, 22,* 3312–3320.

Gerdeman, G. L., Partridge, J. G., Lupica, C. R., & Lovinger, D. M. (2003). It could be habit forming: Drugs of abuse and striatal synaptic plasticity. *Trends in Neurosciences, 26,* 184–192.

Gold, P. E. (2003). Acetylcholine modulation of neural systems involved in learning and memory. *Neurobiology of Learning and Memory, 80,* 194–210.

Haruno, M., Kuroda, T., Doya, K., Toyama, K., Kimura, M., Samejima, K., et al. (2004). A neural correlate of reward-based behavioral learning in caudate nucleus: A functional magnetic resonance imaging study of a stochastic decision task. *Journal of Neuroscience, 24,* 1660–1665.

Hassani, O. K., Cromwell, H. C., & Schultz, W. (2001). Influence of expectation of different rewards on behavior-related neuronal activity in the striatum. *Journal of Neurophysiology, 85,* 2477–2489.

Hershberger, W. A. (1986). An approach through the looking glass. *Animal Learning & Behavior, 14,* 443–451.

Hikosaka, O., Takikawa, Y., & Kawagoe, R. (2000). Role of the basal ganglia in the control of purposive saccadic eye movements. *Physiological Reviews, 80,* 953–978.

Holland, P. C. (1979). Differential effects of omission contingencies on various components of Pavlovian appetitive conditioned responding in rats. *Journal of Experimental Psychology: Animal Behavior Process, 5,* 178–193.

Holland, P. C. (2004). Relations between Pavlovian-instrumental transfer and reinforcer devaluation. *Journal of Experimental Psychology: Animal Behavior Process, 30,* 104–117.

Ito, R., Dalley, J. W., Robbins, T. W., & Everitt, B. J. (2002). Dopamine release in the dorsal striatum during cocaine-seeking behavior under the control of a drug-associated cue. *Journal of Neuroscience, 22,* 6247–6253.

Joel, D., & Weiner, I. (1994). The organization of the basal ganglia-thalamocortical circuits: Open interconnected rather than closed segregated. *Neuroscience, 63,* 363–379.

Joel, D., & Weiner, I. (1997). The connections of the primate subthalamic nucleus: Indirect pathways and the open-interconnected scheme of basal ganglia-thalamocortical circuitry. *Brain Research Reviews, 23,* 62–78.

Joel, D., & Weiner, I. (2000). The connections of the dopaminergic system with the striatum in rats and primates: An analysis with respect to the functional and compartmental organization of the striatum. *Neuroscience, 96,* 451–474.

Jog, M. S., Kubota, Y., Connolly, C. I., Hillegaart, V., & Graybiel, A. M. (1999). Building neural representations of habits. *Science, 286,* 1745–1749.

Jueptner, M., Frith, C. D., Brooks, D. J., Frackowiak, R. S., & Passingham, R. E. (1997). Anatomy of motor learning: II. Subcortical structures and learning by trial and error. *Journal of Neurophysiology, 77,* 1325–1337.

Jueptner, M., Stephan, K. M., Frith, C. D., Brooks, D. J., Frackowiak, R. S., & Passingham, R. E. (1997). Anatomy of motor learning: I. Frontal cortex and attention to action. *Journal of Neurophysiology, 77,* 1313–1324.

Kalivas, P. W. (2004). Glutamate systems in cocaine addiction. *Current Opinions in Pharmacology, 4,* 23–29.

Kanazawa, I., Murata, M., & Kimura, M. (1993). Roles of dopamine and its receptors in generation of choreic movements. *Advances in Neurology, 60,* 107–112.

Kawagoe, R., Takikawa, Y., & Hikosaka, O. (1998). Expectation of reward modulates cognitive signals in the basal ganglia. *Nature Neuroscience, 1,* 411–416.

Kimura, M. (1990). Behaviorally contingent property of movement-related activity of the primate putamen. *Journal of Neurophysiology, 63,* 1277–1296.

Kimura, M., Aosaki, T., Hu, Y., Ishida, A., & Watanabe, K. (1992). Activity of primate putamen neurons is selective to the mode of voluntary movement: Visually guided, self-initiated or memory-guided. *Experimental Brain Research, 89,* 473–477.

Kimura, M., Aosaki, T., & Ishida, A. (1993). Neurophysiological aspects of the differential roles of the putamen and caudate nucleus in voluntary movement. *Advances in Neurology, 60,* 62–70.

Kimura, M., Kato, M., & Shimazaki, H. (1990). Physiological properties of projection neurons in the monkey striatum to the globus pallidus. *Experimental Brain Research, 82,* 672–676.

Knowlton, B. J., Mangels, J. A., & Squire, L. R. (1996). A neostriatal habit learning system in humans. *Science, 273,* 1399–1402.

Konorski, J. (1967). *Integrative activity of the brain.* Chicago: University of Chicago Press.

Lee, I. H., & Assad, J. A. (2003). Putaminal activity for simple reactions or self-timed movements. *Journal of Neurophysiology, 89,* 2528–2537.

Leon, M. I., & Shadlen, M. N. (1999). Effect of expected reward magnitude on the response of neurons in the dorsolateral prefrontal cortex of the macaque. *Neuron, 24,* 415–425.

Levy, R., Friedman, H. R., Davachi, L., & Goldman-Rakic, P. S. (1997). Differential activation of the caudate nucleus in primates performing spatial and nonspatial working memory tasks. *Journal of Neuroscience, 17,* 3870–3882.

Lewis, S. J., Dove, A., Robbins, T. W., Barker, R. A., & Owen, A. M. (2004). Striatal contributions to working memory: A functional magnetic resonance imaging study in humans. *European Journal of Neuroscience, 19,* 755–760.

Miles, F. J., Everitt, B. J., & Dickinson, A. (2003). Oral cocaine seeking by rats: Action or habit? *Behavioral Neuroscience, 117,* 927–938.

Mishkin, M., Malamut, B., & Bachevalier, J. (1984). Memories and habits: Two neural systems. In G. Lynch, J. L. McGaugh, & N. Weinberger (Eds.), *Neurobiology of learning and memory* (pp. 65–77). New York: Guilford.

Nauta, W. J. H. (1989). Reciprocal links of the corpus striatum with the cerebral cortex and limbic system: A common substrate for movement and thought? In J. Mueller (Ed.), *Neurology and psychiatry: A meeting of minds* (pp. 43–63). Basel, Switzerland: Karger.

Olmstead, M. C., Parkinson, J. A., Miles, F. J., Everitt, B. J., & Dickinson, A. (2000). Cocaine-seeking by rats: Regulation, reinforcement and activation. *Psychopharmacology* (Berlin, Germany), *152,* 123–131.

Packard, M. G., & McGaugh, J. L. (1996). Inactivation of hippocampus or caudate nucleus with lidocaine differentially affects expression of place and response learning. *Neurobiology of Learning and Memory, 65,* 65–72.

Packard, M. G., & White, N. M. (1991). Dissociation of hippocampus and caudate nucleus memory systems by posttraining intracerebral injection of dopamine agonists. *Behavioral Neuroscience, 105,* 295–306.

Partridge, J. G., Tang, K. C., & Lovinger, D. M. (2000). Regional and postnatal heterogeneity of activity-dependent long-term changes in synaptic efficacy in the dorsal striatum. *Journal of Neurophysiology, 84,* 1422–1429.

Reep, R. L., Cheatwood, J. L., & Corwin, J. V. (2003). The associative striatum: Organization of cortical projections to the dorsocentral striatum in rats. *Journal of Comparative Neurology, 467,* 271–292.

Restle, F. (1957). Discrimination of cues in mazes: A resolution of the "place-vs.-response" question. *Psychological Review, 64,* 217.

Robinson, T. E., & Berridge, K. C. (2003). Addiction. *Annual Reviews of Psychology, 54,* 25–53.

Rolls, E. T. (2000). The orbitofrontal cortex and reward. *Cerebral Cortex, 10,* 284–294.

Sage, J. R., & Knowlton, B. J. (2000). Effects of US devaluation on win-stay and win-shift radial maze performance in rats. *Behavioral Neuroscience, 114,* 295–306.

Swanson, L. W. (2000). Cerebral hemisphere regulation of motivated behavior. *Brain Research, 886,* 113–164.

Tsujimoto, S., & Sawaguchi, T. (2002). Working memory of action: A comparative study of ability to selecting response based on previous action in New World monkeys (*Saimiri sciureus* and *Callithrix jacchus*). *Behavioral Processes, 58,* 149–155.

Tsujimoto, S., & Sawaguchi, T. (2004a). Neuronal representation of response-outcome in the primate prefrontal cortex. *Cerebral Cortex, 14,* 47–55.

Tsujimoto, S., & Sawaguchi, T. (2004b). Properties of delay-period neuronal activity in the primate prefrontal cortex during memory- and sensory-guided saccade tasks. *European Journal of Neuroscience, 19,* 447–457.

Vanderschuren, L. J., & Everitt, B. J. (2004). Drug seeking becomes compulsive after prolonged cocaine self-administration. *Science, 305,* 1017–1019.

Wallis, J. D., & Miller, E. K. (2003). Neuronal activity in primate dorsolateral and orbital prefrontal cortex during performance of a reward preference task. *European Journal of Neuroscience, 18,* 2069–2081.

West, M. O., Carelli, R. M., Pomerantz, M., Cohen, S. M., Gardner, J. P., & Chapin, J. K., et al. (1990). A region in the dorsolateral striatum of the rat exhibiting single-unit correlations with specific locomotor limb movements. *Journal of Neurophysiology, 64,* 1233–1246.

Wickens, J. R., Reynolds, J. N., & Hyland, B. I. (2003). Neural mechanisms of reward-related motor learning. *Current Opinions in Neurobiology, 13,* 685–690.

Wyvell, C. L., & Berridge, K. C. (2001). Incentive sensitization by previous amphetamine exposure: Increased cue-triggered "wanting" for sucrose reward. *Journal of Neuroscience, 21,* 7831–7840.

Yin, H. H., & Knowlton, B. J. (2004). Contributions of striatal subregions to place and response learning. *Learning & Memory, 11,* 459–463.

Yin, H. H., Knowlton, B. J., & Balleine, B. W. (2004). Lesions of dorsolateral striatum preserve outcome expectancy but disrupt habit formation in instrumental learning. *European Journal of Neuroscience, 19,* 181–189.

Yin, H. H., Ostlund, S. B., Knowlton, B. J., & Balleine, B. W. (in press). The role of the dorsomedial striatum in instrumental conditioning. *European Journal of Neuroscience.*

CHAPTER 13

Imaging the Addicted Brain: Reward, Craving, and Cognitive Processes

INGMAR H. A. FRANKEN, CORIEN ZIJLSTRA, JAN BOOIJ, AND WIM VAN DEN BRINK

Abstract: Functional imaging techniques like functional Magnetic Resonance Imaging (fMRI) and Positron Emission Tomography (PET) make it possible to study the underlying neural substrates of addiction-related phenomena such as the cognitive processing of drug-related stimuli and craving. PET can be also used to image neurotransmitter systems that are involved in addiction. In the present chapter, we will provide a review of studies using neuroimaging techniques to study the neurobiological and pharmacological correlates of addiction-related cognitive processes, including reward and craving processes. From these studies, there are indications that the amygdala and hippocampus are involved in drug-related memories, the anterior cingulate cortex (ACC) is associated with drug-related attentional functions, and that the orbitofrontal cortex is associated with impaired decision making.

INTRODUCTION

In the past decades, there has been growing interest in the role of brain mechanisms in addictive behaviors. The introduction of new imaging techniques has increased significantly our insights into addiction. Functional imaging techniques like functional Magnetic Resonance Imaging (fMRI), Positron Emission Tomography (PET), and Single Photon Emission Computed Tomography (SPECT) made it possible to study the underlying neural substrates of addictive behaviors and addiction-related phenomena such as craving. fMRI makes use of the different magnetic properties of oxygenated and deoxygenated hemoglobin to measure regional brain activity. This technique has been used frequently to measure changes in regional blood flow induced by cues related to addiction. Changes in blood flow could be measured also by PET or SPECT, while PET is also able to measure changes in glucose metabolism. Moreover, both PET and SPECT can be used to image neurotransmitter systems in the brain; for example, dopamine D_2-like receptors.

Imaging techniques can be employed in several ways to visualize neural structures involved in addiction. First, it is known that all drugs of abuse have rewarding properties. By imaging changes in regional brain activity induced by drugs it is becoming clear which structures of the brain are involved in the reward system. Second, by eliciting craving it is possible to study the neural correlates of drug craving by functional neuroimaging. Third, brain-imaging techniques could link specific features of addiction, for example, the activation of implicit memory processes (e.g., Grant et al., 1996) to specific brain structures. This approach increased our insight into the cognitive processes involved in addiction. Fourth, by using PET and SPECT, the role of specific neurotransmitter systems that may be involved in addiction and addiction-related cognitive processes can be studied. The goal of the present chapter is to provide an overview of research that used neuroimaging to study reward, craving, and cognitive processes, that is, attention, memory, and decision making, involved in addiction. The main focus of this chapter will be human neuroimaging studies. Further, when not specified, the term drugs refer to drugs of abuse in general, including alcohol and nicotine.

REWARD

There is an obvious relation between rewarding effects of drugs and their self-administration. When the effect of a drug is experienced to be pleasurable, the likelihood of taking that drug again increases, which is guided by the operant conditioning principles. It is known that all drugs of abuse have rewarding properties. The early neuroscience approaches in addiction research were mainly focused on the neural mechanisms underlying these rewarding effects of self-administration of addictive drugs (Wise & Bozarth, 1987).

Neuroanatomy

The mesolimbic dopaminergic system, and especially its innervations of the ventral striatum, otherwise referred to as the nucleus accumbens, plays a crucial role in the experience of reinforcing effects (Berridge & Robinson, 2003; Di Chiara, 2002). Indeed, imaging studies examining the neural substrates of natural reward show involvement of the ventral striatum (Blood & Zatorre, 2001; Kelley et al., 2002), ventral tegmental area (VTA; Berridge & Robinson, 2003), and orbitofrontal cortex (Blood & Zatorre, 2001; Kringelbach et al., 2003). Not surprisingly, the same areas involved in the experience of natural rewards are also involved in the experience of the pleasurable effects of drugs (Kringelbach & Rolls, 2004; Laviolette et al., 2004; Tzschentke & Schmidt, 2000; Volkow et al., 1997). From these structures, probably the ventral striatum received most attention in the literature (McClure et al., 2004).

Neurotransmitters

Traditionally, it has been hypothesized that the dopaminergic system is involved in the experience of pleasure (Wise & Bozarth, 1987). Several studies indeed showed that striatal dopamine is related to the experience of reward when using drugs of abuse. Several human imaging studies showed that endogenous dopamine release in the striatum was strongly correlated with the experience of pleasure evoked by drugs, that is, drug-induced euphoria (Drevets et al., 2001; Laruelle et al., 1995; Volkow et al., 1997; Volkow, Wang, Fowler, Logan, et al., 1999; Volkow, Wang, Fowler, Hitzemann, et al., 1999). Barrett et al. (2004) showed that the hedonic effects of cigarette smoking, which does not produce extreme pleasurable effects, is also associated with increased dopaminergic activity in the dorsal striatum. Recently, however, it has been acknowledged that dopamine's role goes further than the experience of reward, and that other neurotransmitters are also involved in the experience of reward (Wise, 2004), such as the opioid (Kelley et al., 2002; Pecina & Berridge, 2000), and the GABA system (Berridge & Robinson, 2003).

CRAVING

Pleasurable effects of drugs by themselves cannot solely explain addictive behaviors. Both addicted and nonaddicted persons may experience pleasurable effects and an increase in striatal dopamine concentrations after drug use (Volkow, Fowler, & Wang, 2003). The focus in addiction research is therefore shifting from the rewarding aspects of drug use toward the motivational aspects of addictive behavior (Robinson & Berridge, 1993; Wise, 2004). The motivational properties of drugs last for several years after the termination of drug use, and may even last a lifetime (Hser et al., 2001). Stimuli in the environment associated with drug use are able, by means of Pavlovian conditioning principles, to trigger motivational circuits and elicit a high motivation to use these drugs: so-called cue-elicited craving. This craving contributes to the continuation of drug use in active drug abusers and relapse in detoxified abusers (Everitt, 1997). The idea that craving contributes to relapse resulted in an increased interest to find the neural substrate for craving, and brain-imaging techniques greatly advanced this research.

Neuroanatomy

Functional imaging studies have revealed brain structures crucial to craving and other motivational and reward-related processes. The main structures involved in craving, are involved also in reward, namely, the ventral striatum and connected regions, such as the orbitofrontal cortex and the amygdala. This neural network appears similar for all drugs of abuse (Lingford-Hughes et al., 2003).

One of the problems with the identification of neuroanatomical structures involved in craving is that craving elicited by cue-exposure also coactivates other processes such as memory and attention. From current study designs, it is therefore difficult to assess whether a specific structure is dedicated to craving. The striatum, however, especially the nucleus accumbens, seems involved in craving and other motivational aspects of drug use (e.g., Ikemoto & Panksepp, 1999; Robbins & Everitt, 1996; Robinson & Berridge, 1993). It should be noted that these structures are not only activated in drug craving but also play a role in motivational processes involved in appetitive behaviors in general. Some authors refer to this phenomenon as the "hijacking" of neural circuits by drugs and drug-related stimuli that are usually activated by natural rewards and stimuli (Daglish et al., 2003; Nesse & Berridge, 1997).

Cognitive factors, such as memory processes, expectancies, and attentional processes, have been recently added to the range of cue-elicited reactivities. This supports the idea that there are no dedicated circuits activated, but that several nonspecific brain components are involved in craving. Thus, craving seems to be multidimensional and will be discussed in the following paragraphs, focusing on its relation with attention, memory, and decision making.

Neurotransmitters

Animal studies show that drug craving is associated with an increased dopaminergic activation in the nucleus accumbens (e.g., Di Chiara, 1999). In contrast, recent PET and postmortem studies performed in cocaine and methamphetamine users showed that striatal dopaminergic D_2 receptors are reduced (Kish et al., 2001; Volkow et al., 1993, 1996, 2001). An explanation of these apparently contradictory findings is provided by Pilla et al. (1999) and extended by Childress and O'Brien (2000). These researchers propose that cocaine craving may be the result of two separate neurobiological pathways. First, heightened tonic craving levels may be the result of reduced D_2 receptor densities in the striatum and orbitofrontal cortex and may result in anhedonia. In this case, drugs are used to stimulate the dopamine activity in an attempt to alleviate this chronic anhedonic state. Second, phasic increases in cue-elicited craving may result from an enhanced dopaminergic activity in striatum, amygdala, and anterior cingulate cortex. Although recent PET studies in humans show that dopamine is released in the human striatum during the anticipatory or appetitive phase of motivated behavior (Koepp et al., 1998), no study has addressed this hypothesis in addicted humans.

ATTENTIONAL PROCESSES

During periods of active drug use, stimuli predicting drug use become extremely salient and are more and more capable of attracting attention and eliciting approach behavior (Robinson & Berridge, 2000). For example, it is known that crack cocaine addicts constantly seek out white cocaine-like powder on the floor. Substances that look like cocaine powder immediately attract their attention and their ongoing behavior is interrupted. This "attentional bias" in drug addicts is largely automatic and involuntary. Attentional bias for drugs and drug-related cues has been found in several experimental studies (see Franken, 2003). In addition, several studies found a relation between attentional bias and craving (Field et al., 2004; Franken, Hulstein, et al., 2004; Franken, Kroon, & Hendriks, 2000; Franken, Kroon,

Wiers, et al., 2000; Franken, Stam, et al., 2003; cf. Franken, Hendriks, et al., 2004; Van de Laar et al., 2004), indicating that attentional bias is associated with motivational processes.

Neuroanatomy

The anterior cingulate cortex (ACC) has been implicated in addiction-related attentional processes (Garavan et al., 2000; Wexler et al., 2001). The ACC is relevant for selective attention (Bush et al., 2000; MacLeod & MacDonald, 2000), implying the role of attention in drug-seeking behavior and addiction. The ACC might be responsible for drug-seeking behavior by influencing the direction of the individual's attention toward drug-related stimuli. The ACC has reciprocal connections with the amygdala and nucleus accumbens.

In line with these findings, the study of Wexler and coworkers showed that the increase of activity in the ACC preceded the self-reported onset of craving (Wexler et al., 2001). This supports the idea that the ACC is related to attentive processes directed to drug-related cues and not to the experience of craving itself. Abnormal dopaminergic regulation of the ACC has also been found to be related to the inability to control drug intake and the desire to use drugs (Volkow, Fowler, & Wang, 1999). In addition, ACC activation was shown to be increased in response to drug-related stimuli (Daglish et al., 2001). ACC activation occurred even in subjects who did not report craving in response to stimuli, which strengthens the belief that activation of the ACC is primarily relevant for the direction of attention toward drug-related stimuli.

Neurotransmitters

It is known that noradrenergic, dopaminergic, and cholineric systems are essential elements of the brain's attentional system (Clark et al., 1987; Coull, 1998; Nieoullon, 2002). Bushnell and colleagues (2000) proposed that the attention-consuming preoccupation with incentive stimuli depends on abnormal increase in the reactivity of cortical cholinergic inputs. They showed that cortical acetylcholine (Ach) release mediates the over-processing of a stimulus (Bushnell et al., 2000).

Robinson & Berridge (1993) hypothesized that activation of dopaminergic activity in the corticostriatal reward circuit by reward-cues could contribute to the excessive focusing on stimuli that lead to further drug use. A recent study by Franken, Hendriks, et al. (2004) showed that attentional processes in abstinent heroin addicts can be decreased by a single low dose of a dopamine antagonist, a finding that is supportive for this hypothesis. The role for noradrenaline in addiction-related attentional functioning has not been studied so far in humans.

MEMORY PROCESSES

Simple memories for places, people, music, and even language have been shown to be strong enough to activate the individuals' memory for past drug use, often leading to craving and relapse. Both implicit and explicit memories may lead to relapse in drug use. Memory formation and consolidation is especially influenced by the relevancy of the processed experience, which is largely dependant on reinforcing properties of that experience. Or, as Wise (2004, p. 8) puts it: "Our motivations are motivations to return to the rewards we have experienced in the past, and to cues that mark the way to such rewards." Explicit memories of drug use after a period of abstinence are related to the prior reward experience, and may prompt drug users to seek this reward (i.e., drugs) again. Implicit memory plays a role in addictive behaviors

by means of Pavlovian conditioning, a form of implicit learning in which neutral stimuli become relevant and are able to evoke strong craving and physiological responses. How associative learning mechanisms, such as the encoding and retrieval of memories, may play a role in the maintenance of addictive behaviors has been described by several other authors (e.g., Di Chiara et al., 1999; Grant et al., 1996; Robbins & Everitt, 1999; White, 1996) and shall be discussed elsewhere in this book.

Neuroanatomy

Neuroimaging studies using cue-exposure paradigms, in which abstinent drug abusers are exposed to drug-related stimuli or thoughts, show activations in the amygdala, a structure associated with implicit emotional memory (Childress et al., 1999; Grant et al., 1996). These cue-exposure paradigms trigger implicit (and also explicit) memories of drug use. The amygdala has traditionally been recognized for its role in emotional processing (LeDoux, 1998). Further, the amygdala is known for its traditional role in conditioning and forming stimulus-reward associations. More specifically, it seems that the basolateral amygdala is involved in the perception of emotional cues and appetitive conditioning (Davidson & Irwin, 1999; Holland & Gallagher, 1999). Recent imaging studies show that the amygdala is involved in the encoding and recall of emotional stimuli (Canli et al., 2000; Hamann et al., 1999; Phelps, 2004).

Explicit memory processes are known to involve brain structures including the dorsolateral prefrontal cortex (e.g., Lepage, 2004) and the hippocampus (Phelps, 2004; Rolls, 2000). These areas are also involved when drug addicts are exposed to drug-related cues (Brody et al., 2002; Due et al., 2002; Grant et al., 1996; Kilts et al., 2001; Maas et al., 1998; Schneider et al., 2001). Because it is known that exposure to drug-related stimuli is associated with explicit memories of drug use (Weinstein et al., 1998), it is not a surprise that these structures are activated in drug abusers when exposed to drug-related stimuli.

Neurotransmitters

Drugs of abuse can cause neurochemical changes in the memory circuit in the brain (Nestler, 2001). One important neurotransmitter involved in memory processing is dopamine. Both amygdala and the hippocampus receive dopaminergic innervations from the VTA. Several studies suggest a role for dopamine in memory and learning and show that dopamine may at least facilitate associative learning important for drug-stimulus associations mentioned earlier (Di Chiara, 1999; Pickering & Gray, 2001; Robbins & Everitt, 1999; Wise, 2004). Drugs of abuse that increase dopamine function in these limbic brain regions will thus inherently facilitate consolidation of memory for such rewarding experiences, which contributes to the likelihood of repeated use. Work from cellular and molecular studies point to the similar pathways in drug addiction that include long-term potentiation and long-term depression (Nestler, 2001), both being crucial for learning and memory formation. Up till now, other neurotransmitter systems in this regard have hardly been studied. From animal studies, there is evidence that glutamate (especially the NMDA receptor) is involved in addiction-related memory (see Kelley, 2004). Due to the lack of adequate radiotracers available to image glutamate function, however, the involvement of glutamate in addiction has not been tested yet in humans. It is of interest, however, that recent studies validated the use of [123I]CNS 1261 SPECT to measure NMDA receptors in vivo in the human brain (e.g., Erlandsson et al., 2003).

DECISION-MAKING PROCESSES

Addicted individuals are known to be poor decision makers (Bechara, Damasio, et al., 2000). In spite of the fact that the (long-term) losses the addicts suffer (losing job/friends, risky health situation) due to their behavior are greater than the (short-term) profits they gain (experience of rush, feeling high, loss of anhedonic state), they keep making decisions that are unfavorable in the long run. This even happens when they have been abstinent for a long time—when they have improved their life standard and have the explicit knowledge that drug use is harmful and should not be continued. Their tendency to consume drugs can be regarded as an irrational decision that is harmful to the individual. On specific tasks, addicted subjects keep risking losing more money to win more money; so in spite of the greater punishments, they prefer stronger rewards (e.g., Bechara & Damasio, 2002; Bechara et al., Chapter 15).

Neuroanatomy

There is accumulating evidence that malfunction of frontal neural networks involved in decision making and performance monitoring will lead to repeated self-administration of drugs. This might explain why drug abusers continue to use substances even when they no longer experience pleasurable effects. It appears that individuals with an orbitofrontal cortex/ventromedial (OFC/VM) dysfunction, regardless of its origin, are not capable of making proper associations between present emotions and past (negative) experiences, which results in poor decision making (Bechara et al., 2000). Bolla and coworkers suggested this OFC deficiency (Bolla et al., 2003) is also responsible for the repeated self-administration of drugs. The OFC/VM is a crucial component in the network that subserves positive reinforcement.

It has reciprocal connections with many brain regions that mediate the rewarding effects of drugs as well as decision making and compulsive behaviors. Results from structural imaging studies indicate smaller gray matter volumes in the OFC and surrounding regions in addicted individuals (Franklin et al., 2002). Bolla and coworkers also have found decreased activation of the right dorsolateral prefrontal cortex (DLPFC) and medial prefrontal cortex (MPFC) in drug users and a negative correlation between the amount of cocaine used and activation of the left OFC (Bolla et al., 2003). In contrast, most imaging studies using cue-exposure designs showed an increased activation in the (right) OFC (Childress et al., 1999; Goldstein & Volkow, 2002; Wang et al., 1999). This seems somewhat in contrast with the studies mentioned earlier. Although it might be that the OFC plays several roles in addiction (Goldstein & Volkow, 2002), these discrepancies have to be resolved.

Neurotransmitters

Data from animal studies suggest that decision making is regulated by serotonergic and dopaminergic systems (e.g., King et al., 2003). Only few studies examined the role of neurotransmitters in human decision making. Rogers et al. (1999, 2003) showed that decision making is indeed dependent on the serotonin system. They found that the performance of the subjects with lowered plasma tryptophan (and accordingly lower serotonin levels) was associated with worse decision making (Rogers et al., 2003) and was similar to that associated with amphetamine abuse (Rogers et al., 1999). Anderson et al. (2003), however, could not replicate this finding. O'Carroll et al. (2003) studied the role of noradrenalin on decision making, by challenging the noradrenergic system with a selective noradrenergic reuptake inhibitor, but they were not able to confirm the hypothesis. As far as we know, the role of dopamine on human decision making has not been tested directly. Furthermore, no receptor-imaging studies on the relation between serotonin or dopamine receptor levels in the VM/OFC cortex and decision making are known.

CONCLUSION

Neuroimaging techniques have revealed new insights in the neuroanatomy and neurochemical processes involved in addiction (see Table 13.1 for an overview).

In addition to the well-known involvement of reward and motivational systems such as the mesolimbic dopamine system,

Table 13.1 Major Neuroanatomical and Neurochemical Correlates of Functions Involved in Addiction

	Anatomical structures	*Neurotransmitters*
Reward	Striatum, VTA	Dopamine, opioids, GABA
Craving	Ventral striatum	Dopamine
Memory	Amygdala, hippocampus, dorsolateral frontal cortex	Dopamine, glutamate
Attention	Anterior cingulate cortex	Dopamine, serotonin
Decision making	Ventromedial/orbitofrontal cortex	Dopamine, serotonin

Table 13.2 Studies Addressing the Neuroanatomy of Addiction Processes for Several Substances Employing Cue-Exposure Paradigms

	PET	fMRI	SPECT
Alcohol	Braus et al., 2001	George et al., 2001; Grusser et al., in press; Kareken et al., 2004; Myrick et al., 2004; Schneider et al., 2001; Tapert et al., 2004; Tapert et al., 2003; Wrase et al., 2002	Modell & Mountz, 1995
Nicotine	Brody et al., 2002	Due et al., 2002; Stein et al., 1998	
Opiates	Daglish et al., 2001; Daglish et al., 2003; Sell et al., 1999; Sell et al., 2000		
Cocaine	Bonson et al., 2002; Childress et al., 1999; Grant et al., 1996; Kilts et al., 2001; Wang et al., 1999	Breiter et al., 1997; Garavan et al., 2000; Maas et al., 1998; Wexler et al., 2001	

there are also structures involved in addiction that have been traditionally linked to cognitive functions such as memory, attention, and decision making (see Table 13.2).

This conclusion has first been put forward by Grant et al. (1996) and later by others (Daglish et al., 2003; Garavan et al., 2000; Goldstein & Volkow, 2002). The amygdala and hippocampus are involved in (drug-related) memories, the ACC has been associated with (drug-related) attentional functions, and the OFC has been associated with impaired decision making. There are still several remaining questions concerning the neuroimaging of cognitive processes in addiction. It would be important to study whether it is possible to discern motivational/reward and cognitive processes in addiction. For example, when a subject is exposed to drug-related stimuli, is the ACC activated because the subject is highly motivated (and craves) to take drugs or because the attention is highly focused on these stimuli. Furthermore, most neuroimaging studies do not address the distinction between implicit and explicit cognitions. Most studies only indirectly show an involvement of implicit processes in addiction. New paradigms using implicit memory designs, for example, by employing masked stimuli, should be used to examine the involvement of implicit cognitions directly. In addition, it might be that current functional neuroimaging paradigms are not sophisticated enough to parse these different components of addiction. New and more specific study designs are needed that are capable of studying these distinct brain processes involved in addiction. Since it is becoming more and more clear that dopamine receptors and endogenous dopamine release play a crucial role in addiction (Heinz et al., 2004), and techniques to image this release and receptors are available, this should be high on the research agenda. Other interesting research targets are the NMDA and cannabinoid receptors, as new radioligands become available to image them (e.g., Berding et al., 2004; Erlandsson et al., 2003). Furthermore, as can be observed from Table 13.2, there are still a few "gaps" in the knowledge on the neuroimaging of addiction that have to be filled. Although progress has been made, the use of imaging techniques to study addiction-related problems is still in its infancy and more studies have to be carried out to use neuroimaging for clinical purposes in this field. In the future, however, brain activation patterns could be associated with better prognosis for treatment, or might suggest different treatment approaches.

REFERENCES

Anderson, I. M., Richell, R. A., & Bradshaw, C. M. (2003). The effect of acute tryptophan depletion on probabilistic choice. *Journal of Psychopharmacology, 17*(1), 3–7.

Barrett, S. P., Boileau, I., Okker, J., Pihl, R. O., & Dagher, A. (2004). The hedonic response to cigarette smoking is proportional to dopamine release in the human striatum as measured by positron emission tomography and [11C]raclopride. *Synapse, 54*(2), 65–71.

Bechara, A., & Damasio, H. (2002). Decision-making and addiction (Part 1): Impaired activation of somatic states in substance dependent individuals when pondering decisions with negative future consequences. *Neuropsychologia, 40*, 1675–1689.

Bechara, A., Damasio, H., & Damasio, A. R. (2000). Emotion, decision making and the orbitofrontal cortex. *Cerebral Cortex, 10*(3), 295–307.

Berding, G., Muller-Vahl, K., Schneider, U., Gielow, P., Fitschen, J., Stuhrmann, M., et al. (2004). [123I]AM281 single-photon emission computed tomography imaging of central cannabinoid CB1 receptors before and after delta(9)-tetrahydrocannabinol therapy and whole-body scanning for assessment of radiation dose in Tourette patients. *Biological Psychiatry, 55*(9), 904–915.

Berridge, K. C., & Robinson, T. E. (2003). Parsing reward. *Trends in Neurosciences, 26*(9), 507–513.

Blood, A. J., & Zatorre, R. J. (2001). Intensely pleasurable responses to music correlate with activity in brain regions implicated in reward and emotion. *Proceedings of the National Academy of Sciences, 98*(20), 11818–11823.

Bolla, K. I., Eldreth, D. A., London, E. D., Kiehl, K. A., Mouratidis, M., Contoreggi, C., et al. (2003). Orbitofrontal cortex dysfunction in abstinent cocaine abusers performing a decision-making task. *Neuroimage, 19*(3), 1085–1094.

Bonson, K. R., Grant, S. J., Contoreggi, C. S., Links, J. M., Metcalfe, J., Weyl, H. L., et al. (2002). Neural systems and cue-induced cocaine craving. *Neuropsychopharmacology, 26*(3), 376–386.

Braus, D. F., Wrase, J., Grusser, S., Hermann, D., Ruf, M., Flor, H., et al. (2001). Alcohol-associated stimuli activate the ventral striatum in abstinent alcoholics. *Journal of Neural Transmission, 108*(7), 887–894.

Breiter, H. C., Gollub, R. L., Weisskoff, R. M., Kennedy, D. N., Makris, N., Berke, J. D., et al. (1997). Acute effects of cocaine on human brain activity and emotion. *Neuron, 19*(3), 591–611.

Brody, A. L., Mandelkern, M. A., London, E. D., Childress, A. R., Lee, G. S., Bota, R. G., et al. (2002). Brain metabolic changes during cigarette craving. *Archives of General Psychiatry, 59*(12), 1162–1172.

Bush, G., Luu, P., & Posner, M. I. (2000). Cognitive and emotional influences in anterior cingulate cortex. *Trends in Cognitive Sciences, 4*(6), 215–222.

Bushnell, P. J., Levin, E. D., Marrocco, R. T., Sarter, M. F., Strupp, B. J., & Warburton, D. M. (2000). Attention as a target of intoxication: Insights and methods from studies of drug abuse. *Neurotoxicology and Teratology, 22*, 487–502.

Canli, T., Zhao, Z., Brewer, J., Gabrieli, J. D., & Cahill, L. (2000). Event-related activation in the human amygdala associates with later memory for individual emotional experience. *Journal of Neuroscience, 20*(19), RC99.

Childress, A. R., Mozley, P. D., McElgin, W., Fitzgerald, J., Reivich, M., & O'Brien, C. P. (1999). Limbic activation during cue-induced cocaine craving. *American Journal of Psychiatry, 156*(1), 11–18.

Childress, A. R., & O'Brien, C. P. (2000). Dopamine receptor partial agonists could address the duality of cocaine craving. *Trends in Pharmacological Sciences, 21*(1), 6–9.

Clark, C. R., Geffen, G. M., & Geffen, L. B. (1987). Catecholamines and attention: II. Pharmacological studies in normal humans. *Neuroscience & Biobehavioral Review, 11*(4), 353–364.

Coull, J. T. (1998). Neural correlates of attention and arousal: Insights from electrophysiology, functional neuroimaging and psychopharmacology. *Progress in Neurobiology, 55*, 343–361.

Daglish, M. R. C., Weinstein, A., Malizia, A. L., Wilson, S., Melichar, J. K., Britten, S., et al. (2001). Changes in regional cerebral blood flow elicited by craving memories in abstinent opiate-dependent subjects. *American Journal of Psychiatry, 158*(10), 1680–1686.

Daglish, M. R., Weinstein, A., Malizia, A. L., Wilson, S., Melichar, J. K., Lingford-Hughes, A., et al. (2003). Functional connectivity analysis of the neural circuits of opiate craving: "More" rather than "different"? *Neuroimage, 20*(4), 1964–1970.

Davidson, R. J., & Irwin, W. (1999). The functional neuroanatomy of emotion and affective style. *Trends in Cognitive Sciences, 3*(1), 11–21.

Di Chiara, G. (1999). Drug addiction as dopamine-dependent associative learning disorder. *European Journal of Pharmacology, 375*, 13–30.

Di Chiara, G. (2002). Nucleus accumbens shell and core dopamine: Differential role in behavior and addiction. *Behavioral Brain Research, 137*(1–2), 75–114.

Di Chiara, G., Tanda, G., Bassareo, V., Pontieri, F., Acquas, E., Fenu, S., et al. (1999). Drug addiction as a disorder of associative learning. Role of nucleus accumbens shell/extended amygdala dopamine. *Annals of the New York Academy of Sciences, 877*, 461–485.

Drevets, W. C., Gautier, C., Price, J. C., Kupfer, D. J., Kinahan, P. E., Grace, A. A., et al. (2001). Amphetamine-induced dopamine release in human ventral striatum correlates with euphoria. *Biological Psychiatry, 49*(2), 81–96.

Due, D. L., Huettel, S. A., Hall, W. G., & Rubin, D. C. (2002). Activation in mesolimbic and visuospatial neural circuits elicited by smoking cues: Evidence from functional magnetic resonance imaging. *American Journal of Psychiatry, 159*(6), 954–960.

Erlandsson, K., Bressan, R. A., Mulligan, R. S., Gunn, R. N., Cunningham, V. J., Owens, J., et al. (2003). Kinetic modelling of [123I]CNS 1261—A potential SPET tracer for the NMDA receptor. *Nuclear Medicine Biology, 30*(4), 441–454.

Everitt, B. (1997). Craving cocaine cues: Cognitive neuroscience meets drug addiction research. *Trends in Cognitive Sciences, 1*(1), 1.

Field, M., Mogg, K., & Bradley, B. P. (2004). Cognitive bias and drug craving in recreational cannabis users. *Drug and Alcohol Dependence, 74*(1), 105–111.

Franken, I. H. A. (2003). Drug craving and addiction: Integrating psychological and neuropsychopharmacological approaches. *Progress in Neuro-Psychopharmacology & Biological Psychiatry, 27*(4), 563–579.

Franken, I. H. A., Hendriks, V. M., Stam, C. J., & Van den Brink, W. (2004). A role for dopamine in the processing of drug cues in heroin dependent patients. *European Neuropsychopharmacology, 14,* 503–508.

Franken, I. H. A., Hulstein, K. P., Stam, C. J., Hendriks, V. M., & Van den Brink, W. (2004). Two new neurophysiological indices of cocaine craving: Evoked brain potentials and cue modulated startle reflex. *Journal of Psychopharmacology, 18,* 544–552.

Franken, I. H. A., Kroon, L. Y., & Hendriks, V. M. (2000). Influence of individual differences in craving and obsessive cocaine thoughts on attentional processes in cocaine abuse patients. *Addictive Behaviors, 25*(1), 99–102.

Franken, I. H. A., Kroon, L. Y., Wiers, R. W., & Jansen, A. (2000). Selective cognitive processing of drug cues in heroin dependence. *Journal of Psychopharmacology, 14*(4), 395–400.

Franken, I. H. A., Stam, C. J., Hendriks, V. M., & Van den Brink, W. (2003). Neurophysiological evidence for abnormal cognitive processing of drug cues in heroin dependence. *Psychopharmacology, 170*(2), 205–212.

Franklin, T. R., Acton, P. D., Maldjian, J. A., Gray, J. D., Croft, J. R., Dackis, C. A., et al. (2002). Decreased gray matter concentration in the insular, orbitofrontal, cingulate, and temporal cortices of cocaine patients. *Biological Psychiatry, 51*(2), 134–142.

Garavan, H., Pankiewicz, J., Bloom, A., Cho, J.-K., Sperry, L., Ross, T. J., et al. (2000). Cue-induced cocaine craving: Neuroanatomical specificity for drug users and drug stimuli. *American Journal of Psychiatry, 157*(11), 1789–1798.

George, M. S., Anton, R. F., Bloomer, C., Teneback, C., Drobes, D. J., Lorberbaum, J. P., et al. (2001). Activation of prefrontal cortex and anterior thalamus in alcoholic subjects on exposure to alcohol-specific cues. *Archives of General Psychiatry, 58*(4), 345–352.

Goldstein, R. Z., & Volkow, N. D. (2002). Drug addiction and its underlying neurobiological basis: Neuroimaging evidence for the involvement of the frontal cortex. *American Journal of Psychiatry, 159*(10), 1642–1652.

Grant, S., London, E. D., Newlin, D. B., Villemagne, V. L., Liu, X., Contoreggi, C., et al. (1996). Activation of memory circuits during cue-elicited cocaine craving. *Proceedings of the National Academy of Sciences, 93,* 12040–12045.

Grusser, S. M., Wrase, J., Klein, S., Hermann, D., Smolka, M. N., Ruf, M., et al. (in press). Cue-induced activation of the striatum and medial prefrontal cortex is associated with subsequent relapse in abstinent alcoholics. *Psychopharmacology.*

Hamann, S. B., Ely, T. D., Grafton, S. T., & Kilts, C. D. (1999). Amygdala activity related to enhanced memory for pleasant and aversive stimuli. *Nature Neuroscience, 2*(3), 289–293.

Heinz, A., Siessmeier, T., Wrase, J., Hermann, D., Klein, S., Grusser-Sinopoli, S. M., et al. (2004). Correlation between dopamine d2 receptors in the ventral striatum and central processing of alcohol cues and craving. *American Journal of Psychiatry, 161*(10), 1783–1789.

Holland, P. C., & Gallagher, M. (1999). Amygdala circuitry in attentional and representational processes. *Trends in Cognitive Sciences, 3*(2), 65–73.

Hser, Y. I., Hoffman, V., Grella, C. E., & Anglin, M. D. (2001). A 33-year follow-up of narcotics addicts. *Archives of General Psychiatry, 58,* 503–508.

Ikemoto, S., & Panksepp, J. (1999). The role of nucleus accumbens dopamine in motivated behavior: A unifying interpretation with special reference to reward-seeking. *Brain Research Reviews, 31*(1), 6–41.

Kareken, D. A., Claus, E. D., Sabri, M., Dzemidzic, M., Kosobud, A. E., Radnovich, A. J., et al. (2004). Alcohol-related olfactory cues activate the nucleus accumbens and ventral tegmental area in high-risk drinkers: Preliminary findings. *Alcoholism: Clinical and Experimental Research, 28*(4), 550–557.

Kelley, A. E. (2004). Memory and addiction: Shared neural circuitry and molecular mechanisms. *Neuron, 44,* 161–179.

Kelley, A. E., Bakshi, V. P., Haber, S. N., Steininger, T. L., Will, M. J., & Zhang, M. (2002). Opioid modulation of taste hedonics within the ventral striatum. *Physiology & Behavior, 76*(3), 365–377.

Kilts, C. D., Schweitzer, J. B., Quinn, C. K., Gross, R. E., Faber, T. L., Muhammad, F., et al. (2001). Neural activity related to drug craving in cocaine addiction. *Archives of General Psychiatry, 58*(4), 334–341.

King, J. A., Tenney, J., Rossi, V., Colamussi, L., & Burdick, S. (2003). Neural substrates underlying impulsivity. *Annals of the New York Academy of Science, 1008*(1), 160–169.

Kish, S. J., Kalasinsky, K. S., Derkach, P., Schmunk, G. A., Guttman, M., Ang, L., et al. (2001). Striatal dopaminergic and serotonergic markers in human heroin users. *Neuropsychopharmacology, 24*(5), 561–567.

Koepp, M. J., Gunn, R. N., Lawrence, A. D., Cunningham, V. J., Dagher, A., Jones, T., et al. (1998). Evidence for striatal dopamine release during a video game. *Nature, 393,* 266–268.

Kringelbach, M. L., O'Doherty, J., Rolls, E. T., & Andrews, C. (2003). Activation of the human orbitofrontal cortex to a liquid food stimulus is correlated with its subjective pleasantness. *Cerebral Cortex, 13*(10), 1064–1071.

Kringelbach, M. L., & Rolls, E. T. (2004). The functional neuroanatomy of the human orbitofrontal cortex: Evidence from neuroimaging and neuropsychology. *Progress in Neurobiology, 72*(5), 341–372.

Laruelle, M., Abi-Dargham, A., Van Dyck, C. H., Rosenblatt, W., Zea-Ponce, Y., Zoghbi, S. S., et al. (1995). SPECT imaging of striatal dopamine release after amphetamine challenge. *Journal of Nuclear Medicine, 36*(7), 1182–1190.

Laviolette, S. R., Gallegos, R. A., Henriksen, S. J., & Van der Kooy, D. (2004). Opiate state controls bi-directional reward signaling via GABA-A receptors in the ventral tegmental area. *Nature Neuroscience, 7*(2), 160–169.

LeDoux, J. (1998). Fear and the brain: Where have we been, and where are we going? *Biological Psychiatry, 44*(12), 1229–1238.

Lepage, M. (2004). Differential contribution of left and right prefrontal cortex to associative cued-recall memory: A parametric PET study. *Neuroscience Research, 48*(3), 297–304.

Lingford-Hughes, A. R., Davies, S. J., McIver, S., Williams, T. M., Daglish, M. R., & Nutt, D. J. (2003). Addiction. *British Medical Bulletin, 65,* 209–222.

Maas, L. C., Lukas, S. E., Kaufman, M. J., Weiss, R. D., Daniels, S. L., Rogers, V. W., et al. (1998). Functional magnetic resonance imaging of human brain activation during cue-induced cocaine craving. *American Journal of Psychiatry, 155,* 124–126.

MacLeod, C. M., & MacDonald, P. A. (2000). Interdimensional interference in the Stroop effect: Uncovering the cognitive and neural anatomy of attention. *Trends in Cognitive Sciences, 4*(10), 383–391.

McClure, S. M., York, M. K., & Montague, P. R. (2004). The neural substrates of reward processing in humans: The modern role of fMRI. *Neuroscientist, 10*(3), 260–268.

Modell, J. G., & Mountz, J. M. (1995). Focal cerebral blood flow change during craving for alcohol measured by SPECT. *Journal of Neuropsychiatry & Clinical Neurosciences, 7*(1), 15–22.

Myrick, H., Anton, R. F., Li, X., Henderson, S., Drobes, D., Voronin, K., et al. (2004). Differential brain activity in alcoholics and social drinkers to alcohol cues: Relationship to craving. *Neuropsychopharmacology, 29*(2), 393–402.

Nesse, R. M., & Berridge, K. C. (1997). Psychoactive drug use in evolutionary perspective. *Science, 278*, 63–66.

Nestler, E. J. (2001). Total recall—The memory of addiction. *Science, 292*(5525), 2266.

Nieoullon, A. (2002). Dopamine and the regulation of cognition and attention. *Progress in Neurobiology, 67*(1), 53–83.

O'Carroll, R. E., & Papps, B. P. (2003). Decision making in humans: The effect of manipulating the central noradrenergic system. *Journal of Neurology, Neurosurgery, and Psychiatry, 74*, 376–378.

Pecina, S., & Berridge, K. C. (2000). Opioid site in nucleus accumbens shell mediates eating and hedonic "liking" for food: Map based on microinjection fos plumes. *Brain Research, 863*, 71–86.

Phelps, E. A. (2004). Human emotion and memory: Interactions of the amygdala and hippocampal complex. *Current Opinion in Neurobiology, 14*(2), 198–202.

Pickering, A. D., & Gray, J. A. (2001). Dopamine, appetitive reinforcement, and the neuropsychology of human learning: An individual differences approach. In A. Eliasz & A. Angleitner (Eds.), *Advances in individual differences research* (pp. 113–149). Lengerich, Germany: PABST Science Publishers.

Pilla, M., Perachon, S., Sautel, F., Garrido, F., Mann, A., Wermuth, C. G., et al. (1999). Selective inhibition of cocaine-seeking behaviour by a partial dopamine d 3 receptor agonist. *Nature, 400*(6742), 371–375.

Robbins, T. W., & Everitt, B. J. (1996). Neurobehavioural mechanisms of reward and motivation. *Current Opinion in Neurobiology, 6*(2), 228–236.

Robbins, T. W., & Everitt, B. J. (1999). Interaction of the dopaminergic system with mechanisms of associative learning and cognition: Implications for drug abuse. *Psychological Science, 10*(3), 199–202.

Robinson, T. E., & Berridge, K. C. (1993). The neural basis of drug craving: An incentive-sensitization theory of addiction. *Brain Research Reviews, 18*(3), 247–291.

Robinson, T. E., & Berridge, K. C. (2000). The psychology and neurobiology of addiction: An incentive-sensitization view. *Addiction, 95*(8, Suppl. 2), S91–S117.

Rogers, R. D., Everitt, B. J., Baldacchino, A., Blackshaw, A. J., Swainson, R., Wynne, K., et al. (1999). Dissociable deficits in the decision-making cognition of chronic amphetamine abusers, opiate abusers, patients with focal damage to prefrontal cortex, and tryptophan-depleted normal volunteers: Evidence for monoaminergic mechanisms. *Neuropsychopharmacology, 20*(4), 322–339.

Rogers, R. D., Tunbridge, E. M., Bhagwagar, Z., Drevets, W. C., Sahakian, B. J., & Carter, C. S. (2003). Tryptophan depletion alters the decision-making of healthy volunteers through altered processing of reward cues. *Neuropsychopharmacology, 28*(1), 153–162.

Rolls, E. T. (2000). Memory systems in the brain. *Annual Review of Psychology, 51,* 599–630.

Schneider, F., Habel, U., Wagner, M., Franke, P., Salloum, J. B., Shah, N. J., et al. (2001). Subcortical correlates of craving in recently abstinent alcoholic patients. *American Journal of Psychiatry, 158*(7), 1075–1083.

Sell, L. A., Morris, J. S., Bearn, J., Frackowiak, R. S. J., Friston, K. J., & Dolan, R. J. (1999). Activation of reward circuitry in human opiate addicts. *European Journal of Neuroscience, 11*(3), 1042–1048.

Sell, L. A., Morris, J. S., Bearn, J., Frackowiak, R. S. J., Friston, K. J., & Dolan, R. J. (2000). Neural responses associated with cue evoked emotional states and heroin in opiate addicts. *Drug and Alcohol Dependence, 60*(2), 207–216.

Stein, E. A., Pankiewicz, J., Harsch, H. H., Cho, J.-K., Fuller, S. A., Hoffmann, R. G., et al. (1998). Nicotine-induced limbic cortical activation in the human brain: A functional MRI study. *American Journal of Psychiatry, 155,* 1009–1015.

Tapert, S. F., Brown, G. G., Baratta, M. V., & Brown, S. A. (2004). FMRI bold response to alcohol stimuli in alcohol dependent young women. *Addictive Behaviors, 29*(1), 33–50.

Tapert, S. F., Cheung, E. H., Brown, G. G., Frank, L. R., Paulus, M. P., Schweinsburg, A. D., et al. (2003). Neural response to alcohol stimuli in adolescents with alcohol use disorder. *Archives of General Psychiatry, 60*(7), 727–735.

Tzschentke, T. M., & Schmidt, W. J. (2000). Functional relationship among medial prefrontal cortex, nucleus accumbens, and ventral tegmental area in locomotion and reward. *Critical Review Neurobiology, 14*(2), 131–142.

Van de Laar, M. C., Licht, R., Franken, I. H. A., & Hendriks, V. M. (2004). Event-related potentials indicate motivational relevance of cocaine cues in abstinent cocaine addicts. *Psychopharmacology, 177,* 121–129.

Volkow, N. D., Chang, L., Wang, G. J., Fowler, J. S., Ding, Y.-S., Sedler, M., et al. (2001). Low level of brain dopamine d_2 receptors in methamphetamine abusers: Association with metabolism in the orbitofrontal cortex. *American Journal of Psychiatry, 158*(12), 2015–2021.

Volkow, N. D., Fowler, J. S., Gatley, S. J., Logan, J., Wang, G. J., Ding, Y. S., et al. (1996). PET evaluation of the dopamine system of the human brain. *Journal of Nuclear Medicine, 37*(7), 1242–1256.

Volkow, N. D., Fowler, J. S., & Wang, G. J. (1999). Imaging studies on the role of dopamine in cocaine reinforcement and addiction in humans. *Journal of Psychopharmacology, 13*(4), 337–345.

Volkow, N. D., Fowler, J. S., & Wang, G. J. (2003). The addicted human brain: Insights from imaging studies. *The Journal of Clinical Investigation, 111*(10), 1444–1451.

Volkow, N. D., Fowler, J. S., Wang, G. J., Hitzemann, R., Logan, J., Schlyer, D. J., et al. (1993). Decreased dopamine d2 receptor availability is associated with reduced frontal metabolism in cocaine abusers. *Synapse, 14*(2), 169–177.

Volkow, N. D., Wang, G. J., Fischman, M. W., Foltin, R. W., Fowler, J. S., Abumrad, N. N., et al. (1997). Relationship between subjective effects of cocaine and dopamine transporter occupancy. *Nature, 386*(6627), 827–830.

Volkow, N. D., Wang, G. J., Fowler, J. S., Hitzemann, R., Angrist, B., Gatley, S. J., et al. (1999). Association of methylphenidate-induced craving with changes in right striato-orbitofrontal metabolism in cocaine abusers: Implications in addiction. *American Journal of Psychiatry, 156*(1), 19–26.

Volkow, N. D., Wang, G. J., Fowler, J. S., Logan, J., Gatley, S. J., Wong, C., et al. (1999). Reinforcing effects of psychostimulants in humans are associated with increases in brain dopamine and occupancy of d2 receptors. *Journal of Pharmacological and Experimental Therapeutics, 291*(1), 409–415.

Wang, G. J., Volkow, N. D., Fowler, J. S., Cervany, P., Hitzemann, R. J., Pappas, N. R., et al. (1999). Regional brain metabolic activation during craving elicited by recall of previous drug experiences. *Life Sciences, 64*(9), 775–784.

Weinstein, A., Feldtkeller, B., Malizia, A., Wilson, S., Bailey, J., & Nutt, D. J. (1998). Integrating the cognitive and physiological aspects of craving. *Journal of Psychopharmacology, 12*(1), 31–38.

Wexler, B. E., Gottschalk, C. H., Fulbright, R. K., Prohivnik, I., Lacadie, C. M., Rounsaville, B. J., et al. (2001). Functional magnetic resonance imaging of cocaine craving. *American Journal of Psychiatry, 158,* 86–95.

White, N. M. (1996). Addictive drugs as reinforcers: Multiple partial actions on memory systems. *Addiction, 91*(7), 921–949.

Wise, R. A. (2004). Dopamine, learning and motivation. *Nature Review Neuroscience, 5*(6), 483–494.

Wise, R. A., & Bozarth, M. A. (1987). A psychomotor stimulant theory of addiction. *Psychological Review, 94,* 469–492.

Wrase, J., Grusser, S. M., Klein, S., Diener, C., Hermann, D., Flor, H., et al. (2002). Development of alcohol-associated cues and cue-induced brain activation in alcoholics. *European Psychiatry, 17*(5), 287–291.

CHAPTER 14

Psychophysiology and Implicit Cognition in Drug Use: Significance and Measurement of Motivation for Drug Use With Emphasis on Startle Tests

Ronald F. Mucha, Paul Pauli, and Peter Weyers

Abstract: This chapter addresses the rationale and status of psychophysiological measures of motivation for drug intake. A brief overview of different theories of drug intake indicates that physiological correlates of craving and relapse can be used to provide objective information about motivation for drug use. We then review various experimental designs for applying physiological responses to assess motivation for drug intake. Finally, the acoustic blink reflex is presented and described as a multipurpose method for this assessment. Psychophysiological tests may provide tools for the validation of concepts and methods of implicit cognition in drug intake.

INTRODUCTION

Presented here is a psychophysiological approach to implicit cognition in drug intake. A formal role of implicit cognition in addiction was only recently proposed and considerable work is necessary to determine its exact nature (Wiers et al., 2002; We use the terms "implicit cognition," "addiction," and "drug" generically and wish to acknowledge problems with exact definitions). It is certain that this will be facilitated using traditional psychophysiological techniques, as seen from many examples of their relevance in neurobiological research on mental processes and addictive behavior (see Bechara

AUTHOR'S NOTE: The authors are grateful to E. Wahlen and R. Gerhard for help with the manuscript and to students and colleagues too numerous to mention for help with the data and ideas. Financial support was solely provided by public agencies, including the German Ministry for Education and Research, the German Research Council, the Bavarian Regional Government (Program: Bayernaktiv), and the Regional Government of Baden-Württemberg (Program: Addiction).

et al., Chapter 15; Franken et al., Chapter 13). The concepts and methods of implicit cognition itself, however, are complex and not fully understood. As cogently outlined by De Houwer (Chapter 2), research on this problem may still require a systematic and paradigm-specific validation of putative processes of implicit cognition. One of the essential functional questions in addiction research concerns the motivation for drug, and it is in part for these reasons that we specifically address the rationale and strategy of applying psychophysiology to the measurement of the motivation for drug intake. This will be important for testing any implicit processes of drug-use motivation, but it should also play a role in the probing of accepted nonimplicit processes (e.g., Mucha et al., 1997).

The need for clear and differentiated information on the motivation for drug intake permeates the drug literature. The gold standard tests for verifying processes of motivation for a drug consist of drug self-administration or the secondary reinforcing effects of drugs (see Mucha, 1991). Repeated and prolonged experience with drugs, however, results in a multitude of adaptive processes (see next section and Mucha, 1991). Moreover, such gold standard tests are complex conditioning procedures that are not easily applied, particularly in a drug-experienced human. An alternative option is to infer the motivation for a drug from physiological parameters (see Geier et al., 2000; Mucha, 1991). Indeed, physiological parameters have a long history of providing objective information about the reasons for drug-seeking behavior (see Kolb & Himmelsbach, 1938).

In the first of three related sections, we will briefly overview several theories of drug intake, indicating where and how physiological measures may help to understand the motivation for drug use. In the second section, we will essentially describe three different paradigms using physiological responses as indirect measures of motivation for drug use. This may be particularly helpful when combined with methods examining implicit cognitive processes, given the difficulties of applying direct measures of drug intake in humans (e.g., drug self-administration). In the final section, information is provided on the acoustic blink or Acoustic Startle Response (ASR), which we see as currently the most effective test for indirectly assessing drug motivation.

THEORIES OF DRUG INTAKE AND PSYCHOPHYSIOLOGY

In this section, we describe several physiological and psychological theories with primary and secondary roles of physiological responses for explaining motivation for drug intake.

Physiological Theories

According to traditional understandings of drug motivation, removal of a drug from a dependent individual results in "withdrawal signs." For substances like the opiates, this is a biochemical event that is readily apparent over several hours after withdrawal, and it has been generally assumed that such effects are uncomfortable (Himmelsbach, 1943). Anyone working with opiates in animals can confirm the intense aversive effect of opiate withdrawal even in very mildly treated organisms (see Mucha, 1991). Thus, the escaping or avoidance of withdrawal is assumed to reinforce consumption of even socially acceptable or weak drugs (Griffiths & Woodson, 1988; Hughes et al., 1990). There is compelling evidence, however, that drug consumption is not perfectly correlated with the intensity of withdrawal, and this has led to two weaker versions of this model.

Environmentally Evoked Conditioned Compensatory Responses

Relapse usually occurs in the drug-taking environment and this can be long after withdrawal signs have subsided. Therefore, Wikler (1948) proposed that withdrawal signs are conditioned and give rise to conditioned withdrawal. Siegel (1976) confirmed this and demonstrated the importance of compensatory responses to the acute effect of a drug for the conditioning process. Thus, conditioned compensatory responses (i.e., conditioned withdrawal) evoked by the drug-taking environment are assumed to be the basis of craving and drug intake.

Compensatory Responses and Interoceptive Stimuli

Because compensatory responses are not always seen in the presence of drug-intake environments or stimuli, Siegel et al. (2000) argued that interoceptive stimuli might be the Conditioned Stimuli (CSs) for compensatory conditioned responses. Baker et al. (2004) further suggested that the conditioned responses need only to be an affect; these would not necessarily require any physiological response. These authors, however, also made the interesting proposal that the compensatory responses as discussed by Siegel et al. (2000) may serve as CSs. It is these "secondary CSs" that would then evoke the negative affect of withdrawal, which they also suggested could be implicit (see Curtin et al., Chapter 16).

Psychological Theories

In these views of drug intake, physiological responses play no primary role in the motivational properties of drugs and related events. Therefore, testing of such psychological models actually requires direct measurement of the motivation for drug use. For practical reasons, however, indirect measures of drug motivation could also be used. The following subsections describe categories of psychological processes that may be assessed with psychophysiological measures.

Motivational Theories

These theories postulate that drugs have motivational effects that lead directly to drug intake. Examples would be the opponent motivational process theory of Solomon and Corbit (1973) and theories concerning incentive motivational processes. Stewart et al. (1984) and Wise and Bozarth (1987) first systematically outlined an appetitive model of drug motivation. Robinson and Berridge (1993) then promoted the benefits of an incentive approach. Whereas early incentive models suggest that learned behavior is guided by expectancies for a goal object, Robinson and Berridge proposed properties of drug CSs that extend a simple expectancy notion. Some of these properties underscore distinct implicit and explicit motivational processes (see Berridge, 2001). Thus, different incentive models explain craving and relapse (see Berridge, 2001; Toates, 1986). Moreover, traditional incentive models tend to ignore incentive motivational aspects of withdrawal (see Baker et al., 2004). Withdrawal has negative incentive effects that are independent of appetitive effects (Mucha et al., 1982). A CS for withdrawal also elicits features of goal expectancy (Mucha, 1991). Regardless of incentive model, physiological responses can be applied as correlates of motivational processes.

Arousal or Energizing Theories

The literature recognizes a manifold relation between motivation and general arousal or activation (Duffy, 1962; Lang et al., 1990; Young, 1969). Mucha et al. (1981), for example, used locomotor activation as an index of incentive motivational effects of opiates. Eysenck (1973) and Wise and Bozarth (1987) talked about drug-related psychic activation. Warburton (1988) used terms like relaxing to understand the effects of smoking. Inverted U functions often relate arousal with other psychological processes (Duffy, 1962). Therefore, physiological measures, including cardiovascular, electrodermal, and muscle activity offer insight into activating and relaxing effects of drug-related event, as seen in smoking, for example (see Ashton & Stepney, 1983). Physiological indicators of arousal, however, cannot separate appetitive behavior from withdrawal aversion (Carter & Tiffany, 1999).

Drug Intake as Automatic Behavior

Tiffany (1990) suggested that drug intake occurs automatically. An arithmetic task becomes automatic after only a few hundred trials (Pauli et al., 1998). A smoker, however, would experience this amount of practice in a matter of weeks (Schupp et al., 1999). The automaticity theory contrasts with other theories since the availability of drug is considered to be important: Craving arises when the intake act is interrupted (e.g., depletion of drug); this event triggers arousal, frustration, and drug-seeking. There have been surprisingly few systematic tests of the model using psychophysiological techniques and they are largely circumstantial. Cepeda-Benito and Tiffany (1996) applied a dual task where effects of smoking cues disrupted the reaction time only in the task that required nonautomatic processing; at the same time heart rate and Electrodermal Activation (EDA) were differentially increased by the smoking cues. Schupp et al. (1999) found that smokers showed a significant correlation between the topography of inhaling on an unlit cigarette and real inhaling during smoking. They suggested that this could be explained by the automatic nature of

smoking, which was consistent with the fact that both effects were sensitive to smoke deprivation.

PSYCHOPHYSIOLOGICAL INDICATORS OF DRUG MOTIVATION

In this section, we describe three paradigms for applying physiological measures to assess motivation for drug. They differ in their ease of application but also with regard to the assumptions needed to confirm a motivational process.

Paradigm 1: Cue Reactivity

This is the least demanding test and asks simply whether a cue that evokes craving for drug also triggers a physiological response. Control procedures may confirm that the reactivity to the test stimulus was in fact due to pairing with the drug in question (see Glautier & Tiffany, 1995; Robbins & Ehrman, 1992). A meta-analysis by Carter and Tiffany (1999) revealed a consistent pattern of cue-evoked effects; this comprised heart rate increases, EDA, and finger hypothermia. This pattern, however, was the same over a range of different pharmacological classes of drugs that individually evoke different or even opposite unconditioned physiological effects. Responses were also unspecific to the different motivational processes underlying craving and relapse (see the monograph by Drummond et al., 1995, for many examples). Therefore, there has been a stop to simple reactivity tests for assessing motivational processes.

Cue-reactivity testing could be improved, however, with more specific physiological measures, for example, facial EMG (Dimberg, 1990; Sayette & Hufford, 1995), EEG asymmetry (Zinser et al., 1999), or event-related potentials (Van de Laar et al.,

2004). Two sets of facial muscles are needed to sense appetitive and aversive effects. Thus, Geier et al. (2000) could differentiate smoking cues from negative nonsmoking stimuli on the basis of the corrugator muscle activity, yet needed an additional measurement from the zygomatic muscle to conclude that cues were appetitive. Zinser et al. (1999) used EEG asymmetry in frontal regions as a parameter of motivational valence and were able to conclude that cues for smoking had appetitive effects that did not always parallel self-reports. Such techniques have been successfully applied in other research (Ito & Cacioppo, 1999; Pauli et al., 1999) but only rarely in the addiction field. Franken et al. (2003) looked at heroin cues in opiate-dependent and control individuals but failed to find a pattern of results consistent with that of Zinser et al. (1999). Nevertheless, these and related electrophysiological procedures need to be developed for understanding emotion and motivational components of addictive behavior. Such procedures may be more complex than simple peripheral EMG, but they would be warranted particularly for looking at multiple processes underlying drug cues. For example, the investigation of some models of implicit cognitive processing of cues based on temporal processing of information (see Deutsch & Strack, Chapter 4) could profit from measures of event-related potentials. The reader is also directed to relevant work from various other groups investigating alcohol and smoking cues (e. g., Herrmann et al., 2001; Warren & McDonough, 1999).

Paradigm 2:
Modulated Cue Reactivity

The conditions of testing in this paradigm increase the specificity of the physiological measure to the motivational properties of a cue.

Expectation of Drug, Drug Deprivation, and Actual Drug Availability

Cue reactivity is influenced by several manipulations of a test person that change the need or the opportunity to consume a drug. The simple expectation that a drug can be consumed after a cue reactivity test increases a subject's physiological response to the respective cues (Carter & Tiffany, 2001; Laberg, 1986; Turkkan et al., 1989). Also, deprivation from drug often increases physiological responses to drug cues (e.g., Payne et al., 1996; Turkkan, et al., 1989). This, however, is not always clear (Geier et al., 2000; see Figure 14.1). Also, certain conditioned effects of food do not always respond to deprivation (for references, see Mucha et al., 1999).

Motivational models predict physiological activation as part of the preparation for drug intake (Baker et al., 2004; Robinson & Berridge, 1993; Stewart et al., 1984). This could, however, simply reflect motor activity that would not necessarily index motivation for the goal object (e.g., Mucha et al., 1998). The critical question is whether the motivational effects can be separated from the motor consequences of availability. This seems possible since the availability of drug during a test influences various psychological processes (Wertz & Sayette, 2001). Carter and Tiffany (2001) also showed an effect of availability of smoking material and smoking behavior on cue reactivity that was not present under control conditions with simple motor activation.

The Drug Intake Ritual

There is evidence that goal behavior can be controlled in different ways by the stimuli within the respective goal ritual (e.g., Timberlake, 1993). Thus, craving for cigarettes is high for pictures that depict scenes before the beginning of the smoking ritual relative to those with scenes after the end of consumption (Bushnell et al., 2000; Mucha et al.,

1999). A similar pattern was seen for alcohol pictures in alcohol consumers but not with begin and end smoking pictures in never smokers (Mucha et al., 1999). Begin and end pictures also evoke different physiological responses (Mucha et al., 2000). It is unclear why these different stimuli evoke different effects, as both the begin and end stimuli are signals for drug intake and both activate the "memories" or "networks" of drug consumption (see Baker et al., 2004). Young (1969) suggested that stimuli of the end of consumption simply become irrelevant. Mucha et al. (1999), however, suggested that the end stimuli may signal the lack of a drug goal. Nevertheless, begin and end scenes of the intake ritual do offer useful test and control stimuli, respectively, for investigating cues (see Mucha et al., 2000).

Paradigm 3: Tests Using a Known Motivational Baseline

In this paradigm, the efficacy of a cue is determined by its ability to change a baseline sensitive to an identified motivational state. Estes and Skinner (1941) first showed that rats trained to bar press for a positive reinforcer would press less in presence of a CS eliciting fear. This change from baseline behavior can be used to infer the motivational quality of the test stimulus, as long as the baseline is clearly understood (see also Azrin & Hake, 1969). The ASR provides a well-studied baseline of defensive responses elicited by sudden, high intensity sound and its modulation by drug cues can indicate motivation processes.

STARTLE PARADIGMS FOR ASSESSING MOTIVATIONAL PROCESSES

Although, the ASR is usually measured as the eye blink reflex in humans and as whole body movement in animals (Fendt & Fanselow, 1999; Grillon & Baas, 2003; Koch & Schnitzler, 1997), it can be considered a comparative test for drug motivation (see Fendt & Mucha, 2001). It can be repeatedly applied, allowing for within-subject designs, although good test-retest reliability is currently not possible with all startle paradigms (for data on reliability, see Larson et al., 2000). Nevertheless, within-designs help to overcome problems with between-subjects variability. Important for implicit cognition of drug intake, the acoustic blink reflex itself has a short latency (45 to 50 ms), making it insensitive against voluntarily control by the subject (Hamm & Vaitl, 1996; Lang et al., 1990). This also makes the test well suited for addressing temporal parameters believed to be important for drug cues.

The Raw Startle Response

Baseline ASR

Unusually intense ASRs in patients with Posttraumatic Stress Disorder have been used to infer the presence of chronic fear or anxiety (Grillon et al., 1998). This was tested, in part, with manipulations known to affect fear responses (e.g., darkness; Grillon et al., 1998). Patients in alcohol detoxification also show responses longer than those seen in individuals not dependent on alcohol (Krystal et al., 1997; Mucha et al., 2000). A possibility that this effect was due to the aversive features of withdrawal (Krystal et al., 1997) was not supported, as there was no recovery between two test sessions separated by three weeks (Mucha et al., 2000).

Sensitization and Habituation of the ASR

Upon repeated application of a startling stimulus, there is usually habituation of the startle response. Habituation is reduced or replaced by sensitization, however, when the acoustic signals are intensified and made more aversive (Koch & Schnitzler, 1997). Kumari et al. (1996) indicated a more rapid decrease in startle amplitude after smoking in deprived smokers as opposed to nonsmokers. It was suggested that this effect could reflect relief of smoking withdrawal discomfort. This was not confirmed, however, when order effects and habituation itself were controlled (Müller et al., 1998).

Prepulse Change in the ASR

The startle response is attenuated when a stimulus is given 30 to 500 ms prior to a baseline startle probe; it is suggested that the effect reflects a form of sensorimotor gating (Graham, 1975). Prepulse Inhibition (PPI) is increased by nicotine and cigarette smoking (Acri et al., 1994; Kumari et al., 1996; Orain-Pelissolo et al., 2004), as expected of a cognitive enhancer (Warburton, 1988). Withdrawal from smoking decreases the PPI (Kumari & Gray, 1999). Hutchison et al. (1999) also reported that PPI was decreased after deprived smokers held and looked at a lit cigarette. The authors suggested a possible reduction in attentional processes during withdrawal and a further enhancement of this by smoking cues. Their cues, however, also increased negative affect, which itself could have influenced the PPI (see Hawk et al., 2002).

Affect-Modulated Startle

It is well-known that the startle response in rats is potentiated by fear (Davis, 1979), and is attenuated by appetitive stimuli (e.g., Steidl et al., 2001). This pattern is apparent in humans, as well (e.g., Grillon et al., 1991; Skolnick & Davidson, 2002). Lang and his colleagues (Lang, 1995; Lang et al., 1990) first laid the basis for streamlined testing of momentary motivational states in humans. Their procedure presents standardized pictures

(International Affective Picture System, IAPS) that are pleasurable, neutral, or unpleasant. The slides or computer images are followed shortly after their onset (e.g., 2.5 to 5.5 s) with a startling probe (e.g., 50 ms, 95 dB). The amplitude of the startle responses then show an inverse relation to the degree of momentary pleasure evoked by the pictures. This startle modulation is not due to picture arousal, nature of startle quantification, or amount of testing in the session (see Lang, 1995; Lang et al., 1990). Similar modulation has been seen with other types of motivational stimuli, such as films or periods of imagery (e.g., Schupp et al., 1997). The Lang et al. paradigm, however, can only be modified with caution. Different basic protocols are confounded by arousal produced by the pictures (see Benning et al., 2004; Sabatinelli et al., 2001; Skolnick & Davidson, 2002), which in turn interacts with other effects of drugs (e.g., Stritzke et al., 1995).

Cue-Modulated Startle

Elash et al. (1995) first applied the ASR to test the motivational significance of drug cues; they had subjects imagine smoking. These cues were reported to be aversive and they increased startle magnitude. Imagery, however, may have unclear effects on ASR (Witvliet & Vrana, 1995). The actual application of the Lang et al. (1990) procedure to the study of drug cues was realized in our studies by supplementing IAPS pictures with pictures of smoking for smokers and pictures of drinking for alcoholics (Geier et al., 2000; Mucha et al., 2000). Based on this design, the ASR evoked during a drug cue was significantly lower than the ASR evoked during negatively valenced or neutral, nonsmoking control pictures. With this same procedure, other groups have also confirmed a cue-produced decrease in ASR (e.g., Heinz et al., 2003). To account for the different results of Elash et al. (1995), we may have to address the fact that subjects tested with imagery cues require considerable time for memorizing the specific smoking test cues. Other studies where the subjects have time to deliberate over the drug stimuli (e.g., actual alcoholic drinks) also show a cue-produced increase in the ASR, as if the stimulus is aversive (e.g., Saladin et al., 2002).

Control Conditions and Replications

Geier et al. (2000) confirmed the specificity of smoking cues by using control subjects who had never smoked; the smoking cues actually potentiated the ASR in this population. Mucha et al. (2000) used a within-subject design and control pictures composed of end of alcohol consumption that were matched thematically and technically with the begin alcohol pictures (Mucha et al., 1999). Only the begin alcohol pictures reduced the amplitude of the startle (Mucha et al., 2000). Thus, drug cues (begin stimuli) presented as pictures as in the paradigm of Lang et al. (1990) were concluded to be appetitive.

It has to be noted that in such studies, the modulation of ASR by a cue is a statistical phenomenon that is not seen in every subject. This makes it tempting to interpret those responses above the mean as showing less appetitive effects, or even a cue-aversion (for references see Wiers et al., Chapter 22). Current procedures for studying affect modulation of ASR with cues, however, are typically within-session. They are troubled by low reliability and high subject variability (see Grillon & Bass, 2003; Larson et al., 2000). Therefore, it may be important that outliers be examined in different ways.

Another important question is whether it is sufficient to draw conclusions about drug cues when the only control condition was composed of arbitrarily chosen neutral test material. For example, Orain-Pelissolo et al. (2004) compared ASRs elicited while viewing smoking pictures (developed by themselves) and neutral IAPS pictures. They found no significant differences and concluded

that smoking pictures do not affect ASR. The discrepancy with our findings could be explained in part by arousal produced by the test stimuli. Our smoking and alcohol cues were as arousing as the neutral IAPS material (see Mucha et al., 1999; Geier et al., 2000); the smoking pictures of Orain-Pelissolo et al. (2004) were more arousing. In addition, IAPS pictures with different valence are benchmarks for the Lang et al. (1990) protocol itself. Unfortunately, in the Orain-Pelissolo et al. (2004) data there was no direct information on the validity of their protocol. It might be added that Orain-Pelissolo et al. (2004) also studied minimally dependent smokers (FTQ = 3 ± 0.4, $n = 34$), whereas we examined dependent smokers (FTQ = 5.9 ± 0.3 to 6.4 ± 0.3, $n = 16$).

Effect of Deprivation and Smoking Expectation

Whereas deprivation from smoking appears to affect the PPI (see above), it may have no or only weak effects on the cue-modulated startle. Geier et al. (2000) tested three groups of smokers: one group was smoke satiated and two groups were 12 h smoke deprived, with half of them being informed that they could not or could smoke during the study. The startle data showed no main effect of deprivation and no interaction between picture type and deprivation. Importantly, all groups were dependent and the deprivation manipulations could be confirmed.

Given the significance of this, we (unpublished data) replicated this with two groups of subjects who had abstained from smoking for 12 h. One group was tested deprived and a second smoked before and during the study. The ASR results in Figure 14.1 indicate, on the one hand, no significant group differences; the expected deprivation effect was not appreciable relative to the high between-group variance. On the other hand, both the valance of IAPS pictures and the different smoking stimuli modulated the startle

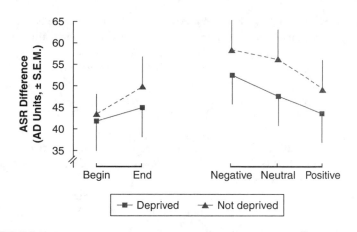

Figure 14.1   Mean ASR during presentation of smoking (begin or end pictures), or negative, neutral, or positive nonsmoking IAPS pictures in dependent smokers who were required ($n = 14$) or not required ($n = 15$) to abstain from smoking for 12 hours (confirmed by differences in CO levels). No overall effect of group was significant (both F values < 0.7); however, there was an effect of test picture, $F_{(4, 108)} = 11.3$, $p < .001$. Separate analyses collapsed over groups confirmed a linear trend over the IAPS pictures, $F_{(2, 54)} = 17.1$, $p < .001$, and a difference between begin and end pictures, $F_{(1, 27)} = 7.8$, $p < .01$. The matched smoking pictures and the IAPS nonsmoking pictures were derived from Mucha et al. (1999) and (2000), respectively; the protocols were from Geier et al. (2000).

response. The data confirmed a pattern of consistency for cue-modulated startle and further indicate that there may be differences in the sensitivity of cue-modulated and PPI paradigms to drug deprivation.

SUMMARY AND CONCLUSIONS

A clear and differentiated measurement of motivation for drug intake is an essential goal of research on addiction in general and on implicit cognition in drug intake in particular.

A psychophysiological approach is seen to be effective for theoretical and methodological strategies to reach this goal. Different tests using the acoustic blink reflex as a baseline to measure motivational effects of drug and drug cues seem to be especially valuable. The features of these tests and the data available confirm several phenomena of drug motivation. Application of psychophysiological measures of motivation for drug intake may help integrate understandings of implicit and automatic cognitive processes of drug motivation with the traditional literature on addictive behavior.

REFERENCES

Acri, J. B., Morse, D. E., Popke, E. J., & Grunberg, N. E. (1994). Nicotine increases sensory gating measured as inhibition of the acoustic startle reflex in rats. *Psychopharmacology, 114,* 369–374.

Ashton, H., & Stepney, R. (1983). *Smoking, psychology and pharmacology.* London and New York: Tavistock Publications.

Azrin, N. H., & Hake, D. F. (1969). Positive conditioned suppression: Conditioned suppression using positive reinforcers as the unconditioned stimulus. *Journal of Experimental Analysis of Behavior, 12,* 167–173.

Baker, T. B., Piper, M. E., McCarthy, D. E., Majeskie, M. R., & Fiore, M. C. (2004). Addiction motivation reformulated: An affective processing model of negative reinforcement. *Psychological Review, 111,* 33–51.

Benning, S. D., Patrick, C. J., & Lang, A. R. (2004). Emotional modulation of the post-auricular reflex. *Psychophysiology, 41,* 426–432.

Berridge, K. C. (2001). Reward learning: Reinforcement, incentives, and expectations. In D. L. Medin (Ed.), *The psychology of learning and motivation* (Vol. 40, pp. 223–278). San Diego, CA: Academic Press.

Bushnell, P. J., Levin, E. D., Marrocco, R. T., Sarter, M. F., Strupp, B. J., & Warburton, D. M. (2000). Attention as a target of intoxication: Insights and methods from studies of drug abuse. *Neurotoxicity and Teratology, 22,* 487–502.

Carter, B. L., & Tiffany, S. T. (1999). Meta-analysis of cue-reactivity in addiction research. *Addiction, 94,* 327–340.

Carter, B. L., & Tiffany, S. T. (2001). The cue-availability paradigm: The effects of cigarette availability on cue reactivity in smokers. *Experimental & Clinical Psychopharmacology, 9,* 183–190.

Cepeda-Benito, A., & Tiffany, S. T. (1996). The use of a dual-task procedure for the assessment of cognitive effort associated with cigarette craving. *Psychopharmacology, 127,* 155–163.

Davis, M. (1979). Diazepam and flurazepam: Effects on conditioned fear as measured with the potentiated startle paradigm. *Psychopharmacology, 62,* 1–7.

Dimberg, U. (1990). Facial electromyography and emotional reactions. *Psychophysiology, 27,* 481–494.

Drummond, D. C., Tiffany, S. T., Glautier, S., & Remington, B. (1995). *Addictive behaviour: Cue exposure theory and practice.* Oxford, UK: Wiley.

Duffy, E. (1962). *Activation and behavior.* New York and London: John Wiley.

Elash, C. A., Tiffany, S. T., & Vrana, S. R. (1995). Manipulation of smoking urges and affect through a brief-imagery procedure: Self-report, psychophysiological, and startle probe responses. *Experimental & Clinical Psychopharmacology, 3,* 156–162.

Estes, W. K., & Skinner, B. F. (1941). Some quantitative properties of anxiety. *Journal of Experimental Psychology, 29,* 390–400.

Eysenck, H. J. (1973). Personality and the law of effect. In D. E. Berlyne & K. B. Madsen (Eds.), *Pleasure, reward, preference: Their nature, determinants, and role in behavior* (pp. 133–166). New York: Academic Press.

Fendt, M., & Fanselow, M. S. (1999). The neuroanatomical and neurochemical basis of conditioned fear. *Neuroscience & Biobehavioral Reviews, 23,* 743–760.

Fendt, M., & Mucha, R. F. (2001). Anxiogenic-like effects of opiate withdrawal seen in the fear-potentiated startle test, an interdisciplinary probe for drug-related motivational states. *Psychopharmacology, 155,* 242–250.

Franken, I. H. A., Stam, C. J., Hendriks, V. M., & Van den Brink, W. (2003). Neurophysiological evidence for abnormal cognitive processing of drug cues in heroin dependence. *Psychopharmacology, 170,* 205–212.

Geier, A., Mucha, R. F., & Pauli, P. (2000). Appetitive nature of drug cues confirmed with physiological measures in a model using pictures of smoking. *Psychopharmacology, 150,* 283–291.

Glautier, S., & Tiffany, S. T. (1995). Methodological issues in cue reactivity research. In D. C. Drummond, S. T. Tiffany, S. Glautier, & B. Remington (Eds.), *Addictive behaviors: Cue exposure theory and practice* (pp. 75–97). Chichester, UK: Wiley.

Graham, F. (1975). The more or less startling effects of weak prestimulation. *Psychophysiology, 12,* 238–248.

Griffiths, R. R., & Woodson, P. P. (1988). Caffeine physical dependence: A review of human and laboratory animal studies. *Psychopharmacology, 94,* 437–451.

Grillon, C., Ameli, R., Woods, S. W., Merikangas, K., & Davis, M. (1991). Fear-potentiated startle in humans: Effects of anticipatory anxiety on the acoustic blink reflex. *Psychophysiology, 28,* 588–595.

Grillon, C., & Baas, J. (2003). A review of the modulation of the startle reflex by affective states and its application in psychiatry. *Clinical Neurophysiology, 114,* 1557–1579.

Grillon, C., Morgan, C. A., Davis, M., & Southwick, S. M. (1998). Effect of darkness on acoustic startle in Vietnam veterans with PTSD. *American Journal of Psychiatry, 155,* 812–817.

Hamm, A. O., & Vaitl, D. (1996). Affective learning: Awareness and aversion. *Psychophysiology, 33,* 698–710.

Hawk, L. W., Redford, J. S., & Baschnagel, J. S. (2002). Influence of a monetary incentive upon attentional modification of short-lead prepulse inhibition and long-lead prepulse facilitation of acoustic startle. *Psychophysiology, 39,* 674–677.

Heinz, A., Loeber, S., Georgi, A., Wrase, J., Hermann, D., Rey, E. R., et al. (2003). Reward craving and withdrawal relief craving: Assessment of different motivational pathways to alcohol intake. *Alcohol and Alcoholism, 38,* 35–39.

Herrmann, M. J., Weijers, H. G., Wiesbeck, G. A., Boning, J., & Fallgatter, A. J. (2001). Alcohol cue-reactivity in heavy and light social drinkers as revealed by event-related potentials. *Alcohol and Alcoholism, 36,* 588–593.

Himmelsbach, C. K. (1943). IV. With reference to physical dependence. *Federal Proceedings of American Societies for Experimental Biology, 3,* 187–203.

Hughes, J. R., Higgins, S. T., & Hatsukami, D. (1990). Effects of abstinence from tobacco: A critical review. *Research Advances in Alcohol and Drug Problems, 10,* 317–398.

Hutchison, K. E., Niaura, R., & Swift, R. (1999). Smoking cues decrease prepulse inhibition of the startle response and increase subjective craving in humans. *Experimental & Clinical Psychopharmacology, 7,* 250–256.

Ito, T. A., & Cacioppo, J. T. (1999). The psychophysiology of utility appraisals. In D. Kahneman, E. Diener, & N. Schwarz (Eds.), *Well-being: The foundations of hedonic psychology* (pp. 470–488). New York: Russell Sage.

Koch, M., & Schnitzler, H. U. (1997). The acoustic startle response in rats: Circuits mediating evocation, inhibition and potentiation. *Behavioral Brain Research, 89,* 35–49.

Kolb, L., & Himmelsbach, C. K. (1938). Clinical studies of drug addiction: III. A critical review of the withdrawal treatments with method of evaluating abstinence syndromes. *The American Journal of Psychiatry, 94,* 759–799.

Krystal, J. H., Webb, E., Grillon, C., Cooney, N., Casal, L., Morgan, C., III, et al. (1997). Evidence of acoustic startle hyperreflexia in recently detoxified early onset male alcoholics: Modulation by yohimbine and m-chlorophenylpiperazine (mCPP). *Psychopharmacology, 131,* 207–215.

Kumari, V., Checkley, S. A., & Gray, J. A. (1996). Effect of cigarette smoking on prepulse inhibition of the acoustic startle reflex in healthy male smokers. *Psychopharmacology, 128,* 54–60.

Kumari, V., & Gray, J. A. (1999). Smoking withdrawal, nicotine dependence and prepulse inhibition of the acoustic startle reflex. *Psychopharmacology, 141,* 11–15.

Laberg, J. C. (1986). Alcohol and expectancy: Subjective, psychophysiological and behavioral responses to alcohol stimuli in severely, moderately and non-dependent drinkers. *British Journal of Addiction, 81,* 797–808.

Lang, P. J. (1995). The emotion probe: Studies of motivation and attention. *American Psychologist, 50,* 372–385.

Lang, P. J., Bradley, M. M., & Cuthbert, B. N. (1990). Emotion, attention, and the startle reflex. *Physiological Reviews, 97,* 377–395.

Larson, C. L., Ruffalo, D., Nietert, J. Y., & Davidson, R. J. (2000). Temporal stability of the emotion-modulated startle response. *Psychophysiology, 37,* 92–101.

Mucha, R. F. (1991). Opiate withdrawal dysphoria. In A. Boulton, G. Baker, & P. H. Wu (Eds.), *Animal models of drug addiction* (pp. 271–314). Totowa, NJ: Humana.

Mucha, R. F., Geier, A., & Pauli, P. (1999). Modulation of craving by cues having differential overlap with pharmacological effect: Evidence for cue approach in smokers and social drinkers. *Psychopharmacology, 147,* 306–313.

Mucha, R. F., Geier, A., Stuhlinger, M., & Mundle, G. (2000). Appetitive effects of drug cues modelled by pictures of the intake ritual: Generality of cue-modulated startle examined with inpatient alcoholics. *Psychopharmacology, 151,* 428–432.

Mucha, R. F., & Iversen, S. D. (1984). Reinforcing properties of morphine and naloxone revealed by conditioned place preferences: A procedural examination. *Psychopharmacology, 82,* 241–247.

Mucha, R. F., Pauli, P., & Angrilli, A. (1998). Conditioned responses elicited by experimentally produced cues for smoking. *Canadian Journal of Physiology and Pharmacology, 76,* 259–268.

Mucha, R. F., Van der Kooy, D., O'Shaughnessy, M., & Bucenieks, P. (1982). Drug reinforcement studied by the use of place conditioning in rat. *Brain Research, 243,* 91–105.

Mucha, R. F., Volkovskis, C., & Kalant, H. (1981). Conditioned increases in locomotor activity produced with morphine as an unconditioned stimulus, and the relation of conditioning to acute morphine effect and tolerance. *Journal of Comparative and Physiological Psychology, 95,* 351–362.

Mucha, R. F., Weiss, R. V., & Mutz, G. (1997). Detection of the erect position in the freely moving human: Sensor characteristics, reliability, and validity. *Physiology & Behavior, 61,* 293–300.

Müller, V., Mucha, R. F., & Pauli, P. (1998). Dependence on smoking and the acoustic startle response in healthy smokers. *Pharmacology Biochemistry & Behavior, 59,* 1031–1038.

Orain-Pelissolo, S., Grillon, C., Perez-Diaz, F., & Jouvent, R. (2004). Lack of startle modulation by smoking cues in smokers. *Psychopharmacology, 173,* 160–166.

Pauli, P., Bourne, L. E., & Birbaumer, N. (1998). Extensive practice in mental arithmetic and practice transfer over a ten-month retention interval. *Mathematical Cognition, 4,* 21–46.

Pauli, P., Wiedemann, G., & Nickola, M. (1999). Pain sensitivity, cerebral laterality, and negative affect. *Pain, 4,* 21–46.

Payne, T. J., Smith, P. O., Sturges, L. V., & Holleran, S. A. (1996). Reactivity to smoking cues: Mediating roles of nicotine dependence and duration of deprivation. *Addictive Behaviors, 21,* 139–154.

Robbins, S. J., & Ehrman, R. N. (1992). Designing studies of drug conditioning in humans. *Psychopharmacology, 106,* 143–153.

Robinson, T. E., & Berridge, K. C. (1993). The neural basis of drug craving: An incentive-sensitization theory of addiction. *Brain Research Reviews, 18,* 247–291.

Sabatinelli, D., Bradley, M. M., & Lang, P. J. (2001). Affective startle modulation in anticipation and perception. *Psychophysiology, 38,* 719–722.

Saladin, M. E., Drobes, D. J., Libet, J. M., & Coffey, S. F. (2002). The human startle reflex and alcohol cue reactivity: Effects of early versus late abstinence. *Psychology of Addictive Behaviors, 16,* 98–105.

Sayette, M. A., & Hufford, M. R. (1995). Urge and affect: A facial coding analysis of smokers. *Experimental & Clinical Psychopharmacology, 3,* 417–423.

Schupp, H. T., Cuthbert, B. N., Bradley, M. M., & Birbaumer, N. (1997). Probe P3 and blinks: Two measures of affective startle modulation. *Psychophysiology, 34,* 1–6.

Schupp, P. E., Mucha, R. F., & Pauli, P. (1999). Topography of sham and real puffing examined using a paced smoking regimen. *Addictive Behaviors, 24,* 695–699.

Siegel, S. (1976). Morphine analgesic tolerance: Its situation specificity supports a Pavlovian conditioning model. *Science, 193,* 323–325.

Siegel, S., Baptista, M. A., Kim, J. A., McDonald, R. V., & Weise-Kelly, L. (2000). Pavlovian psychopharmacology: The associative basis of tolerance. *Experimental & Clinical Psychopharmacology, 8,* 276–293.

Skolnick, A. J., & Davidson, R. J. (2002). Affective modulation of eyeblink startle with reward and threat. *Psychophysiology, 39,* 835–850.

Solomon, R. L., & Corbit, J. D. (1973). An opponent-process theory of motivation: II. Cigarette addiction. *Journal of Abnormal Psychology, 81,* 158–171.

Steidl, S., Li, L., & Yeomans, J. S. (2001). Conditioned brain-stimulation reward attenuates the acoustic startle reflex in rats. *Behavioral Neuroscience, 115,* 710–717.

Stewart, J., de Wit, H., & Eikelboom, R. (1984). Role of unconditioned and conditioned drug effects in the self-administration of opiates and stimulants. *Psychological Review, 91,* 251–268.

Stritzke, W. G., Patrick, C. J., & Lang, A. R. (1995). Alcohol and human emotion: A multidimensional analysis incorporating startle-probe methodology. *Journal of Abnormal Psychology, 104,* 114–122.

Tiffany, S. T. (1990). A cognitive model of drug urges and drug-use behavior: Role of automatic and nonautomatic processes. *Psychological Reviews, 97,* 147–168.

Timberlake, W. (1993). Behavior systems and reinforcement: An integrative approach. *Journal of the Experimental Analysis of Behavior, 60,* 105–128.

Toates, F. M. (1986). *Motivational systems.* Cambridge, UK: Cambridge University Press.

Turkkan, J. S., McCaul, M. E., & Stitzer, M. L. (1989). Psychophysiological effects of alcohol-related stimuli: II. Enhancement with alcohol availability. *Alcoholism: Clinical and Experimental Research, 13,* 392–398.

Van de Laar, M. C., Licht, R., Franken, I. H. A., & Hendriks, V. M. (2004). Event-related potentials indicate motivational relevance of cocaine cues in abstinent cocaine addicts. *Psychopharmacology, 177,* 121–129.

Warburton, D. M. (1988). The puzzle of nicotine use. In M. Lader (Ed.), *Psychopharmacology of addiction* (pp. 27–49). Oxford, UK: Oxford University Press.

Warren, C. A., & McDonough, B. E. (1999). Event-related brain potentials as indicators of smoking cue-reactivity. *Clinical Neurophysiology, 110,* 1570–1584.

Wertz, J. M., & Sayette, M. A. (2001). A review of the effects of perceived drug use opportunity on self-reported urge. *Experimental & Clinical Psychopharmacology, 9,* 3–13.

Wiers, R. W., Stacy, A. W., Ames, S. L., Noll, J. A., Sayette, M. A., Zack, M., et al. (2002). Implicit and explicit alcohol-related cognitions. *Alcoholism: Clinical and Experimental Research, 26,* 129–137.

Wikler, A. (1948). Recent progress in research on the neuropsychological basis of morphine addiction. *American Journal of Psychiatry, 67,* 672–684.

Wise, R. A., & Bozarth, M. A. (1987). A psychomotor stimulant theory of addiction. *Psychological Review, 94,* 469–492.

Witvliet, C., & Vrana, S. R. (1995). Psychophysiological responses as indices of affective dimensions. *Psychophysiology, 32,* 436–443.

Young, P. T. (1969). *Motivation and emotion.* New York: John Wiley.

Zinser, M. C., Fiore, M. C., Davidson, R. J., & Baker, T. B. (1999). Manipulating smoking motivation: Impact on an electrophysiological index of approach motivation. *Journal of Abnormal Psychology, 108,* 240–254.

CHAPTER 15

Loss of Willpower: Abnormal Neural Mechanisms of Impulse Control and Decision Making in Addiction

ANTOINE BECHARA, XAVIER NOEL,
AND EVELINE A. CRONE

Abstract: Addiction is a condition in which the person becomes unable to choose according to long-term outcomes when it comes to drugs. We will argue that this is the product of an imbalance between two separate, but interacting, neural systems: (1) an *impulsive, amygdala-dependent* system for signaling the pain or pleasure of *immediate* prospects and (2) a *reflective, orbitofrontal-dependent* system for signaling the prospects of the *future*. The conditions that lead to this imbalance include (1) a dysfunctional reflective system and (2) a hyperactive impulsive system. In other words, drugs can acquire properties of triggering bottom-up, involuntary signals through the amygdala that modulate, bias, or even "hijack," top-down, goal-driven attentional resources needed for the normal operation of the reflective system and exercising the will.

Imagine yourself at a party during your first year in college, and you see your friends drinking, using drugs, and engaging in sexual activities. In the back of your mind, you hear the voices of your parents, warning you and asking you not to engage in such activities. What would you do? This is a hard decision, but you are the one who will ultimately decide, with a clear sense of deciding and exercising free will.

Willpower, as defined by the *Encarta® World English Dictionary*, is a combination of determination and self-discipline that enables somebody to do something despite the difficulties involved. This is the mechanism that enables one to endure sacrifices now to obtain benefits later. Otherwise, how would one accept the pain of surgery? On the other hand, why would someone resist the temptation to have something so irresistible, or delay the gratification from something that is so appealing? We will argue that these complex and apparently indeterminist behaviors are the product of a complex cognitive process subserved by two separate, but interacting, neural systems: (1) an *impulsive*, amygdala-dependent, neural system for signaling the pain or pleasure of the *immediate* prospects of an option and (2) a *reflective*, prefrontal-dependent, neural system for signaling the pain or pleasure of the *future* prospects of an option. The final decision is determined by the relative strengths of the pain or pleasure signals associated with immediate or future prospects. When the immediate prospect is unpleasant, but the future is more pleasant, then the positive signal of future prospects forms the basis for enduring the unpleasantness of immediate prospects. This also occurs when the future prospect is even more pleasant than the immediate one. Otherwise, the immediate prospects predominate, and decisions shift toward short-term horizons. As suggested by Damasio (1994, p. 175): "Willpower is just another name for the idea of choosing according to long-term outcomes rather than short-term ones."

We have used the term *somatic* (Damasio, 1994) to refer to the collection of body-related responses that hallmark these affective and emotional responses. Somatic is derived from the Greek word "soma," that is, body. Although during the process of weighing somatic (affective) responses, the immediate and future prospects of an option may trigger numerous somatic responses that conflict with each other, the end result is that an overall positive or negative somatic state emerges. We have proposed that the mechanisms that determine the nature of this overall somatic state (i.e., being positive or negative) are consistent with the principles of natural selection, that is, survival of the fittest (Bechara & Damasio, 2004). In other words, numerous and often conflicting somatic states may be triggered at the same time, but stronger ones gain selective advantage over weaker ones. With each "thought" brought to working memory, the strength of the somatic state triggered by that "thought" determines whether the same "thought" is likely to recur (i.e., will be brought back to memory so that it triggers another somatic state that reinforces the previous one), or whether that "thought" is likely to be eliminated. Thus, over the course of pondering a decision, positive and negative somatic markers that are strong are reinforced, whereas weak ones are eliminated. This process of elimination can be very fast. Ultimately, a winner takes all; an overall, more dominant, somatic state emerges (a "gut feeling" or "a hunch," so to speak), which then provides signals to the telencephalon that modulate activity in neural structures involved in biasing decisions (Figure 15.1). This "winner takes all" view is consistent with the conception of Strack and Deutsch (2004) on competition between motor schemata (see also Deutsch & Strack, Chapter 4).

Addiction is a condition in which the person becomes unable to choose according to long-term outcomes. Choosing according to long-term outcomes rather than short-term ones requires that the pain or pleasure signals triggered by the reflective system dominate those triggered by the impulsive system. Two broad types of conditions could alter this relationship and lead to loss of willpower: (1) a dysfunctional reflective system, which has lost its ability to process and trigger somatic signals associated with future prospects; and (2) a hyperactive impulsive system, which exaggerates the somatic signals from immediate prospects. When drug cues acquire properties for triggering bottom-up, automatic, and involuntary somatic states through the amygdala, this bottom-up somatic bias can modulate top-down cognitive mechanisms, in which the prefrontal cortex is a critical substrate. If strong enough, this bottom-up influence can interfere or "hijack" the top-down cognitive mechanisms necessary for triggering somatic states about future outcomes.

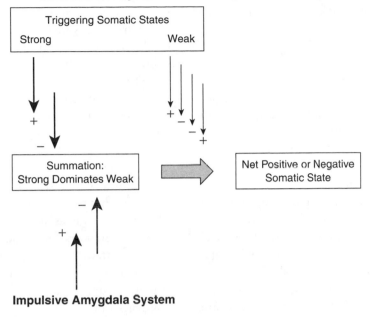

Figure 15.1 Diagram illustrating the interaction of the reflective and impulsive systems in relation to their triggering of somatic states and the ultimate emergence of a net or overall somatic state that plays a critical role in biasing decisions.

A SOMATIC MARKER MODEL OF DRUG ADDICTION

The somatic marker framework provides a systems-level neuroanatomical and cognitive framework for decision making, and for choosing according to long-term outcomes rather than short-term ones, and it suggests that the process of decision making depends in many important ways on neural substrates that regulate homeostasis, emotion, and feeling (Damasio, 1994).

1. *Induction of somatic states*: Somatic states can be induced from (1) primary inducers, and (2) secondary inducers (Damasio, 1995). *Primary inducers* are innate or learned stimuli that cause pleasurable or aversive states. Once present in the immediate environment, they automatically and obligatorily elicit a somatic response. The actual encounter of a drug by an addicted individual is an example of a primary inducer (Bechara et al., 2003). It is important to note that unlike stimuli such as food and sex, the sensations stimulated by drugs are not innately pleasant. Through learning, however, drugs acquire properties that are characteristics of a "primary inducer." The process by which a foreign substance, such as a drug, acquires these primary inducer properties, that is, a capacity to trigger somatic states automatically and obligatorily like food and sex, is beyond the scope of this discussion.

Secondary inducers, on the other hand, are entities generated by the recall of a personal or hypothetical emotional event, that is, "thoughts" and "memories" of the primary inducer, which elicit a somatic response. The recall or imagination of a drug experience by an addicted individual is one example of a secondary inducer (Bechara et al., 2003).

We have argued that the amygdala is a critical substrate in the neural system necessary for triggering somatic states from primary inducers. It couples the features of primary inducers with the somatic state associated with the inducer. This somatic state is evoked via effector structures such as the hypothalamus and autonomic brainstem nuclei that produce changes in internal milieu and visceral structures along with other effector structures such as the ventral striatum, periacqueductal grey (PAG), and other brainstem nuclei, which produce changes in facial expression and specific approach or withdrawal behaviors (Bechara et al., 2003). In the case of drugs, several lines of direct and indirect evidence support the view that addiction relates to abnormal activity in the amygdala-ventral striatum system, thereby resulting in exaggerated processing of the incentive values of substance-related stimuli (Everitt et al., 1999; Jentsch & Taylor, 1999). Alcoholics showed exaggerated autonomic responses to alcohol cues (Glautier & Drummond, 1994), and so did cocaine addicts (Ehrman et al., 1992; O'Brien et al., 1992). Similarly, smokers showed exaggerated increase in heart rate to cues associated with smoking (Abrams et al., 1988). Functional neuroimaging studies have revealed increased amygdala activity in response to drug-related cues (Grant et al., 1996). We have shown that individuals with alcohol and/or stimulant dependence showed exaggerated autonomic responses to reward in general, for example, winning a large sum of play money during the Iowa Gambling Task (IGT; Bechara et al., 2002), autonomic responses that we have shown to be dependent on the integrity of the amygdala (Bechara et al., 1999).

Once somatic states from primary inducers are induced, signals from these somatic states are relayed to the brain. Signals from activated somatic states lead to the development of somatic state patterns in brainstem nuclei (e.g., the parabrachial nuclei [PBN]), and in somatosensing cortices (e.g., insular and somatosensory I and II cortices, and cingulate cortices). After a somatic state has been triggered by a primary inducer and experienced at least once, a pattern for this somatic state is formed. The subsequent presentation of a stimulus that evokes memories about a specific primary inducer will then operate as a secondary inducer. Secondary inducers are presumed to reactivate the pattern of somatic state belonging to a specific primary inducer. For example, recalling or imagining the experience of a drug reactivates the pattern of somatic state belonging to the actual previous encounter with that drug. The somatic state generated by the recall or imagination of using a drug (secondary inducer), however, is usually fainter than one triggered by an actual use of that drug (primary inducer).

Provided that somatic state representations in somatosensing cortices develop normally, triggering somatic states from secondary inducers becomes dependent on cortical circuitry in which the ventromedial prefrontal cortex plays a critical role. The ventromedial prefrontal cortex (which includes the orbitofrontal region) is a *trigger* structure for somatic states from secondary inducers. It serves as a convergence-divergence zone, which neuron ensembles can couple (1) a certain category of event based on memory records in high-order association cortices to (2) the effector structures that execute the somatic state (Bechara et al., 2003).

It is important to note that the anticipatory skin conductance responses acquired during the Iowa Gambling Task are examples of instances where the ventromedial prefrontal cortex couples knowledge of secondary inducer events to covert response effectors (Bechara et al., 1997). Pondering on which deck to choose from is a conscious process, which elicits a covert somatic response, regardless of how much factual knowledge the person has about the goodness or badness of the choices they are making. This covert somatic response is an expression of the *bias* process that leads the subject to choose the correct deck without necessarily knowing why they made that choice. Perhaps in the case of drugs, conscious deliberation on whether to use drugs in an addicted individual may elicit covert somatic responses that implicitly *bias* cognition in such a way to propel the person to seek drugs, perhaps without much awareness of the choice being made.

2. *Operation of somatic states*: During the pondering of a decision, somatic states are triggered by primary (drug cues) or secondary inducers (thoughts about taking drugs). Once induced, they participate in two functions (see Figure 15.2). In one (i), they provide a substrate for feeling the emotional state, and in the other (ii) they provide a substrate for biasing decisions:

(i) *Feeling the emotional state*: The insular and Somatosensory I and II cortices are necessary, although they may not be sufficient, for feelings of an emotion to occur (Damasio, 1995, 1999). Evidence suggests that there may be two variant forms of feelings dependent on partially separate neural sectors. This evidence is derived from studies on pain showing dissociation between two sensory aspects of pain. One is related to feeling the pain itself, so-called "pain sensation," and the other is related to discomfort and the desire to avoid the pain, so called "pain affect" (Rainville et al., 1997). In the case of drugs, Berridge and Robinson (1995, 1998) have proposed a model that dissociates the "liking" from the "wanting" effects of drugs. The "liking" effects include

feelings of pleasure and affective facial reactions during the pleasurable state. The "wanting" effects include the desire and urge to obtain the drug. We suggest that the insular/ somatosensory cortices are necessary substrates for the feeling of euphoria (not action-related). On the other hand, the supracallosal sector of the anterior cingulate cortex is necessary for the feeling of craving (related to the action of seeking, obtaining, and consuming the drug). In support, studies have revealed changes in activity in the insular and somatosensory cortices in association with euphoric experience of acute doses of opiate and stimulant drugs (Breiter et al., 1997; London et al., 2000; Volkow & Fowler, 2000). Craving has also been linked to activity in the supracallosal sector of the anterior cingulate cortex in functional neuroimaging studies (Childress et al., 1999).

(ii) *Biasing the decision to select a response*: In order for somatic signals to influence cognition and behavior, they must act on appropriate neural systems:

One target for somatic state action is the striatum. Evidence suggests that in the striatum, the operation of somatic states is implicit, that is, the subject learns to select a correct response, but without awareness of whether the response is correct. Studies of patients with Parkinson's disease (PD), and patients whose brain damage involved both medial temporal lobes, a portion of the orbital prefrontal cortex, and the anterior cingulate, but spared the striatum/basal ganglia completely, suggest that the striatum is both necessary (Knowlton et al., 1996) and sufficient (Tranel & Damasio, 1993) to modify behavior through the influence of somatic states at a covert (implicit) level. This supports the notion that this region plays a role in "knowledge without awareness." This is consistent with several investigations that suggested that the amygdala-ventral striatum

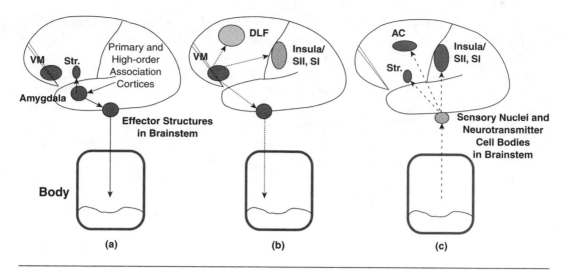

Figure 15.2 A schematic model of somatic state activation and decision making. In diagram (a), the amygdala is a trigger structure for emotional (somatic) states from primary inducers. It couples the features of primary inducers, which can be processed subliminally (e.g., via the thalamus) or explicitly (e.g., via early sensory and high-order association cortices), with effector structures that trigger the emotional/somatic response. In diagram (b), the ventromedial prefrontal (VM) cortex is a trigger structure for emotional (somatic) states from secondary inducers. It couples knowledge of events held temporarily in working memory (which is dependent on dorsolateral prefrontal [DLF] cortices) to effector structures that induce the somatic responses, and to structures holding representations of previous feeling states (e.g., insula, and Somatosensory I [SI] and Somatosensory II [SII] cortices).

system is important for drug stimulus-reward (incentive) learning (White, 1996), and the control of drug-related cues over behavior (Cador et al., 1989).

In the supracallosal sector of the anterior cingulate, and perhaps the adjacent supplementary motor area (SMA), the biasing mechanism of response selection is conscious or explicit, that is, there is "action with awareness of what is right or wrong"; the decisions are "voluntary" or "willful," and guided by knowledge, awareness, and premeditation. Evidence shows that the anterior cingulate plays a role in the implementation of "voluntary" or "willful" decisions, decisions that are guided by "knowledge with awareness." Studies have shown that performance on target detection tasks and the Stroop interference task is associated with activity in the anterior cingulate (Pardo et al., 1990; Posner &

Petersen, 1990; Posner et al., 1988). Another study (Frith et al., 1991) compared willed acts requiring explicit deliberate choice to automatic/routine acts and detected significant increase in activity in the supracallosal anterior cingulate during the willed acts. These results suggest that the supracallosal anterior cingulate is involved in response selection when a wide range of novel choices is required, and when the response selection is driven by conscious/explicit knowledge.

There are other neural sites where ascending somatic signals exert influence on cognition. At the level of the lateral orbitofrontal and dorsolateral prefrontal region, the biasing mechanism of somatic states is explicit, but it is at the level of "thought" or "memory," and not behavioral action. In other words, as one is deliberating on several options and scenarios held in their working memory, the biasing effect of somatic states is to endorse some options and reject other ones, before any of these options are translated into actions.

NEURAL MECHANISMS OF WILLPOWER

Based on the somatic marker framework, willpower (or lack of) emerges from the dynamic interaction between two separate, but interacting, neural systems: (1) an *impulsive* system that triggers somatic states from primary inducers, and (2) a *reflective* system that triggers somatic states from secondary inducers.

The reflective system controls the impulsive system via several mechanisms of impulse control. This control of the reflective system is not, however, absolute: Hyperactivity of the impulsive system can overwhelm or "hijack" the influence of the reflective system. This model is consistent with the Berridge and Robinson model (1995, 1998) in that reward systems (e.g., dopamine) become sensitized to the incentive effects of drugs, so that drug cues become capable of eliciting more intense "wanting" effects that override any conscious attempt by the reflective system to suppress or control that urge.

It is important to note that at the process level, the characteristics of the "impulsive" and "reflective" neural systems are similar to the two-system view of Kahneman and Tversky (1979) on "intuition" versus "reasoning," or that of Strack and Deutsch (2004) on reflective and impulsive determinants of social behavior (see also Deutsch & Strack, Chapter 4). In all cases, the distinction is between the operations of one system that are typically fast, automatic, effortless, implicit, and habitual, and the operations of another system that are slow, deliberate, effortful, explicit, and rule-governed. The distinct characteristic of our model is

the assignment of neural substrates and physiological mechanisms for the operations of these systems.

More specifically, exposure to primary inducers (e.g., drugs) triggers fast, automatic, and obligatory somatic states via the amygdala system. Somatic states triggered by the amygdala are short-lived and habituate very quickly (Buchel et al., 1998; Dolan et al., 1996; LaBar et al., 1998). Secondary inducers trigger somatic states via the ventromedial prefrontal cortex from perceived or recalled mental images. While the amygdala is engaged in emotional situations requiring a rapid response, that is, "low-order" emotional reactions arising from relatively automatic processes (Berkowitz, 1993; LeDoux, 1996), the ventromedial prefrontal cortex is engaged in emotional situations driven by thoughts and reflection. Once this initial amygdala emotional response is over, "high-order" emotional reactions begin to arise from relatively more controlled, higher-order processes involved in thinking, reasoning, and consciousness (Schneider & Shiffrin, 1977). Unlike the amygdala response, which is sudden and habituates quickly, the ventromedial prefrontal cortex response is deliberate, slow, and lasts for a long time.

Thus, the prefrontal cortex, especially the ventromedial prefrontal cortex part, helps predict the emotion of the future, thereby forecasting the consequences of one's own actions. The forecasting properties of this reflective system are also consistent with the view of Deutsch and Strack (see Chapter 4). Neurally speaking, the ventromedial prefrontal cortices contain convergence-divergence neuron ensembles, which hold a record of temporal conjunctions of activity in varied regions (i.e., sensory cortices and limbic structures) caused by external and internal stimuli. When parts of certain exteroceptive-interoceptive conjunctions are reprocessed, consciously or nonconsciously, their activation is signaled to ventromedial prefrontal cortices, which in turn activate somatic effectors in hypothalamus, and brainstem nuclei. This latter activity is an attempt to reconstitute the kind of somatic state that belonged to the original conjunction.

A large number of channels convey body information to the central nervous system (e.g., spinal cord, vagus nerve, humoral signals). Evidence suggests that the vagal route is especially critical for relaying somatic signals (Martin et al., 2004). Although research in this area is still in progress, early evidence suggests that the biasing action of somatic states on behavior and cognition is mediated by the release of neurotransmitters in neural structures belonging to the reflective system. Indeed, the cell bodies of the neurotransmitter dopamine (DA), serotonin (5-HT), noreadrenaline (NA), and acetylcholine (Ach) are located in the brainstem; the axon terminals of these neurotransmitter neurons synapse on cells and/or terminals all over the cortex (Blessing, 1997). When somatic state signals are transmitted to the cell bodies of serotonin neurons, for example, the signaling influences the pattern of serotonin release at the terminals. In turn, changes in serotonin release will modulate synaptic activities of neurons subserving behavior and cognition within the reflective system. This chain of neural mechanisms provides a way for somatic states to exert a biasing effect on decisions (Figure 15.3).

Thus, once somatic states are enacted, in the body (body-loop) or in the brain stem (as-if-body-loop) via direct and indirect connections between the amygdala and the ventromedial prefrontal cortex, and the neurotransmitter nuclei within the brainstem (Blessing, 1997; Nauta, 1971), they can then influence activity in (1) regions involved in *body mapping*, that is, holding patterns of somatic states that help generate *feelings*; (2) regions involved in the triggering of somatic states (e.g., amygdala and ventromedial prefrontal cortex), so that the threshold for

triggering subsequent somatic states is increased or decreased; (3) regions involved in *working memory* (e.g., lateral orbitofrontal, dorsolateral prefrontal, and other high-order association cortices), so that a particular representation is strengthened or weakened; and finally (4) somatic state signals influence activity in regions concerned with motor responses and behavioral actions (e.g., striatum and anterior cingulate/supplementary motor area [SMA]).

The significance of this neural arrangement is that regardless of how somatic states are triggered, that is, impulsively (primary induction) or reflectively (secondary induction), once they are triggered they can gain access to cortical and subcortical neurons subserving cognition. Thus, depending on their strength, they have the capacity to modify and influence cognition.

LOSS OF WILLPOWER

Early in life, the reflective system is poorly developed, and willpower is relatively weak; behavior is more dominated by the impulsive system—children tend to behave in a manner that they do what they feel like doing right now, without much thought about the future. Through learning, however, they learn to constrain many desires and behaviors that conflict with social rules, and which lead to negative consequences. This is the first sign of the development of willpower, and an example of how the reflective system gains control over the impulsive system. This ability, that is, to choose according to long-term outcomes, and resist immediate desires, requires the normal development and normal triggering of somatic states by the reflective system, which signal the value of long-term outcomes. Deprived of these somatic states, the reflective system loses its control, and willpower breaks down. Indeed, this is what happens when areas of the ventromedial

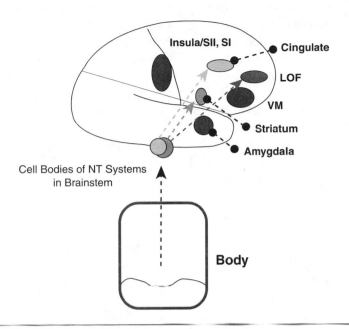

Figure 15.3 A diagram illustrating three different levels at which somatic states can bias decisions via the release of neurotransmitters (NT): (1) Dopamine biases decisions covertly (perhaps through action in the striatum and affective sector of anterior cingulate (Brodmann Area (BA) 25 and lower 24, 32); (2) Serotonin biases decisions overtly (perhaps through action in the cognitive sector of anterior cingulate and probably the adjacent SMA [supplementary motor area]); and (3) Somatic states also bias working memory in the LOF (lateral orbitofrontal and dorsolateral regions of the prefrontal cortex). They help endorse or reject "thoughts," "options," or "scenarios" brought to mind during the pondering of decisions, that is, before their translation into action. The neurotransmitter system that mediates this biasing function remains to be determined.

prefrontal cortex are damaged, as described in the case of Phineas Gage who became impatient of restraint or advice when it conflicted with his desires (Damasio, 1994). It appears, however, that there is more than one mechanism through which the reflective system exerts control over the impulsive system.

The functional evolution of the prefrontal cortex appears to involve an incremental increase in its capacity to access representations of events that occur in the more distant future. This enhanced "futuristic" capacity coincides with the development of more rostral/anterior regions of the ventromedial prefrontal cortex. Comparative studies of the frontal lobes in humans and nonhuman primates have revealed that the major

advancement in the size, complexity, and connectivity of the frontal lobes in humans relates primarily to Brodmann Area 10, that is, the frontal pole (Semendeferi et al., 2001), and not so much to the more posterior areas of the ventromedial prefrontal cortex (Semendeferi et al., 2002). For this reason, we have argued that there is a distinction between two broad mechanisms of behavioral and cognitive control:

1. Decision making, which reflects a tendency to think about the consequences of a planned act before engaging in that act. It requires knowledge about facts and values, and it involves conscious, slow, and effortful deliberation about consequences that may or may not happen in a distant future. To give

an example requiring decision making is finding a briefcase with $100,000 in a dark alley. The decision to take or not take the money may require some deliberation about the ethics, morality, and consequences of such an action. The critical neural region for this mechanism of control is the more anterior region of the ventromedial prefrontal cortex, that is, those involving the frontal pole and Brodmann Area 10 (Bechara, 2004). We have shown that this decision-making function can be taxed by the Iowa Gambling Task (Bechara, 2004).

2. Impulse control reflects inhibition of a pre-potent act (motor impulse control), or a pre-potent mental image/thought (perceptual impulse control). Learning to quickly and automatically inhibit such a pre-potent act (or thought) is due, in large part, to the triggering of a somatic state (as-if-body-loop), which signals the immediate and certain nature of the consequences. An example of this quick, automatic, and implicit mechanism of impulse control is finding a similar amount of $100,000 spread out on a table inside a bank. Normally, any thought, intention, or impulse to grab the money is inhibited automatically and effortlessly. The critical neural region for the mechanism of motor impulse control is the more posterior region of the ventromedial prefrontal cortex, that is, those involving the anterior cingulate (Bechara, 2003, 2004). The Stroop Continuous Performance Task (CPT), Stop Signal, Go/No-Go, delayed alternation, and reversal learning tasks are examples of paradigms that detect deficits in this type of behavioral/motor impulse control. The critical neural region for the mechanism of perceptual impulse control is the lateral orbitofrontal and dorsolateral (inferior frontal gyrus) regions (Bechara, 2003, 2004). Perseveration on the Wisconsin Card Sorting Task (WCST) and inability to shift attentional sets (Intradimensional-Extradimensional [ID-ED]

shift), as well as other tasks that require shifting attention from one perception to another are laboratory measures that detect this type of deficit in perceptual impulse control.

It is very important to realize that although these different cognitive and behavioral mechanisms can be dissociated under controlled experimental conditions, they are all interrelated and act together in a functioning brain. Injuries or diseases that affect a single or a combination of any of these mechanisms will have a devastating impact on judgment, decision making, and the whole social and real-life behavior of the affected individual.

Thus, an addict may have abnormalities in any of these top-down control mechanisms of the reflective system, that is, decision making and impulse control (motor and/or perceptual). For instance, the choice between another drug-use episode and the family pressure not to use drugs presents a dilemma to individuals with substance dependence, and the choice depends on mechanisms of decision making. When this mechanism fails, the addict decides to seek the drug, regardless of the consequences. On the other hand, the ability to put a stop to and resist another drug use when exposed to an environment with many drug cues depends on intact mechanisms of impulse control. When these mechanisms fail, the individual with substance dependence becomes unable to suppress the "thought" of taking the drug (perceptual impulsiveness), or may actually act quickly, without thinking, and take the drug (motor impulsiveness).

Although dysfunction within these top-down control mechanisms of the reflective system can be responsible for maintaining drug use, the problem can also arise from bottom-up mechanisms of the impulsive system, where hyperactivity in the impulsive system can weaken control of the reflective system. In other words, choosing according to long-term outcomes rather than short-term ones requires that the somatic states triggered by the reflective system dominate those triggered by the impulsive system. Two broad types of conditions could alter this relationship and lead to loss of willpower: (1) a dysfunctional reflective system, and (2) a hyperactive impulsive system. The neural regions of the reflective system, which exert "top-down" control on decision making (anterior ventromedial prefrontal cortex), motor impulse control (anterior cingulate), and perceptual impulse control (lateral orbitofrontal and dorsolateral) are all targets for the neural systems that convey "bottom-up" influence of somatic signals. The influence of these somatic signals could be nonconscious and implicit, or conscious and explicit, that is, accompanied by a certain feeling of urge. Addiction to drugs provides examples of disorders that affect each type of these mechanisms:

1. *A dysfunctional reflective system:* Patients with bilateral ventromedial prefrontal cortex damage and individuals with substance dependence show similar behaviors: (1) They often deny, or they are not aware, that they have a problem. (2) When faced with a choice to pursue a course of action that brings an immediate reward, at the risk of incurring future negative consequences, including the loss of reputation, job, home, and family, they choose the immediate reward and ignore the future consequences. Research has shown a link between the "myopia" for future consequences seen in ventromedial prefrontal cortex lesion patients and that seen in individuals with substance dependence by finding a relationship between substance abuse and poor decision making as measured by the Iowa Gambling Task, as well as other similar decision-making tasks (Bartzokis et al., 2000; Grant et al., 1999; Grant et al., 1997, 2000; Mazas et al., 2000; Petry et al., 1998; Rogers et al., 1999).

Studies have shown that the abnormal mechanisms of processing drug reward in individuals with substance dependence generalize to other rewards, including monetary reward (Breiter et al., 2001; Breiter & Rosen, 1999). Therefore, we predicted that the abnormalities of individuals with substance dependence in processing somatic states would apply not only to drugs, but also to reward in general, such as the monetary reward used in the Iowa Gambling Task paradigm. We conducted experiments in which we tested three groups of subjects: individuals with substance dependence, normal controls, and ventromedial prefrontal cortex lesion patients on the Iowa Gambling Task (Bechara et al., 1994; Bechara et al., 2000). All individuals with substance dependence met the DSM-IV criteria for dependence, with either alcohol or stimulants (methamphetamine or cocaine) as the primary substance of choice. The results revealed a significant impairment in the performance of individuals with substance dependence relative to normal controls on the Iowa Gambling Task.

Measuring skin conductance response activity of subjects after receiving reward or punishment (Reward or Punishment skin conductance responses), and before making a choice (Anticipatory skin conductance responses), revealed that a subgroup of individuals with substance dependence was similar to ventromedial prefrontal cortex lesion patients. These individuals with substance dependence triggered normal Reward and Punishment skin conductance responses, but they failed to trigger skin conductance responses (Anticipatory) when they pondered choices associated with high immediate gains, but also with more delayed and more severe losses (Bechara et al., 2002). This showed that individuals with substance dependence, like ventromedial prefrontal cortex lesion patients, were deprived of a mechanism for triggering somatic states that implicitly (or explicitly) help bias and guide decisions in favor of long-term outcomes.

In addition to decision making, we examined the integrity of the other impulse control mechanisms of the reflective system in individuals with substance dependence. We assessed response inhibition using the stop-signal task (Crone et al., 2003). In the stop-signal paradigm, the participant performs a choice reaction time task requiring responses to left and right pointing arrows. Occasionally and unpredictably the color of the arrows change, instructing participants to inhibit responses. The main dependent variables in this task are the response time (RT) and the estimate of the covert response to the stop signal, by inferring the stop-signal reaction time (SSRT). Relative to normal controls, individuals with substance dependence had significantly longer SSRTs, but shorter RTs, thus reflecting difficulties or impairments in impulse control.

In another experiment, we used a task-switch paradigm requiring participants to rapidly switch between two reaction time tasks, requiring left or right hand responses to squares and rectangles that could appear as local or global figures (Crone et al., 2003). The main dependent variable was the difference in reaction time between task-repetition trials and task-alternation trials. Individuals with substance dependence showed significantly larger switch costs than controls, although there was no difference in accuracy of responding.

In a separate study (Noel et al., 2003, 2005), we tested the hypotheses that alcoholics suffer from deficits in their cognitive control mechanisms of "stopping" and of "shifting" and that these deficits are exacerbated by cognitive biases for alcohol-related stimuli. Noel et al. designed a laboratory task called the Alcohol Shifting Task, to examine distinctly motor inhibition, shifting attention, and the influence of alcohol-related stimuli on these functions in detoxified poly-substance abusers with alcoholism. The Alcohol Shifting Task involves the presentation of alcohol-related versus nonalcohol-related words on a computer screen. The subject is instructed to press the bar key when a nonalcohol-related word appears on the screen and withhold the response if an alcohol-related word appeared instead. After

establishing a habit for responding this way, the contingencies would reverse unexpectedly in the task so that the subject must now withhold responding to nonalcohol-related words and respond to alcohol-related words. In a second cycle, there is a return to the first contingency, that is, respond to nonalcohol and withhold responding to alcohol cues followed by a reversal. Relative to control subjects, we found that alcoholics were slower to respond to neutral, but not alcohol, stimuli in both stopping and shifting conditions. In addition, when subjects were supposed to withhold responding to an alcohol or neutral stimulus, alcoholics made more errors than controls in both "stopping" and "shifting" conditions. Most important, the failure of alcoholics to inhibit their responses ("stopping" condition) was significant when alcoholics had to suppress their response to an alcohol stimulus, but not when they had to withhold their response to a neutral stimulus. In contrast, in "shifting" condition, alcoholics made more errors in both neutral and alcohol words conditions. The deficit was much more pronounced, however, when alcoholics had to shift attention from alcohol to neutral cues, but not so much when they shifted attention from neutral to alcohol cues.

Together, the results reflect disorders in the reflective system of individuals with substance dependence at both the level of decision making as well as the ability to control impulses.

2. *A hyperactive impulsive system:* Somatic states work through neurotransmitter systems, and neurotransmitters modulate synapses of cortical neurons within the reflective system. Therefore, a hyperactive impulsive system subserved by an amygdala-ventral striatal (nucleus accumbens) neural circuit, which exaggerates the somatic response of reward stimuli, can weaken the reflective/prefrontal system, thus gaining control over behavior and cognition.

We have shown that many individuals with substance dependence may suffer from a hyperactive amygdala system that exaggerates the processing of reward, which results in poor decision making as measured by the Iowa Gambling Task (Bechara, 2003). We have described this condition as "hypersensitivity to reward," in which a subgroup of individuals with substance dependence expressed exaggerated responses to reward and relatively weak responses to punishment (Bechara, 2003). Specifically, we used different versions of the Iowa Gambling Task, where the contingencies were reversed, so that the punishment was immediate and the reward was delayed. When testing individuals with substance dependence on this variant task, a subgroup of individuals with substance dependence behaved on the original and variant versions of the Iowa Gambling Task in such a way that they were drawn to choices that yielded larger gains, irrespective of the losses that were encountered. This subgroup showed higher magnitude Reward skin conductance responses, in comparison to normal controls. Furthermore, during the anticipation of a reward, this subgroup of individuals with substance dependence showed higher Anticipatory skin conductance responses, in comparison to controls (Bechara et al., 2002). On the basis of these behavioral and physiological results, we have described this subpopulation of individuals with substance dependence as hypersensitive to reward, so that the presence or the prospect of receiving reward dominates their choice and behavior.

CONCLUSIONS: IMPLICATIONS FOR TREATMENT AND DIRECTIONS FOR FUTURE RESEARCH

Advances in the study of cognition and emotion can improve our understanding of the implicit and explicit mechanisms that govern decisions to abuse drugs. This chapter began with addressing the role of willpower in the decision to use substances. Although the act of using substances can be resisted under extreme conditions (e.g., a gun to the head), in most cases there is no gun to the head. The research discussed provides evidence that the loss of willpower in individuals with substance dependence is likely the result of their experiencing the world differently. Addiction is a condition in which the person becomes unable to choose according to long-term outcomes. This inability, however, can result from a dysfunction of one or more of several mechanisms of cognitive and behavioral control within the reflective system, or hyperactivity of the impulsive system. The breakdown of one or more of these cognitive and emotional mechanisms constitutes one of the principal mechanisms responsible for the switch from controlled to uncontrolled and compulsive behavior. Thus, future research should address the reasons for why these mechanisms break down: Is it genetic, for example, abnormal neurotransmitter transporters? Is it developmental, for example, environmental stress or exposure to drugs during a time window in adolescence where the prefrontal cortex has not yet developed completely? Other questions should address the mechanisms of "predisposition" versus "specificity." Acquisition of addictive behaviors may depend on at least two steps: (1) a predisposition to becoming addicted to anything, and (2) specificity to an addictive stimulus. Breakdown in the mechanisms of decision making and impulse control may explain the issue of predisposition. But what determines the specificity of an addiction? For instance, why do certain people become pathological gamblers but not drug addicts?

We have suggested that the different mechanisms of cognitive and impulse control of the reflective system could be assessed by different sets of cognitive tasks, and linked to abnormalities in different neural sectors.

Characterization of individuals with substance dependence on the basis of neurocognitive criteria has strong implications for prognosis and rehabilitation. For instance, many individuals with substance dependence do not show signs of prefrontal impairment, and it is possible that these are the individuals who decide at some point to quit their addiction habit and they succeed. These individuals seem in full control of their behavior and this is why they possess the capability to control their addiction. On the other hand, individuals who show profiles of cognitive deficits similar to ventromedial prefrontal cortex lesion patients probably have the worst prognosis. Such individuals may fall into one trouble after the other and repeat one mistake after the other and can never shift their behavior toward long-term thinking and avoiding future negative consequences on their own. Individuals who show only signs of hypersensitivity to reward may fall somewhere in between. We speculate that the weakness of these individuals and their loss of behavioral control are precipitated primarily in the presence of reward or irresistible cues. In other words, they may have the cognitive capacity to learn to stay away from the situations that make them vulnerable to succumbing to their addiction.

We have begun pharmacological research aimed at understanding the chemical deficiency in the reflective/prefrontal system of individuals with substance dependence, which underlies their decision-making impairment and loss of control over their behavior. We found that the stimulation or blockade of both dopamine and serotonin interfere with the ability to make advantageous decisions in the Iowa Gambling Task, but the dopamine effect seemed restricted to decisions guided by covert knowledge, that is, decisions under ambiguity. In contrast, the serotonin effect seemed restricted to decisions guided by conscious knowledge of which choices are good or bad, that is, decisions under risk (Bechara et al., 2001). The results suggest that covert biasing of decisions might be dopaminergic, whereas overt biasing might be serotonergic. These findings have implications for the treatment of addictive disorders in that more than one neurotransmitter system may be involved in the addictive process, and thus different aspects of the addictive process may need different pharmacological treatments. Most important, pharmacological treatments may never work alone, that is, without cognitive and behavioral rehabilitation. The idea is that the poor prefrontal mechanisms of decision making in individuals with substance dependence are in part related to learning in the presence of a deficiency in the chemicals that modulate nonconscious (e.g., at the level of the striatum) or conscious (e.g., at the level of the cortex) decisions. Thus decision making and poor learning to control certain behaviors are flawed in part because of this deficiency. Reversal of this chemical deficiency alone is not sufficient for learning to decide advantageously. The individual must relearn how to think and behave in a particular situation related to drugs or gambling while being treated with medications, which correct the chemical imbalance. Thus, only relearning (i.e., rehabilitation) in the presence of normal pharmacology (i.e., drug treatment) is perhaps the most effective way to restore advantageous decisions in an addicted individual.

REFERENCES

Abrams, D. B., Monti, P. M., Carey, K. B., Pinto, R. P., & Jacobus, S. I. (1988). Reactivity to smoking cues and relapse: 2 studies of discriminant validity. *Behaviour Research and Therapy, 26*(3), 225–233.

Bartzokis, G., Lu, P. H., Beckson, M., Rapoport, R., Grant, S., Wiseman, E. J., et al. (2000). Abstinence from cocaine reduces high-risk responses on a gambling task. *Neuropsychopharmacology, 22*(1), 102–103.

Bechara, A. (2003). Risky business: Emotion, decision-making and addiction. *Journal of Gambling Studies, 19*(1), 23–51.

Bechara, A. (2004). Separate neural substrates underlie different mechanisms of performance monitoring and behavioral control. In M. Ullsperger & M. Falkenstein (Eds.), *Errors, conflicts, and the brain: Current opinions on performance monitoring* (pp. 55–63). Dortmund, Germany: Max Planck Institute for Human Cognitive and Brain Sciences, Leipzig-München.

Bechara, A., & Damasio, A. R. (2004). The somatic marker hypothesis: A neural theory of economic decision [Electronic version]. *Games and Economic Behavior,* doi: 10.1016/j.geb.2004.1006.1010.

Bechara, A., Damasio, A. R., Damasio, H., & Anderson, S. W. (1994). Insensitivity to future consequences following damage to human prefrontal cortex. *Cognition, 50,* 7–15.

Bechara, A., Damasio, H., & Damasio, A. R. (2001). Manipulation of dopamine and serotonin causes different effects on covert and overt decision-making. *Society for Neuroscience Abstracts, 27,* 126.

Bechara, A., Damasio, H., & Damasio, A. R. (2003). The role of the amygdala in decision-making. In P. Shinnick-Gallagher, A. Pitkanen, A. Shekhar, & L. Cahill (Eds.), *The amygdala in brain function: Basic and clinical approaches. Annals of the New York Academy of Science, 985,* 356–369.

Bechara, A., Damasio, H., Damasio, A. R., & Lee, G. P. (1999). Different contributions of the human amygdala and ventromedial prefrontal cortex to decision-making. *The Journal of Neuroscience, 19*(13), 5473–5481.

Bechara, A., Damasio, H., Tranel, D., & Damasio, A. R. (1997). Deciding advantageously before knowing the advantageous strategy. *Science, 275,* 1293–1295.

Bechara, A., Dolan, S., & Hindes, A. (2002). Decision-making and addiction: Part 2. Myopia for the future or hypersensitivity to reward? *Neuropsychologia, 40*(10), 1690–1705.

Bechara, A., Tranel, D., & Damasio, H. (2000). Characterization of the decision-making impairment of patients with bilateral lesions of the ventromedial prefrontal cortex. *Brain, 123,* 2189–2202.

Berkowitz, L. (1993). Towards a general theory of anger and emotional aggression: Implications of the cognitive-neoassociationistic perspective for the analysis of anger and other emotions. In R. S. Wyer & T. K. Srull (Eds.), *Advances in social cognition* (Vol. 6, pp. 1–46). Hillsdale, NJ: Lawrence Erlbaum.

Berridge, K. C., & Robinson, T. E. (1995). The mind of an addicted brain: Neural sensitization of wanting versus liking. *Current Directions in Psychological Science, 4,* 71–75.

Berridge, K. C., & Robinson, T. E. (1998). What is the role of dopamine in reward: Hedonic impact, reward learning, or incentive salience? *Brain Research Reviews, 28,* 309–369.

Blessing, W. W. (1997). Anatomy of the lower brainstem. In *The lower brainstem and bodily homeostasis* (pp. 29–99). New York and Oxford, UK: Oxford University Press.

Breiter, H. C., Aharon, I., Kahneman, D., Dale, A., & Shizgal, P. (2001). Functional imaging of neural responses to expectancy and experience of monetary gains and losses. *Neuron, 30*(2), 619–639.

Breiter, H. C., Gollub, R. L., Weisskoff, R. M., Kennedy, D. N., Makris, N., Berke, J. D., et al. (1997). Acute effects of cocaine on human brain activity and emotion. *Neuron, 19*(3), 591–611.

Breiter, H. C., & Rosen, B. R. (1999). Functional magnetic resonance imaging of brain reward circuitry in the human. In J. F. McGinty (Ed.), Advancing from the ventral striatum to the extended amygdala. *Annals of the New York Academy of Sciences, 877,* 523–547.

Buchel, C., Morris, J., Dolan, R. J., & Friston, K. J. (1998). Brain systems mediating aversive conditioning: An event-related fMRI study. *Neuron, 20*(5), 947–957.

Cador, M., Robbins, T. W., & Everitt, B. J. (1989). Involvement of the amygdala in stimulus-reward associations: Interaction with the ventral striatum. *Neuroscience, 30,* 77–86.

Childress, A. R., Mozley, P. D., McElgin, W., Fitzgerald, J., Reivich, M., & O'Brien, C. P. (1999). Limbic activation during cue-induced cocaine craving. *American Journal of Psychiatry, 156,* 11–18.

Crone, E. A., Cutshall, C., Recknor, E., Van den Wildenberg, W. P. M., & Bechara, A. (2003, November). *Impaired executive function performance in substance abusers: Evidence from inhibition, set-shifting, and working memory measures.* Paper presented at the 33rd annual meeting of the Society for Neuroscience, New Orleans, LA.

Damasio, A. R. (1994). *Descartes' error: Emotion, reason, and the human brain.* New York: Grosset/Putnam.

Damasio, A. R. (1995). Toward a neurobiology of emotion and feeling: Operational concepts and hypotheses. *The Neuroscientist, 1,* 19–25.

Damasio, A. R. (1999). *The feeling of what happens: Body and emotion in the making of consciousness.* New York: Harcourt Brace.

Dolan, R. J., Fletcher, P., Morris, J., Kapur, N., Deakin, J. F. W., & Frith, C. D. (1996). Neural activation during covert processing of positive emotional facial expressions. *Neuroimage, 4*(3), 194–200.

Ehrman, R., Ternes, J., O'Brien, C. P., & McLellan, A. T. (1992). Conditioned tolerance in human opiate addicts. *Psychopharmacology, 108*(1–2), 218–224.

Everitt, B. J., Parkinson, J. A., Olmstead, M. C., Arroyo, M., Robledo, P., & Robbins, T. W. (1999). Associative processes in addiction and reward: The role of amygdala and ventral striatal subsystems. In J. F. McGinty (Ed.), Advancing from the ventral striatum to the extended amygdala. *Annals of the New York Academy of Science, 877,* 412–438.

Frith, C. D., Friston, K., Liddle, P. F., & Frackowiak, R. S. J. (1991). Willed action and the prefrontal cortex in man: A study with PET. *Proceedings of the Royal Society of London: Series B. Biological Sciences, 244*(1311), 241–246.

Glautier, S., & Drummond, D. C. (1994). Alcohol dependence and cue reactivity. *Journal of Studies on Alcohol, 55*(2), 224–229.

Grant, S., Bonson, K. R., Contoreggi, C. C., & London, E. D. (1999). Activation of the ventromedial prefrontal cortex correlates with gambling task performance: A FDG-PET study. *Society for Neuroscience Abstracts, 25*(2), 1551.

Grant, S., Contoreggi, C., & London, E. D. (1997). Drug abusers show impaired performance on a test of orbitofrontal function. *Society for Neuroscience Abstracts, 23,* 1943.

Grant, S., Contoreggi, C., & London, E. D. (2000). Drug abusers show impaired performance in a laboratory test of decision-making. *Neuropsychologia, 38*(8), 1180–1187.

Grant, S., London, E. D., Newlin, D. B., Villemagne, V. L., Liu, X., Contoreggi, C., et al. (1996). Activation of memory circuits during cue-elicited cocaine craving. *Proceedings of the National Academy of Sciences, 93*, 12040–12045.

Jentsch, J. D., & Taylor, J. R. (1999). Impulsivity resulting from frontostraital dysfunction in drug abuse: Implications for the control of behavior by reward-related stimuli. *Psychopharmacology, 146*(4), 373–390.

Kahneman, D., & Tversky, A. (1979). Prospect theory: An analysis of decision under risk. *Econometrica, 47*, 263–291.

Knowlton, B. J., Mangels, J. A., & Squire, L. R. (1996). A neostriatal habit learning system in humans. *Science, 273*, 1399–1402.

LaBar, K. S., Gatenby, J. C., Gore, J. C., LeDoux, J. E., & Phelps, E. A. (1998). Human amygdala activation during conditioned fear acquisition and extinction: A mixed-trial fMRI study. *Neuron, 20*, 937–945.

LeDoux, J. (1996). *The emotional brain: The mysterious underpinnings of emotional life.* New York: Simon & Schuster.

London, E. D., Ernst, M., Grant, S., Bonson, K., & Weinstein, A. (2000). Orbitofrontal cortex and human drug abuse: Functional imaging. *Cerebral Cortex, 10*(3), 334–342.

Martin, C., Denburg, N., Tranel, D., Granner, M., & Bechara, A. (2004). The effects of vagal nerve stimulation on decision-making. *Cortex, 40*, 1–8.

Mazas, C. A., Finn, P. R., & Steinmetz, J. E. (2000). Decision making biases, antisocial personality, and early-onset alcoholism. *Alcoholism: Clinical and Experimental Research, 24*(7), 1036–1040.

Nauta, W. J. H. (1971). The problem of the frontal lobes: A reinterpretation. *Journal of Psychiatric Research, 8*, 167–187.

Noel, X., Van der Linden, M., Verbanck, P., Pelc, I., & Bechara, A. (2003). Attentional bias and inhibitory control processes in substance-dependent individuals with alcoholism. *Journal of Psychophysiology, 17*, S8.

Noel, X., Van der Linden, M., Verbanck, P., Pelc, I., & Bechara, A. (2005). Deficits of inhibitory control and of shifting associated with cognitive bias in polysubstance abusers with alcoholism. *Addiction*, doi: 10.1111/j.1360-0443.2005.01125.

O'Brien, C. P., Childress, A. R., McLellan, A. T., & Ehrman, R. (1992). Classical conditioning in drug-dependent humans. *Annals of the New York Academy of Science, 654*, 400–415.

Pardo, J. V., Pardo, P. J., Janer, K. W., & Raichle, M. E. (1990). The anterior cingulate cortex mediates processing selection in the Stroop attentional conflict paradigm. *Proceedings of the National Academy of Sciences, 87*(1), 256–259.

Petry, N. M., Bickel, W. K., & Arnett, M. (1998). Shortened time horizons and insensitivity to future consequences in heroin addicts. *Addiction, 93*(5), 729–738.

Posner, M. I., & Petersen, S. E. (1990). The attention system of the human brain. *Annual Review of Neuroscience, 13*, 25–42.

Posner, M. I., Petersen, S. E., Fox, P. T., & Raichle, M. E. (1988). Localization of cognitive operations in the human brain. *Science, 240*(4859), 1627–1631.

Rainville, P., Duncan, G. H., Price, D. D., Carrier, B., & Bushnell, M. C. (1997). Pain affect encoded in human anterior cingulate but not somatosensory cortex. *Science, 277*(5328), 968–971.

Rogers, R. D., Everitt, B. J., Baldacchino, A., Blackshaw, A. J., Swainson, R., Wynne, K., et al. (1999). Dissociable deficits in the decision-making cognition of chronic amphetamine abusers, opiate abusers, patients with focal damage to prefrontal cortex, and tryptophan-depleted normal volunteers: Evidence for monoaminergic mechanisms. *Neuropsychopharmacology, 20*(4), 322–339.

Schneider, W., & Shiffrin, R. M. (1977). Controlled and automatic human information processing. *Psychological Reviews, 84,* 1–66.

Semendeferi, K., Armstrong, E., Schleicher, A., Zilles, K., & Van Hoesen, G. W. (2001). Prefrontal cortex in humans and apes: A comparative study of area 10. *American Journal of Physical Anthropology, 114*(3), 224–241.

Semendeferi, K., Lu, A., Schenker, N., & Damasio, H. (2002). Humans and great apes share a large frontal cortex. *Nature Neuroscience, 5*(3), 272–276.

Strack, F., & Deutsch, R. (2004). Reflective and impulsive determinants of social behavior. *Personality and Social Psychology Review, 8*(3), 220–247.

Tranel, D., & Damasio, A. R. (1993). The covert learning of affective valence does not require structures in hippocampal system or amygdala. *Journal of Cognitive Neuroscience, 5,* 79–88.

Volkow, N. D., & Fowler, J. S. (2000). Addiction, a disease of compulsion and drive: Involvement of the orbitofrontal cortex. *Cerebral Cortex, 10*(3), 318–325.

White, N. M. (1996). Addictive drugs as reinforcers: Multiple partial actions on memory systems. *Addiction, 91*(7), 921–949.

CHAPTER 16

Implicit and Explicit Drug Motivational Processes: A Model of Boundary Conditions

JOHN J. CURTIN, DANIELLE E. MCCARTHY,
MEGAN E. PIPER, AND TIMOTHY B. BAKER

Abstract: The model proposed in this paper is an attempt to suggest mechanisms and structures that are involved in both implicit and explicit processing of drug motivational information, and to propose when and how these mechanisms are recruited. To support this model, we first review research on negative and positive reinforcement mechanisms that establish the potent but often-implicit drug-use motivation in drug-dependent users. Next, we integrate basic cognitive neuroscience research on the cognitive control of behavior to understand how boundary conditions are imposed on these implicit motivational processes via the recruitment of attention (i.e., what constrains their occurrence and influence). Finally, model implications are proposed to guide theory and research on drug-use motivation and craving.

INTRODUCTION

The inveterate smoker may smoke cigarette after cigarette without being aware of deciding to smoke or without paying much attention to the act of smoking (Tiffany, 1990). Conversely, when making a quit attempt, the individual may agonize over whether or not to smoke and even go to elaborate lengths to secure a cigarette. Indeed, relapse cigarettes are often stolen (Brandon et al., 1990). Similarly, an alcohol-dependent individual may rather automatically consume a drink set in front of him or her, or go to elaborate lengths to distill or ferment alcohol to drink.

These observations are consistent with the notion that addictive behavior is supported by different types of information processing. Some of this information processing must be implicit: that is, occur fairly automatically without significant awareness. Other processing, however, must be explicit: that is, be planful and available to awareness. The model proposed in this paper is an attempt to suggest mechanisms and structures that are involved in both implicit and explicit processing of drug motivational information, and to propose when and how these mechanisms are recruited. In what follows, we first present a brief outline of our proposed model. Following this, we review research on negative and positive reinforcement mechanisms that establish the potent but often implicit, drug-use motivation among dependent drug users. Next, we integrate basic cognitive neuroscience research on the cognitive control of behavior to understand how boundary conditions are imposed on these implicit motivational processes via the recruitment of attention (i.e., what constrains their occurrence and influence). Finally, model implications are proposed to guide theory and research on drug-use motivation and craving.

BRIEF OUTLINE OF MODEL TENETS

We propose the following five tenets about drug-use motivation, drug-craving, and actual drug use:

1. Drug-use motivation is established via both negative and positive reinforcement mechanisms.

2. Once established, drug-use motivational processes often operate implicitly. In other words, the activation of drug-seeking or administration behaviors can occur automatically without the need for attention or extensive conscious awareness. The drug user may not necessarily be aware of the motivation to use drugs, the cues that elicited the motivation, or even the drug-administration behavior itself.

3. Drug-use motivational processes will become explicit (i.e., the person will be aware of the urge to use drugs) in situations where cognitive control attentional resources are recruited. We will reserve the term "drug-craving" to describe this conscious awareness of an urge to use drugs.

4. Basic research elucidates setting events for the recruitment of cognitive control. These include response conflict (i.e., concurrent activation of competing behavior responses), unfavorable outcomes (e.g.,

performance errors, negative feedback, pain, or other conscious distress), unexpected reward or punishment, and novel situations in which stimulus-response associations have not been previously established.

5. Cognitive control can be recruited to either support or inhibit drug use. When pursuing either drug abstinence or restriction of drug use, however, cognitive control is critical to overcome drug-use motivation and bias behavior toward nondrug-use behaviors. Therefore, explication of the factors that affect the cognitive control of drug-use motivation is clinically important.

"IMPLICIT" DRUG MOTIVATION

Negative Reinforcement

Evidence suggests that physical dependence, as inferred from the capacity to experience withdrawal symptoms, can develop quite early in the course of addictive drug use (Heischman et al., 1989). Moreover, it is clear that withdrawal is aversive, with negative affect being a core feature common to the withdrawal syndromes of all addictive drugs (Kelsey & Arnold, 1994; Malin, 2001). An extensive body of research shows that withdrawal is a powerful instigator of urges and self-administration (see Baker et al., 2004). In particular, negative affect is the element of withdrawal that appears most highly associated with later relapse (Kenford et al., 2002; Piasecki et al., 2000).

Baker et al. (2004) proposed that, over repeated drug-use episodes, addicted organisms learn that discontinuation of drug use (or a mere drop in drug blood levels [Mello & Mendelson, 1970]) leads to escalating withdrawal with associated affective distress, and that resumption of drug intake dramatically ameliorates these aversive affective symptoms. This leads to withdrawal-elicited affective distress becoming a key setting event for drug self-administration (Baker et al., 1987; Baker et al., 2004). Moreover, drug responding may generalize across similar internal states elicited by nondrug negative affect eliciting stimuli (e.g., stressful events; Gauvin et al., 1993; Gauvin et al., 1989).

There is copious evidence that unconscious processing of affect has the capacity to affect not only attitudes, but also behavior (e.g., Murphy & Zajonc, 1993; Öhman & Mineka, 2001). We argue that internal states or cues associated with negative affect can be detected automatically and without awareness, are afforded processing priority, and can trigger drug-use motivation implicitly. Of particular relevance, there is suggestive evidence that withdrawal and negative affect can implicitly activate processing of drug information. For instance, there is evidence that for regular smokers, abstinence enhances the salience of smoking cues (Gross et al., 1993; Sayette & Hufford, 1994; Waters & Feyerabend, 2000). Further, using a first-associates method, McKee et al. (2003) showed that negative mood induction via music led smokers to generate negative reinforcement expectancies regarding smoking (see also Birch et al., Chapter 18). In general, research suggests that manipulations of both withdrawal status and affect result in the greatest interference by drug cues. There is also evidence that implicit or automatized processing has motivational significance (e.g., Stacy, 1995, 1997). For instance, Waters et al. (2003) found that the behavioral interference produced by smoking cues, as assessed via a Stroop task, predicted early relapse among smokers trying to quit smoking.

Research performed by Siegel and his colleagues shows that the initial manifestations of a mounting interoceptive response can effectively signal the later elements of that same reaction (Sokowloska et al., 2002). This research suggests that interoceptive cues have especially great associative strength relative to exteroceptive signals; overshadowing them as effective conditioned stimuli (CS) for

interoceptive reinforcers. As such, inchoate or fledgling interoceptive signs of withdrawal may serve as effective discriminative stimuli for the addicted organism's renewed self-administration of addictive drugs. This could account for drug use in the absence of marked or notable distress.

We propose that, over the course of addiction, the organism learns that initial elements of the withdrawal syndrome—or cues that typically signal incipient withdrawal—predict escalating distress. Such signals serve as potent stimuli that elicit drug self-administration. Over countless drug-use episodes, this information processing routine is proceduralized (Tiffany, 1990), so that the organism may perform this with little or no awareness, or manifestation, of the distress that served as a setting event for self-administration. In keeping with current theory regarding overlearned response patterns, we adopt the assumption from connectionist models that nodes representing repeatedly executed and reinforced responses develop low thresholds for future activation (Yeung et al., 2004). Thus, drug self-administration is likely to recur in the context of stimulus conditions (i.e., negative affect, distress) that previously signaled substantial drug reward and that frequently preceded previous self-administration.

Avoidance/withdrawal models of addiction motivation hold that addicted organisms show especially high levels of motivation for drug when suffering from withdrawal-induced distress. Some question, however, whether the mechanism of such an increase in motivation can be attributed to avoidance/withdrawal motivation (Hutcheson et al., 2001; Robinson & Berridge, 1993). We emphasize the role of avoidance/withdrawal motivation for several reasons (Baker et al., 2004). In classic motivational models, approach and avoidance motivation are distinguished on the basis of the instigating stimulus (Elliot & Thrash, 2002). We contend that many instances of drug self-administration, especially after periods of deprivation, are occasioned by the detection of distress, or detection of cues signaling distress. Mesoaccumbens dopamine activity may mediate the salience of drug cues (Robinson & Berridge, 1993), but we believe the motivational instigator is distress. In addition, it is important to distinguish between conditions of origin versus conditions of well-practiced execution, when evaluating the role of avoidance/withdrawal in addiction motivation. Thus, we believe that early in the development of addiction, drug acquires stronger incentive properties than it otherwise would because of negative reinforcement: that is, it alleviates withdrawal distress (Baker et al., 2004).

Positive Reinforcement

Considerable research shows that drugs have strong reinforcing value even in the absence of physical dependence. For instance, organisms can acquire conditioned place preferences for environments paired with initial doses of psychomotor stimulants. Also, addicted individuals report strong desires to take drugs even when experiencing positive affect (Zinser et al., 1992), suggesting significant drug-motivational processing in the absence of even mild or incipient withdrawal. Thus, not all drug motivation is spurred by withdrawal or distress.

There are reasons to question the importance of positive reinforcement as a motive for drug use (Robinson & Berridge, 1993). For instance, due to tolerance, heavy drug users may experience pleasure or reward infrequently. Although tolerance to appetitive drug effects does occur, however, it is possible that positive reinforcement remains a formative and influential factor. Addictive agents do yield strong appetitive effects even in heavy users, effects that are described by users as a "high," "rush," or "elation" (Seecof & Tennant, 1986). It is true that

these effects do not occur routinely. Evidence suggests, however, that addictive agents are especially likely to produce strong stimulus-response (S-R) connections that render the organism relatively immune to extinction, nonreinforcement, or deflation of the reinforcer (Miles et al., 2003). Moreover, one must recognize that reinforcers do not occur in isolation. It is important to ask what other reinforcers available to an addicted individual match or exceed addictive drugs in terms of intensity, availability/controllability, and rapid onset of appetitive effects (Vuchinich & Tucker, 1996).

We assert that approach motivation may be directly engaged (without prior activation of withdrawal/negative affect) via cues associated with rewarding drug effects. We assume (Baker et al., 1987) that the cues that are most effective in this regard are ones that have been associated with direct drug effects. For instance, positive affective states, produced either pharmacologically or nonpharmacologically, might prime further drug self-administration since these may serve as effective reminder cues of prior appetitive drug effects such as elation. This supposition is consistent with research showing effective reinstatement of drug self-administration by small "priming" doses of drug (Stewart et al., 1984; Stewart & Wise, 1992). It is also consistent with the observation that urges to use drug are often correlated with positive affect when drug users are using ad libitum (Zinser et al., 1992).

It is important to note that affect need not be engaged in order for self-administration to occur. For instance, drug self-administration may be elicited by cues previously contingent with self-administration, cues that do not by themselves evoke strong affective reaction. To the extent that the cues strongly evoke approach systems, however, it is likely that affective change will be observed. This is because cues may associatively elicit drug agonist effects (e.g., Kenny et al., 2003; Stewart et al., 1984), and the approach system comprises "hardwired" affective response components such as heightened arousal.

Bottom-Up Motivational Processes

There is considerable evidence that processes necessary and sufficient for drug motivation are subcortical, and that such "bottom-up" processes can serve to spur drug pursuit via implicit processes. Thus, we believe that the signals of withdrawal, or the incentive value of drug cues, reflect the operations of subcortical systems and activate motivational processes that *may* remain implicit in the absence of environmental obstacles to self-administration.

There is ample evidence across a variety of agents that withdrawal is mediated by subcortical structures. For instance, the structures that appear to mediate opiate withdrawal responses include the periaqueductal gray (Wise, 1988), the amygdala and extended amygdala, (Harris & Gewirtz, 2004; Reti & Baraban, 2003), and the locus coeruleus (e.g., Nestler & Aghajanian, 1997). In addition, other researchers (Frenois et al., 2002) used in situ hybridization to characterize c-fos mRNA expression in dependent rats in which opiate withdrawal was precipitated by different doses of naloxone. These researchers revealed a set of structures that responded to a low dose of naloxone (e.g., extended amygdala, lateral septal nucleus, basolateral amygdala, and field CA1 of the hippocampus) and another set of structures that responded to a higher dose of naloxone (motor striatal areas, dopaminergic and noradrenergic nuclei, hypothalamic nuclei, and periaqueductal grey). The authors speculate the former structures may mediate the motivational influence of the withdrawal syndrome, while the latter structures mediate the somatic elements of withdrawal. Finally, research suggests the involvement of brain stem mechanisms in opiate withdrawal: For example, the classic signs of opiate withdrawal can be obtained in decerebrate cats (De Andres et al., 2004).

The rewarding and incentive effects of psychomotor stimulants also appear to be mediated subcortically. Brain regions such as the nucleus accumbens and ventral tegmentum, once thought to mediate reward, may be more intimately involved in marking incentive value (Berridge & Robinson, 1998). Imaging data show correlations between subjective pleasure and activity in regions such as the bilateral ventral tegmentum, the right cingulate gyrus, the insula, bilateral thalamus, bilateral striatum, and the bilateral pontine brainstem (Holstege et al., 2003). Indeed, research also implicates the cerebellum in intense pleasurable reactions to pharmacologic and nonpharmacologic stimuli (Hostege et al., 2003; Sell et al., 1999). Research with drug and nondrug reinforcers suggests that the central nucleus of the amygdala and the basolateral amygdala are necessary for either the acquisition or expression of appetitively consequated instrumental behaviors (Cardinal et al., 2002). Finally, Koob and his colleagues suggest that the nucleus accumbens may be critical to nonassociative cocaine reward, but that associative reward effects may involve the basolateral amygdala (Koob & Le Moal, 2001; See et al., 2001; Whitelaw et al., 1996).

In sum, a great deal of evidence supports the assertion that drug reinforcement and incentive processes are mediated by activity in subcortical regions. We believe that in the inveterate user, such processing may remain implicit in the absence of obstacles or countervailing influences.

Flow of Information Processing

We propose that internal and external cues may activate incentive systems either by activating approach or withdrawal systems. These systems provide cues that signal the availability and potential magnitude of reinforcement, and activate attentional-incentive mechanisms that mediate the organism's pursuit of drug (Berridge & Robinson, 1998; Miles et al., 2003; Robinson & Berridge, 1993). Due to the extensive reinforcement history of addicted organisms, it is likely that drug cues can also directly activate incentive systems, but indicants of drug motivation will be weaker than when approach or withdrawal systems are engaged. Strong activation of drug motivation requires significant activation of either the approach or withdrawal system.

It is likely that approach and withdrawal systems cannot be simultaneously highly activated (Baker et al., 1987). This supposition is consistent with the observation that amygdala activity is suppressed during intense pleasure produced by either heroin, ejaculation, or viewing pictures of loved ones (Bartels & Zeki, 2000; Holstege et al., 2003). It is possible, however, that incentive mechanisms may first be activated via the withdrawal motivational system, and the approach system then activates approach motivational processing.

To review: Addictive drug-use results in the development of physical dependence, manifested as the tendency to display withdrawal signs contingent upon falling levels of drug in the body. In addition, addictive agents produce potent rewarding effects, even in inveterate users. Although the brain loci of these effects cannot be localized to discrete brain regions, there is substantial evidence that withdrawal and reward processes depend upon subcortical, meso- and meta-telencephalic structures. It is certainly the case that learning about strategies to acquire and use drug may involve much more widely distributed brain systems. Withdrawal, drug reward, and incentive effects, the central determinants of addictive drug motivation, however, reflect necessary and sufficient involvement of bottom-up neuropharmacologic mechanisms. Finally,

prior positive and negative reinforcement do affect the incentive value associated with drug and withdrawal cues (e.g., Berridge & Robinson, 1998; Hutcheson et al., 2001) and the activation of motivational processes and their impact on incentive systems typically unfolds implicitly in the absence of obstacles.

COGNITIVE CONTROL, DRUG USE, AND CRAVING

The preceding sections reviewed and integrated evidence about the positive and negative reinforcement mechanisms underlying the establishment of well-learned drug-seeking and administration behaviors. It is difficult, however, to understand the role and contribution of these often-implicit drug-motivational processes without understanding their boundary conditions; that is, what constrains their occurrence and influence. Therefore, we now review theory and empirical evidence from cognitive neuroscience research on the factors and mechanisms responsible for the elicitation of cognitive control processes as they constrain implicit information processing, with reference to their potential influence on drug use.

Cognitive control has been defined as effortful, controlled activation and allocation of attention to select and process goal-relevant information to behave adaptively in tasks involving high difficulty, novelty, decision uncertainty, or response conflict (Botvinick et al., 2001; Miller & Cohen, 2001). Cognitive control resources are also critical to modify behavior after unfavorable outcomes such as response errors, or unexpected outcomes including unpredicted reward or punishment (Holroyd & Coles, 2002; Ridderinkhof et al., 2004). We focus first on research that clarifies the contribution of cognitive control processes to adaptive behavior during *response conflict* because of its relevance to the conflict that dependent drug users experience when attempting to refrain from drug use. We will return to other functions of cognitive control, however, in the concluding "Model Implications" section.

Cognitive control is crucial to overcome well learned, habitual, or prepotent responses that are not adaptive, goal-relevant, or contextually appropriate. These prepotent responses often conflict with alternative weaker responses that are more adaptive but require additional support to compete successfully with this strong activation. Cognitive control provides this support by biasing processing in favor of the weaker, adaptive responses in the service of the individual's current goals. This cognitive control system is a general-purpose executive attention system that is recruited to guide adaptive behavior across diverse contexts, eliciting stimuli, and S-R complexes, often with no connection to drug use. It seems clear, however, that cognitive control may be recruited to regulate drug-seeking or -administration behaviors that have been well learned through repeated positive or negative reinforcement.

The Stroop task (see MacCleod, 1991) provides an experimental analogue to investigate cognitive control processes during response conflict. In this task, participants are presented with color words in varying ink colors. Participants are instructed to either read the word or name the ink color and trials can be *congruent* (ink color and word meaning match), *incongruent* (ink color and word meaning conflict), or *neutral* (one attribute does not contain color information). The robust "Stroop interference" effect refers to the relative increase in response time and error rate observed on incongruent trials when participants are instructed to name the ink color. Theory and experimental evidence suggest that this interference results from response conflict between the task-appropriate ink color-name response and the incorrect but strongly activated word-reading response (Cohen et al., 1990; MacCleod, 1991).

Basic cognitive neuroscience research with Stroop and similar attentionally demanding paradigms (e.g., flanker task, n-back) indicate that cognitive control is implemented in an anterior attention system that includes structures such as anterior cingulate cortex (ACC) and prefrontal cortex (PFC) that receive dopaminergic projections from the ventral tegmental area (Botvinick et al., 2001; Holroyd & Coles, 2002; Miller & Cohen, 2001). Furthermore, it appears that cognitive control and the brain systems that govern it can be subdivided into at least two separate components referred to as *evaluative* and *regulative* control (Carter et al., 2000; MacDonald et al, 2000).

The evaluative component provides an important action-monitoring function and serves to recruit additional attention when necessary to support adequate task performance or, more generally, adaptive goal-directed behavior. ACC monitoring for *response conflict* is believed to provide one mechanism through which the evaluative component can detect the need to recruit additional attention (Botvinick et al., 2001). For example, in computational models of the Stroop task (e.g., Cohen et al., 1990), correct color-naming response on incongruent trials requires biasing input from the cognitive control system to successfully compete with the word-reading response. The evaluative control component detects this need for attention by observing the strong activation of conflicting responses units (i.e., saying "red" vs. "green"), which subsequently recruits the regulative control component to positively bias the goal-relevant, color-naming response. Strong activation of ACC on incongruent color-naming trials has been empirically verified (e.g., Carter et al., 2000; Pardo et al., 1990). In addition to response conflict, evidence suggests that ACC also responds to other indicants that additional attention is necessary: viz. unfavorable outcomes, error feedback, and unexpected reward or punishment (Holroyd & Coles, 2002; Ridderinkhof et al., 2004; see "Model Implications" section).

Once recruited, the regulative control component is responsible for both the representation and integration of information regarding context and goals, and the actual implementation of top-down attentional control. Clearly, as task-inappropriate responses become more potent or reinforcement contingencies change, the importance of regulative control for guiding novel or weaker, but adaptive, responses increases (Botvinick et al., 2001; Yeung et al., 2004). These regulative control functions have been found to be closely associated with activation in sectors of the prefrontal cortex. Nonhuman primate lesion studies and human neuroimaging research strongly implicate dorsolateral prefrontal cortex (DLPFC) in the working memory processes that are critical for the active maintenance and utilization of both goal and context representations to guide adaptive behavior (Goldman-Rakic, 1987; Jonides et al., 1997; Miller & Cohen, 2001). Orbital frontal cortex (OFC) integrates information about future consequences (e.g., stimulus-reinforcement associations) and may be particularly critical for adaptive behavior when reinforcement contingencies in the environment change (Bechara et al., 2000; Rogers et al., 1999).

Cognitive Control of Drug-Use Motivation

The foregoing description indicates that cognitive control is crucial to overcome potent S-R mappings that are not adaptive in the current context. For the dependent drug user who is pursuing a drug-abstinence goal, cognitive control becomes critical to overcome strong implicit drug-use motivation elicited by negative affect or drug cues in favor of alternative but weaker nondrug-use behaviors in these contexts. The Stroop task provides a useful conceptual analogue to understand the interaction of implicit drug-use motivation with cognitive control mechanisms in the dependent user. Negative affect and drug cues are strongly mapped to associated drug-seeking and administration behaviors much as Stroop color words are strongly mapped to word reading responses. Operation of positive and negative reinforcement mechanisms and repetition across the drug user's career established this strong mapping much as extensive practice has strongly established word reading. Cognitive control allows the weaker color-naming response to effectively compete against the otherwise more potent word-reading response when color-naming has been established as the task-goal. Similarly, when the drug user establishes a drug-abstinence goal, cognitive control becomes critical for nondrug behaviors to successful compete with drug use that is strongly activated by drug cues. Finally, when color-naming, the research participant is often explicitly aware of both the effort (i.e., use of cognitive control resources) to inhibit word-reading, as well as the inclination to read (the person notes that she or he "wants" to read—a feeling that is not noted when reading occurs automatically). Similarly, the drug user will be explicitly aware of the formerly implicit drug-use motivation as cognitive control is used to support alternative behaviors, resulting in the conscious experience of drug-craving.

Cognitive control processes allow weaker responses to compete effectively against well learned and more potently activated behaviors during response conflict. Cognitive scontrol, however, is also recruited in other situations. Consideration of the various situations and consequences associated with the recruitment of cognitive control provides an explanatory mechanism for many observations about drug use and craving. Moreover, consideration of the tenets of this model also results in some novel and not entirely intuitive predictions.

MODEL IMPLICATIONS

1. *Self-report of drug-craving will covary with the recruitment of the cognitive control system and its neural substrates.* Research using neuroimaging techniques to examine the neural substrates of drug-craving in the cue-reactivity paradigm offers preliminary support for this model prediction. In this paradigm, drug-craving is elicited in drug-dependent users by exposing them to various cues that typically co-occur with drug administration (e.g., drug paraphernalia, photographs or video of drug administration). Neuroimaging research has demonstrated increased activation of key neural structures associated with the recruitment and implementation of cognitive control in this paradigm (see also Franken et al., Chapter 13). In fact, recent reviews of this literature have concluded that ACC and sectors of prefrontal cortex (primarily DLPFC and OFC) are the most reliably activated neural structures across experiments (See, 2002; Wilson et al., 2004). Moreover, several studies have documented that the degree of activation of these neural substrata of the cognitive control system covaries directly with craving self-report (e.g., Bonson et al., 2002; Brody et al., 2002; Grant et al., 1996).

In other research, a modified version of the Stroop task was used to examine implicit, drug-cue-related information processing and the top-down attentional control of this processing (see Birch et al., Chapter 18, for further review of this literature). In this "drug-cue" Stroop task, drug-use-related words are substituted for the color words and presentation of these drug cues activates drug-use motivational processes that conflict with performance of the color-naming task. Analogous to the interference observed on incongruent trials in the traditional Stroop task, drug-cue interference (i.e., relative increased color-naming response time to drug cues) is used to index the conflict caused by implicit drug-related responses, and indirectly, the activation of the cognitive control system that is recruited to resolve this conflict and successfully color-name.

Research with the drug-cue Stroop task has generally supported primary assertions from our model. The drug-cue interference resulting from the predicted response conflict between implicitly activated drug motivation versus task-relevant color-naming has been verified for individuals who are dependent on alcohol (e.g., Johnsen et al., 1994, Stormark et al., 2000), cigarettes (Munafo et al., 2003; Zack et al., 2001), cocaine (Franken, Kroon, Wiers, et al., 2000), and heroin (Franken, Kroon, & Hendriks, 2000). Moreover, manipulation of acute nicotine deprivation increases this drug-cue interference (Gross et al., 1993; Waters & Feyerabend, 2000; Zack et al., 2001). Similarly, increased severity of subjective withdrawal distress during deprivation covaries positively with this interference (Zack et al., 2001) and treatments that alleviate withdrawal symptoms reduce this response conflict (i.e., nicotine patch in smokers [Waters et al., 2003]). Finally, if the cognitive control system is recruited to resolve this response conflict in Stroop, our model predicts that drug-cue interference should covary with self-reported craving. Recent research has confirmed this predicted correlation among users dependent on cocaine (Franken, Kroon, & Hendriks, 2000) and heroin (Franken, Kroon, Wiers, et al., 2000).

2. Response conflict *surrounding drug use will recruit cognitive control and precipitate drug-craving.* Our model predicts that

response conflict surrounding drug use will be one potential indicant that spurs recruitment of the cognitive control system, with resultant drug-craving. In the drug-dependent user, this response conflict will frequently occur when strong bottom-up drug motivational processes elicited by exposure to drug cues or drug-deprivation conflict with a drug-abstinence goal. In particular, the early stages of quitting are often characterized by both significant withdrawal-related distress, which strongly primes drug-use responses, and strong motivation to sustain drug abstinence. The arguably potent conflict between these competing motivations may strongly recruit cognitive control and explain the high levels of self-reported craving during early abstinence (McCarthy et al., in press).

Response conflict surrounding drug use may be observed in nonabstinent drug users as well. In fact, many theorists have argued that conflict or ambivalence surrounding drug use should be the basis of the definition of addictive behavior (Breiner et al., 1999; Heather, 1998). This conflict is clearly reflected in the diagnostic criteria for substance dependence (e.g., persistent desire for the substance despite efforts to cut down or control use).

Unfortunately, explicit, well-controlled manipulations of response conflict in research on drug-craving have not yet been conducted. Instead, only weaker, post hoc support is available. For example, a recent review of neuroimaging research concluded that activation of DLPFC and OFC in response to drug cues was moderated by treatment status (Wilson et al., 2004). Thus, only those dependent subjects who presumably intended to use drugs following the experiment (i.e., were not in treatment) showed such activation. Similarly, recent data reveal that drug availability moderates the self-report of craving. This may occur because information that drug is not available reduces response conflict by shutting down implicit drug motivation (Wertz &

Sayette, 2001b). Preliminary evidence that drug unavailability reduces response conflict is available (Wertz & Sayette, 2001a), but stronger evidence would involve direct manipulation of response conflict with resultant effects on self-report of craving, regional brain activity, and behavioral indices of cognitive control activation.

In the presence of strong motives to abstain, increasing the strength of bottom-up activation of drug-use motivation would be expected to produce strong response conflict and greater requirement for cognitive control to support abstinence behaviors. As indicated above, drug cues appear to produce response conflict when color-naming in the Stroop task and the magnitude of this conflict covaries with drug-craving (Franken, Kroon, & Hendriks, 2000; Franken, Kroon, Wiers, et al., 2000). In addition, factors that may mark the strength of the implicitly activated drug-use S-R complex (e.g., measures of dependence, frequency of drug use that may mark opportunity for implicit learning) do covary with the magnitude of response conflict produced by drug cues in Stroop (e.g., latency to first cigarette in the morning [Waters & Feyerabend, 2000]; level of cigarette consumption [Zack et al., 2001]; frequency of alcohol use [Cox et al., 2003]).

3. Novel *or* unexpected outcomes *may recruit cognitive control and precipitate drug-craving*. If craving is caused largely by conflict, why is it that addicts sometimes report craving immediately after drug use (e.g., Jaffe et al., 1989; Zinser et al., 1992)? In addition to responding to response conflict, cognitive control is involved in the acquisition of new behaviors in novel or difficult tasks (Botvinick et al., 2001; Holroyd & Coles, 2002). In particular, anterior cingulate cortex responds to mesencephalic dopaminergic activity involved in reinforcement learning when outcomes are better (unpredicted reward) or worse (absence of predicted

reward) than expected (Holroyd & Coles, 2002; Holroyd et al., 2004; Schultz, 1997). Thus, drug effects that are stronger or weaker than anticipated (e.g., because of tolerance), or unexpected/unusual, may recruit cognitive control and perhaps result in drug-craving.

4. Unfavorable outcomes *such as unsuccessful coping strategies and withdrawal distress will recruit cognitive control and precipitate drug-craving.* Considerable research suggests that the evaluative component of cognitive control serves a critical action monitoring function and is activated in response to indicants that current behavior is not adaptive. For example, electrophysiological and functional imaging studies indicate that both explicit task errors and evaluative feedback about task performance strongly activate anterior cingulate cortex and that this activation is associated with recruitment of prefrontal cortex and the execution of corrective behavior on the current or subsequent task trials (Gehring et al., 1993; Luu et al., 2003). Similarly, pain is often a salient indicant that corrective action is necessary and ACC is strongly recruited in response to manipulations that produce both physical pain (Sewards & Sewards, 2002) and psychological "pain" or distress (Eisenberger et al., 2003).

These observations may have relevance to the occurrence of drug-craving. For instance, if an individual executes a coping response (in lieu of drug use) according to our model one should expect to see *increased* drug-craving if the coping response did not "work." There is evidence, in fact, that nondrug-coping responses that are executed to avoid drug use may increase a person's craving and subsequent drug use (Shiffman, 1984). Our model would attribute increased craving in this instance to monitoring of the disappointing outcomes of coping (e.g., inadequate reduction in negative affect). One important implication is that a nondrug-coping response

that does not produce desired or expected effects may be worse than not executing a coping response. In addition, if distressing events such as pain and stressors have the capacity to engage cognitive control directly, this may account, in part, for the strong relations between stressors, thoughts about drug, and desire to use drug (Kassel et al., 2003). (In a sense, the need to exercise cognitive control or problem-solve elicits thoughts about drug.)

5. *Compromised or deficient cognitive control resources will result in a lack of craving and an inability of cognitive control to inhibit drug self-administration.* If the dependent drug user's goal is to inhibit drug use and engage in other behaviors, our model predicts that individual differences and other factors that mark impaired recruitment or implementation of cognitive control will be associated with increased probability of drug use when exposed to negative affect or drug cues (i.e., trait or state reductions in cognitive control activation are associated with increased drug-use probability when pursuing drug abstinence). In fact, several varied literatures provide preliminary support for this prediction. In the drug-cue Stroop paradigm, the drug user's task is to color-name. Thus, regardless of their current drug-use status (e.g., treatment seeking, drug-abstinent, actively using drug), to color-name successfully they must inhibit competition from implicitly activated drug motivation. Recent research has demonstrated that individuals that exhibit decreased ability to behave adaptively in this task, presumably because of inferior cognitive control, have more difficulty in subsequent abstinence attempts. Specifically, increased drug-cue interference prospectively predicted decreased abstinence rates at 1-week posttreatment among dependent smokers (Waters et al., 2003) and at 3 months posttreatment among alcoholics

(Cox et al., 2002). Of course, the indirect measurement of cognitive control activation via response time interference prevents stronger conclusions. Subsequent research must control for potential alternative accounts (e.g., stronger implicit motivation rather than weaker control among unsuccessful abstainers) and/or provide more direct measurement of cognitive control activation (e.g., functional imaging, ERPs).

Research on distress tolerance also provides data that link individual differences in cognitive control with drug-use probability. Across these studies, drug users are instructed to perform stressful behavioral or mental tasks (e.g., solving difficult anagrams or performing challenging mental arithmetic, mirror tracing). Presumably, drug users experience conflict between adhering to instructions to persist at the task versus motivation to terminate the aversive experience. Thus, duration of task persistence may be a proxy for successful application of top-down control. Consistent with this, decreased ability to persist on the aversive tasks is associated with decreased duration of cigarette abstinence among smokers (Brandon et al., 2003; Brown et al., 2002). Similarly, decreased task persistence also predicts decreased previous drug- or alcohol-abstinence duration and probability of treatment completion (Daughters et al., in press).

Behavioral and electrophysiological evidence indicates that acute alcohol intoxication impairs cognitive control (Casbon et al., 2003; Curtin & Fairchild, 2003). This impairment in top-down attentional control process has been implicated in the general increase in behavior regulation problems observed among intoxicated individuals (e.g., aggression, impulsive risk taking; Steele & Josephs, 1990). This acute impairment in cognitive control, however, has important implications for individuals attempting to abstain from other drugs. For example, this alcohol-impaired cognitive control may account for the increased risk for relapse to smoking when intoxicated (Krall et al., 2002). Abstaining smokers who are in a bar or drinking context will frequently encounter smoking cues that activate strong motivation to smoke. If cognitive control processes are acutely compromised due to alcohol intoxication, these smokers will not be successful in inhibiting this smoking motivation and will fail to maintain their abstinence goal. If the intoxication is severe enough, smokers may smoke without ever experiencing urges to do so because of their compromised recruitment of control resources.

6. *The interplay between implicit drug motivation, components of cognitive control, and craving is dynamic.* When measuring neurobiological response, attentional or behavioral consequences, or self-report of drug-craving, the timing of these measurements relative to presentation of the eliciting stimulus is critical. For example, subcortical structures (e.g., amygdala, nucleus accumbens) that support implicit drug-motivation processes may respond relatively quickly and automatically following exposure to negative affect or drug cues. Our model predicts that cognitive control processes that are recruited to regulate or support implicit drug-use motivation and precipitate the self-report of craving will lag behind these earlier implicit processes—and should persist as long as the conflict is unresolved.

Similarly, theory on cognitive control reviewed previously also implies a dynamic interplay between evaluative and regulative control and recent basic research on cognitive control has confirmed this temporal ordering. For example, Kerns et al. (2004) demonstrated that ACC activation on any specific incongruent trial in the traditional Stroop task predicted increased PFC activation on subsequent trials. In other research, Curtin and Fairchild (2003) used the increased temporal resolution of event-related brain potentials to confirm this temporal ordering of evaluative and regulative control within a single incongruent Stroop trial.

In fact, intriguing preliminary evidence of the temporal ordering of these processes as drug-craving unfolds has been provided in a recent neuroimaging study (Wexler et al., 2001). In a cue-reactivity paradigm, cocaine-dependent participants reported real-time, self-report of drug-craving with concurrent functional MRI measurement of neural response. Consistent with other neuroimaging reports, drug-cue-specific responding was observed in ACC and sectors of PFC. The timing, however, of neural response activation relative to the onset of participants' self-report of craving varied across neural structures. Activation in anterior cingulate was observed immediately preceding report of craving, whereas PFC activation was not detected until a subsequent sampling epoch.

It would be possible to test some model elements via studies that track the evolution of drug-motivation processes across dependence development. In theory, one should observe a strong temporal congruence between the development of strong motivational responses (e.g., reflected in nucleus accumbens activity or cerebral asymmetry [Zinser et al., 1999]) and the development of activation of the ACC and associated prefrontal regions in response to blocked drug access. This would highlight the interdependence between the basic motivational processes and setting events for recruitment of cognitive control. Further, the capacity of non-drug stressors to elicit drug urges should develop only after individuals have developed physical dependence, which would allow them to appreciate the stimulus overlap between withdrawal and nonpharmacologic distress.

REFERENCES

Baker, T. B., Morse, E., & Sherman, J. E. (1987). The motivation to use drugs: A psychobiological analysis. In C. Rivers (Ed.), *Nebraska Symposium on Motivation.* (Vol. 34, pp. 257–323). Lincoln: University of Nebraska Press.

Baker, T. B., Piper, M. E., McCarthy, D. E., Majeskie, M. R., & Fiore, M. C. (2004). Addiction motivation reformulated: An affective processing model of negative reinforcement. *Psychological Review, 111*, 33–51.

Bartels, A., & Zeki, S. (2000). The neural basis of romantic love. *NeuroReport, 11(17)*, 3829–3834.

Bechara, A., Damasio, H., & Damasio, A. (2000). Emotion, decision making and the orbitofrontal cortex. *Cerebral Cortex, 10*, 295–307.

Berridge, K., & Robinson, T. (1998). What is the role of dopamine in reward: Hedonic impact, reward learning, or incentive salience? *Brain Research Reviews, 28*, 309–369.

Bonson, K., Grant, S., Contoreggi, C., Links, J., Metcalfe, J., & Weyl, H. (2002). Neural systems and cue-induced cocaine craving. *Neuropsychopharmacology, 26*, 376–386.

Botvinick, M., Braver, T., Barch, D., Carter, C., & Cohen, J. (2001). Conflict monitoring and cognitive control. *Psychological Review, 108(3)*, 624–652.

Brandon, T., Herzog, T., Juliano, L., Irvin, J., Lazev, A., & Simmons, N. (2003). Pretreatment task-persistence predicts smoking cessation outcome. *Journal of Abnormal Psychology, 112*, 448–456.

Brandon, T., Tiffany, S., Obremski, K., & Baker, T. (1990). Postcessation cigarette use: The process of relapse. *Addictive Behaviors, 15,* 105–114.

Breiner, M., Stritzke, W., & Lang, A. (1999). Approaching avoidance: A step essential to the understanding of craving. *Alcohol Research & Health, 23*(3), 197–206.

Brody, A., Mandelkern, M., London, E., Childress, A., Lee, G., Bota, R., et al. (2002). Brain metabolic changes during cigarette craving. *Archives of General Psychiatry, 59,* 1162–1172.

Brown, R., Lejuez, C., Kahler, C., & Strong, D. (2002). Distress tolerance and duration of past smoking cessation attempts. *Journal of Abnormal Psychology, 111,* 180–185.

Cardinal, R., Parkinson, J., Lachenal, G., Halkerston, K., Rudarakanchana, N., Hall, J., et al. (2002). Effects of selective excitotoxic lesions of the nucleus accumbens core, anterior congulate cortex, and central nucleus of the amygdala on autoshaping performance in rats. *Behavioral Neuroscience, 116,* 553–567.

Carter, C., Macdonald, A., Botvinick, M., Ross, L., Stenger, V., & Noll, D. (2000). Parsing executive processes: Strategic vs. evaluative functions of the anterior cingulate cortex. *Proceedings of the National Academy of Sciences, 97,* 1944–1948.

Casbon, T., Curtin, J., Lang, A., & Patrick, C. (2003). Deleterious effects of alcohol intoxication: Diminished cognitive control and its behavioral consequences. *Journal of Abnormal Psychology, 112,* 476–487.

Cohen, J., Dunbar, K., & McClelland, J. (1990). On the control of automatic processes: A parallel distributed processing account of the Stroop effect. *Psychological Review, 97,* 332–361.

Cox, W., Brown, M., & Rowlands, L. (2003). The effects of alcohol cue exposure on non-dependent drinkers' attentional bias for alcohol-related stimuli. *Alcohol and Alcoholism, 38,* 45–49.

Cox, W., Hogan, L., Kristian, M., & Race, J. (2002). Alcohol attentional bias as a predictor of alcohol abusers' treatment outcome. *Drug and Alcohol Dependence, 68*(3), 237–243.

Curtin, J., & Fairchild, B. (2003). Alcohol and cognitive control: Implications for regulation of behavior during response conflict. *Journal of Abnormal Psychology, 112*(3), 424–436.

Daughters, S., Lejuez, C., Kahler, C., Strong, D., & Brown, R. (in press). Psychological distress tolerance and duration of most recent abstinence attempt among residential treatment seeking substance abusers. *Addictive Behaviors.*

De Andres, I., Garzon, M., & Villablanca, J. (2004). The brain stem but not forebrain independently supports morphine tolerance and dependence effects in cats. *Behavioural Brain Research, 148,* 133–144.

Eisenberger, N., Lieberman, M., & Williams, K. (2003). Does rejection hurt? An fMRI study of social exclusion. *Science, 302*(5643), 290–292.

Elliot, A., & Thrash, T. (2002). Approach-avoidance motivation in personality approach and avoidance temperaments and goals. *Journal of Personality and Social Psychology, 82,* 804–818.

Franken, I., Kroon, L., & Hendriks, V. (2000). Influence of individual differences in craving and obsessive cocaine thoughts on attentional processes in cocaine abuse patients. *Addictive Behaviors, 24*(1), 99–102.

Franken, I., Kroon, L., Wiers, R., & Jansen, A. (2000). Selective cognitive processing of drug cues in heroin dependence. *Journal of Psychopharmacology, 14*(4), 395–400.

Frenois, F., Cador, M., Caille, S., Stinus, L., & Le Moine, C. (2002). Neural correlates of the motivational and somatic components of naloxone-precipitated morphine withdrawal. *European Journal of Neuroscience, 16,* 1377–1389.

Gauvin, D., Carl, K., Goulden, K., & Holloway, F. (1993). Cross-generalization between drug discriminative stimuli and condition safety and danger cues. *Experimental & Clinical Psychopharmacology, 1,* 133–141.

Gauvin, D., Harland, R., & Holloway, F. (1989). The discriminative stimulus properties of ethanol and acute ethanol withdrawal states in rats. *Drug and Alcohol Dependence, 24,* 103–113.

Gehring, W., Goss, B., Coles, M., Meyer, D., & Donchin, E. (1993). A neural system for error detection and compensation. *Psychological Science, 4*(6), 385–390.

Goldman-Rakic P. S. (1987). Circuitry of primate prefrontal cortex and regulation of behavior by representation knowledge. In F. Plum & V. Mountcastle (Eds.), *The handbook of physiology* (Vol. 5, pp. 373–417). Bethesda, MD: American Physiological Society.

Grant, S., London, E., Newlin, D., Villemagne, V., Liu, X., & Contoreggi, C. (1996). Activation of memory circuits during cue-elicited cocaine craving. *Proceedings of the National Academy of Sciences, 93,* 12040–12045.

Gross, T., Jarvik, M., & Rosenblatt, M. (1993). Nicotine abstinence produces content-specific Stroop interference. *Psychopharmacology, 110,* 333–336.

Harris, A., & Gewirtz, J. (2004). Elevated startle during withdrawal from acute morphine: A model of opiate withdrawal and anxiety. *Psychopharmacology, 171,* 140–147.

Heather, N. (1998). A conceptual framework for explaining drug addiction. *Journal of Psychopharmacology, 12*(1), 3–7.

Heischman, S., Stitzer, M., Bigelow, G., & Liebson, I. (1989). Acute opioid physical dependence in postaddict humans: Naloxone dose effects after brief morphine exposure. *Journal of Pharmacology and Experimental Therapeutics, 248,* 127–134.

Holroyd, C., & Coles, M. (2002). The neural basis of human error processing: Reinforcement learning, dopamine, and the error-related negativity. *Psychological Review, 109,* 679–709.

Holroyd, C., Larsen, J., & Cohen, J. (2004). Context dependence of the event-related brain potential associated with reward and punishment. *Psychophysiology, 41*(2), 245–253.

Holstege, G., Geordiadis, J., Paans, A., Meineres, L., Van der Graaf, F., & Reinders, A. (2003). Brain activation during human male ejaculation. *The Journal of Neuroscience, 23,* 9185–9193.

Hutcheson, D., Everitt, B., Robbins, T., & Dickinson, A. (2001). The role of withdrawal in heroin addiction: Enhances reward or promotes avoidance? *Nature Neuroscience, 4,* 943–947.

Jaffe, J., Cascella, N., Kumor, K., & Sherer, M. (1989). Cocaine-induced cocaine craving. *Psychopharmacology, 97,* 59–64.

Johnsen, B., Laberg, J., Cox, W., Vaksdal, A., & Hugdahl, K. (1994). Alcoholic subjects' attentional bias in the processing of alcohol-related words. *Psychology of Addictive Behaviors, 8,* 111–115.

Jonides, J., Schumacher, E., Smith, E., Lauber, E., Awh, E., & Minoshima, S. (1997). Verbal working memory load affects regional brain activation as measured by PET. *Journal of Cognitive Neuroscience, 9*(4), 462–475.

Kassel, J., Stroud, L., & Paronis, C. (2003). Smoking, stress, and negative affect: Correlation, causation, and context across stages of smoking. *Psychological Bulletin, 127*, 270–304.

Kelsey, J. E., & Arnold, S. R. (1994). Lesions of the dorsomedial amygdale, but not the nucleus accumbens, reduce the aversiveness of morphine withdrawal in rats. *Behavioral Neuroscience, 108*, 1119–1127.

Kenford, S., Smith, S., Wetter, D., Jorenby, D., Fiore, M., & Baker, T. (2002). Predicting relapse back to smoking: Contrasting affective and physical models of dependence. *Journal of Consulting and Clinical Psychology, 70*, 216–227.

Kenny, P., Koob, G., & Markou, A. (2003). Conditioned facilitation of brain reward function after repeated cocaine administration. *Behavioral Neuroscience, 117*, 1103–1107.

Kerns, J., Cohen, J., MacDonald, A., Cho, R., Stenger, V., & Carter, C. (2004). Anterior cingulate conflict monitoring and adjustments in control. *Science, 303*(5660), 1023–1026.

Koob, G., & Le Moal, M. (2001). Drug addiction, dysregulation of reward, and allostasis. *Neuropsychopharmacology, 24*, 97–129.

Krall, E., Garvey, A., & Garcia, R. (2002). Smoking relapse after 2 years of abstinence: Findings from the VA Normative Aging Study. *Nicotine & Tobacco Research, 4*(1), 95–100.

Luu, P., Tucker, D., Derryberry, D., Reed, M., & Poulsen, C. (2003). Electrophysiological responses to errors and feedback in the process of action regulation. *Psychological Science, 14*(1), 47–53.

MacDonald, A., Cohen, J., Stenger, V., & Carter, C. (2000). Dissociating the role of the dorsolateral prefrontal and anterior cingulate cortex in cognitive control. *Science, 288*, 1835–1838.

MacCleod, C. (1991). Half a century of research on the Stroop effect: An integrative review. *Psychological Bulletin, 109*(2), 163–203.

Malin, D. (2001). Nicotine dependence studies with a laboratory model. *Pharmacology Biochemistry and Behavior, 70*, 551–559.

McCarthy, D., Piasecki, T., Fiore, M., & Baker, T. (in press). Life before and after quitting smoking: An electronic diary study. *Journal of Abnormal Psychology.*

McKee, S., Wall, A., Hinson, R., Goldstein, A., & Bissonnette, M. (2003). Effects of an implicit mood prime on the accessibility of smoking expectancies in college women. *Psychology of Addictive Behaviors, 17*, 219–225.

Mello, N., & Mendelson, J. (1970). Experimentally induced intoxication in alcoholics: A comparison between programmed and spontaneous drinking. *Journal of Pharmacology and Experimental Therapeutics, 173*, 101–116.

Miles, F., Everitt, B., & Dickinson, A. (2003). Oral cocaine seeking by rats: Action or habit? *Behavioral Neuroscience, 117*, 927–938.

Miller, E., & Cohen, J. (2001). An integrative theory of prefrontal cortex function. *Annual Review of Neuroscience, 24*, 167–202.

Munafo, M., Mogg, K., Roberts, S., Bradley, B., & Murphy, M. (2003). Selective processing of smoking-related cues in current smokers, ex-smokers and never-smokers on the modified Stroop task. *Journal of Psychopharmacology, 17*(3), 310–316.

Murphy, S., & Zajonc, R. (1993). Affect, cognition, and awareness: Affective priming with optional and suboptimal stimulus exposures. *Journal of Personality and Social Psychology, 64*, 723–739.

Nestler, E., & Aghajanian, G. (1997). Molecular and cellular basis of addiction. *Science, 278*, 58–63.

Öhman, A., & Mineka, S. (2001). Fears, phobias, and preparedness: Toward an evolved module of fear and fear learning. *Psychological Review, 108,* 483–522.

Pardo, J., Pardo, P., Janer, K., & Raichle, M. (1990). The anterior cingulate cortex mediates processing selection in the Stroop attentional conflict paradigm. *Proceedings of the National Academy of Sciences, 87,* 256–259.

Piasecki, T., Niaura, R., Shadel, W., & Baker, T. B. (2000). Smoking withdrawal dynamics in unaided quitters. *Journal of Abnormal Psychology, 109,* 74–86.

Reti, I., & Baraban, J. (2003). Opiate withdrawal induces Narp in the extended amygdala. *Neuropsychopharmacology, 28,* 1606–1613.

Ridderinkhof, K., Ullsperger, M., Crone, E., & Nieuwenhuis, S. (2004). The role of the medial frontal cortex in cognitive control. *Science, 306*(5695), 443–447.

Robinson, T., & Berridge, K. (1993). The neural basis of drug craving: An incentive sensitization theory of addiction. *Brain Research Reviews, 18,* 247–291.

Rogers, R., Owen, A., Middleton, H., Williams, E., Pickard, J., Sahakian, B., et al. (1999). Choosing between small, likely rewards and large, unlikely rewards activates inferior and orbital prefrontal cortex. *Journal of Neuroscience, 19,* 9029–9038.

Sayette, M., & Hufford, M. (1994). Effects of cue-exposure and deprivation on cognitive resources in smokers. *Journal of Abnormal Psychology, 103,* 812–818.

Schultz, W. (1997). Dopamine neurons and their role in reward mechanisms. *Current Opinion in Neurobiology, 7,* 191–197.

See, R. (2002). Neural substrates of conditioned-cued relapse to drug-seeking behavior. *Pharmacology Biochemistry and Behavior, 71*(3), 517–529.

See, R., Kruzich, P., & Grimm, J. (2001). Dopamine, but not glutamate, receptor blockade in the basolateral amygdala attenuates conditioned reward in a rat model of relapse to cocaine-seeking behavior. *Psychopharmacology, 154,* 301–310.

Seecof, R., & Tennant, F., Jr. (1986). Subjective perceptions to the intravenous "rush" of heroin and cocaine in opioid addicts. *American Journal of Drug and Alcohol Abuse, 12,* 79–87.

Sell, L., Morris, J., Bearn, J., Frackowiak, R., Friston, K., & Dolan, R. (1999). Activation of reward circuitry in human opiate addicts. *European Journal of Neuroscience, 11,* 1042–1048.

Sewards, T., & Sewards, M. (2002). The medial pain system: Neural representations of the motivational aspect of pain. *Brain Research Bulletin, 59*(3), 163–180.

Shiffman, S. (1984). Cognitive antecedents and sequelae of smoking relapse crises. *Journal of Applied Social Psychology, 14,* 296–309.

Sokowloska, M., Siegel, S., & Kim, J. A. (2002). Intra-administration associations: Conditional hyperalgesia elicited by morphine onset cues. *Journal of Experimental Psychology: Animal Behavior Processes, 28,* 309–320.

Stacy, A. (1995). Memory association and ambiguous cues in models of alcohol and marijuana use. *Experimental & Clinical Psychopharmacology, 3,* 183–194.

Stacy, A. (1997). Memory activation and expectancy as prospective predictors of alcohol and marijuana use. *Journal of Abnormal Psychology, 106,* 61–73.

Steele, C., & Josephs, R. (1990). Alcohol myopia: Its prized and dangerous effects. *American Psychologist, 45*(8), 921–933.

Stewart, J., de Wit, H., & Eikelboom, R. (1984). Role of unconditioned and conditioned drug effects in the self-administration of opiates and stimulants. *Psychological Review, 91,* 251–268.

Stewart, J., & Wise, R. (1992). Reinstatement of heroin self-administration habits: Morphine promotes and naltrexone discourages renewed responding after extinction. *Psychopharmacology, 108,* 79–84.

Stormark, K., Bergen, N., Laberg, J., Nordby, H., & Hugdahl, K. (2000). Alcoholics' selective attention to alcohol stimuli: Automated processing? *Journal of Studies on Alcohol, 61,* 18–23.

Tiffany, S. (1990). A cognitive model of drug urges and drug-use behavior: Role of automatic and nonautomatic processes. *Psychological Review, 97*(2), 147–168.

Vuchinich, R., & Tucker, J. (1996). Alcoholic relapse, life events, and behavioral theories of choice: A prospective analysis. *Experimental & Clinical Psychopharmacology, 4,* 19–28.

Waters, A., & Feyerabend, C. (2000). Determinants and effects of attentional bias in smokers. *Psychology of Addictive Behaviors, 14,* 111–120.

Waters, A., Shiffman, S., Sayette, M., Paty, J. A., Gwaltney, C., & Balabanis, M. (2003). Attentional bias predicts outcome in smoking cessation. *Health Psychology, 22,* 378–387.

Wertz, J., & Sayette, M. (2001a). Effects of smoking opportunity on attentional bias in smokers. *Psychology of Addictive Behavior, 15*(3), 268–271.

Wertz, J., & Sayette, M. (2001b). A review of the effects of perceived drug use opportunity on self-reported urge. *Experimental & Clinical Psychopharmacology, 9*(1), 3–13.

Wexler, B., Gottschalk, C., & Fulbright, R. (2001). Functional magnetic resonance imaging of cocaine craving. *American Journal of Psychiatry, 158,* 86–95.

Whitelaw, R., Markou, A., Robbins, T., & Everitt, B. (1996). Excitotoxic lesions of the basolateral amygdala impair the acquisition of cocaine-seeking behaviour under a second-order schedule of reinforcement. *Psychopharmacology, 127,* 213–224.

Wilson, S., Sayette, M., & Fiez, J. (2004). Prefrontal responses to drug cues: A neurocognitive analysis. *Nature Neuroscience, 7*(3), 211–214.

Wise, R. (1988). The neurobiology of craving: Implications for the understanding and treatment of addiction. *Journal of Abnormal Psychology, 97,* 118–132.

Yeung, N., Botvinick, M., & Cohen, J. (2004). The neural basis of error detection: Conflict monitoring and the error-related negativity. *Psychological Review, 111,* 939–959.

Zack, M., Belsito, L., Scher, R., Eissenberg, T., & Corrigall, W. (2001). Effects of abstinence and smoking on information processing in adolescent smokers. *Psychopharmacology, 153,* 249–257.

Zinser, M., Baker, T., & Sherman, J. (1992). Relation between self-reported affect and drug urges and cravings in continuing and withdrawing smokers. *Journal of Abnormal Psychology, 101,* 617–629.

Zinser, M., Fiore, M., Davidson, R., & Baker, T. (1999). Manipulating smoking motivation: Impact of an electrophysiological index of approach motivation. *Journal of Abnormal Psychology, 108,* 240–254.

Section IV

EMOTION, MOTIVATION, CONTEXT, AND ACUTE DRUG EFFECTS ON IMPLICIT COGNITION

CHAPTER 17

Motivational Processes Underlying Implicit Cognition in Addiction

W. Miles Cox, Javad S. Fadardi, and Eric Klinger

Abstract: The motivational theory of current concerns accounts for attentional focus on stimuli related to a person's goal pursuits. When people actively pursue a goal of using addictive substances in order to regulate their affective states, they have a current concern for procuring and using the substance. A current concern is a latent, time-binding, goal-lurking motivational state that sensitizes the person's attentional and other cognitive processes related to the goal of using the substance. Such hyper-sensitivity to substance-related stimuli both implicitly and explicitly influences a substance abuser's decision-making processes. Attentional bias for substance-related stimuli is one of the implicit processes that make addictive behaviors hard to control. The chapter discusses motivational and attentional interventions for curbing addictive behaviors.

This chapter presents a motivational theory in which an implicit motivational process (a *current concern*) exerts an implicit influence on cognitive processing, in that it biases attention, recall, and explicit thought toward goal-related cues. This is a normal, inescapable process with regard to any kind of goal. As applied to goals involving addictive substances, it may become part of a vicious circle that helps to maintain the addiction. The current-concerns conceptualization, however, also provides ideas for countering this effect and hence helping addicted individuals to break out of the circle.

SOME TERMINOLOGICAL AND THEORETICAL ISSUES

As used here, *implicit cognitions* are those thought processes that fall beyond one's conscious awareness but nevertheless influence a wide variety of everyday behaviors in automatized ways, including addictive behaviors (see Bruce & Jones, Chapter 10). The motivational processes that underlie implicit cognition in addiction are best understood in light of some basic principles of motivation in general. We define *motivation* as "the internal states of the organism that lead to the instigation, persistence, energy, and direction of behavior towards a goal" (Klinger & Cox, 2004, pp. 4–5).

How does goal-directed behavior come about? In our view, people are motivated to get (and hence they want) things when they anticipate that having them will bring a positive emotional payoff, and they are motivated to get rid of or avoid things when they anticipate that having these things will bring a negative emotional payoff. We call the things that people want *positive incentives* and the things that they want to get rid of or avoid *negative incentives*. That is, positive incentives are those things (objects or events) that people expect will make them feel good or better. Negative incentives are those that people expect will make them feel bad or worse. Thus, an incentive is defined as any object or event that a person expects will change his or her *affect,* and its value depends on the valence and magnitude of that emotional payoff. *Affective change,* therefore, is a central motivational concept, because it is the essence of what people are motivated to achieve.

People are not, of course, motivated to get or get rid of all of the incentives that could potentially bring about desirable affective changes. There are a number of variables in addition to expected affective change—that is, in addition to incentive *value*—that determine whether or not an incentive will become the object of a person's goal-directed behavior, and, if it does, the intensity of the motivation. One of the most important of these variables, according to *Value X Expectancy* formulations (e.g., Feather, 1982; Van Eerde & Thierry, 1996), is the person's expected *chance of success* (i.e., *expectancy*) of being able to acquire the desired incentive or to get rid of the unwanted one. If people expect both (1) that particular incentives will bring about strong, desirable affective changes (i.e., if they place great value on them) *and* (2) that they have a strong likelihood of getting what they want or getting rid of what they do not

want, they likely will be motivated to do so. That is, their goal-directed behavior will be instigated, and it might become persistent and energetic—depending, in part, on the value of other motivational variables that we introduce later.

CURRENT CONCERNS AND THEIR COGNITIVE EFFECTS AS IMPLICIT PROCESSES

Klinger (1975, 1977) formulated the *current-concern* construct as part of a general theory of motivation to refer to the motivational state of an individual during each goal pursuit (see also Klinger & Cox, 2004). The construct refers to a time-binding process that begins when the individual becomes committed to pursuing a particular goal and continues until either the goal is attained or the person gives up the pursuit. Both attaining a goal and giving up the pursuit are associated with affective changes, that is, either happiness from achieving the goal or sadness from relinquishing it (Klinger & Cox, 2004).

In this definition of current concern, two components need explanation. *Commitment* indicates that the person has decided to pursue the selected goal. This constitutes a change in the person's emotional reactivity from which there is no turning back without psychological cost. That is, although people often change their minds and relinquish goals to which they had once been committed, disengaging from such goals always entails a degree of negative emotion—anger, disappointment, sadness, perhaps depression—unless the goal is dropped in favor of another goal that provides similar or greater satisfaction (Klinger, 1975, 1977).

Time-binding means that the current concern is an enduring neural process over the interval of the goal pursuit, one that implicitly biases cognitive processing toward goal-related cues and most likely periodically injects goal-related ideation into the person's stream of consciousness. This is a much more encompassing conception than those of stimulus salience and prepotent responses, but goal-related cues gain salience and goal-directed responses are potentiated. Thus, after a current concern has been established, it does not vanish even if it is not in the focus of one's attention at a given point in time. Rather, it remains active and directed toward attainment of the goal at a nonconscious level, competing with various other current concerns for access to the center of the person's conscious awareness (Klinger, 1975, 1977, 1990; Klinger & Cox, 2004). Hence, the implicit current concern keeps the individual on track toward a goal by inducing cognitive reminders of the goal pursuit and keeping the individual oriented toward cues and actions that advance attainment of the goal.

Although the concept of current concern refers to the underlying, *nonconscious process* of having a goal, people are usually conscious of the goals that undergird their current concerns. People's current concerns determine what they think and recall, what they pay attention to, and the activities that they engage in. Therefore, when a person makes a commitment to pursue a particular goal, he or she becomes a motivationally and cognitively changed individual.

The following section describes the process through which some people develop current concerns for drinking alcohol (or using other addictive substances), and how having such a concern influences their implicit cognitions as part of the cognitive-motivational factors underlying addictive goal-seeking behavior.

A MOTIVATIONAL MODEL OF ADDICTION IN ALCOHOL USE

Drinking alcohol (or using another addictive substance) can become a goal that a person actively pursues, just like any other goal except for the chemical influences of such substances on a person's motivational state. Problems arise, however, when drinking alcohol becomes a goal that overshadows the other goal pursuits in a person's life and conflicts with their attainment. When this happens, the person's concern about drinking alcohol is reflected in his or her implicit cognitive processes. For example, he or she might become preoccupied with alcohol or might selectively attend to alcohol-related stimuli in the environment. These cognitive processes might further fuel the motivation to drink and make it more difficult for the person to change his or her abusive drinking. Current concerns, therefore, provide an avenue for studying how a given incentive such as drinking alcohol or using other addictive substances can become a goal that is intermeshed with the other incentives, goals, and current concerns in a person's life.

There are, of course, complex determinants of alcohol use and abuse and of other addictive behaviors. These determinants include biological, psychological, and sociocultural variables that contribute to the motivation to drink or not to do so. Cox and Klinger's (1988, 1990, 2004a) motivational model of alcohol use shows how each variable that contributes to drinking is channeled through a motivational pathway, thereby affecting individuals' expectations of affective change from drinking versus not doing so. In other words, each variable influences the *incentive value* that the person attributes to drinking alcohol. In turn, whether or not a person sets a goal of regulating his or her affect by drinking alcohol depends vitally on the incentives and goal strivings in other life areas that might compete with the satisfaction derived from drinking alcohol. We introduce the motivational model here to show how implicit cognitive processes that underlie addictive behaviors are affected by basic motivational principles.

Components of the Motivational Model

An abridged version of Cox and Klinger's (1988, 1990, 2004a) motivational model of alcohol use is shown in Figure 17.1. The flow diagram in Figure 17.1 ends with the decision to drink or not to drink a particular drink of alcohol on a particular occasion. That decision is made on the basis of the balance between the expected positive and negative affective changes from drinking. If the positive expected changes outweigh the negative, the decision will be to drink. Many proximal

and distal factors feed into that apparently simple decision. Some of these might add weight to the decision to drink; others might add weight to the decision not to drink.

Distal Determinants

Past drinking experiences. The types of drinking experiences (e.g., positive, negative) that people have had in the past are important determinants of their current expectations of affective change from drinking. In fact, those experiences appear to be essential to

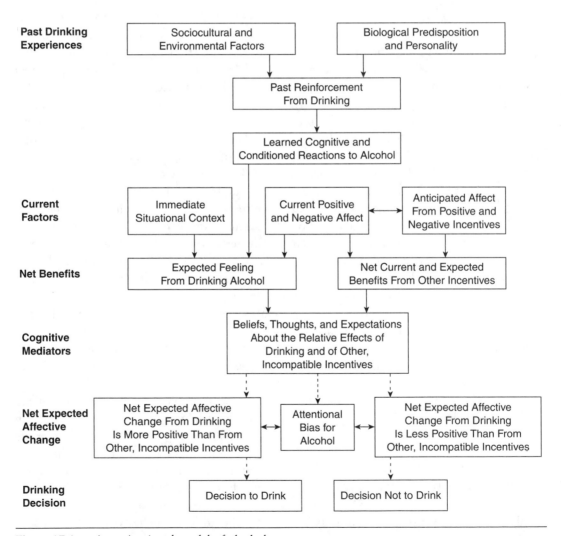

Figure 17.1   A motivational model of alcohol use

establishing the incentive value of alcohol for an individual, including its value in relation to withdrawal symptoms (Glasner, 2004). The major determinants of past drinking experiences include (1) the person's neurochemical reactions to alcohol and the manner in which the body metabolizes alcohol, (2) personality characteristics, and (3) the drinking practices in the society in which the person lives.

Each person's pharmacological reactions to alcohol are largely determined by genetic factors (Cook & Gurling, 2001; McGue, 1999). Some people will have had negative drinking experiences in the past that should detract from the incentive value that they attribute to drinking alcohol and add weight to their current decisions *not* to drink. Other people will have had positive pharmacological reactions to alcohol (see Fromme & D'Amico, 1999; Robinson & Berridge, 1993, 2001, 2003). These reactions are likely to increase the incentive value of drinking alcohol and contribute to people's current decisions to drink.

Personality characteristics are another determinant of past drinking experiences. These might either place people at risk for excessive drinking or protect them from it (Cox et al., 2001; Sher et al., 1999). The antecedent characteristics that seem to promote excessive drinking are antisocial, aggressive, and impulsive behaviors (Cox et al., 2001; Finn et al., 2000). People with these antecedent personality characteristics are more likely than other people to value drinking alcohol and to disregard the negative consequences of drinking excessively.

Finally, people's drinking experiences are strongly influenced by the society in which they live (see Partanen & Simpura, 2001). People learn to imitate the drinking behavior of other people in the same society; they are socially reinforced for doing so (Heath, 2000). For instance, if a person has learned that it is socially acceptable to drink heavily, he or she will have formed expectancies about positive affective changes from drinking, and will be likely to continue drinking heavily in the future.

Current factors. Expectations about drinking from past drinking experiences can be modified by the situation that the person is currently in. One critical factor is the (1) positive incentives in other areas of the person's life and the positive affect that the person derives from these incentives, and (2) the negative incentives that burden the person and intensify his or her negative affect. In other words, the positive and negative affective changes that the person expects to get from drinking alcohol are balanced against those expected from positive and negative incentives in other areas of life (Cox & Klinger, 2004a, pp. 129–130). Correia (2004) and Heather and Vuchinich (2003) present similar evidence from a behavioral-economic model of choice behavior.

Cognitive mediators. Cognitive mediators, which are depicted near the center of the flow diagram in Figure 17.1, include the beliefs, thoughts, and expectations about affective changes from drinking alcohol versus those from other, incompatible incentives. In turn, the cognitive mediators give rise to the net affective changes from drinking alcohol, which are immediately proximal to the decision to drink or not to drink.

Attentional Bias for alcohol-related stimuli is positioned adjacent to the *Net Expected Affective Change* in the diagram. This is because being motivated to change one's affect by drinking alcohol should increase the person's attentional sensitivity to alcohol-related cues. The two cognitive processes are expected to have reciprocal effects on each other. *Net Expected Affective Change* from drinking is divided into two categories—*More Positive* and *Less Positive* change than is expected from other incentives. *Attentional Bias* is positioned between the *More Positive* and *Less Positive* expected affective change from drinking because (1) sometimes automatic processes activated by alcohol-related cues override the drinker's expected negative affective consequences from drinking, or they cause such consequences to be underestimated, and (2) urges to drink triggered automatically by alcohol cues do not necessarily lead to the act of drinking (Tiffany, 1990, 1991).

In a recent study in our laboratory (Shamloo et al., 2004), a sample of participants randomly assigned to one of four groups completed experimental tasks that varied in terms of their difficulty for each group. There was a control group and three experimental groups in which task-specific sense of control was either enhanced or reduced from manipulations of participants' rate of success or failure in completing the task. Unlike the control group, the groups whose sense of control was reduced reported postexperimental increases in urges to drink, and the group whose sense of control was increased showed decreases in urges to drink. In addition, posttest urges to drink predicted participants' degree of attentional bias for alcohol-related stimuli after habitual alcohol consumption had been controlled. These results support the idea that there is a reciprocal relationship between expected affective changes from drinking and attentional bias for alcohol-related stimuli.

Development of Implicit Cognitions

Implicit cognitions occur when past experiences influence one's judgment in a covert way, such that one cannot introspectively realize their existence and influence. Many aspects of humans' judgments and behaviors are automatic; the automaticity is not limited to individual behaviors, but it extends to various types of higher mental processes, social judgments, and reactions (Bargh & Ferguson, 2000; Fadardi et al., Chapter 9; Greenwald & Banaji, 1995). Research indicates that implicit

learning occurs even when people pursue unclear goals and are not sure about their performance on them (Tunney & Shanks, 2003). Such learning is necessary not only from an economic viewpoint, but it also often provides people with adequate behavioral reactions when they encounter dangerous situations. Such ready-to-use cognitive-behavioral units do not, however, always provide optimal solutions.

Regarding the development of implicit cognitions in addictive behaviors, Wiers et al. (2002) summarized the results of the empirical research as follows: (1) implicit cognitions are powerful predictors and cross-sectional correlates of alcohol use, (2) the activation of implicit processes affects both drinking outcome expectancies and alcohol consumption, and (3) negative affect exacerbates the retrieval of implicit cognitions in problem drinkers. As McCusker (2001) pointed out, findings on implicit cognitions related to addictive behaviors provide a firm ground for understanding alcohol abuse and other addictive behaviors, both from a theoretical and an applied point of view.

There are various explanations of the origins of implicit cognitions, including attentional bias, the most popular of which we briefly name here. One explanation is that direct experience with drinking alcohol or using other substances causes a person to develop conditioned and learned cognitive reactions to alcohol-related or other substance-related stimuli (e.g., Shapiro & Nathan, 1986). This kind of classically conditioned implicit reaction to alcohol cues can be elicited by both craving-related and withdrawal-related stimuli (Feldtkeller et al., 2001). Another explanation is Stacy's (1997) Implicit Cognition Theory (ICT), which emphasizes the important effect of activating the alcohol-related concept in memory on drinking behavior. Such alcohol-related associations in a person's memory can be established and strengthened through frequent experience with alcohol. According to Stacy, strong associations between drinking and both its outcomes (e.g., feeling relaxed) and drinking-related cues have important motivational implications. Stacy (1997) found that measures of implicit cognition were stronger predictors of drinking than were outcome expectancies. A third explanation is McClelland's (1998) connectionist model, which explains the role of particular brain regions—the neocortex, forebrain, hippocampus, and related areas in the medial temporal lobes—in the development of learning and memory associations classified as implicit cognitions.

A fourth explanation is based on evidence that the brain becomes sensitized to concern-related stimuli. In the case of substance-related goals, such sensitization may in part be due to the chemical effects of the addictive substance on the brain's reward system. For example, *sensitization* of the dopaminergic neural system (Franken, 2003; Robinson & Berridge, 1993, 2001, 2003) suggests that neurochemical changes in the brain are due to chemical effects of alcohol that sensitize the brain's reward loci and networks to alcohol; this leads to urges to drink alcohol.

The latter supposition has found support in research by Myrick et al. (2004). Given a sip of alcohol, alcohol-dependent participants responded to alcoholic-beverage cues, but not to other beverage cues, with increased fMRI activity in the prefrontal cortex and anterior limbic system. These investigators also established a correlation between craving self-ratings and fMRI activity levels in the left nucleus accumbens, anterior cingulate, and left orbitofrontal cortex, which have previously been found associated with craving and with other goal-related processing and decision making (Banfield et al., 2004; Bechara et al., 2000). These effects, found in alcoholic participants, did not occur in social drinkers. These findings have important implications for adaptive behavior.

An impaired cortical system followed by neurocognitive changes imposed by addictive substances alters the efficiency of decision-making processes and behavioral control in addicts when they encounter addiction-related cues and situations.

None of the views discussed so far about how implicit cognitions develop encompasses the full pathway through which the motivation to abuse alcohol or other drugs sustains a particularly vicious cycle. We now consider the path through which a current concern acts as a specialized cognitive-motivational entity, perpetuating this cycle.

Current Concerns and Implicit Cognitions

As discussed earlier, the theory of current concerns suggests that being committed to a goal pursuit is associated with developing a nonconscious cognitive hypersensitivity to goal-related stimuli. Increasing the frequency of using an abusive substance as a tool to regulate one's emotions will gradually cause substance use to become a nonconscious, automatized goal. This feature is embedded in the concept of current concerns as a time-binding, goal-lurking motivational entity. By "goal-lurking," we mean that a current concern causes a person's attentional system to locate and focus on stimuli that will facilitate attainment of goals.

A current concern acts as a prominent schema in modulating attention to and selection of wanted over unwanted stimuli. With increases in the value and expectancy of an incentive as the object of a goal pursuit, chances increase that the current concern will win out in the competition for the focus of attention among other current concerns. Therefore, a current concern is not an *idle* entity waiting to be fulfilled; rather, it actively gravitates toward the center of a person's attention. For example, current concerns control thought content in both waking and dream states (Klinger, 1990; Nikles et al., 1998). There is evidence that sleeping on a problem facilitates achieving a solution despite the fact that during the period of *sleep* the person has not been consciously thinking about the problem (Barrett, 1993; Wagner, 2004). Therefore, as a motivational entity, a current concern is not merely dependent on a person's conscious efforts. Neither is it a permanent supervisory system because current concerns change from one point in time to another. Nonetheless, the underlying mechanism—which makes the nonconscious, time-binding, and automatic effects of current concerns possible—remains stable across time. We suggest that each specific current concern corresponds to a specific set of cognitive functions. The process through which these functions allow a current concern to exert its effects can be formulated as follows.

Having a current concern first causes stimuli related to the concern to become salient. Perceptual pathways for analyzing the relevant structural features of stimuli then become sensitized; this analysis is confined to a global emotional evaluation (i.e., goal-lurking), which interacts with the general executive cognitive system that is responsible for cognitive processes related to goal attainment. Those stimuli that are evaluated as emotionally important will become the focus of attention and further emotional evaluation.

There are various methods for studying implicit cognitions relevant to current concerns, especially the role of a biased attentional system in addictive behaviors. Among these methods, modified versions of the classic Stroop test have been widely used (see Bruce & Jones, Chapter 10). In the classic Stroop test, participants are asked to respond as quickly and accurately as possible to two sets of color words: one set that is congruent with its font color (red in *red*); the other that is incongruent with its font color (red in *green*). Interference scores are calculated by subtracting participants' mean reaction time (RT) to the congruent color words from their mean RT to the incongruent color words. In emotional versions of the Stroop test, interference scores are calculated by subtracting participants' mean RT to an emotionally neutral category of words (e.g., items found in a house) from their mean RT to an emotionally salient category of words—usually related to their psychopathology. An emotional Stroop test, therefore, is intended to measure attentional bias for the emotionally salient stimuli. For example, an alcohol-Stroop test includes alcohol-related words as the salient category. Recently, Fadardi and Cox (2004b) showed that alcohol-attentional bias is not an artifact of participants' general cognitive flexibility and inhibitory processes, lending additional support to the validity of attentional bias for alcohol-related stimuli. In addition, Fadardi and Cox (2004a) found that alcohol attentional bias was a more potent predictor of the amount of alcohol that university students habitually consumed than was a set of demographic characteristics and motivational variables.

The convergent evidence from emotional Stroop studies supports the view that each current concern activates a specific cognitive circuit that is different from the circuits for other current concerns. For example, attentional bias in clinical samples is not limited to mood-congruent stimuli (e.g., Bauer & Cox, 1998; Crombez et al., 2000; de Ruiter & Brosschot, 1994; Kinderman, 1994) or mood-congruent states (e.g., Riemann & McNally, 1995; Spinks & Dalgleish, 2001), and participants show greater attentional bias for alcohol-related words than for other concern-related words (Cox et al., 2000), and greater attentional bias for alcohol-related words than for more emotionally positive and negative words that are unrelated to alcohol (Bauer & Cox, 1998).

IMPLICATIONS FOR TREATMENT

As a result of the impact of the variables shown in the motivational model, many people drink alcohol excessively. Excessive drinkers, however, vary widely in their ability to reduce their drinking. We now consider some factors that affect people's motivation to change their drinking and how this change can affect their attentional allocation to alcohol-related stimuli. These are factors addressed by Systematic Motivational Counseling (Cox & Klinger, 2004b), a technique to help substance abusers develop adaptive motivational patterns.

Changing the Motivation to Drink

One important step in overcoming the automatic nature of substance use is for the person to set, become committed to, and successfully attain alternative, positive goals, which are compatible with his or her core values. Establishing attractive nonsubstance goals is a central principle of Systematic Motivational Counseling.

A number of factors come into play to influence the relative attractiveness of nonsubstance goals. For example, one needs to enhance his or her motivational system by becoming more appetitive in goal selection and pursuit. Research has shown that an aversive motivational style, characterized by a larger than average proportion of goals addressed at negative things in one's life instead of at positive outcomes, is associated with negative emotional states (Cooper et al., 2000; Roberson, 1989).

Examples of other substance-abuse factors addressed by Systematic Motivational Counseling are as follows:

Gaining knowledge about how to pursue a goal will enhance one's sense of control and self-confidence (Baldwin, 1992; Goodie, 2001). Little hope is expected for attaining a goal when one does not have sufficient information about how to do so, relying instead on chance and other external factors. Intervention can include providing information and directing clients toward appropriate training and education.

People also need to be realistic in setting their goals. Setting goals that are beyond a person's capability may lead to frustration and other negative emotions that underlie one's motivation to abuse alcohol or another substance. Assessing feasibility of goals is part of a sound motivational-intervention process.

In addition, people need to set goals that will cause them to become emotionally involved. If one feels emotionally blasé about either attaining or failing to attain a goal, there will be little motivation to pursue it. On the other hand, the effective pursuit of meaningful, realistic goals enhances positive emotions, thereby reducing the need to resort to a substance to regulate one's emotions. Systematic Motivational Counseling tries to help clients find emotionally compelling nonsubstance goals.

Changing the Attentional System

Without a need to ingest abusive substances, there would be no current concern for doing so, and substance use would lose its importance for the person. Nevertheless, although a client in treatment may have explicitly decided to stop using the substance, the hypersensitivity to substance-related cues might continue for a time and still adversely affect the person's conscious decisions to remain abstinent. For example, there is considerable evidence that when abusers encounter substance-related cues, they show increased craving for the substance, and that the craving is accompanied by increased physiological arousal (Childress et al., 1993). This could lead to impulsive resumption of use.

Greeley et al. (1993) found that in-treatment alcohol abusers' desire to consume alcohol increased in the presence of alcohol-related cues, suggesting that automatized alcohol-related implicit cognitions might adversely influence conscious decisions about drinking. In Greeley et al.'s study, stronger negative expectancies in the presence of alcohol cues were associated with self-reports of greater resistance to future drinking; however, the extent to which this relationship can be translated into actual drinking situations is unknown. To date, there has been no research to indicate the extent to which negative expectancies about drinking are reflected in implicit measures of concerns about using alcohol or other substances of abuse. Cox et al. (2000) and Cox et al. (2002) reported, however, that alcohol abusers with greater alcohol attentional bias had poorer treatment outcomes.

On the basis of this evidence, it would seem reasonable to develop interventions to train the sensitized brain—which seeks out addiction-related cues nonconsciously—to quickly and efficiently overcome this tendency. Some techniques have been used to reduce alcohol abusers' reactivity to alcohol-related cues. Cue exposure combined with urge-control techniques (Monti et al., 1993) and Naltrexone administration (Monti et al., 2000; Monti et al., 1999; Monti et al., 2001) have been associated with reductions in alcohol-abusers' urges to drink when exposed to alcohol-related cues.

Evidence on the effectiveness of these methods is mixed. The effect of Naltrexone on reducing cue reactivity has been reported only after a high frequency of exposure to alcohol cues (Rohsenow et al., 2000). From their review of the literature on cue-exposure addiction treatments, Conklin and Tiffany (2002) concluded that the evidence does not consistently support the efficacy of cue-exposure treatments as they are currently practiced. Drummond (2002), however,

pointed out that Conklin and Tiffany's conclusions were based on studies with methodological shortcomings and that other evidence shows that cue-exposure treatment is efficacious. Finally, Niaura (2002) asserted that cue-exposure treatment is feasible, provided that it involves higher-order learning mechanisms and that two conditions hold. First, the training should include real-world stimuli, such as virtual simulation of drug-using environments. Second, the training should extend over a long period of time and with sufficient practice.

In contrast to the techniques referred to so far, the Alcohol Attention Control Training Program (AACTP; Fadardi, 2003; Cox & Fadardi, 2004) requires excessive drinkers to become actively involved in overcoming their attentional bias for alcohol-related stimuli. The AACTP involves three phases. *First*, it assesses drinkers' uncontrollable attention to alcohol-related stimuli, and helps them understand the meaning and consequences of the distraction and whether or not they could benefit from changing their distractibility. *Second*, it helps drinkers to set goals for controlling their distractions by strengthening inhibitory processes that enable them to ignore alcohol-related stimuli. *Third*, it evaluates drinkers' progress while taking part in the program and provides them with immediate feedback. Preliminary results from a project to evaluate the effectiveness of the AACTP suggest that it reduces excessive drinkers' alcohol-specific attentional bias and helps them overcome their temptations to drink.

In conclusion, then, implicit attentional bias toward substance-related stimuli is an integral part of normal goal-striving processes. One can divert clients from continued substance use by helping them to adopt attractive nonsubstance goals and by direct modification of attentional processes.

REFERENCES

Baldwin, T. T. (1992). Effects of alternative modelling strategies on outcomes of interpersonal skills training. *Journal of Applied Psychology, 77*(2), 147–154.

Banfield, J. F., Wyland, C. L., Macrae, C. N., Munte, T. F., & Heatherton, T. F. (2004). The cognitive neuroscience of self-regulation. In R. F. Baumeister & K. D. Vohs (Eds.), *Handbook of self-regulation: Research, theory, and applications* (pp. 62–83). New York: Guilford.

Bargh, J. A., & Ferguson, M. J. (2000). Beyond behaviorism: On the automaticity of higher mental processes. *Psychological Bulletin, 126*, 925–945.

Barrett, D. (1993). The "Committee of Sleep": A study of dream incubation for problem solving. *Dreaming, 3*(2), 115–122.

Bauer, D., & Cox, W. M. (1998). Alcohol-related words are distracting to both alcohol abusers and non-abusers in the Stroop colour-naming task. *Addiction, 93*(10), 1539–1542.

Bechara, A., Damasio, H., & Damasio, A. R. (2000). Emotion, decision making and the orbitofrontal cortex. *Cerebral Cortex, 10*, 295–307.

Childress, A. R., Hole, A. V., Ehrman, R. N., Robbins, S. J., McLellan, A. T., & O'Brien, C. P. (1993). Cue reactivity and cue reactivity interventions in drug dependence. *NIDA Research Monograph, 137*, 73–95.

Conklin, C. A., & Tiffany, S. T. (2002). Cue-exposure treatment: Time for change. *Addiction, 97*(9), 1219–1221.

Cook, C. C. H., & Gurling, H. H. D. (2001). Genetic predisposition to alcohol dependence and problems. In N. Heather, T. J. Peters, & T. Stockwell (Eds.), *International handbook of alcohol dependence and problems* (pp. 257–279). New York: John Wiley.

Cooper, M. L., Agocha, V. B., & Sheldon, M. S. (2000). A motivational perspective on risky behaviors: The role of personality and affect regulatory processes. *Journal of Personality, 68*(6), 1059–1088.

Correia, C. J. (2004). Behavioral economics: Basic concepts and clinical applications. In W. M. Cox & E. Klinger (Eds.), *Handbook of motivational counseling: Concepts, approaches, and assessment* (pp. 49–64). Chichester, UK: Wiley.

Cox, W. M., Blount, J. P., & Rozak, A. M. (2000). Alcohol abusers' and non-abusers' distraction by alcohol and concern-related stimuli. *American Journal of Drug and Alcohol Abuse, 26*(3), 489–495.

Cox, W. M., & Fadardi, J. S. (2004, September). *A cognitive-motivational model of alcohol use*. Paper presented at the World Congress of Biomedical Alcohol Research, Mannheim, Germany.

Cox, W. M., Hogan, L. M., Kristian, M. R., & Race, J. H. (2002). Alcohol attentional bias as a predictor of alcohol abusers' treatment outcome. *Drug and Alcohol Dependence, 68*, 237–243.

Cox, W. M., & Klinger, E. (1988). A motivational model of alcohol use. *Journal of Abnormal Psychology, 97*(2), 168–180.

Cox, W. M., & Klinger, E. (1990). Incentive motivation, affective change, and alcohol use: A model. In W. M. Cox (Ed.), *Why people drink: Parameters of alcohol as a reinforcer*. New York: Gardner Press.

Cox, W. M., & Klinger, E. (2004a). A motivational model of alcohol use: Determinants of use and change. In W. M. Cox & E. Klinger (Eds.), *Handbook of motivational counseling: Concepts, approaches, and assessment* (pp. 121–138). Chichester, UK: Wiley.

Cox, W. M., & Klinger, E. (2004b). Systematic Motivational Counseling: The Motivational Structure Questionnaire in action. In W. M. Cox & E. Klinger (Eds.), *Handbook of motivational counseling: Concepts, approaches, and assessment* (pp. 217–237). Chichester, UK: Wiley.

Cox, W. M., Yeates, G. N., Gilligan, P. A. T., & Hoiser, S. G. (2001). Individual differences. In N. Heather, T. J. Peters, & T. Stockwell (Eds.), *International handbook of alcohol dependence and problems* (pp. 357–374). Chichester, UK: Wiley.

Crombez, G., Hermans, D., & Adriaensen, H. (2000). The emotional Stroop task and chronic pain: What is threatening for chronic pain sufferers? *European Journal of Pain, 4*(1), 37–44.

de Ruiter, C., & Brosschot, J. F. (1994). The emotional Stroop interference effect in anxiety: Attentional bias or cognitive avoidance? *Behaviour Research and Therapy, 32*(3), 315–319.

Drummond, D. C. (2002). Is cue exposure cure exposure? *Addiction, 97*(3), 357–359.

Fadardi, J. S. (2003). *Cognitive-motivational determinants of attentional bias for alcohol-related stimuli: Implications for a new attentional-training intervention.* Unpublished doctoral dissertation, University of Wales, Bangor, UK.

Fadardi, J. S., & Cox, W. M. (2004a). *Can university students' alcohol-attentional bias and motivational structure predict their alcohol consumption?* Manuscript submitted for publication.

Fadardi, J. S., & Cox, W. M. (2004b). *Alcohol attentional bias: Drinking salience or cognitive impairment?* Manuscript submitted for publication.

Feather, N. T. (Ed.). (1982). *Expectations and actions: Expectancy-value models in psychology.* Hillsdale, NJ: Lawrence Erlbaum.

Feldtkeller, B., Weinstein, A., Cox, W. M., & Nutt, D. (2001). Effects of contextual priming on reactions to craving and withdrawal stimuli in alcohol-dependent participants. *Experimental & Clinical Psychopharmacology, 9*(3), 343–351.

Finn, P. R., Sharkansky, E. J., Brandt, K. M., & Turcotte, N. (2000). The effects of familial risk, personality, and expectancies on alcohol use and abuse. *Journal of Abnormal Psychology, 109*(1), 122–133.

Franken, I. H. (2003). Drug craving and addiction: Integrating psychological and neuropsychopharmacological approaches. *Progress in Neuro-Psychopharmacology & Biological Psychiatry, 27*(4), 563–579.

Fromme, K., & D'Amico, E. J. (1999). Neurobiological bases of alcohol's psychological effects. In K. E. Leonardo & H. T. Blane (Eds.), Psychological theories of drinking and alcoholism (2nd ed., pp. 422–455). New York: Guilford.

Glasner, S. V. (2004). Motivation and addiction: The role of incentive processes in understanding and treating addictive disorders. In W. M. Cox & E. Klinger (Eds.), *Handbook of motivational counseling: Concepts, approaches, and assessment* (pp. 29–47). Chichester, UK: Wiley.

Goodie, A. S. (2001). The effects of control on betting: Paradoxical betting on items of high confidence with low value. *Journal of Experimental Psychology: Learning, Memory, and Cognition, 29,* 598–610.

Greeley, J. D., Swift, W., & Heather, N. (1993). To drink or not to drink? Assessing conflicting desires in dependent drinkers in treatment. *Drug and Alcohol Dependence, 32*(2), 169–179.

Greenwald, A. G., & Banaji, M. R. (1995). Implicit social cognition: Attitudes, self-esteem, and stereotypes. *Psychological Review, 102*(1), 4–27.

Heath, D. B. (2000). *Drinking occasions: Comparative perspectives on alcohol and culture*. Philadelphia: Brunner/Mazel.

Heather, N., & Vuchinich, R. E. (Eds.). (2003). *Choice, behavioural economics and addiction*. New York: Pergamon.

Kinderman, P. (1994). Attentional bias, persecutory delusions and the self-concept. *British Journal of Medical Psychology, 67*(Pt. 1), 53–66.

Klinger, E. (1975). Consequences of commitment to and disengagement from incentives. *Psychological Review, 82*, 1–25.

Klinger, E. (1977). *Meaning and void: Inner experience and the incentives in people's lives*. Minneapolis: University of Minnesota Press.

Klinger, E. (1990). *Daydreaming*. Los Angeles: Tarcher (Putnam).

Klinger, E., & Cox, W. M. (2004). Motivation and the theory of current concerns. In W. M. Cox & E. Klinger (Eds.), *Handbook of motivational counseling: Concepts, approaches, and assessment* (pp. 3–27). Chichester, UK: Wiley.

McClelland, J. L. (1998). Complementary learning systems in the brain. A connectionist approach to explicit and implicit cognition and memory. *Annals of the New York Academy of Sciences, 843*, 153–169.

McCusker, C. G. (2001). Cognitive biases and addiction: An evolution in theory and method. *Addiction, 96*(1), 47–56.

McGue, M. (1999). Behavioral genetic models of alcoholism and drinking. In K. E. Leonard & H. T. Blanc (Eds.), *Psychological theories of drinking and alcoholism* (2nd ed., pp. 372–421). New York: Guilford.

Monti, P. M., Rohsenow, D. J., & Hutchison, K. E. (2000). Toward bridging the gap between biological, psychobiological and psychosocial models of alcohol craving. *Addiction, 95*(Suppl. 2), S229–S236.

Monti, P. M., Rohsenow, D. J., Hutchison, K. E., Swift, R. M., Mueller, T. I., Colby, S. M., et al. (1999). Naltrexone's effect on cue-elicited craving among alcoholics in treatment. *Alcoholism: Clinical and Experimental Research, 23*(8), 1386–1394.

Monti, P. M., Rohsenow, D. J., Rubonis, A. V., Niaura, R. S., Sirota, A. D., Colby, S. M., et al. (1993). Cue exposure with coping skills treatment for male alcoholics: A preliminary investigation. *Journal of Consulting and Clinical Psychology, 61*(6), 1011–1019.

Monti, P. M., Rohsenow, D. J., Swift, R. M., Gulliver, S. B., Colby, S. M., Mueller, T. I., et at. (2001). Naltrexone and cue exposure with coping and communication skills training for alcoholics: Treatment process and 1-year outcomes. *Alcoholism: Clinical and Experimental Research, 25*(11), 1634–1647.

Myrick, H., Anton, R. F., Li, X., Henderson, S., Drobes, D., Voronin, K., et al. (2004). Differential brain activity in alcoholics and social drinkers to alcohol cues: Relationship to craving. *Neuropsychopharmacology, 29*(2), 393–402.

Niaura, R. (2002). Does "unlearning" ever really occur: Comment on Conklin & Tiffany. *Addiction, 97*(3), 357.

Nikles, C. D., II, Brecht, D. L., Klinger, E., & Bursell, A. L. (1998). The effects of current-concern- and nonconcern-related waking suggestions on nocturnal dream content. *Journal of Personality and Social Psychology, 75*, 242–255.

Partanen, J., & Simpura, J. (2001). International trends in alcohol production and consumption. In N. Heather, T. J. Peters, & T. Stockwell (Eds.), *International handbook of alcohol dependence and problems* (pp. 379–394). Chichester, UK: Wiley.

Riemann, B. C., & McNally, R. J. (1995). Cognitive processing of personally relevant information. *Cognition & Emotion, 9*(4), 325–340.

Roberson, L. (1989). Assessing personal work goals in the organizational setting: Development and evaluation of the Work Concerns Inventory. *Organizational Behavior and Human Decision Processes, 44,* 345–367.

Robinson, T. E., & Berridge, K. C. (1993). The neural basis of drug craving: An incentive-sensitization theory of addiction. *Brain Research Reviews, 18*(3), 247–291.

Robinson, T. E., & Berridge, K. C. (2001). Incentive-sensitization and addiction. *Addiction, 96*(1), 103–114.

Robinson, T. E., & Berridge, K. C. (2003). Addiction. *Annual Review of Psychology, 54*(1), 25–53.

Rohsenow, D. J., Monti, P. M., Hutchison, K. E., Swift, R. M., Colby, S. M., & Kaplan, G. B. (2000). Naltrexone's effects on reactivity to alcohol cues among alcoholic men. *Journal of Abnormal Psychology, 109*(4), 738–742.

Shamloo, Z. S., Cox, W. M., & Fadardi, J. S. (2004). *Effects of manipulated sense of control on urges to drink and alcohol attentional bias.* Unpublished manuscript.

Shapiro, A. P., & Nathan, P. E. (1986). Human tolerance to alcohol: The role of Pavlovian conditioning processes. *Psychopharmacology, 88*(1), 90–95.

Sher, K. J., Trull, T. J., Bartholow, B. D., & Vieth, A. (1999). Personality and alcoholism: Issues, methods, and etiological processes. In K. E. Leonardo & H. T. Blane (Eds.), *Psychological theories of drinking and alcoholism* (2nd ed., pp. 422–455). New York: Guilford.

Spinks, H., & Dalgleish, T. (2001). Attentional processing and levels of symptomatology in Seasonal Affective Disorder (SAD): A preliminary longitudinal study. *Journal of Affective Disorders, 62*(3), 229–232.

Stacy, A. W. (1997). Memory activation and expectancy as prospective predictors of alcohol and marijuana use. *Journal of Abnormal Psychology, 106*(1), 61–73.

Tiffany, S. T. (1990). A cognitive model of drug urges and drug-use behavior: Role of automatic and nonautomatic processes. *Psychological Review, 97*(2), 147–168.

Tiffany, S. T. (1991). The application of 1980s psychology to 1990s smoking research. *British Journal of Addictions, 86*(5), 617–620.

Tunney, R. J., & Shanks, D. R. (2003). Subjective measures of awareness and implicit cognition. *Memory & Cognition, 31*(7), 1060–1071.

Van Eerde, W., & Thierry, H. (1996). Vroom's expectancy models and work-related criteria: A meta-analysis. *Journal of Applied Psychology, 81,* 575–586.

Wagner, U., Gais, S., Haider, H., Verleger, R., & Born, J. (2004). Sleep inspires insight. *Nature, 427*(6972), 352–355.

Wiers, R. W., Stacy, A. W., Ames, S. L., Noll, J. A., Sayette, M. A., Zack, M., et al. (2002). Implicit and explicit alcohol-related cognitions. *Alcoholism: Clinical and Experimental Research, 26*(1), 129–137.

CHAPTER 18

Emotion and Motive Effects on Drug-Related Cognition

CHERYL D. BIRCH, SHERRY H. STEWART,
AND MARTIN ZACK

Abstract: This chapter reviews theories and evidence on the possible main effect of emotions in triggering explicit and implicit drug cognitions. The findings are highly variable, suggesting that a state x trait approach, taking moderators like drug-use motives into account, might better explain the link between emotions and drug cognitions. Accordingly, subsequent research is reviewed showing that drinking motives, specifically, moderate emotion-alcohol cognition relations. Whereas positive emotions trigger both explicit and implicit alcohol cognitions in enhancement-motivated drinkers, negative emotions primarily trigger explicit cognitions in coping-motivated drinkers. Further research on emotion-alcohol cognition relations is called for to explain the disparate moderating effects of enhancement versus coping motives. Incorporating drug-use motives into cognitive interventions may improve outcomes of addiction treatment.

INTRODUCTION

Substance use often occurs in the context of positive or negative emotions. The first half of this chapter reviews theories explaining how emotions may exert a causal influence on, or "trigger," drug cognition and behavior, and provides an overview of the empirical evidence that emotions have a main (unmoderated)

effect in triggering drug-related cognition, specifically. The second half of this chapter reviews theories and evidence suggesting that individual differences, such as substance-use motives, must be taken into account to best explain the causal influence of emotions on drug cognition. We conclude with a summary and integration of findings reviewed that highlights important areas for future research, as

AUTHOR'S NOTE: The authors gratefully acknowledge the support they have received from different agencies in supporting some of the research reviewed in this paper. The first author is supported by a Social Sciences and Humanities Research Council (SSHRC) Doctoral Fellowship. The second author acknowledges operating grant support from SSHRC, and an Investigator Award from the Canadian Institutes of Health Research. The third author acknowledges grant support from the Alcoholic Beverage Medical Research Foundation.

well as key implications for understanding and managing substance misuse.

Several reviews have examined the impact of emotions on substance-use behaviors, such as alcohol consumption (e.g., Greeley & Oei, 1999; Sher, 1987), but the unique goal for this chapter was to review the experimental research available to date on some of the cognitions and individual differences thought to underlie this mood-drug-use association (cf. Maisto et al., 1999). Although we have made an effort to review the effects of emotions on substance cognition in general, most relevant research has examined drinking cognition, specifically; and so our review reflects this bias in the literature. We separately discuss studies below that have purported to measure explicit versus implicit processing. The functional features of cognitions measured in these studies generally appear consistent with their categorization as either explicit or implicit. The explicit (vs. implicit) cognitions, for example, appear to be more conscious, voluntary, deliberate, or goal-dependent (De Houwer, Chapter 2).

We propose a model that consists of three main parts (see Figure 18.1). These are Emotions, Cognitions, and Drug-Use Behavior. Emotions are broadly categorized into Positive (Panel a) and Negative (Panel b), and are the main antecedent stimuli. The target behavior, irrespective of the emotion, is drug use itself. As depicted by the first horizontal arrow in both panels of our figure, we assume that cognitions mediate the emotion/drug-use relationship (cf. Maisto et al., 1999). These cognitions can be explicit or implicit, and these two types of cognition may operate as mediators through different processes (see Wiers et al., Chapter 22). As we discuss, specific trait-like individual difference variables, such as motives for drug use (i.e., enhancement or coping motives; EM or CM), or anxiety-related variables (e.g., anxiety sensitivity; AS), appear to be proximal moderators of the relationship between emotions and drug

cognition, whereas variables such as gender and drug-abuse severity may be more distal moderators of this relationship. This is illustrated by the variables at the bottom of each panel in our figure with upward arrows depicting their moderating influence on the emotion-drug-cognition pathways.

We first specify how the term "emotion" is used in this chapter. We primarily review the effects of state (acute), rather than trait (chronic), emotions, as it is the state versus trait emotions that can be manipulated in the laboratory (cf. Martin, 1990). Experimental results provide the most compelling evidence about the causal effects of emotions on drug cognition. The term "emotion" is also used interchangeably with "mood" and "affect." Whereas some have argued that emotional, and affective, states have a somewhat shorter duration and stronger intensity than mood states (cf. Forgas, 1995), the intensity of all three of these states can presumably be altered in the laboratory (cf. Martin, 1990), and they are all thought to be shorter in duration than chronic emotional conditions (e.g., depressive disorder characterized by enduring, recurrent sad mood states) (cf. Barlow et al., in press; Kozma et al., 1990). There is also a general assumption in extant research that all types of positive (e.g., happy, relaxed), and negative (e.g., sad, tense), emotions should have similar effects. Although it is important to first establish and summarize any main effects of emotions that may exist overall, further research should evaluate whether different types of positive, or negative, emotions have distinct effects.

THE MAIN EFFECT OF EMOTIONS

Theoretical Accounts

The first theory linking mood and substance-related outcomes was the Tension Reduction

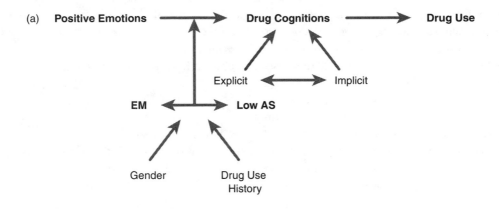

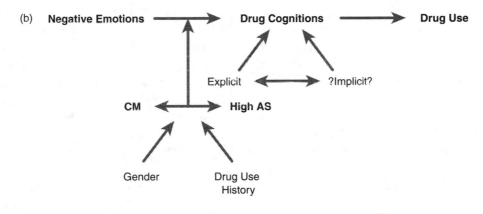

Figure 18.1   Panel (a) displays our hypothesized model for the relation of positive emotions to drug cognitions and drug-use behavior, whereas panel (b) displays our hypothesized model for the relation of negative emotions to drug cognitions and drug-use behavior.

Hypothesis (TRH; cf. Greeley & Oei, 1999). The formal articulation of the TRH (Conger, 1956) prompted decades of research to determine whether negative affective states, like stress and tension, initiate alcohol-seeking (and that alcohol actually dampens unpleasant emotions). The theoretical explanation, offered by proponents of the TRH, for why negative affect should stimulate alcohol-seeking, is a straightforward behavioral account based on principles of operant learning. According to this explanation, unpleasant emotions create an aversive drive state within an individual, and serve as discriminative stimuli signaling that drinking will result in drive-reduction by the negatively reinforcing properties of alcohol (cf. Greeley & Oei, 1999).

Other learning-based theories have been applied to explain how moods trigger alcohol cognition and consumption. According to observational learning accounts, sociocultural factors (e.g., peer or parental models) primarily shape individual learning about whether it is acceptable or useful to drink in response to various mood states (Maisto et al., 1999). As well, classical conditioning has been suggested as a mechanism through which mood cues can trigger alcohol cognitions, which then in turn increase the probability of drinking (cf. Cooney et al., 1997). According to this account, alcohol is the unconditioned stimulus and its physiological effects are the unconditioned response. After the repeated pairing of a specific mood cue with drinking, the mood cue preceding drinking can eventually become a conditioned stimulus independently capable of eliciting conditioned responses, like alcohol-related cognitive processing. This processing can either be nonautomatic (e.g., craving; see Tiffany, 1990) or automatic (cf. Zack et al., 1999). Alcohol expectancies (AE's) are specific cognitions that may also be elicited by affective cues through mechanisms like classical conditioning. AE's are learned beliefs about the consequences of drinking (cf. Goldman et al., 1999). If individuals hold many, strong beliefs about the positive effects of alcohol, this has been shown to operate as a potent incentive for drinking (cf. Darkes & Goldman, 1998).

Integrative, information-processing theories have also been applied to explain how affective cues influence drug use through the triggering of drug-related neural processing and cognition. Baker et al. (1987) propose that there are two countervailing neural networks: a positive-affect and a negative-affect urge network. The positive-affect network is most likely to be activated by prevailing positive affect stimulus conditions, and in contrast, the negative affect network is most likely to be activated by negative affect or drug withdrawal. Baker et al. (1987) suggest that once activated, each network will influence urges or cravings, and conscious drug-seeking. Others have proposed that automatic drug processing or drug-use action plans, rather than nonautomatic urge responding, can also be triggered when affective cues activate drug-related neural networks (cf. Baker et al., 2004; Tiffany, 1990).

To this point, we have provided an overview of some theories that have been offered to account for how affect might exert a main, causal influence on drug cognition and drug use. The empirical research reviewed below partly confirms, but also refines, these initial formulations.

Empirical Evidence

Fourteen experiments, of which we are aware, have examined the main effects of mood on drug cognitions. Most examined specific cognitions (e.g., craving or expectancies), and only one examined cognitions that are clearly more implicit (vs. explicit) in nature.

Five experiments investigated whether there is a main effect of mood in triggering alcohol-craving. Relative to a neutral mood, higher ratings of the subjective desire to drink have been found among alcoholics following exposure to a guided imagery negative mood induction (Cooney et al., 1997). In contrast, Jansma et al. (2000) found that negative mood, induced with either false feedback or Musical Mood Induction Procedures (MMIP), did not increase the desire to drink among alcoholics any more than a neutral mood. Rubonis et al. (1994) induced either a happy, sad, angry, or nervous state among alcoholics and found that self-reported craving increased significantly from baseline, for all participants on average. They did not, however, analyze whether there were different effects for the different moods induced. Willner et al. (1998) employed MMIP among undergraduates and found that, relative to elated and neutral moods, depressed moods increased craving, but decreased ratings of alcohol-liking. Overall, these findings are not entirely consistent, implying the existence of uncontrolled factors that influenced the experimental outcome.

Five experiments examined relations between mood and the craving for drugs other than alcohol. In the study conducted by Tiffany and Drobes (1990), cigarette-craving reports among smokers were found to be significantly stronger following exposure to negative versus positive affect guided imagery scripts; however, they were also found to be significantly stronger following exposure to positive affect versus neutral scripts. In contrast, Baker et al. (1987) review evidence that levels of negative affect are inversely associated (and levels of positive affect are directly associated) with cigarette-urge ratings following an aversive noise blast. Three studies examined opiate cravings before and after manipulating affect. One found an increase in craving following exposure to either anxiety-provoking or boring videotapes (Sherman et al., 1985); another found no increase in craving following exposure to imagery and Velten negative mood induction procedures (Hillebrand, 2000); and a final experiment found increases in craving only following hypnotically induced depression, but not anger or euphoria (Childress et al., 1994). It appears that the effects of various positive and negative affective states overall are not consistent enough to suggest they have a main effect in triggering craving for drugs other than alcohol.

Three studies examined the impact of mood on drug expectancies. Hufford (2001) measured AE's with a questionnaire, after inducing positive or negative emotions with a combination of musical and visual manipulations. Participants in the negative (vs. positive) mood group endorsed significantly more total positive AE's (and specifically, global positive change, and tension-reduction AE's). Goldstein et al. (2004) measured self-generated AE's after randomly assigning undergraduates to a neutral mood condition, or to listen to either positive or negative MMIP. They found that negative (vs. positive and neutral) mood did not predict increased self-generation of any specific AE's, whereas positive (vs. negative and neutral) mood predicted increased self-generation of AE's coded as social/situational enhancement outcomes, and neutral (vs. positive and negative) mood

predicted increased relaxation/tension-reduction AE's. Although some argue that first self-generated AE's are relatively more automatic than AE's assessed on questionnaires (see Noll in Wiers et al., 2002), in the self-generation task, participants are instructed to consciously reflect on their past learning about alcohol's effects. Reflective retrospection has been associated with explicit (rather than implicit) cognition (cf. Stacy et al., Chapter 6). Therefore, the respective contribution of explicit versus implicit processes in Goldstein et al.'s findings cannot be clearly established.

McKee et al. (2003) conducted a similar study on smoking expectancies and found that positive (vs. negative and neutral) mood predicted increased self-generation of positive reinforcement smoking expectancies, whereas negative and neutral (vs. positive) mood predicted increased self-generation of negative reinforcement expectancies. Thus, as in the case of craving cognitions, a consistent main effect of mood is not evident in these studies on drug expectancies.

A final experiment (Zack et al., 2003) assessed the main effect of mood cues on drug cognitions. In this study, a semantic priming task assessed priming of implicit alcohol concepts by verbal positive and negative mood (vs. neutral) cues. Priming was operationalized as a faster response time (RT) to read an alcohol target word aloud (e.g., B*E*E*R) following the presentation of a sentence stem containing either a positive, or negative, affect (vs. neutral) word. Overall, negative (but not positive) affect cues primed alcohol targets relative to neutral control cues. It should be noted that in this study the effects of exposure to affectively valenced prime words on mood state were not examined. As prior research (Stein et al., 2000) suggests that exposure to positive AE words (which are primarily affect words) does not change affect, we cannot conclude that the negative affect word priming observed in the Zack et al. (2003) study was due to the impact of induced negative mood on alcohol cognition.

Although there is a particular need to conduct further research examining the effects of mood on implicit (vs. explicit) cognition, the variability of effects seen in the literature implies it is doubtful that evidence will emerge that a particular mood state or cue reliably triggers any type of drug cognition, irrespective of moderating factors. As reviews on similar topics have found equally contradictory results, there has been a growing recognition of the need to take important moderators into account, such as individual differences, that can help explain the relationship between affect and drug-related outcomes (cf. Greeley & Oei, 1999). Research to date that has considered the combined effects of mood and individual differences has been largely restricted to alcohol, as opposed to other drugs, and it has particularly focused on subtypes of drinking motives. Accordingly, our review focuses on this literature. Brief descriptions of other important individual differences that may help explain complex relations between mood and addiction-related cognition or behavior (see Figure 18.1) are provided at the end of the chapter.

THE EFFECTS OF EMOTIONS MODERATED BY DRINKING MOTIVES

Theoretical Accounts

In this section we first define drinking motives and why they are important in the prediction of drinking. Drinking motives and AE's have been found to be conceptually and empirically distinct in part because drinking motives are considered to be trait-like, whereas much current thinking conceptualizes AE's as more state-like (cf. Birch et al., 2004). Cooper (1994) identified four important motives for drinking, and her Drinking Motives Questionnaire-Revised (DMQ-R) assesses the self-reported frequency of drinking for each motive. The classes of motives in this model reflect the assumption that people drink to improve either their emotional (internal) or social (external) well-being, and that within these levels of motivation people are specifically seeking either positive or negative reinforcement. Thus, for example, there are two types of internal motives: (1) enhancement motives (EM: drinking to enhance positive affect), and (2) coping motives (CM: drinking to alleviate negative affect).

Research has reliably revealed that drinking for internal, affect regulation reasons (either EM or CM) is associated with more heavy and/or problem drinking than drinking for external or social reasons (cf. Cooper, 1994). Thus, there has been an increasing amount of research in recent years conducted to identify the unique antecedents (e.g., emotional antecedents) associated with each of these "risky" motives for drinking. We outline below theoretical reasons for why positive affect might trigger alcohol cognition and drinking for EM drinkers specifically, and for why negative affect might trigger alcohol cognition and drinking for CM drinkers.

First of all, it is likely there are important individual (e.g., drinking motive) differences in the sensitivity to various reinforcing effects of alcohol, and these could influence operant learning about the reinforcement value of drinking in response to various mood states. Some individuals (possibly EM drinkers) may be particularly sensitive to euphoric effects of alcohol, whereas others (possibly CM drinkers) may be more likely to achieve tension reduction (cf. Verheul et al., 1999). Though further research is needed, there is some evidence that individuals, at least similar to CM drinkers using Cooper's (1994) terminology, are particularly sensitive to pain-dampening effects of alcohol (e.g., Brown & Cutter, 1977).

If there are drinking-motive differences in sensitivity to various effects of alcohol, there may also be drinking-motive differences in the pattern of alcohol cognitions activated in response to emotions. According to the mood-dependent memory theory (cf. Eich & Forgas, 2003), information retrieval is primed in memory if there is a concordance between the encoding and retrieval mood states. By definition, enhancement entails an increase in a preexisting positive mood state. Therefore, EM drinkers would be most likely to develop reward AE's when experiencing positive emotions. Thus, reward AE's should be primed for EM drinkers when a positive mood is reinstated. In contrast, CM drinkers may be most likely to experience tension-reduction from alcohol and to develop relief AE's when experiencing negative emotions. Clearly, emotionally relieving effects are only possible with a preexisting negative mood. Thus, in CM drinkers, relief AE's should be primed when a negative mood is reinstated. Therefore, drinking-motive differences in sensitivity to various effects of alcohol could explain drinking-motive specificity in the initial conscious use of alcohol, which in turn would dictate the class of mood cues that trigger alcohol cognitions after a period of mood-specific drinking.

Dispositional drinking-motive differences in positive versus negative affect neural networks (cf. Baker et al., 1987) or in sensitivity to different motivational systems (cf. Gray, 1990) could also explain why EM drinkers might tend to drink in response to positive affect, and CM drinkers in response to negative affect. For example, EM drinkers may be predisposed to have their positive-affect network activated or to have sensitivity to approach-related cues, whereas CM drinkers may be predisposed to have their negative-affect network activated or to have sensitivity to avoidance or threat-related cues (cf. Birch et al., 2004; Verheul et al., 1999). This possibility is consistent with a number of published reports indicating there are reliable relations between personality and internal drinking motives (e.g., Stewart & Devine, 2000).

Empirical Evidence

Two experiments measured the effects of negative mood cues, and a construct similar to CM, on explicit alcohol cognitions. As mentioned, Cooney et al. (1997) found a main effect for negative mood in triggering craving. They also found that those who reported frequent drinking in situations involving unpleasant emotions (likely CM drinkers) reported the strongest cravings following the negative versus neutral mood induction. Zack et al. (2002) found that the self-reported tendency to drink in negative moods predicted better explicit recall of alcohol targets when they were cued by negative affect (vs. neutral) words.

In two additional studies, Zack and colleagues examined how implicit alcohol cognitions vary as a function of CM-type motives for drinking and mood cues. In the Zack et al. (2003) study described above, the main effect was qualified by a significant interaction for female participants. Only those women who did (vs. did not) report a tendency to drink in bad moods showed the negative-mood-phrase priming of alcohol concepts. It is not clear why only the main effect, and not the interaction, was significant for men. In another study, Zack et al. (1999) used a lexical decision task in which a series of word-word and word-nonword, prime-target trials were presented, and participants categorized targets as words or nonwords. Prime words were negative affect (e.g., HOPELESS) versus neutral (CHIMNEY) words, whereas targets were alcohol-related (BEER), neutral (SHIRT), and nonwords (e.g., SLORE). Participants who reported a bias to drink in negative (vs. positive) mood states showed greater priming of alcohol concepts by negative affect (vs. neutral) words.

Thus, negative mood cues trigger both explicit (Cooney et al., 1997; Zack et al., 2002) and implicit (Zack et al., 1999, 2003) alcohol cognitions only among individuals who are at least very similar to CM (and not EM) drinkers (using Cooper's, 1994, terminology). There have been five experiments conducted to date, of which we are aware, that examined how drinking motives, as measured specifically by the DMQ-R (Cooper, 1994), influence the relationship between both positive and negative mood cues and alcohol cognition.

Birch et al. (2004) examined the effects of mood on explicit AE's. Undergraduates with extreme screening scores on either the EM or CM subscale of the DMQ-R were randomly assigned to either a positive or negative MMIP. The self-reported strength of AE's for emotional reward and relief was measured with a questionnaire before and after MMIP. As predicted, the strength of reward AE's only increased significantly from baseline for EM (and not CM) drinkers in the positive mood group, whereas the strength of relief AE's only increased significantly from baseline for CM (and not EM) drinkers in the negative mood group. These symmetrical and selective mood-AE priming effects provide clear evidence of theoretically predictable drinking motive specificity in the mood triggers for alcohol cognitions.

As mentioned above, Goldstein et al. (2004) found a main effect for positive and neutral (but not negative) affect in predicting the memory-accessibility of AE's that are likely explicit (and not implicit) in nature. Contrary to Birch et al. (2004), however, they did not find that EM or CM moderated the relationship between mood and AE's. Goldstein et al. performed a median split on drinking motives scores to identify groups relatively high and low in EM and CM, rather than specifically selecting participants with extreme drinking motives (cf. Birch et al., 2004). It is possible that motives exert a reliable moderating influence only when they are extreme.

Only three studies have investigated if drinking motives, as measured specifically by the DMQ-R (Cooper, 1994), moderate relations between mood cues and implicit alcohol cognition. Stewart et al. (2002) preselected participants with extreme EM or CM scores. The mood cues were neutral, positive, and negative prime words, presented during a primed Stroop computer task, just prior to alcohol, or nonalcohol, target words. Alcohol cognitions were considered activated when participants had longer color-naming latencies for alcohol versus nonalcohol targets. Consistent with the mood-specific priming hypothesis, positive (but not negative) affect primes activated alcohol cognitions for EM drinkers, and negative affect (but not neutral) primes activated alcohol cognitions for CM drinkers. Unexpectedly, however, neutral primes also activated alcohol cognitions for EM drinkers, and positive affect primes also activated alcohol cognitions for CM drinkers. It is unclear why these unexpected findings were obtained. As well, this study is similar to the Zack et al. studies (1999, 2003) in that the effects of mood cues on state affect were not assessed, and hence results do not address whether drinking motives moderate relations between actual mood states and implicit alcohol-related cognition.

Two experiments were conducted (Birch et al., 2005) to address interpretive limitations of previous experiments on affect, drinking motives, and implicit alcohol cognitions. Both experiments employed MMIP and preselected participants according to their status as EM or CM drinkers. The first experiment involved the administration of a computerized Stroop task. Participants were randomly assigned to either a positive or negative MMIP. Implicit alcohol-related cognitive processing on the Stroop task was indexed as a slower RT to color-name alcohol versus clothing (control) targets. Consistent with hypotheses, EM (and not CM) drinkers in the positive (but not negative) mood condition had slower RTs to color-name alcohol (vs. clothing) targets after the MMIP. Inconsistent with hypotheses, however, there was no evidence that CM (vs. EM) drinkers in the negative mood condition displayed interference for alcohol versus clothing targets after the MMIP. Variability in the results could be due to the fact that the congruency effect among motives and the cue-induced activation of alcohol concepts has not been fully defined. The relative importance of group effects (EM vs. CM), prime effects (positive vs. negative affect), and target effects (alcohol vs. nonalcohol) has not been established.

In the second experiment (Birch et al., 2005), the effects of mood and motives on implicit AE's for emotional reward and relief were measured with a modified version of a sophisticated computerized RT task called the Extrinsic Affective Simon Task (EAST; De Houwer, 2003). The EAST compares the strength of association between various attribute-target pairs. Stronger associations are indexed by a relatively faster RT to associate a specific attribute-target pair. For this study, the attribute concepts were reward (e.g., EXCITED) and relief (CONSOLED) AE words that always appeared in white lettering and were always categorized explicitly, according to semantic meaning. The targets were alcohol (e.g., BEER) and nonalcohol (e.g., SODA) beverage words that always appeared in color (blue or green) and were categorized implicitly, according to color. Consistent with hypotheses, following the positive MMIP, EM (and not CM) drinkers were faster to make reward-alcohol, than relief-alcohol, associations. This effect appeared to be due to the tendency to associate reward (vs. relief) AE's specifically with alcohol

concepts, and not with beverage concepts in general, because (as hypothesized) there were no mood or motive group differences in the speed to associate reward-nonalcohol versus relief-nonalcohol attribute-target pairs. Inconsistent with hypotheses, however, CM drinkers in the negative mood group were not faster to make relief-alcohol, than reward-alcohol, associations. Thus, findings from these two experiments are consistent in suggesting that positive mood states trigger implicit alcohol cognitions for EM (and not CM) drinkers. They cast doubt, however, on the suggestion that negative mood states trigger implicit alcohol cognitions for CM drinkers.

Overall positive moods seem to reliably trigger both cognitions that could be considered explicit and implicit among EM drinkers, but negative moods only reliably trigger explicit, and not implicit, alcohol cognitions among CM drinkers (see Figure 18.1 for a schematic summary of these results). Our finding that negative mood only reliably triggers explicit, and not implicit, alcohol cognitions among CM drinkers could be accurate, or a function of our unique methods or undergraduate sample. Alternatively, social learning may have augmented the effects of positive cues for EM drinkers but attenuated the effects of negative cues for CM drinkers because drinking in positive moods is more normative than drinking to cope. Findings for the effects of negative (vs. positive) mood may also be less reliable because the negative MMIP employed, like many negative mood inductions (e.g., Cooney et al., 1997), does not result in higher overall levels of negative versus positive affect. It could also be more difficult to measure a negative mood activation of implicit relief cognition than a positive mood activation of implicit reward cognition (see Wiers et al., Chapter 22). For example, positive mood-drinking relations may be mediated by two bidirectional, implicit associations (feel happy < > alcohol < > feel happier) that are both positive AE's. In contrast, negative mood-drinking relations may be mediated by two different associations: one that reflects a negative, and one a positive, AE (feel sad < > alcohol < > feel less sad). Finally, the role of other moderators, in addition to drinking motives, may need to be specified in order to interpret complex findings and more fully understand relations between affect and alcohol cognition (see Figure 18.1 and discussion below).

SUMMARY AND CONCLUSIONS

In this chapter, we first provided an overview of theories and evidence, accumulated within the past half century, suggesting that mood states have a main or unmoderated influence on drug processing. We concluded that this literature is replete with inconsistency and that research designs were limited to the extent they assumed that mood states would have a uniform impact on the drug-processing of all people. There is an increasing recognition in this area that cognitions and behaviors have multiple determinants, and are best explained by an interactionist state × trait approach (cf. Mischel, 1986). In the second section of this chapter, we reviewed evidence indicating that drinking motives moderate affect-alcohol cognition relations. Despite some limitations and inconsistent findings within this research, there is sufficient evidence to suggest that future research on mood as a determinant of drinking cognition or behavior should assess, or control for, variation introduced by individual differences in drinking motives.

Methodological limitations of this research as a whole mostly stem from the need for improved manipulation and measurement of mood and drinking-motive independent variables. As noted above, there is concern about the efficacy of various mood inductions.

Research in this area should consistently evaluate the efficacy of mood manipulations, as well as variations in mood state that could result from affect-word exposure (e.g., Stewart et al., 2002). The mood-effects of exposure to verbal affective stimuli could be measured using a Velten (1968) mood induction. Prospective research (e.g., Swendsen et al., 2000) would also be useful to examine if different intensities of naturally existing moods have different effects on drug cognition. As well, further research is needed on how drinking motives moderate the effects of qualitatively different positive and negative states (e.g., sad vs. anxious; happy vs. excited).

There is a need for further research that measures substance use (both alcohol and nonalcohol) motives in a consistent manner, to more systematically examine how this important variable moderates relations between affect and drug cognition or behavior. For the measurement of drinking motives, the DMQ-R (Cooper, 1994) provides a more valid and reliable assessment than other tools (cf. MacLean & Lecci, 2000). A methodological concern is that the relevant research to date has neglected to compare how internal (i.e., EM and CM) versus external (e.g., social) drug-use motives moderate the effects of mood on drug cognition or behavior.

It is important to acknowledge that there are several other individual differences, such as level of anxiety-related characteristics, gender, or drug-abuse severity that may moderate the effects of mood on drug processing and drug use (see Figure 18.1). Negative mood, for example, has been found to more reliably trigger alcohol cognition and drinking among individuals with high versus low levels of anxiety-related characteristics (e.g., anxiety sensitivity [AS], psychiatric distress, social anxiety; see, e.g., Cooney et al., 1997; Zack et al., 1999, 2002). There have, however, been contrary findings (e.g., Zack et al., 2003). Findings relating to the possible moderator role of gender and drug-abuse severity have been even more inconsistent, and so their effects may be qualified by other variables, such as drug-use motives or AS. Further research is needed to determine which moderators exert a proximal versus distal influence, as well as the extent to which moderators are correlated and exert an overlapping or additive influence (e.g., AS and CM).

Treatments for substance abuse can be enhanced by well-designed research that identifies important cognitive targets for intervention. Accordingly, there is a need for high-quality research to investigate, in the same study, how both explicit and implicit drug cognitions and behaviors vary as a function of positive and negative affective states, substance-use motives, and other dispositional correlates of substance abuse. There has been scant research in this area investigating implicit cognition. Research on implicit cognition may yield particularly valuable insights, however, because it is less prone to confounds associated with experiments involving explicit self-reports (demand characteristics, biased self-perception, etc.). Further research should also test whether the cognitions measured by various tasks are primarily explicit or implicit (see De Houwer, Chapter 2) Finally, there is clear need for studies that assess both cognition and behavior in the same study to test the hypothesized mediating role of cognition.

If research continues to suggest there are specific mood states and substance-use motives that interact to trigger drug cognitions and behaviors, this knowledge could be applied to improve drug-abuse prevention and intervention programs. Individuals with "risky" EM or CM for substance use could be identified with a screening and given feedback about their drug use motives (cf. Conrod et al., 2000). Training could help them recognize the unique mood triggers that may increase their likelihood of substance misuse, and the cognitive processes through which this might occur. Both the unique explicit (cf. Darkes & Goldman, 1998), and implicit (Wiers et al., 2004), drug-related cognitions that tend to be triggered by specific mood states for these individuals could be directly targeted for reduction. Procedures that enhance self-awareness and detachment from emotional triggers, like mindfulness-based cognitive behavior therapy, can also be applied to control mood-induced, substance-related cognition and behavior (Breslin et al., 2002). Finally, both explicit and implicit measures of substance-related cognitive reactivity to mood cues could be employed to evaluate the efficacy of treatment in changing these underlying cognitive processes (cf. Zack et al., 1997).

REFERENCES

Baker, T. B., Morse, E., & Sherman, J. E. (1987). The motivation to use drugs: A psychobiological analysis of urges. In P. C. Rivers (Ed.), *The Nebraska Symposium on Motivation: Alcohol use and abuse* (pp. 257–323). Lincoln: University of Nebraska Press.

Baker, T. B., Piper, M. E., McCarthy, D. E., Majeskie, M. R., & Fiore, M. C. (2004). Addiction motivation reformulated. *Psychological Review, 111*, 33–51.

Barlow, D. H., Durand, V. M., & Stewart, S. H. (in press). *Abnormal psychology* (1st Canadian ed.). Toronto, ON: Nelson-Thomson.

Birch, C. D., Stewart, S. H., Wall, A. M., McKee, S. A., Eisnor, S. J., & Theakston, J. A. (2004). Mood-induced increases in alcohol expectancy strength in internally motivated drinkers. *Psychology of Addictive Behaviors, 18*, 231–238.

Birch, C. D., Stewart, S. H., Wiers, R. W., Klein, R., & MacLean, A. (2005). *The mood-activation of alcohol expectancies in internally motivated drinkers.* Manuscript in preparation.

Breslin, F. C., Zack, M., & McMain, S. (2002). An information-processing analysis of mindfulness: Implications for relapse prevention in the treatment of substance abuse. *Clinical Psychology: Science and Practice, 9,* 275–312.

Brown, R. A., & Cutter, H. S. G. (1977). Alcohol, customary drinking behavior, and pain. *Journal of Abnormal Psychology, 86,* 179–188.

Childress, A. R., Ehrman, R., McLellan, A. T., MacRae, J., Natale, M., & O'Brien, C. P. (1994). Can induced moods trigger drug-related responses in opiate abuse patients? *Journal of Substance Abuse Treatment, 11,* 17–23.

Conger, J. J. (1956). Alcoholism: Theory, problem and challenge: II. Reinforcement theory and the dynamics of alcoholism. *Quarterly Journal of Studies on Alcohol, 13,* 296–305.

Conrod, P. J., Stewart, S. H., Pihl, R. O., Côté, S., Fontaine, V., & Dongier, M. (2000). Efficacy of brief coping skills interventions that match different personality profiles of female substance abusers. *Psychology of Addictive Behaviors, 14,* 231–242.

Cooney, N. L., Litt, M. D., Morse, P. A., Bauer, L. O., & Gaupp, L. (1997). Alcohol cue reactivity, negative mood reactivity, and relapse in treated alcoholic men. *Journal of Abnormal Psychology, 106,* 243–250.

Cooper, M. L. (1994). Motivations for alcohol use among adolescents: Development and validation of a four-factor model. *Psychological Assessment, 6,* 117–128.

Darkes, J., & Goldman, M. S. (1998). Expectancy challenge and drinking reduction: Process and structure in the alcohol expectancy network. *Experimental & Clinical Psychopharmacology, 6,* 64–76.

De Houwer, J. (2003). The Extrinsic Affective Simon Task. *Experimental Psychology, 50,* 77–85.

Eich, E., & Forgas, J. P. (2003). Mood, cognition and memory. In A. F. Healy & R. W. Proctor (Eds.), *Handbook of psychology* (Vol. 4, pp. 61–83). New York: John Wiley.

Forgas, J. P. (1995). Mood and judgment. *Psychological Bulletin, 117,* 39–66.

Goldman, M. S., Del Boca, F., & Darkes, J. (1999). Alcohol expectancy theory: The application of cognitive neuroscience. In K. E. Leonard & H. T. Blane (Eds.), *Psychological theories of drinking and alcoholism* (2nd ed., pp. 203–246). New York: Guilford.

Goldstein, A. L., Wall, A. M., McKee, S. A., & Hinson, R. E. (2004). Accessibility of alcohol expectancies from memory: Impact of mood and motives in college student drinkers. *Journal of Studies on Alcohol, 65,* 95–104.

Gray, J. A. (1990). Brain systems that mediate both emotion and cognition. *Cognition & Emotion, 4,* 269–288.

Greeley, J., & Oei, T. (1999). Alcohol and tension reduction. In K. E. Leonard & H. T. Blane (Eds.), *Psychological theories of drinking and alcoholism* (2nd ed., pp. 14–53). New York: Guilford.

Hillebrand, J. (2000). New perspectives on the manipulation of opiate urges and the assessment of cognitive effort associated with opiate urges. *Addictive Behaviors, 25,* 139–143.

Hufford, M. R. (2001). An examination of mood effects on positive alcohol expectancies among undergraduate drinkers. *Cognition & Emotion, 15,* 593–613.

Jansma, A., Breteler, M. H., Schippers, G. M., de Jong, C. A. J., & Van der Staak, C. P. F. (2000). No effect of negative mood on the alcohol cue reactivity of in-patient alcoholics. *Addictive Behaviors, 25,* 619–624.

Kozma, A., Stone, S., Stones, M. J., Hannah, T. E., & McNeil, K. (1990). Long- and short-term affective states in happiness. *Social Indicator Research, 22,* 119–138.

MacLean, M. G., & Lecci, L. (2000). A comparison of models of drinking motives in a university sample. *Psychology of Addictive Behaviors, 14,* 83–87.

Maisto, S. A., Carey, K. B., & Bradizza, C. M. (1999). Social learning theory. In K. E. Leonard & H. T. Blane (Eds.), *Psychological theories of drinking and alcoholism* (2nd ed., pp. 328–371). New York: Guilford.

Martin, M. (1990). On the induction of mood. *Clinical Psychology Review, 10,* 669–697.

McKee, S. A., Wall, A. M., Hinson, R. E., Goldstein, A., & Bissonnette, M. (2003). Effects of an implicit mood prime on the accessibility of smoking expectancies in college women. *Psychology of Addictive Behaviors, 17,* 219–225.

Mischel, W. (1986). Introduction to personality (4th ed.). New York: Holt, Rinehart & Winston.

Rubonis, A. V., Colby, S. M., Monti, P. M., Rohsenow, D. J., Gulliver, S. B., & Sirota, A. D. (1994). Alcohol cue reactivity and mood induction in male and female alcoholics. *Journal of Studies on Alcohol, 55,* 487–494.

Sher, K. J. (1987). Stress response dampening. In H. Blane & K. Leonard (Eds.), *Psychological theories of drinking and alcoholism* (pp. 227–271). New York: Guilford.

Sherman, J. E., Zinser, M. C., & Sideroff, S. (1985, August). *Subjective reports of craving, withdrawal sickness and mood.* Paper presented at the American Psychological Association meeting, Los Angeles, CA.

Stein, K. D., Goldman, M. S., & Del Boca, F. K. (2000). The influence of alcohol expectancy priming and mood manipulation on subsequent alcohol consumption. *Journal of Abnormal Psychology, 109,* 106–115.

Stewart, S. H., & Devine, H. (2000). Relations between personality and drinking motives in young adults. *Personality and Individual Differences, 29,* 495–511.

Stewart, S. H., Hall, E., Wilkie, H., & Birch, C. (2002). Affective priming of alcohol schema in coping and enhancement motivated drinkers. *Cognitive Behaviour Therapy, 31,* 68–80.

Swendsen, J. D., Tennen, H., Carney, M. A., Affleck, G., Willard, A., & Hromi, A. (2000). Mood and alcohol consumption: An experience sampling test of the self-medication hypothesis. *Journal of Abnormal Psychology, 109,* 198–204.

Tiffany, S. T. (1990). A cognitive model of drug urges and drug-use behavior: Role of automatic and nonautomatic processes. *Psychological Review, 97,* 147–168.

Tiffany, S. T., & Drobes, D. J. (1990). Imagery and smoking urges: The manipulation of affective content. *Addictive Behaviors, 15,* 531–539.

Velten, E. (1968). A laboratory task for induction of mood states. *Behaviour Research and Therapy, 6,* 473–482.

Verheul, R., van den Brink, W., & Geerlings, P. (1999). A three-way pathway psychobiological model of craving for alcohol. *Alcohol and Alcoholism, 34,* 197–222.

Wiers, R. W., de Jong, P. J., Havermans, R., & Jelicic, M. (2004). How to change implicit drug-related cognitions in prevention: A transdisciplinary integration of findings from experimental psychopathology, social cognition, memory and experimental learning psychology. *Substance Use & Misuse, 39,* 1625–1684.

Wiers, R. W., Stacy, A. W., Ames, S. L., Noll, J. A., Sayette, M. A., Zack, M., et al. (2002). Implicit and explicit alcohol-related cognitions. *Alcoholism: Clinical and Experimental Research, 26,* 129–137.

Willner, P., Field, K., Pitts, K., & Reeve, G. (1998). Mood, cue, and gender influences on motivation, craving, and liking for alcohol in recreational drinkers. *Behavioural Pharmacology, 9,* 631–642.

Zack, M., Poulos, C. X., Fragopulos, F., & MacLeod, C. M. (2003). Effects of negative and positive mood phrases on priming of alcohol words in young drinkers with high and low anxiety sensitivity. *Experimental & Clinical Psychopharmacology, 11,* 176–185.

Zack, M., Toneatto, T., & Calderwood, K. (1997, November). *Automatic alcohol-distress associations decline after cognitive behavioural therapy.* Paper presented at the co-occuring Substance Use and Mental Disorders Conference, Toronto, ON.

Zack, M., Toneatto, T., & MacLeod, C. M. (1999). Implicit activation of alcohol concepts by negative affective cues distinguishes between problem drinkers with high and low psychiatric distress. *Journal of Abnormal Psychology, 108,* 518–531.

Zack, M., Toneatto, T., & MacLeod, C. M. (2002). Anxiety and explicit alcohol-related memory in problem drinkers. *Addictive Behaviors, 27,* 331–343.

CHAPTER 19

Context and Retrieval Effects on Implicit Cognitions for Substance Use

MARVIN D. KRANK AND ANNE-MARIE WALL

Abstract: This chapter reviews context effects on substance use and substance-use associations. We interpret these ubiquitous effects as a natural consequence of memory retrieval processes that influence the accessibility of substance-use associations. Further, accessibility of memories about substance-use outcomes and behaviors potentially mediates substance-use behaviors by determining what behavioral options are considered and what outcomes are anticipated. Context effects may have unconscious influences and impact on implicit memories about substance use. The implicit memory effects of context may be uniquely relevant to developing more effective prevention and intervention approaches by encouraging procedures that reduce or replace the retrieval of substance-use memories that influence behavioral decisions.

Context has its roots in the Latin word, con*textus,* literally meaning to weave together. In psychology, context refers to the tapestry of external or internal events interwoven around a target behavior or cognitive process. Context shapes our experience, is encoded in our memories, and sets the options for our thoughts and actions. In the true sense of its Latin meaning, context is the ubiquitous background integrated with the foreground of our interest. The impact of context is twofold. First, it provides the setting for current thoughts and actions. Second, context wraps our memories in a rich array of detail that is often the means of memory retrieval and the material of meaning. Context is most important when meaning is ambiguous: a word with multiple meanings, a subtle shading of intention, or the choice point in a maze. Context implicitly reduces ambiguity, defines the options, and forces choices. This chapter explores how context influences memories, associations, and expectancies about substance use, with the goal of improving our understanding of the cognitive processes underlying substance-use behavior.

Before reviewing the role of context in substance use, it is useful to distinguish between content and context. In studying memory processes, researchers often focus on a defined content item and measure performance against that item. For example, an individual may read a word and respond with a "free" associate. This may appear to be an isolated task, tapping into the association between two words in memory, but contextual background is always part of the equation: What kinds of words were seen before the current word, are you happy or sad, who is listening? The content is the focus, but it cannot be divorced from its background setting. Moreover, the content is only the arbitrary locus of attention. One could examine the situation from a different angle with a different lens; content defines the question of interest, whereas context provides the interpretive setting. The content focus of the present chapter is substance use, specifically cognitions (expectancies and associations) that predict current and subsequent substance use (Goldman et al., 1999; Krank et al., 2005; Stacy, 1995, 1997).

When applied to substance use, context includes the myriad of social, cognitive, affective, and environmental events that might be associated with substance use. Specific contextual features are not necessarily intrinsic to substance use. Indeed, the context of substance use may be quite idiosyncratic; some smokers never smoke in their car, whereas others smoke immediately when they are behind the wheel. Some people drink when upset; others do not. The result is that context affects substance-use cognitions in two main ways that combine to influence the gist of substance use itself. First, current context provides the setting, the stimulus conditions, and the tone for current behavior. The choices and resources available are largely determined by the individual's current setting (Vuchinich & Tucker, 1988, 1996). Second, context may be an integral part of memory processing (Smith & Vela, 2001) and be encoded as part of memory representation of substance-use cognitions. That is, contextual features will often be processed and encoded with information

about substance use. Indeed, the principle of encoding specificity purports that such contexts will be important to memory retrieval (Tulving & Thomson, 1973). Thus, context influences the retrieval and accessibility of the substance-use content focus. Context can determine when and what content is retrieved from memory. Most important, context assists in defining content. In this second and critical role, memory retrieval is the means for context effects; interpretation of meaning is the outcome.

Careful observation and research indicate that context influences substance use, dependence, and treatment. This should not be surprising as context is a defining feature of psychological and social functions. Context may influence substance use directly in a number of plausible ways, including the availability of drugs and alternative activities, social support systems, and social influence (Maddux & Desmond, 1982; Tucker et al., 2002). Our focus in this chapter, however, is on the second effect of context, the psychological impact of context on memory processing (Smith & Vela, 2001). In short, the evidence that context-dependent memory retrieval modifies the accessibility of both implicit and explicit substance-use associations will be reviewed and it will be argued that this accessibility provides an explanation for many of the effects of context on substance-use behavior and the effectiveness of treatment.

CONTEXT AND MEMORY RETRIEVAL

Many theories of memory are guided by two main principles: encoding specificity (Tulving & Thomson, 1973) and similarity-based retrieval (Hintzman, 1986, 1988; Roediger, 1990). The key notion in encoding specificity is that memory representations comprise specific details about the cognitive elements encoded at the time of learning. Retrieval of these memories involves the partial reinstatement of the cognitive conditions that were present during encoding. The more similar the retrieval conditions, the more likely an individual memory representation will be retrieved. The types of context shown to influence memory retrieval include environmental (Smith & Vela, 2001), social (Von Hecker, 2004), mood (Bower & Forgas, 2001), drug state (Weingartner et al., 1995), and cognitive processing (Roediger, 1990) conditions. Each of these conditions may be associated with substance use and social learning about substance use. Substance use often occurs in unique physical settings (bars) and social occasions (with friends, at a party), in emotional or mood states (sad, angry, or celebrating), unique drug states, or with a specific cognitive set or expectations. In each case, the context may not only modify the experience of substance use, but also may be encoded in the memory representation.

From a memory perspective, the main impact of context on content is determining when and what is retrieved from memory. If contextual features form part of the substance-use memory representation, then they will influence the retrieval of substance-use cognitions. Models of encoding specificity and similarity-based retrieval are important to understanding addictive behavior because they predict the accessibility of associative memories relevant to substance use. Such accessibility may be critical to when and what we think about substance use. Critically, such memory retrieval provides the mechanism for interpreting meaning and reducing ambiguity. The interpretation arises from the retrieval of specific substance-use memory associations. Our contention is that the accessibility of particular substance-use and competing associations defines the context and influences substance-use choice behavior.

We propose that retrieval factors such as context determine when and which behavioral

associations are accessed and that this in turn determines behavioral choice. Specifically, retrieval of positive substance-use associations would increase the likelihood of choosing substance-use behaviors. Conditions that reduce such retrieval or enhance the retrieval of negative associations or positive associations with alternative behaviors would reduce the selection of substance-use behaviors (for a discussion of substance use and behavioral choice, see Krank & Goldstein, Chapter 28). In direct support of cognitive mediation of substance use, Palfai et al. (2000) used reaction time as an indicator of positive alcohol outcome expectancy accessibility and demonstrated that accessibility mediated college students' consumption levels on a taste-rating task. Although many studies have shown context effects on substance use, only a few studies have shown that context influences substance-use cognitions and these cognitions mediate higher levels of consumption (see Krank et al., 2005, for one recent example).

Implicit Cognition and Context

Before reviewing the evidence for context effects on substance use and substance-use cognitions, it is worth considering how context effects relate to implicit memory. We have not restricted our review of data supporting context effects to studies that meet stringent criteria for implicit memory because our goal here is to demonstrate the range of context affects on memory accessibility and substance use. Some of the studies reviewed measured context effects on implicit measures, others measures effects on more explicit measures such as outcome expectancies. The studies of implicit measures are obviously relevant to implicit cognition. Certain context manipulations such as mood induction are also likely to be implicit. These observations indicate that context and retrieval effects are relevant to implicit memory. Given the powerful nature of context effects and the unique contribution of implicit memory associations to understanding substance use, our hope is that the studies reviewed here will set the stage for research delimiting (1) the range of context effects on implicit memories for substance-use associations, and (2) the extent that these effects represent unconscious influences.

CONTEXT AND SUBSTANCE ABUSE

Evidence showing the effects of environmental context on substance use and relapse to substance use comes from both animal and human experimental studies, as well as natural studies of spontaneous remission of substance use. In animal research, environmental contexts associated with drugs elicit conditioned responses that increase incentive or drug-seeking behaviors, elicit withdrawal symptoms and, most important, increase the likelihood of drug-taking behavior (Berridge & Robinson, 1995; Krank, 1989; Krank & O'Neill, 2002; Krank & Wall, 1990; Siegel, 1999; Stewart et al., 1984; see Crombag & Robinson, 2004, and Krank, 2003, for recent summaries). The conditioning approach has also been applied extensively in human cue-reactivity research revealing a variety of physiological and motivational effects of drug-associated cues, such as the taste, smell, or physical features of alcoholic beverages, or contexts, such as simulated bars (Niaura et al., 1988).

Siegel (1999) reviewed several lines of evidence of environmental context effects on addictive behavior. Perhaps the most dramatic example is the Vietnam experiment. The number of U.S. soldiers stationed in Vietnam that used heroin was so great that concerns were raised about how to deal with addiction on their return home. Although Vietnam veterans suffered many problems on their return, heroin addiction did not materialize at the feared level. Siegel (1999) argues that this is because the change in context reduced the effect of past learning. Maddux and Desmond (1982) followed 248 opiate addicts for 20 years, also demonstrating the role of context in remission form addiction to heroin. Physical relocation supported levels of abstinence three times greater than treatment or correctional interactions. Moreover, 81 percent of abstinent individuals relapsed within 1 month of return to the location of past drug use. Tucker and her colleagues (2002) also argue that environmental context, defined by the mix of positive and negative life events, influences the success of spontaneous abstinence and interacts with intervention success. Finally, Marlatt and Gordon (1985) describe a number of high-risk situations for relapse to substance use following a period of abstinence. Emotional contexts including both negative and positive affective states were among the most frequent relapse triggers. The general importance of situational antecedents has been documented by Turner et al. (1997).

Distinctive contexts may be associated with substance use and abstinence success for several reasons. Some of the effects of context include the attainability of drugs and alcohol, options for alternative activities and reinforcers, and social expectations such as peer influence. From a cognitive processing perspective, context may also selectively retrieve or activate past associations related to substance use. In the present discussion, Pavlovian conditioning can be viewed as a special case of retrieval effects where the condition stimulus (e.g., environmental context) is a retrieval cue for memory of the unconditioned stimulus (see Rescorla, 1988). Conditioning is a special case of memory retrieval as its effects are measured in changes in behavior and physiology. Memory retrieval, however, provides a broader umbrella for context effects that extends to substance-use associations, in general, and implicit cognitions, in particular. Context-based memory retrieval processes will be particularly important to addiction under the following conditions: (1) Context is processed with and influences the retrieval of substance-use cognitions and (2) retrieval of substance-use cognitions influences behavioral choice. The next section describes initial evidence for the first condition that context does influence the retrieval of substance-use cognitions. The second condition remains more speculative, but deserves attention given the growing linkage between substance use and cognitive measures of substance-use associations and expectancies.

CONTEXT EFFECTS ON SUBSTANCE-USE COGNITIONS

The range of context variables that affect substance-use associations parallels the range of retrieval conditions studied in cognitive studies of context effects on memory. Most of the available studies have used alcohol as the target, but a few have also considered marijuana use and smoking. With respect to alcohol, physical and socially defined locations, induced mood, and cognitive processing manipulations modify the accessibility of outcome expectancies and implicit memories of alcohol associations (Krank et al., 2005). Generally, context enhances the accessibility of alcohol- and drug-related associations. To date, however, this line of inquiry is in its infancy. Of the limited work that has been done, evidence in support of memory-based explanations of substance use has been found.

Social and Physical Context Determinants

Cognitions regarding alcohol vary when individuals are either categorized according to where and with whom they usually drink (Brown, 1985; Sher, 1985) or when they are presented with vignettes that vary along social and physical dimensions of drinking (Levine & Goldman, 1989; MacLatchy-Gaudet & Stewart, 2001). Employing an unrelated studies paradigm, Roehrich and Goldman (1995) found that undergraduate women undergoing implicit priming of alcohol-related cues (i.e., videotaped bar setting and alcohol expectancy word primes) consumed more placebo beer, in comparison to their female counterparts who were presented with control primes. Using similar methodology, Stein et al. (2000) found that male undergraduates consumed significantly more alcoholic beer when they were exposed to alcohol expectancy word primes. Consistent with current learning and memory-based conceptualizations of alcohol outcome expectancies, this priming effect was greatest among undergraduates with heavy, as opposed to light, drinking histories.

In one of the first investigations involving exposure to environmental cues associated with alcohol use, Fromme and Dunn (1992) found no evidence to support the effect of context on explicit measures of alcohol-related cognitions. More recent research suggests, however, that when individuals are exposed to naturalistic barroom cues, they endorse more positive cognitions in a laboratory context, and they tend to evaluate alcohol-related outcomes more positively in this naturalistic drinking environment (Wall et al., 2000). Alcohol-related cognitions are also more readily accessed from memory in the presence of naturalistic barroom cues (Wall et al., 2001). In keeping with our conceptualization of context, retrieval, and drinking behavior, the ease with which alcohol-related cognitions are accessed mediates higher consumption patterns in naturalistic bar settings (Krank et al., 2005). This effect is moderated by gender and drinking history and requires further study.

Affective Influences

With respect to both alcohol- and smoking-related cognitions, individuals' affective states serve as a context that influences the retrieval of specific expectations. Using a musical induction procedure, Goldstein et al. (2004) found that the accessibility of specific cognitions about alcohol varied as a function of mood state with positive mood inductions leading to greater accessibility. Using similar methodology, Birch et al. (in press) report similar results; however, unlike Goldstein et al., these investigators demonstrated that the effect of affective context on the retrieval of alcohol-related cognitions was moderated by individual differences in drinking motives. They classified drinkers into enhancement-motivated, drinking to enhance positive outcomes, and coping-motivated, drinking to reduce negative affect. Positive inductions increased retrieval of implicit alcohol related cognitions in enhancement-motivated drinkers and, somewhat surprisingly, in coping-motivated drinkers. As expected, negative mood induction increased implicit memory accessibility only in coping-motivated drinkers. Among women, the accessibility of specific beliefs about the positive effects of smoking are increased as a function of positive mood state induction (McKee, et al., in press).

Cognitive Procedures That Prime or Bias Memory Processing

Cognitive manipulation of retrieval factors can be accomplished by several methods. For example, written vignettes can be used to describe settings either associated with substance use or not. Such vignettes can be presented in advance of a measure as an unrelated task to effectively enhance the accessibility of alcohol-outcome expectancies (Levine & Goldman, 1989; MacLatchy-Gaudet & Stewart, 2001). Similarly, verbal or imagined situational contexts associated with alcohol use increase the accessibility of alcohol associations (Stacy et al., 1994). As Schwarz and Sudman (1994) have argued convincingly for survey research methods, engaging in one kind of cognitive task sets the context and biases memory for subsequent tasks. For example, Krank and Johnson (1999) asked adolescents to complete a survey that included implicit measures of alcohol associations and explicit outcome expectancies. They prefaced this survey with a brainstorming task designed to bias autobiographical memories about alcohol effects by listing either the positive or negative effects of alcohol on themselves or others. They found that biasing toward self-referent negative events increased the endorsement of negative outcome expectancies. Although positive expectancies were not affected, implicit alcohol responses to outcome associates or ambiguous words were more likely following biasing toward positive alcohol events.

Vignettes can also be used to set the context more explicitly by framing the question itself. We asked college students a series of open-ended alcohol-outcome expectancy questions, where each question was immediately preceded by a scenario that varied in its association with alcohol: low, medium, or high. The low associates were situations that would not normally be associated with alcohol (e.g., studying for a test), the medium associates were situations where some students would drink (on a date), and the high associates were situations where many students would drink (at a party with friends). In addition to listing three or four expected effects of a moderate amount of alcohol, the students were asked to indicate whether they would like or not like the effect. Our primary dependent variable was the alcohol outcome likability score. This score represents the number of responses endorsed as like outcomes (range 0 to 4).

Figure 19.1 shows the mean alcohol outcome likability score as a function of the alcohol-associated context of the question. In addition, the students were divided into two groups, heavier and lighter drinkers, based on a median split. As the degree of alcohol association increased, the expectancy liking score also increased. Not surprisingly, heavier drinkers had higher liking scores than lighter drinkers. Heavier drinkers, however, were more affected by the context manipulation with a steeper slope of change than lighter drinkers.

The differential effect of vignette association on this measure of outcome expectancy is important for two reasons. First, it supports the retrieval interpretation of context effects. Retrieval manipulations should only be effective if the memory is present. Consistent with this view, expectancy liking scores increase more with alcohol associations in drinkers who generally hold stronger positive outcome expectancies. Second, the results suggest a practical implication: Alcohol-context effects should improve the predictive value of alcohol cognitions. That is, assuming that alcohol cognitions predict future alcohol use (Krank et al., 2003, 2005; Stacy, 1997), then to the extent that context supports better retrieval of preexisting alcohol associations, the better these measures should predict current and future drinking behavior. In a recent symposium, we presented data from a longitudinal study of adolescents showing precisely this effect (Krank et al., 2005). Using a variation on cognitive biasing, we measured implicit memory associations (behavioral associate or ambiguous word associates) either before or after questions about alcohol and drug use. We found that the context manipulation increased the number of alcohol associations produced. In addition, both implicit measures predicted alcohol use over and above demographic variables not only on the immediate survey (concurrently) but

also when tested a year later (prospectively). Directly relevant to the present argument, both the concurrent and prospective predictive powers of the implicit measures were improved by obtaining the measure after setting an alcohol context.

Media Effects

Observation of substance use in the popular media provides both a vicarious learning experience and another potential source of context effects. Settings involving alcoholic beverages are common in television advertisements. References to drinking, smoking, and illicit drug use are also common in movies and music. Media portray more frequent and more positive alcohol use than is true in real life (Grube, 1993; McIntosh et al., 1999), and exposure to such media portrayals is a significant risk for substance use (Villani, 2001). Analyzing natural exposure patterns, Stacy and colleagues (2004) provide evidence that cognitive changes predictive of substance use in youth are influenced by the messages in popular media (see also Fleming et al., 2004). Consistent with a context analysis where alcohol advertisements are viewed as retrieval cues, experimental studies are also beginning to demonstrate that advertising can have a direct effect on the accessibility of alcohol-related cognitions. Dunn and Yniguez (1999) have reported evidence showing that exposure to alcohol advertisements increases positive outcome expectancies in fourth- and fifth-grade students. In addition, Krank and Kreklewetz (2003) found that exposure to alcohol advertisements in grades six and ten students increased alcohol responses on both the behavioral associate and ambiguous word associate tasks. Moreover, consistent with the pattern shown in Figure 19.1, only drinkers were affected by the exposure. This finding also supports a retrieval interpretation of advertising priming effects.

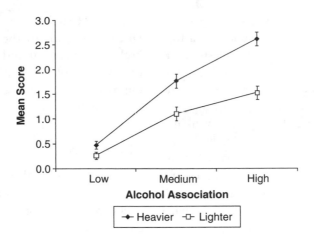

Figure 19.1 Alcohol outcome likability. The figure shows the effect of question-framing context as a function of alcohol association and a median split of heavier and lighter college student drinkers. The dependent measure is the alcohol outcome likability score, which represents the number of responses endorsed as like outcomes (range 0 to 4). The data were obtained from a sample of 116 university students. The data were analyzed by a two-way mixed design on three levels of the within-subject factor (alcohol association) and two levels of the between-subject factor (drinking level). Consistent with other cognitive measures of alcohol associations, drinking level had significant effects with heavier drinkers revealing higher alcohol-outcome likability scores than lighter drinkers, $F(1, 110) = 26.8$, $p < .001$. In addition, the effect of alcohol association was highly significant, $F(2, 220) = 243.7$, $p < .001$, demonstrating a context effect. Finally, as predicted, the interaction effect was also significant, $F(2, 220) = 20.9$, $p < .001$, with heavier drinkers increasing likability scores more than lighter drinkers as the question context had a greater association with drinking. See text for theoretical discussion.

In summary, a variety of contextual manipulations influence the accessibility of alcohol cognitions. These manipulations run the gamut of variables used to demonstrate context effects on memory retrieval. In addition, context selectively enhances alcohol associations in heavier drinkers. Given that evidence shows that heavier drinkers have more underlying alcohol-memory associations, this finding also supports a retrieval interpretation. Finally, contextual enhancement of alcohol associations improves their predictive value. This outcome is a natural consequence of retrieval-based enhancement with potential applications to prevention and treatment of substance abuse.

Implications for Substance Abuse Intervention

In our review of context effects on substance use, we present evidence that substance-use context is associated with greater relapse to substance use. Although there are several plausible sources for these effects, our analysis of context effects on substance-use cognitions suggests that memory retrieval is one outcome that bears attention. As there is a strong predictive link between substance-use associations and substance use and a strong theoretical link to incentive motivation and behavioral choice theory (see Krank & Goldstein, Chapter 28), these observations indicate that context-induced accessibility of substance-use cognitions, especially implicit cognitions, is a risk factor for initiating an episode of substance use. Context variables, therefore, should be front and center in identifying high-risk situations both for prevention of and treatment for substance abuse. This observation also suggests that effective interventions should target drug-associated contexts to assist the user to prepare for or replace memory retrieval of these risky associations. This approach would be similar to expectancy challenge studies that explicitly target alcohol-related cognitions within a drinking-related environment (e.g., see Darkes & Goldman, 1993, 1998; Dunn et al., 2000; Jones et al., 2001; Wiers et al., 2003). Implicit memory measures may also be used diagnostically to target the level and nature of intervention used (Krank & Goldstein, Chapter 28). In this capacity, context may be a stimulant to more effective memory retrieval analogous to a more powerful diagnostic microscope. Finally, understanding the role of memory-retrieval processes in substance use may lead to more effective interventions employing cognitive processes to support alternative memories and behavioral choices.

Future Directions

The future directions pointed to by this chapter are guided by the assumption that the expression of addictive behavior is largely mediated by enduring cognitive representations. This cognitive expression must be viewed as part of an overall complex of biological and environmental risk factors (Goldman, 2002). Genetic, personality, and social factors are all important to determining the relative risk of acquiring an addictive pattern of behavior toward any given substance, but the learned associations and expectancies stored in memory lay down the paths that guide future behavior. Context is one of many variables that may influence the selection of a particular path. Context is a common form of retrieval cue for selecting which memory representations are active and when. The result is that the path ahead is lighted and the choice becomes clear. Unfortunately, in addiction the maladaptive and self-destructive paths become all too clear and well-worn. The choices not taken become obscure and unseen. Fully appreciating the potential role of cognitive processing in general, and retrieval in particular, should reveal alternative and more adaptive paths and create new avenues of escape from the ruts of addiction.

REFERENCES

Berridge, K. C., & Robinson, T. E. (1995). The mind of an addicted brain: Neural sensitization of wanting versus liking. *Current Directions in Psychological Science, 4,* 71–76.

Birch, C. D., Stewart, S. H., Wall, A.-M., McKee, S. A., Eisoner, S. J., & Theakston, J. A. (in press). The mood-induced activation of alcohol expectancies in internally motivated drinkers. *Psychology of Addictive Behaviors.*

Bower, G. H., & Forgas, J. P. (2001). Mood and social memory. In J. P. Forgas (Ed.), *Handbook of affect and social cognition* (pp. 95–120). Mahwah, NJ: Lawrence Erlbaum.

Brown, S. A. (1985). Context of drinking and reinforcement from alcohol: Alcoholic patterns. *Addictive Behaviors, 10,* 191–196.

Crombag, H. S., & Robinson, T. E. (2004). Drugs, environment, brain, and behavior. *Current Directions in Psychological Science, 13*(3), 107–111.

Darkes, J., & Goldman, M. S. (1993). Expectancy challenge and drinking reduction: Experimental evidence for a mediational process. *Journal of Consulting and Clinical Psychology, 61,* 344–353.

Darkes, J., & Goldman, M. S. (1998). Expectancy challenge and drinking reduction: Process and structure in the alcohol expectancy network. *Experimental & Clinical Psychopharmacology, 6,* 64–76.

Dunn, M. E., Lau, C. H., & Cruz, I. Y. (2000). Changes in activation of alcohol expectancies in memory in relation to changes in alcohol use after participation in an expectancy challenge program. *Experimental & Clinical Psychopharmacology, 8,* 566–575.

Dunn, M. E., & Yniguez, R. M. (1999). Experimental demonstration of the influence of alcohol advertising on the activation of alcohol expectancies in memory among fourth- and fifth-grade children. *Experimental & Clinical Psychopharmacology, 7,* 473–483.

Fleming, K., Thorson, E., & Atkin, C. K. (2004). Alcohol advertising exposure and perceptions: Links with alcohol expectancies and intentions to drink or drinking in underaged youth and young adults. *Journal of Health Communication, 9*(1), 3–29.

Fromme, K., & Dunn, M. E. (1992). Alcohol expectancies, social and environmental cues as determinants of drinking and perceived reinforcement. *Addictive Behaviors, 17,* 167–177.

Goldman, M. S. (2002). Expectancy and risk for alcoholism: The unfortunate exploitation of a fundamental characteristic of neurobehavioral adaptation. *Alcoholism: Clinical and Experimental Research, 26,* 737–746.

Goldman, M. S., Del Boca, F. K., & Darkes, J. (1999). Alcohol expectancy theory: The application of cognitive neuroscience. In K. E. Leonard & H. T. Blane (Eds.), *Psychological theories of drinking and alcoholism* (2nd ed., pp. 233–262). New York: Guilford.

Goldstein, A. L., Wall, A.-M., McKee, S. A., & Hinson, R. E. (2004). Accessibility of alcohol expectancies from memory: Impact of mood and motives in college student drinkers. *Journal of Studies on Alcohol, 65,* 95–104.

Grube, J. W. (1993). Alcohol portrayals and alcohol advertising on television: Content and effects on children and adolescents. *Alcohol Health & Research World, 17*(1), 54–60.

Hintzman, D. L. (1986). "Schema abstraction" in a multiple-trace memory model. *Psychological Review, 93,* 411–428.

Hintzman, D. L. (1988). Judgments of frequency and recognition memory in a multiple-trace memory model. *Psychological Review, 95,* 528–551.

Jones, B. T., Corbin, W., & Fromme, K. (2001). A review of expectancy theory and alcohol consumption. *Addiction, 96,* 57–72.

Krank, M. D. (1989). Environmental signals for ethanol enhance free-choice ethanol consumption. *Behavioral Neuroscience, 103*(2), 365–372.

Krank, M. D. (2003). Pavlovian conditioning with ethanol: Sign-tracking (autoshaping), conditioned incentive, and ethanol self-administration. *Alcoholism: Clinical and Experimental Research, 27*(10), 1592–1598.

Krank, M. D., & Johnson, T. (1999). Retrieval and implicit memory for alcohol associations. *Alcoholism: Clinical and Experimental Research, 23*(5), 187A. Presented at the annual meeting of the Research Society on Alcoholism, Santa Barbara, CA.

Krank, M. D. & Kreklewetz, K. L. (2003). Exposure to alcohol advertising increases implicit alcohol cognitions in adolescents. *Alcoholism: Clinical and Experimental Research, 27*(5), 135A. Presented at the annual meeting of the Research Society on Alcoholism, Fort Lauderdale, FL.

Krank, M. D., & O'Neill, S. O. (2002). Environmental context conditioning with ethanol reduces the aversive effects of ethanol in the acquisition of self-administration in rats. *Psychopharmacology, 159,* 258–265.

Krank, M. D., & Wall, A.-M. (1990). Cue exposure during a period of abstinence reduces the resumption of operant behaviour for oral ethanol reinforcement. *Behavioral Neuroscience, 104,* 725–733.

Krank, M. D., Wall, A.-M., Lai, D., Wekerle, C., & Johnson, T. (2003). Implicit and explicit cognitions predict alcohol use, abuse and intentions in young adolescents. *Alcoholism: Clinical and Experimental Research, 27*(5), 135A. Presented at the annual meeting of the Research Society on Alcoholism, Fort Lauderdale, FL.

Krank, M. D., Wall, A.-M., Stewart, S. H., Wiers, R.W., & Goldman, M. S. (2005). Context effects on alcohol cognitions. *Alcoholism: Clinical and Experimental Research, 29,* 196–206.

Levine, B., & Goldman, M. S. (1989). Situational variations in expectancies. Paper presented at the 97th annual convention of the American Psychological Association, New Orleans, LA.

MacLatchy-Gaudet, H. A., & Stewart, S. H. (2001). Context-specific positive alcohol outcome expectancies of university women. *Addictive Behaviors, 26,* 31–49.

Maddux, J. F., & Desmond, D. P. (1982) Residence relocation inhibits opioid dependence. *Archives of General Psychiatry, 39*(11), 1313–1317.

Marlatt, G. A., & Gordon, J. R. (1985). *Relapse prevention.* New York: Guildford.

McIntosh, W. D., Smith, S. M., & Bazzini, D. G. (1999) Alcohol in the movies: Characteristics of drinkers and nondrinkers in films from 1940 to 1989. *Journal of Applied Social Psychology, 29*(6), 1191–1199.

McKee, S. A., Wall, A.-M., Hinson, R. E., Goldstein, A., & Bissonnette, M. (in press). Effects of an implicit mood prime on the accessibility of smoking expectancies. *Psychology of Addictive Behaviors.*

Niaura, R. S., Rohsenow, D. J., Binkoff, J. A., Monti, P. M., Pedraza, M., & Abrams, D. B. (1988). The relevance of cue reactivity to understanding alcohol and smoking relapse. *Journal of Abnormal Psychology, 97,* 133–152.

Palfai, T. P., Monti, P. M., Ostafin, B., & Hutchison, K. (2000). Effects of nicotine deprivation on alcohol-related information processing and drinking behavior. *Journal of Abnormal Psychology, 109,* 96–105.

Rescorla, R. A. (1988). Pavlovian conditioning: It's not what you think it is. *American Psychologist, 43,* 151–160.

Roediger, H. L. (1990). Implicit memory: Retention without remembering. *American Psychologist, 45,* 1043–1056.

Roehrich, L., & Goldman, M. S. (1995). Implicit priming of alcohol expectancy memory processes and subsequent drinking behavior. *Experimental & Clinical Psychopharmacology, 3,* 402–410.

Schwarz, N., & Sudman, S. (1994). *Autobiographical memory and the validity of retrospective reports.* New York: Springer-Verlag.

Sher, K. J. (1985). Subjective effects of alcohol: The influence of setting and individual differences in alcohol expectancies. *Journal of Studies on Alcohol, 46*(2), 137–146.

Siegel, S. (1999). Drug anticipation and drug addiction. *Addiction, 94,* 1113–1124.

Smith, S. M., & Vela, E. (2001). Environmental context-dependent memory: A review and meta-analysis. *Psychonomic Bulletin & Review, 8*(2), 203–220.

Stacy, A. W. (1995). Memory association and ambiguous cues in models of alcohol and marijuana use. *Experimental & Clinical Psychopharmacology, 3,* 183–194.

Stacy, A. W. (1997). Memory activation and expectancy as prospective predictors of alcohol and marijuana use. *Journal of Abnormal Psychology, 106,* 61–73.

Stacy, A. W., Leigh, B. C., & Weingardt, K. (1994). Memory accessibility and association of alcohol use and its positive outcomes. *Experimental & Clinical Psychopharmacology, 2,* 1–14.

Stacy, A.W., Pearce, S. G., Zogg, J. B., Unger, J., & Dent, C. W. (2004). A non-verbal test of naturalistic memory for alcohol commercials. *Psychology & Marketing, 21*(4), 295–322.

Stein, K. D., Goldman, M. S., & Del Boca, F. K. (2000). The influence of alcohol expectancy priming and mood manipulation on subsequent alcohol consumption. *Journal of Abnormal Psychology, 109,* 106–115.

Stewart, J., de Wit, H., & Eikelboom, R. (1984). Role of unconditioned and conditioned drug effects in the self-administration of opiates and stimulants. *Psychological Review, 91,* 251–268.

Tucker, J. A., Vuchinich, R. E., & Rippens, P. D. (2002). Environmental contexts surrounding resolution of drinking problems among problem drinkers with different help-seeking experiences. *Journal of Studies on Alcohol, 63,* 334–341.

Tulving, E., & Thomson, D. M. (1973). Encoding specificity and retrieval processes in episodic memory. *Psychological Review, 80*(5), 359–380.

Turner, N. E., Annis, H. M., & Sklar, S. M. (1997). Measurement of antecedents to drug and alcohol use: Psychometric properties of the Inventory of Drug-Taking Situations (IDTS). *Behaviour Research and Therapy, 35*(5), 465–483.

Villani, S. (2001). Impact of media on children and adolescents: A 10-year review of the research. *Journal of the American Academy of Child & Adolescent Psychiatry, 40,* 392–401.

Von Hecker, U. (2004). Disambiguating a mental model: Influence of social context. *Psychological Record, 54*(1), 27–43.

Vuchinich, R. E., & Tucker, J. A. (1988). Contributions from behavioural theories of choice to an analysis of alcohol abuse. *Journal of Abnormal Psychology, 97,* 181–195.

Vuchinich, R. E., & Tucker, J. A. (1996). The molar context of alcohol abuse. In L. Green & J. H. Kagel (Eds.), *Advances in behavioural economics: Vol. 3. Substance use and abuse* (pp. 133–162). Norwood, NJ: Ablex Publishing

Wall, A.-M., McKee, S. A., & Hinson, R. E. (2000). Assessing variation in alcohol outcome expectancies across environmental contexts: An examination of the situational-specificity hypothesis. *Psychology of Addictive Behaviors, 14,* 367–375.

Wall, A.-M., McKee, S. A., Hinson, R. E., & Goldstein, A. (2001). Examining alcohol outcome expectancies in laboratory and naturalistic bar settings: A within-subject analysis. *Psychology of Addictive Behaviors, 15,* 219–226.

Weingartner, H. J., Putnam, F., & George, D. T. (1995). Drug state-dependent autobiographical knowledge. *Experimental & Clinical Psychopharmacology, 3*(3), 304–307.

Wiers, R. W., Wood, M. D., Darkes, J., Corbin, W. R., Jones, B. T., & Sher, K. J. (2003). Changing expectancies: Cognitive mechanisms and context effects. *Alcoholism: Clinical and Experimental Research, 27,* 186–197.

CHAPTER 20

Acute Effects of Alcohol and Other Drugs on Automatic and Intentional Control

MARK T. FILLMORE AND MURIEL VOGEL-SPROTT

Abstract: Research in substance abuse has witnessed increased application of cognitive theories and methodologies and there is growing interest in the role of automatic (i.e., implicit) processes. This chapter explains how process-dissociation models distinguish between automatic and controlled processes and considers how drugs alter the degree to which behavior is influenced by automatic processes. The chapter reviews findings from studies that used process-dissociation models to examine acute effects of alcohol, and other drugs. It is argued that the ability of drugs to promote a reliance on automatic influences could explain a broad range of behavioral effects observed in the drugged state, and provide new insights into factors that contribute to drug-taking and drug abuse.

INTRODUCTION

A central puzzle in drug addiction, such as alcoholism, is the seeming inability to refrain from taking a drink, or halting consumption. While this problematic behavior is complex and likely influenced by many factors, one important consideration stems from the theory that learning is a process of acquiring information that is retained in the form of expectancies that instigate and guide behavior appropriate to the expected outcome (e.g., Bolles, 1979). The application of this theory to alcohol abuse suggests that individual differences in learned expectancies about alcohol and the consequences of behavior under the drug may, in part, explain why only some individuals use the drug to extreme and why some relapse while attempting to retain sobriety (e.g., Vogel-Sprott, 1995). Additional evidence on the behavioral influence of learned information in the form of expectancies has been obtained in studies showing that individuals' self-reported expectancies about alcohol and other drugs are related to their drug use (e.g.,

AUTHOR'S NOTE: Preparation of this chapter was supported by the National Institute on Alcohol Abuse and Alcoholism (AA12895), the National Institute on Drug Abuse (DA14079), and by a grant from the Alcoholic Beverage Medical Research Foundation.

Brown, 1993; Goldman et al., 1999). Research in cognition has shown that learned information can be retained and guide behavior consciously or unconsciously. The influence of unconscious processes on alcohol- related behavior is a longstanding notion in North American society where it is expressed variously. "Alcohol weakens self-control." "Alcohol loosens the tongue." It is not uncommon for drinkers to report that they acted unintentionally "without thinking" because they had too much to drink. The slogan of Alcoholics Anonymous, "one drink, one drunk," also implies that consumption of any amount of alcohol lessens self-control, and is consistent with abstinence as a crucial component of treatment for alcohol abuse.

Whereas most applications of cognitive concepts in drug-abuse research concern cognitive events that precede drug use, some researchers have begun to consider that drugs themselves may produce acute changes in cognitive functions that might contribute to their abuse potential. One such application concerns the general distinction between controlled and automatic cognitive processes. Controlled processes are considered to represent explicit cognitions that operate at the level of awareness to influence effortful goal-directed behavior. Explicit memory is considered to provide a measure of controlled, intentional processes, and is tested by tasks, such as recall or recollection, that directly require people to remember and to respond on the basis of earlier events. By contrast, automatic processes are considered to represent implicit cognitions, and are revealed when past experiences unconsciously influence behavior (e.g., Greenwald & Banaji, 1995). Acts committed without attention or awareness, such as well-learned habitual behaviors, are commonly thought to be guided by automatic, implicit influences (e.g., Hasher & Zacks, 1979). Implicit memory is assumed to be unintentional, and is tested by asking people to perform a task that

indirectly requires information about a previous event.

Research equating measures from direct tests with controlled processes, and indirect tests with automatic processes has fairly consistently shown that performance on direct tests of recall and recollection is impaired by alcohol, whereas indirect tests are essentially unchanged (e.g., Tracy & Bates, 1999). But these relationships are clouded by basic research in cognition that indicates the two processes seldom work alone, and both processes may affect the performance of a given task (e.g., Jacoby et al., 1993). Thus, when an indirect test of implicit memory is used to estimate automatic influences on performance, the result may reflect some combination of automatic and controlled processes. Furthermore, when performance on direct tests of recall or recollection is impaired by alcohol, the degree to which this reflects an increase in the strength of automatic processes, and/or a reduction in controlled processes cannot be determined.

The need for separate measures of the influence of automatic and controlled processes on the performance of a task has been addressed in cognitive research by the use of a "process-dissociation" paradigm (Jacoby, 1991). This chapter reviews the experimental procedures that provide these measures, and the factors that have been found to affect one or other process. Results of research distinguishing the effect of alcohol on automatic and controlled processes are described, along with the role these effects may play in contributing to drug abuse. Directions for future research are considered with special reference to integrating the evidence from alcohol-related expectancies, drinking history, and aggression.

DISTINGUISHING THE PROCESSES

The use of either implicit or explicit tasks as pure measures of automatic or controlled retrieval processes has been criticized on the grounds that the two processes rarely act in isolation (e.g., Jacoby et al., 1993; Reingold & Merikle, 1988). The problem of measuring the relative influence of automatic and controlled processes led to the development of a process-dissociation paradigm to separate their influence on the performance of a given task (Jacoby, 1991). The paradigm is based on the rationale that if an action is as likely to occur when one is trying not to do it, as compared to when one is trying to do it, then the individual displays no intentional control. Thus, the experimental procedure measures the difference between performance when one is *trying to*, as compared with *trying not to* engage in some act.

In a process-dissociation paradigm, an individual performs a task under two conditions: (1) when automatic and controlled processes act in concert, and (2) when they act in opposition. When automatic and controlled processes operate in concert to achieve the same goal, task performance is facilitated. When the two processes are in opposition, however, automatic processes generate responses that oppose those of controlled processes, so that errors, or "action slips" are displayed and intentional behavior is compromised. The difference between a person's performance under these two conditions reveals the degree of cognitive control over the behavior, and provides estimates of the degree to which automatic and controlled cognitive processes operate to influence the behavior.

The relative influence of controlled and automatic processes is estimated algebraically. The influence of conscious controlled processes is the difference between the probability of responding when one is trying to make a response (i.e., intentional response) and the probability of responding when one is trying not to make the response (i.e., an action slip). This is calculated by the equation $CP = IR - AS$, where CP = estimate of controlled processes; IR = probability of the intentional response; and AS = probability of

an action slip. A higher value of CP indicates a greater influence of consciously controlled processes.

The influence of automatic processes is estimated by the probability of an action slip (AS) when the controlled processes fail to influence the response (i.e., $1 - CP$). Thus, the estimated influence of the automatic process (AP) can be determined as: $AP = AS/(1 - CP)$

Given that distinctions between automatic and controlled processes have been particularly central to theories of human memory, applications of the process-dissociation paradigm have been largely based on memory tests, such as a stem-completion task. A detailed explanation is available elsewhere (e.g., Jacoby et al., 1993), and is briefly described here. After individuals study a list of five-letter nouns (e.g., motor), they are presented with the first three letters of each word with the remaining two letter spaces represented by dashes (e.g., mot _ _). They are to complete half of these word-stems with the studied word. Under this condition, controlled and automatic processes act in concert to facilitate performance because each process operates to increase the likelihood of completing a stem with a studied word. The other half of the word-stems are to be completed with a word that was not from the study list. Here, controlled and automatic influences are in opposition. Conscious controlled processes are required to retrieve the study list words to offer a different word as a response. If controlled retrieval fails, any unconscious automatic influences evoked by the stem should result in the completion of the stem with a studied word (i.e., an action slip).

The process-dissociation procedure has enjoyed widespread application in recent years. Studies have shown that these processes are affected by different factors, and can make independent contributions to performance. Strengthening a habit increases the influence of automatic processes, but leaves controlled processes unchanged (e.g., Hay &

Jacoby, 1996). In contrast, the passage of time diminishes the influence of controlled processes but does not affect automatic processes (Stolz & Merikle, 2001). Moreover, there is growing evidence that controlled processes are particularly compromised in conditions commonly characterized by the display of poor self-control, such as age-related cognitive decline (Jacoby et al., 1996; Zelazo et al., 2004), schizophrenia (Kazes et al., 1999), severe head injury (Schmitter-Edgecombe & Nissley, 2000), and major depression (MacQueen et al., 2002). The influence of controlled processes also is reduced by environmental factors that impose constraints on information-processing capacity, such as speeded responding, distraction, and divided attention (Jacoby et al., 2001; Shapiro & Krishnan, 2001). By contrast, estimates of automatic processes tend to be unaffected by these conditions, and thus appear remarkably impervious to pathologically and environmentally based disturbances of behavioral control. As a consequence, the net result is a relative increase in the overall reliance on automatic influences to guide behavior.

ACUTE EFFECTS OF ABUSED DRUGS

Studies have used the process-dissociation paradigm to test the acute effects of alcohol and other CNS depressant drugs on controlled and automatic processes. Fillmore et al. (1999) had social drinkers study a list of words prior to receiving either 0.56 g/kg alcohol or a placebo. The subjects were then tested on a word-stem completion task that provided estimates of controlled influences and of automatic influences on their responses. The results showed that alcohol reduced the influence of controlled processes on behavior compared with placebo and no-vehicle control treatments. In contrast, the influence of automatic processes was unaffected by alcohol (Figure 20.1). Other studies of alcohol

effects have since replicated this pattern of results using the same basic measures of stem-completion (Grattan & Vogel-Sprott, 2001; Grattan-Miscio & Vogel-Sprott, 2005; Kirchner & Sayette, 2003). What is particularly remarkable about these findings is the selectivity and the magnitude of the impairing effect of alcohol on controlled processes despite the comparatively mild alcohol doses administered. These impairments were observed at average blood alcohol concentrations ranging between 60 and 70 mg/100 ml. This is less than the legally-sanctioned limit of 80 mg/100 ml, used to prosecute drunk drivers throughout most of the United States and Canada.

The process-dissociation paradigm also has been used to study the effects of benzodiazepines (BZPs). BZPs can produce a wide range of behavioral and cognitive impairment. Their amnestic effects are especially well-known, and are of particular theoretical interest. Numerous studies have reported amnestic effects of BZPs in healthy human volunteers (for reviews, see Curran, 1991, 2000). The majority of studies have demonstrated anterograde amnesia by showing impairment of memory for information that was both studied and recalled in the drugged state. Studies using the process-dissociation paradigm find the effects of BZPs to be remarkably similar to those of alcohol, in that behavior under the drug is characterized by a relative dominance of automatic influences (e.g., Fillmore et al, 2001; Mintzer et al., 2003; Vidailhet et al., 1996). The manner in which BZPs increase automatic influences, however, might differ from alcohol. For example, Fillmore et al. (2001) found that the short-acting BZP, triazolam, directly increased automatic influences without affecting (i.e., reducing) the influence of controlled processes. Mintzer et al. (2003) found that midazolam produced an increase in automatic influences coupled with a decrease of controlled influences. The evidence to date

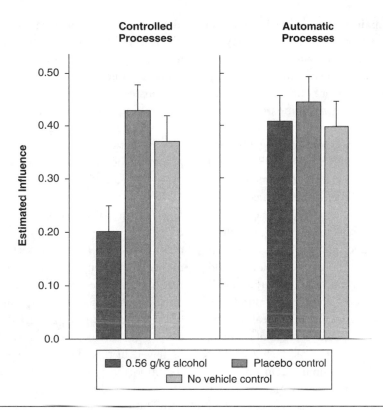

Figure 20.1   Mean estimated influence of controlled and automatic processes under 0.56 g/kg alcohol compared with placebo and no-vehicle control conditions. From Fillmore et al. (1999).

suggests that alcohol and BZPs both promote a dominance of automatic influences, but BZPs are more likely to achieve this net effect by directly increasing the influence of automatic processes. Presently, however, only a few studies have applied process-dissociation techniques in BZP research and many cross-study procedural differences exist, making any clear distinctions between BZPs and alcohol difficult.

Some research has applied the process-dissociation model to study factors known to counteract the impairing effects of alcohol on behavioral control. Stimulant drugs are generally known to reduce many of the impairing effects of alcohol. Considerable evidence indicates that caffeine acts as a functional antagonist to the impairing effects of moderate doses of alcohol on the performance of humans.

Several studies have shown that the coadministration of caffeine can reduce the impairing effect of alcohol on psychomotor performance (Burns & Moskowitz, 1990; Fillmore & Vogel-Sprott, 1995). At a process level, a counteracting effect of a stimulant, such as caffeine, might reflect an increase in controlled influences, a reduction of automatic influences, or a combination of these outcomes. A recent study examined the alcohol-antagonist effects of caffeine in terms of automatic and controlled influences as measured by a stem-completion task (Grattan-Miscio & Vogel-Sprott, 2005). The study found that when a moderate caffeine dose (4 mg/kg) was coadministered with 0.56 g/kg alcohol, controlled processes did not differ from placebo control and thus appeared to be unaffected.

Alcohol impairment also can be reduced by incentives or rewards for the display of unimpaired, sober behavior. Laboratory studies show that drinkers can purposefully display sober behavior under alcohol in drinking situations where unimpaired behavior is reinforced (e.g., Fillmore & Vogel-Sprott, 1997; Sdao-Jarvie & Vogel-Sprott, 1991; Zack & Vogel-Sprott, 1997). Field observations by law enforcement officers also point to the role of reinforcement in suppressing alcohol impairment. Before the Breathalyzer was available, a medical examination of suspected intoxicated drivers was required to support the charge. Goldberg and Havard (1968) reported that the field-sobriety tests were completely unreliable because suspects faced with a doctor called in by the police often were quite capable of "pulling themselves together" to pass all the tests.

Two studies have examined reinforcement of appropriate sober performance under alcohol in terms of its effects on controlled and automatic processes (Grattan & Vogel-Sprott, 2001; Grattan-Miscio & Vogel-Sprott, 2005). These studies showed that positive reinforcement for correct stem-completions under a moderate dose of alcohol (0.56 g/kg) increased the influence of controlled processes on behavior, reestablishing intentional control to sober levels under the drug. These findings are consistent with a growing body of evidence that refutes the notion that impaired self-control is an inevitable consequence of alcohol intoxication. Moreover, the application of process-dissociation techniques indicate that controlled processes might be particularly receptive to environmental factors known to reduce behavioral impairment under alcohol.

RELEVANCE TO ABUSE POTENTIAL

Although there is little dispute that reward mechanisms play an important role in the abuse potential of a drug, cognitive mechanisms have become another focus of research in recent years. Many drinkers report intentions to limit their alcohol use, only to fail and instead drink excessively. Terminating a drinking episode requires control that inhibits ongoing alcohol self-administration. Any reduction in the influence of controlled processes occasioned by an initial dose of alcohol could diminish the ability to halt additional drinking. Thus, acute alcohol impairment of controlled processes might represent an important cognitive mechanism by which an initial alcohol dose promotes subsequent self-administration. Much research to date concerns the link between alcohol use and cognitive processes that operate immediately prior to self-administration (e.g., craving and urges). The research reviewed in this chapter, however, indicates the importance of considering how the acute effects of alcohol, themselves, might directly contribute to abuse by altering cognitive mechanisms involved in the regulation and self-control of behavior.

It has been proposed that automatic and controlled processes might mediate drug-taking, and play a role in "craving" for drugs (Tiffany, 1990). Evidence that drugs, such as alcohol, promote a dominance of automatic influences fits well with the view that drug-abuse behavior comprises highly cue-dependent and stimulus-bound patterns of action (Tiffany & Conklin, 2000). In addition, memory-based models of addiction assume that individuals have memories about the positive effects of alcohol that might be retrieved automatically by alcohol-associated cues that prompt drug-taking behavior (Goldman et al., 1991; Stacy et al., 1994; Weingardt et al., 1996). The alcohol-associated cues in those models typically refer to stimuli that precede actual alcohol consumption (e.g., the sight of a bar), and thus represent a "trigger" mechanism that initiates the drinking episode. Our evidence for increased reliance on automatic processes, as an acute drug effect, suggests that the accessibility of such automatic memories about positive alcohol effects might be further enhanced after drinking has actually begun. Such an effect might operate as a second mechanism that sustains the drinking episode, once it has begun.

Evidence that alcohol increases reliance on automatic influences is also relevant to cue-reactivity research. This approach is based on the assumption that prior drug use results in learning predictive relationships involving pre-drug cues in the environment (O'Brien, 1976; Vogel-Sprott & Fillmore, 1999; Wikler, 1948). For alcohol, pre-drug cues might be the sight or smell of alcohol or the general locale of a drinker's favorite bar. The working hypothesis is that the pre-drug cues gain control over the individual and lead to drug self-administration. The experimental procedure usually involves the presentation of some pre-drug cue to an abstinent drug user followed by a measure of the response (i.e., the reactivity). The response could be some physiological (e.g., heart rate) or behavioral reaction, or some self-reported subjective state (e.g., craving). The principle characteristic of this model is its emphasis on cues that precede actual drug administration, and the underlying assumption that these pre-drug cues can reduce an individual's ability to refrain from drug use. In this respect, cue-reactivity models also concern the issue of intentional self-control over drug-use behavior. Our evidence for increased reliance on automatic processes, as an acute drug effect, suggests that responsiveness to these pre-drug cues might actually increase when drinking has begun. Simply put, the same cues that lead a person to initiate a drug-use episode, might gain further stimulus control over the individual when drug use has begun. The use of a process-dissociation paradigm to assess behavior before and after drug administration could provide a more complete picture of how drug users are influenced by environmental cues that precede or follow drug self-administration. Such evidence would be useful in understanding prolonged drug-use episodes, such as binge drinking.

FUTURE DIRECTIONS: INTEGRATING THE EVIDENCE

Expectancy Effects

The expectancy concept has received considerable attention in studies concerning drinking practices and alcohol abuse. Research has shown that individuals report expectations about alcohol effects on a variety of social, affective, cognitive, and motor behaviors (e.g., Goldman et al., 1999). Studies have obtained both implicit and explicit measures of alcohol expectancies (for a review, see Jones et al., 2001). Measures of explicit expectancies are those obtained by direct, self-report of anticipated alcohol effects. Implicit measures are derived from word-association techniques, such as implicit association tasks and tests of semantic priming, in which subjects respond to associations between alcohol-related words (e.g., beer) and descriptors of specific outcomes (e.g., enjoyable). Fast responses indicate strong associations between alcohol-related words and outcomes, suggesting implicit expectancies (Wiers et al., 2002).

Alcohol expectancies have been of particular interest because of their relationship to alcohol use, and the possibility that they might predict potential alcohol-related problems, such as risk for alcoholism (Jones et al., 2001). Research has also investigated the effect of changing alcohol expectancies as a potential treatment to reduce heavy drinking. These expectancy challenge procedures are designed to reduce expectancies of positive alcohol effects (e.g., euphoria, arousal) by providing brief education that highlights the negative effects (e.g., dysphoria, sedation). The treatments have been found to yield some beneficial outcomes with respect to alcohol-related behaviors. Challenging drinkers' positive expectations has been shown to reduce heavy drinkers' alcohol consumption (e.g., Darkes & Goldman, 1993, 1998; Wiers et al., 2003). These treatments also appear to alter drinkers' expectancies as measured by explicit, self-report techniques, but not by implicit indicators. Reasons for this dissociation are unclear, but could highlight an important difference in the degree to which implicit and explicit alcohol expectancies are amenable to change.

Another important property of alcohol expectations concerns their direct influence on the drinker's acute behavioral response to alcohol. Studies have shown that certain expectancies produce adaptive responses to alcohol that reduce the degree of behavioral impairment displayed (Fillmore & Blackburn, 2002; Fillmore, Mulvihill, & Vogel-Sprott, 1994; Fillmore & Vogel-Sprott, 1996). When individuals are given prior information that leads them to expect strong performance-impairing effects from alcohol, the degree of impairment they display under the drug is reduced. These observations suggest that an expectation of intense impairment has adaptive value for a drinker. It may strengthen intentional controlled processes to occasion a compensatory response that counteracts the impairing behavioral effects of the drug. The ability to change drinkers' expectations of mild alcohol impairment has important implications for harm reduction (Fillmore et al.; Vogel-Sprott & Fillmore, 1999). High-risk behaviors, such as drinking and driving, are hazardous because alcohol impairs the cognitive and motor skills required for safety. Individuals who expect little impairment from alcohol, however, may readily decide to engage in risky behaviors despite having consumed the drug.

Moreover, because automatic influences on behavior may dominate under alcohol, such decisions might occur with little or no conscious deliberation. Changing drinkers' expectancies about the effect of alcohol on their behavior might strengthen intentional control of behavior under the drug. To date, however, no research has examined the effects of changing expectancies in terms of the changes in controlled and automatic influences on behavior under alcohol.

Drinking History

The extent of alcohol use also may contribute to the relative influences of automatic and controlled processes on behavior under alcohol. Learning about alcohol effects appears to be a normal process that develops with prior experience using the drug. The initial use of alcohol is associated with a number of effects, and as drinking is repeated, an individual can learn to identify the effects that occur reliably. This learning provides a basis for expecting particular effects, and as alcohol use continues, these expectancies become well learned, occurring more "automatically," with little conscious deliberation (Vogel-Sprott & Fillmore, 1999). Studies have produced findings that are consistent with this notion (Fillmore & Vogel-Sprott, 1995, 1996). Research has shown that the expectation of alcohol is more likely to affect the behavior of "experienced" drinkers (i.e., those who have been drinking regularly for more than 2 years) than the behavior of "novice" drinkers (i.e., those who have been using alcohol less than one year). Moreover, the drinkers in that research appeared unable to accurately assess changes in their behavior when they expected alcohol, and so the effects seemed to occur without awareness, and may represent automatic influences on behavior. Studies comparing alcohol effects on automatic and controlled processes in novice and experienced drinkers are needed to test the hypothesis that the extent of regular alcohol use may increase automatic influences on behavior when the drug is consumed.

Aggression

Alcohol-related violence is a serious social problem that has prompted a wide range of studies. A review of predisposing factors has identified personal characteristics such as impulsivity and weak inhibitory control, as well as social situations, like crowding, rivalries, threats, and provocation (e.g., Lang, 1993). Laboratory experiments have generally found that alcohol consumption intensifies aggression in predisposing situations, such as provocation (for reviews, see Bushman & Cooper, 1990; Taylor & Chermack, 1993).

Numerous investigators have speculated about the relationship of aggression to the alcohol impairment of various cognitive processes (e.g., Hoaken et al., 1998; Pernanen, 1976; Taylor & Leonard, 1983). Although little is yet known about these relationships, cognitive processes governing the inhibition of undesirable responses are likely to play an important role in aggressive responding. An acute dose of alcohol has been found to selectively weaken inhibitory control without affecting the ability to display an appropriate response (Mulvihill et al., 1997). In contrast, the provision of a reward for inhibiting inappropriate responses under alcohol strengthens inhibitory control (Fillmore & Vogel-Sprott, 1999). More generally, alcohol increases a drinker's reliance on the environmental context for the maintenance of inhibitory control (Fillmore, 2004). Although this evidence does not indicate the degree to which a failure of inhibition under alcohol is inadvertent or deliberate, drinkers often report that it is unintentional. This important issue may be more directly addressed by research based on a distinction between controlled and automatic influences offered by a process-dissociation model.

Evidence cited earlier in this chapter suggests that an acute dose of alcohol increases a reliance on automatic processes and responsiveness to environmental cues. This may also apply to inhibitory control: A relative increase in the influence of automatic processes should increase responsiveness to environmental signals for the response, or its inhibition. The framework of a process-dissociation paradigm could study how the acute effects of alcohol alter automatic and controlled cognitive processes that influence the inhibition of aggression. Conceptualizing alcohol-related aggression in terms of changes in the influence of automatic and controlled processes would also allow predictions about how other factors that specifically affect one or other process might mediate aggression under alcohol.

CONCLUSIONS

Recent years have seen an increased application of cognitive theories and methodologies in substance-abuse research. In particular, there is growing recognition and interest in implicit cognitive processes associated with substance abuse and addictive behavior. The distinction between actions that result from explicit, controlled influences and those that are governed by implicit, automatic processes, is a fundamental concept in cognitive psychology. With regard to substance abuse, research has been primarily concerned with the role of these processes as antecedent influences that precede and possibly contribute to drug use. By contrast, this chapter considers how drugs themselves can alter the degree to which these processes determine behavior that might contribute to abuse potential. The ability of drugs, such as alcohol, to promote a reliance on automatic influences could explain a broad range of behavioral effects that are observed in the drugged state, and provide new insights into factors that contribute to drug-taking and drug abuse. This chapter explained how process-dissociation models can be used to gain a better understanding of how alcohol and other drugs affect basic cognitive processes influencing intentional control of behavior. The chapter also described how a distinction between controlled and automatic processes can be integrated within other theories of substance abuse, such as models of addiction based on expectancy or memory. Integration of these approaches should provide important new insights into how intentional control over drug use might be mediated by drug-related expectancies and prior learning.

The study of acute drug effects on controlled and automatic influences is at an early stage and many questions remain. With respect to alcohol abuse, it is unclear how controlled and automatic influences might be involved in factors traditionally associated with risk for alcohol abuse, such as disorders characterized by behavioral under-control, or genetic-based risks, such as a family history of alcoholism. The role of these processes in abuse of drugs other than alcohol is also of interest. To date, the majority of research has concerned CNS depressant effects produced by alcohol or benzodiazepines. Little is known about how stimulants of abuse, such as cocaine and methamphetamine, might alter behavioral control in terms of changes in controlled and automatic influences.

The limitations and boundary conditions of the process-dissociation paradigm also need to be better understood (Jacoby, 1998). The model assumes that automatic and controlled processes represent independent influences on behavior. As such, the model is ideal as an initial strategy to study potentially selective effects of a drug on one process. There is debate, however, with regard to this independence assumption (e.g., Joordens & Merikle, 1993). A better understanding of how automatic and controlled processes influence drugged behavior might be gained by comparing the conclusions obtained from process-dissociation measures with other techniques for measuring implicit cognition, such as semantic priming and implicit association tests. Finally, it is important to note that process-dissociation models of memory-based behaviors have focused on verbal responses, such as word recollection. Adapting these models to other behavioral domains, such as motor responses, would broaden our understanding of implicit influences on substance abuse and allow us to better characterize addictive behavior.

REFERENCES

Bolles, R. C. (1979). *Learning theory* (2nd ed.). New York: Holt, Reinhart & Winston.

Brown, S. A. (1993). Drug effect expectancies and addictive behavior change. *Experimental & Clinical Psychopharmacology, 1,* 55–67.

Burns, M., & Moskowitz, H. (1990). Two experiments on alcohol-caffeine interaction. *Alcohol, Drugs, and Driving, 5,* 303–315.

Bushman, B. J., & Cooper, H. M. (1990). Effects of alcohol on human aggression: An integrative review. *Psychological Bulletin, 107,* 341–354.

Curran, H. V. (1991). Benzodiazepines, memory, and mood: A review. *Psychopharmacology, 105,* 1–8.

Curran, H. V. (2000). Psychopharmacological perspectives on memory. In E. Tulving & F. M. Craik (Eds.), *The Oxford handbook of memory* (pp. 539–554). New York: Oxford University Press.

Darkes, J., & Goldman, M. S. (1993). Expectancy challenge and drinking reduction: Experimental evidence for a mediational process. *Journal of Consulting and Clinical Psychology, 61,* 344–353.

Darkes, J., & Goldman, M. S. (1998). Expectancy challenge and drinking reduction: Process and structure in the alcohol expectancy network. *Experimental & Clinical Psychopharmacology, 6,* 64–76.

Fillmore, M. T. (2004). Environmental dependence of behavioral control mechanisms: Effects of alcohol and information processing demands. *Experimental & Clinical Psychopharmacology, 12,* 216–223.

Fillmore, M. T., & Blackburn, J. (2002). Compensating for alcohol-induced impairment: Alcohol expectancies and behavioral disinhibition. *Journal of Studies on Alcohol, 63,* 237–246.

Fillmore, M. T., Carscadden, J. L., & Vogel-Sprott, M. (1998). Alcohol, cognitive impairment, and expectancies. *Journal of Studies on Alcohol, 59,* 174–179.

Fillmore, M. T., Kelly, T. H., Rush, C. R., & Hays, L. (2001). Retrograde facilitation of memory by triazolam: Effects on automatic processes. *Psychopharmacology, 158,* 314–321.

Fillmore, M. T., Mulvihill, L. E., & Vogel-Sprott, M. (1994). The expected drug and its expected effect interact to determine placebo responses to alcohol and caffeine. *Psychopharmacology, 115,* 383–388.

Fillmore, M. T., & Vogel-Sprott, M. (1995). Behavioral effects of combining alcohol and caffeine: Contribution of drug-related expectancies. *Experimental & Clinical Psychopharmacology, 3,* 33–38.

Fillmore, M. T., & Vogel-Sprott, M. (1996). Evidence that expectancies mediate behavioral impairment under alcohol. *Journal of Studies on Alcohol, 57,* 598–603.

Fillmore, M. T., & Vogel-Sprott, M. (1997). Resistance to cognitive impairment under alcohol: The role of environmental consequences. *Experimental & Clinical Psychopharmacology, 5*(3), 251–255.

Fillmore, M. T., & Vogel-Sprott, M. (1999). An alcohol model of impaired inhibitory control and its treatment in humans. *Experimental & Clinical Psychopharmacology, 7,* 49–55.

Fillmore, M. T., Vogel-Sprott, M., & Gavrilescu, D. (1999). Alcohol effects on intentional behavior: Dissociating controlled and automatic influences. *Experimental & Clinical Psychopharmacology, 7,* 372–378.

Goldberg, L., & Havard, J. (1968). *Research on the effect of alcohol and drugs on driver behavior and their importance as a cause of road accidents.* Paris, France: Organization for Economic Cooperation and Development.

Goldman, M. S., Brown, S. A., Christiansen, B. A., & Smith, G. T. (1991). Alcoholism and memory: Broadening the scope of alcohol expectancy research. *Psychological Bulletin, 110,* 137–146.

Goldman, M. S., Darkes, J., & Del Boca, F. (1999). Expectancy mediation of biopsychosocial risk for alcohol use and alcoholism. In I. Kirsch (Ed.), *How expectancies shape experience* (pp. 215–232). Washington, DC: American Psychological Association.

Grattan, K. E., & Vogel-Sprott, M. (2001). Maintaining intentional control of behavior under alcohol. *Alcoholism: Clinical and Experimental Research, 25,* 192–197.

Grattan-Miscio, K. E., & Vogel-Sprott, M. (2005). Alcohol, intentional control and inappropriate behavior: Regulation by caffeine or an incentive. *Experimental & Clinical Psychopharmacology, 13*, 48–55.

Greenwald, A. G., & Banaji, M. R. (1995). Implicit social cognition: Attitudes, self-esteem, and stereotypes. *Psychological Review, 102*, 4–27.

Hasher, L., & Zacks, R. T. (1979). Automatic and effortful processes in memory. *Journal of Experimental Psychology: General, 108*, 356–388.

Hay, J. F., & Jacoby, L. L. (1996). Separating habit and recollection: Memory slips, process dissociations and probability matching. *Journal of Experimental Psychology: Learning, Memory, and Cognition, 22*, 1323–1335.

Hoaken, P. N. S., Giancola, P. R., & Pihl, R. O. (1998). Executive Cognitive Functions as mediators of alcohol-related aggression. *Alcohol and Alcoholism, 33*, 47–54.

Jacoby, L. L. (1991). A process dissociation framework: Separating automatic from intentional uses of memory. *Journal of Memory and Language, 30*, 513–541.

Jacoby, L. L. (1998). Invariance in automatic influences of memory: Toward a user's guide for the process-dissociation procedure. *Journal of Experimental Psychology: Learning, Memory, and Cognition, 24*, 3–26.

Jacoby, L. L., Debner, J. A., & Hay, J. F. (2001). Proactive interference, accessibility bias, and process dissociations: Valid subjective reports of memory. *Journal of Experimental Psychology: Learning, Memory, and Cognition, 27*, 686–700.

Jacoby, L. L., Jennings, J. M., & Hay, J. F. (1996). Dissociating automatic and consciously controlled processes: Implications for diagnosis and rehabilitation of memory deficits. In D. Herrmann, C. McEroy, C. Hertzog, P. Hertel, & M. K. Johnson (Eds.), *Basic & applied memory research: Theory in context* (Vol. 1, pp. 161–193). Hillsdale, NJ: Lawrence Erlbaum.

Jacoby, L. L., Toth, J. P., & Yonelinas, A. P. (1993). Separating conscious and unconscious influences of memory. Measuring recollection. *Journal of Experimental Psychology: General, 122*, 139–154.

Jones, B. T., Corbin, W., & Fromme, K. (2001). A review of expectancy theory and alcohol consumption. *Addiction, 96*, 57–72.

Joordens, S., & Merikle, P. M. (1993). Independence or redundancy? Two models of conscious and unconscious influences. *Journal of Experimental Psychology: General, 122*, 462–467.

Kazes, M., Danion, J. M., Robert, P., Berthet, L., Amado, I., Willard, D., et al. (1999). Impairment of consciously controlled use of memory in schizophrenia. *Neuropsychology, 13*, 54–61.

Kirchner, T. R., & Sayette, M. A. (2003). Effects of alcohol on controlled and automatic memory processes. *Experimental & Clinical Psychopharmacology, 11*, 167–175.

Lang, A. R. (1993). Alcohol-related violence: Psychological perspectives. In S. Martin (Ed.), *Alcohol and interpersonal violence: Fostering multidisciplinary perspectives* (pp. 121–148). (NIAAA Research Monograph 24; DHHS Pub. No. (ADM) 93-3496). Washington, DC: Government Printing Office.

MacQueen, G. M., Galway, T. M., Hay, J., Young, L. T., & Joffe, R. T. (2002). Recollection memory deficits in patients with major depressive disorder predicted by past depressions but not current mood state or treatment status. *Psychological Medicine, 32*, 251–258.

Mintzer, M. Z., Griffiths, R. R., & Hirshman, E. (2003). A paradoxical dissociation in the effects of midazolam on recollection and automatic processes in the process dissociation procedure. *American Journal of Psychology, 116*, 213–237.

Mulvihill, L., Skilling, T., & Vogel-Sprott, M. (1997). Alcohol and the ability to inhibit behavior of men and women. *Journal of Studies on Alcohol, 58,* 600–605.

O'Brien, C. P. (1976). Experimental analysis of conditioning factors in human narcotic addiction. *Pharmacological Reviews, 27,* 533–543.

Pernanen, K. (1976). Alcohol and crimes of violence. In B. Kissin & H. Beigleiter (Eds.), *The biology of alcoholism* (Vol. 4, pp. 344–351). New York: Plenum.

Reingold, E. M., & Merikle, P. M. (1988). Using direct and indirect measures to study perception without awareness. *Perception & Psychophysics, 44,* 563–575.

Schmitter-Edgecombe, M., & Nissley, H. M. (2000). Effects of divided attention on automatic and controlled components of memory after severe closed-head injury. *Neuropsychology, 14,* 559–569.

Sdao-Jarvie, K., & Vogel-Sprott, M. (1991). Response expectancies affect the acquisition and display of behavioral tolerance to alcohol. *Alcohol, 78,* 491–498.

Shapiro, S., & Krishnan, H. S. (2001). Memory-based measures for assessing advertising effects: A comparison of explicit and implicit memory effects. *Journal of Advertising, 30,* 1–13.

Stacy, A. W., Leigh, B. C., & Weingardt, K. R. (1994). Memory accessibility and association of alcohol use and its positive outcomes. *Experimental & Clinical Psychopharmacology, 2,* 269–282.

Stolz, J., & Merikle, P. M. (2001). Conscious and unconscious influences of memory: Temporal dynamics. *Memory, 8,* 333–343.

Taylor, S. P., & Chermack, S. T. (1993). Alcohol, drugs, and human physical aggression. *Journal of Studies on Alcohol,* (Suppl. 11), 78–88.

Taylor, S. P., & Leonard, K. (1983). Alcohol and aggression. In R. Green & E. Donnerstein (Eds.), *Aggression: Theoretical and empirical reviews* (pp. 77–102). New York: Academic Press.

Tiffany, S. T. (1990). A cognitive model of drug urges and drug-use behavior: Role of automatic and nonautomatic processes. *Psychological Review, 97,* 147–168.

Tiffany, S. T., & Conklin, C. A. (2000). A cognitive processing model of alcohol craving and compulsive alcohol use. *Addiction, 95*(Suppl. 2), S145–S153.

Tracy, J. I., & Bates, M. E. (1999). The selective effects of alcohol on automatic and effortful memory processes. *Neuropsychology, 13,* 282–290.

Vidailhet, P., Kazes, M., Danion, J. M., Kauffman-Muller, F., & Grange, D. (1996). Effects of lorazepam and diazepam on conscious and automatic memory processes. *Psychopharmacology, 127,* 63–72.

Vogel-Sprott, M. (1995). The psychobiology of conditioning, reinforcement and craving. In B. Tabakoff & P. Hoffman (Eds.), *Biological aspects of alcoholism* (pp. 225–244) [WHO Expert Series on Biological Psychiatry]. Geneva, Switzerland: Hogrefe & Huber.

Vogel-Sprott, M., & Fillmore, M. T. (1999). Learning theory and research. In K. E. Leonard & H. T. Blane (Eds.), *Psychological theories of drinking and alcoholism* (2nd ed., pp. 292–327). New York: Guilford.

Weingardt, K. R., Stacy, A. W., & Leigh, B. C. (1996). Automatic activation of alcohol concepts in response to positive outcomes of alcohol use. *Alcoholism: Clinical and Experimental Research, 20,* 25–30.

Wiers, R. W., van Woerden, N., Smulders, F. T. Y., & de Jong, P. J. (2002). Implicit and explicit alcohol-related cognitions in heavy and light drinkers. *Journal of Abnormal Psychology, 111,* 648–658.

Wiers, R. W., Wood, M. D., Darkes, J., Corbin, W. R., Jones, B. T., & Sher, K. J. (2003). Changing expectancies: Cognitive mechanisms and context effects. *Alcoholism: Clinical and Experimental Research, 27,* 186–197.

Wikler, A. (1948). Recent progress in research on the neurophysiological basis of morphine addiction. *American Journal of Psychiatry, 105,* 329–338.

Zack, M., & Vogel-Sprott, M. (1997). Drunk or sober? Learned conformity to a behavioural standard. *Journal of Studies on Alcohol, 58,* 475–501.

Zelazo, P. D., Craik, F. I. M., & Booth, L. (2004). Executive function across the life span. *Acta Psychologica, 115,* 167–183.

Section V

IMPLICIT COGNITIONS AND DIFFERENT ADDICTIONS

CHAPTER 21

Implicit Cognition and Tobacco Addiction

ANDREW J. WATERS AND MICHAEL A. SAYETTE

Abstract: Much recent research has used implicit assessment techniques to examine automatic motivational and affective processes relevant to tobacco addiction. We review this literature. We review reaction time studies using the modified Stroop task, visual dot-probe task, dual-task paradigm, implicit association task, priming task, and the expectancy accessibility task. We also briefly review memory association studies, facial coding studies, and startle probe studies. We assess whether each implicit measure is (1) associated with smoking status (smokers vs. nonsmokers), (2) associated with heaviness of smoking, (3) prospectively related to cessation outcomes, (4) associated with self-reported craving, and (5) moderated by abstinence from smoking or perceived availability of smoking. Research in implicit cognition and tobacco addiction is in its infancy, but this early research suggests some promising research avenues.

Smoking is an important risk factor for cancer and heart disease. Smoking cessation results in considerable health benefits (U.S. Department of Health and Human Services, 1990). The majority of smokers are motivated to quit. Most quit attempts, however, end in failure (Hughes et al., 1992). Relapse to smoking is also rapid, with many relapses occurring in the first few days (Garvey et al., 1992). Medications such as nicotine replacement and bupropion improve cessation outcomes (Jorenby et al., 1999; Silagy et al., 2000) but even with treatment, the majority of cessation efforts fail. It is therefore important to understand the psychological mechanisms underlying tobacco addiction, so that more effective interventions can be developed.

Psychological Processes Underlying Tobacco Dependence

It has been argued that tobacco dependence is strongly associated with affective processes (e.g., Baker et al., 2004; Stewart et al., 1984). For example, smokers feel acute discomfort when abstaining, and may relapse to avoid this aversive state (the "withdrawal-relief" hypothesis). Smokers also experience pleasure from smoking, lay down memories of these pleasurable experiences, and may therefore relapse to reexperience those pleasurable feelings (the "memory of past pleasure" hypothesis). Robinson and Berridge (1993) offered an alternative perspective. They argued that the motivational (or "wanting") system of addicts becomes sensitized by drug-taking. According to this view (described in more detail later), addicts assign too much motivational salience to drugs, drug-related stimuli, and the act of drug-taking.

Limitations of Self-Report Measures of Affective and Motivational Processes

Historically, much research on the affective and motivational mechanisms underlying smoking cessation has been conducted using self-report measures. Self-report measures, however, have a number of well-known limitations that have been noted elsewhere in this volume. In addition, as described below, it has become clear that self-report measures of affect and craving do not predict all, or even most, of the variance in smoking behavior.

Self-Reported Negative Affect and Smoking

Although smokers often report that they smoke more when in a bad mood, data collected using ecological momentary assessment methodologies have demonstrated that the association between self-reported negative affect and ad libitum smoking is, at best, weak (Shiffman et al., 2002). Furthermore, although a sudden rise of negative affect is an important risk factor for some relapse episodes (Shiffman & Waters, 2004), most lapses occur when participants report being in a neutral or positive mood (Shiffman et al., 1996). Moreover, background levels of self-reported stress or negative affect do not appear to be related to risk of relapse (Shiffman & Waters, 2004). The association between severity of withdrawal and cessation outcome is not as strong as might be predicted by withdrawal-relief accounts (e.g., Patten & Martin, 1996).

Self-Reported Craving and Smoking

Although some studies have documented associations between self-reported craving and smoking behavior (e.g., Shiffman et al., 1997; Shiffman et al., 1996), Tiffany (1990) has argued that these two variables are generally not tightly coupled. Other researchers have noted limitations with self-reported craving as a measure of motivation to smoke (Sayette et al., 2000).

Automatic Psychological Processes in Addiction

An important distinction has been drawn in cognitive psychology between controlled and automatic psychological processes (e.g., Schneider & Shiffrin, 1977). Controlled processes are typically slow, serial, effortful, and driven by a conscious appraisal of events. These types of processes may be captured reasonably well by self-report measures. In contrast, automatic processes are fast, parallel, effortless, and may not engage conscious awareness. As noted elsewhere, a number of authors have highlighted the role of automatic processes in drug addiction (Robinson & Berridge, 1993; Stacy, 1997; Tiffany, 1990).

Implicit Processes in Tobacco Addiction

To summarize: (1) There has been growing interest in automatic processes in addiction and (2) research has suggested that measures of self-reported affect/motivation are not tightly coupled with smoking behavior. The net effect of these two developments has been to stimulate interest in alternative measures that may index automatic affective and motivational processes. Thus, recent articles have stressed the importance of automatic affective and motivational processes (Baker et al., 2004; Robinson & Berridge, 1993). Automatic processes can be assessed using implicit assessment techniques, which are useful for theory development and clinical research.

Theoretical Utility of Implicit Measures

Implicit measures may provide insight into automatic affective and motivational processes. This facilitates testing of psychological theory.

Clinical Utility of Implicit Measures

If an implicit measure were associated with smoking cessation and other dependence-relevant measures, then it could provide a valuable laboratory tool for evaluating the effectiveness of an intervention. For example, a treatment that attenuates both an implicit measure and self-reported craving might do better than a treatment that reduces only self-reported craving.

Scope of Chapter

The main aim of this chapter is to review the literature on implicit cognition and tobacco addiction. We focus on tasks that assess the impact of smoking stimuli (vs. control stimuli) on cognition. Thus, we do not review studies that examined the effects of acute nicotine (e.g., Heishman et al., 1994), nicotine abstinence (e.g., Sherwood, 1993), or craving (e.g., Zwann et al., 2000) on general measures of cognitive performance. Due to space limitations, we also do not review the literature that assesses the impact of imaginal smoking stimuli (vs. imaginal control stimuli) on cognition (e.g., Cepeda-Benito & Tiffany, 1996). Because most research has been conducted in adult smokers, our review mainly addresses the relation between implicit cognition and smoking dependence/cessation, rather than the relation between implicit cognition and smoking initiation.

ATTENTIONAL BIAS

The importance of attentional bias to smoking cues is highlighted in Robinson and Berridge's (1993) incentive-sensitization theory of addiction. They argue that mental representations of stimuli consistently paired with pleasure become the targets of incentive salience. These "incentive stimuli" become attractive and wanted, and "grab attention" (Robinson & Berridge, 1993, p. 261). Ordinarily, incentive salience is only assigned to stimuli that are consistently paired with pleasure. They argue, however, that certain brain manipulations, such as drugs, can circumvent pleasure, and cause the attribution of incentive salience to drug-related stimuli even in the absence of pleasure. Critically, in some individuals, the effect of the drug becomes more pronounced over time (i.e., sensitization occurs). The drug-related cues become pathologically wanted ("craved") and exert a strong influence over behavior. This may be an important index of dependence.

Anecdotally, we have noted that smokers attempting to quit often report that they notice cigarettes and people smoking much more than they did while smoking normally. More theoretically, some authors have interpreted Robinson and Berridge's (1993) theory to predict that acute nicotine deprivation should potentiate the incentive salience of smoking cues (e.g., Field et al., 2004; Waters & Feyerabend, 2000; but see Powell et al., 2002, for an alternative hypothesis). Toates (1986) argued that drive states such as hunger do not motivate behavior directly (i.e., by eliciting escape behavior). Rather, these states serve to potentiate the incentive value of food stimuli and prompt consumption through this route. Drug deprivation states may work in a similar way.

The primary consequence of the drug-induced neuro-adaptations is excessive salience attribution to drug-related stimuli. It has also been suggested, however, that the neuro-adaptations may also impair smokers' motivation for other, nonsmoking related, reinforcers, and that this should be revealed when smokers are abstinent (Powell et al., 2002). A couple of studies have examined attentional bias for positively and negatively valenced stimuli.

Modified Stroop Task

Task Overview

Studies have used a modified Stroop task to assess attentional bias to smoking cues. Participants are required to classify the colors of neutral and smoking-related words as quickly and as accurately as possible. The difference in reaction times—the smoking Stroop effect—indexes attentional bias to smoking cues. Table 12.1 presents a review of modified Stroop studies.

Association with smoking status. One study has documented that smokers exhibit greater smoking Stroop effects than nonsmokers on the smoking Stroop task (Munafo et al., 2003). The same study reported that the smoking Stroop effects of never-smokers and ex-smokers did not significantly differ.

Associations with cigarettes per day (CSD). One study has reported a significant correlation between CSD and smoking Stroop effects in a student sample (Mogg & Bradley, 2002), whereas another reported no correlation in a clinical sample (Waters, Shiffman, Sayette, et al., 2003). Among adolescent smokers, one study has documented associations between CSD and smoking Stroop effects (Zack et al., 2001).

Associations with clinical outcome. The one study that assessed the prospective relations between smoking Stroop effects and short-term cessation outcomes reported significant associations (Waters, Shiffman, Sayette, et al., 2003).

Associations with self-reported craving. Two studies have reported significant correlations between self-reported craving and smoking Stroop effects in adult and adolescent smokers, respectively (Mogg & Bradley, 2002; Zack et al., 2001). Another study (Waters, Shiffman, Sayette, et al., 2003) reported a marginally significant correlation between urge ratings and the acute Stroop effect. There was no association between self-reported craving and the smoking Stroop effect in the Wertz and Sayette (2001) study.

Effects of abstinence and perceived availability. One study reported that participants who expected to smoke soon showed elevated smoking Stroop effects compared with those who did not (Wertz & Sayette, 2001). Although some earlier studies using the smoking Stroop task reported that smoking Stroop effects are potentiated in abstinence (Gross et al., 1993; Waters & Feyerabend, 2000; Zack et al., 2001), these results have not been replicated (Rusted et al., 2000; Mogg & Bradley, 2002; Munafo et al., 2003).

Other effects. Waters, Sayette, et al. (2003) reported secondary analyses of two data sets that used a mixed smoking Stroop task. These demonstrated that smokers are slower to color-name words occurring after smoking-related words than words occurring after neutral words (see also Waters, Sayette, et al., 2004). Carryover effects may capture the difficulty in disengaging attention from smoking stimuli. Further research is required to understand their significance.

Limitations of the Modified Stroop Task

Despite the widespread use of the modified Stroop task, the psychological processes

Table 21.1 Summary of Published Studies Using the Modified Stroop Task

Study	Participants	Mean age	Stroop task	Independent variables	Word types	Smoking Stroop effects	Significant effects	Correlational analyses
Gross et al. (1993)	10 AB, 10 NON-AB	39	Cards	Abstinence (12-hr vs. NON-AB)	Smoking, Neutral	AB = 88 ms*; NON-AB = −92 ms*	Main Effect Abstinence	
Johnsen et al. (1997)	11 AB, 11 NON-AB, 11 Nonsmokers	40, 40, 45	Computer, Blocked, VR + MR	Group Status (3-days AB vs. NON-AB vs. Nonsmokers)	Smoking, Neutral, Incongruent	AB ≈ 100 ms; NON-AB ≈ 60 ms; Nonsmokers ≈ −10 ms		
Waters & Feyerabend (2000)	48 AB, 48 NON-AB	25, 27	Computer, Blocked + Mixed, VR	Abstinence (24-hr vs. NON-AB) Format (Blocked vs. Mixed) Word Type (Smoking vs. Withdrawal)	Smoking, Neutral vs. Withdrawal, Neutral	AB: Blocked = 37 ms*, Mixed = −11 ms*; NON-AB: Blocked = 6 ms, Mixed = 9 ms	Blocked: Main Effect Abstinence	Blocked, Smoking-word: correlation between Stroop and time to first cigarette
Rusted et al. (2000)	28 Smokers, complete AB, NON-AB sessions	25	Cards	Abstinence (2-hr vs. just smoked; within-S)	Smoking, Neutral	AB = 50 ms*; NON-AB = 60 ms*		
Zack et al. (2001)	16 AB Adolescent Smokers (8 HEAVY, 12 + cigs/day; 8 LIGHT, <12 cigs/day)	17	Computer, Mixed, VR	Acute Smoking (pre-cig vs. post-cig); Heaviness of Smoking	Smoking, Positive, Negative, Neutral	HEAVY: AB = 56 ms*; Post-Smoking ≈ −4 ms; LIGHT: AB = 19 ms; Post-Smoking ≈ 39 ms	Heaviness of Smoking by Acute Smoking Interaction	Correlation between Stroop and (1) Factor 2 craving (r = .52), and (2) CSD (r = .69)

(Continued)

Table 21.1 (Continued)

Study	Participants	Mean age	Stroop task	Independent variables	Word types	Smoking Stroop effects	Significant effects	Correlational analyses
Wertz & Sayette (2001)	92 AB	20	Computer, Mixed, VR	Perceived Opportunity to Smoke ("YES" vs. "MAYBE" vs. "NO"; between-S)	Smoking Neutral	YES = 24 ms*; MAYBE = 3 ms; NO = 11 ms*	Main Effect Perceived Opportunity	
Mogg & Bradley (2002)	27 Smokers, complete AB, NON-AB sessions	33	Computer, Blocked, VR	Exposure (Supra. vs. Sub., within-S) Abstinence (within-S)	Smoking Neutral Incongruent	AB: Supra. = 24 ms*; Sub. = 3 ms NON-AB: Supra. = 24 ms*; Sub. = −12 ms		Supra.: Correlation between Stroop and (1) CSD (rs = .39, .56), (2) Urge (rs = .58, .43), on NON-AB, AB sessions, respectively
Powell et al. (2002)	21 Smokers, complete AB, NON-AB sessions 10 NEVER	23 22	Cards	Group Status (overnight deprived vs. "just smoked" vs. NEVER)	Positive Negative Neutral	AB: Pos. Stroop ≈ 5 ms; Neg. Stroop ≈ 10 ms NON-AB: Pos. Stroop ≈ 60 ms*; Neg. Stroop ≈ 70 ms* NEVER: Pos. Stroop ≈ 60 ms; Neg. Stroop ≈ 50 ms	Main Effect Abstinence for Pos., Neg. Stroop Effects	

314

Study	Participants	Mean age	Stroop task	Independent variables	Word types	Smoking Stroop effects	Significant effects	Correlational analyses
Munafo et al. (2003)	43 Smokers 22 EX 30 NEVER	28 38 22	Computer, Blocked, VR	Exposure (Supra. vs. Sub.) Abstinence (between-S) Smoking Status	Smoking Neutral	NEVER = 10 ms, 5 ms, − 6 ms, − 1 ms EX = 7 ms, 7 ms, 4 ms, − 1 ms NON-AB = 19 ms[#], 8 ms[#], 10 ms[#], 13 ms[#] AB = 23 ms[#], 16 ms[#], − 1 ms[#], 3 ms[#] (Supra. Se 1, Se 2; Sub. Se 1, Se 2, respectively)	Main Effect Smoking Status (Smokers vs. Nonsmokers)	Supra.: Correlation between Stroop and sensitivity to reward ($r = .36$)
Waters, Shiffman, Sayette, et al. (2003)	158 AB	39	Computer, Blocked, MR	Nicotine Replacement (NICOTINE vs. PLACEBO) Relapse	Smoking Neutral	NICOTINE = 66 ms* PLACEBO = 72 ms*		Acute Stroop effect predicts 1-week lapse, time to first lapse

NOTE: Smoking Stroop Effect = RT on smoking trials – RT on neutral trials. Larger (more positive) smoking Stroop effects reflect greater attentional bias. Participants in Gross et al. (1993) were undergoing treatment for drug or alcohol addiction. AB participants in Johnsen et al. (1997) were attending a smoking-cessation program and reported that they had been 3 days abstinent at test. In Zack et al. (2001), participants were (1) 17 ms faster to color-name the positive words than the neutral words before smoking, and 20 ms faster after smoking; and (2) 14 ms slower to color-name the negative words before smoking, and 6 ms slower after smoking (not shown in Table 21.1). There were no significant effects for positive and negative word types. In Wertz and Sayette (2001), "YES" group participants were told they would be able to smoke during the study; "NO" group participants were told they would not; and "MAYBE" group participants were told that a coin would be tossed to determine if they would be able to smoke. In Munafo et al. (2003) each participant was tested twice, 24 hours apart. Smokers smoked normally before the first session, and were subsequently randomly assigned to smoke normally or abstain from smoking before the second session. In Waters et al. (2003), participants were randomly assigned to wear a high-dose nicotine patch (35 mg) or a placebo patch. They completed the smoking Stroop task on the first day of a quit attempt, after roughly 18 hours of abstinence. All participants completed the neutral block before the smoking block. The acute Stroop effect reflects slowed responses on the first 11 trials of the smoking block (vs. neutral trials).

Key: Supra. = Supraliminal; Sub. = Subliminal; NEVER = never-smokers; EX = ex-smokers; AB = abstinent smokers; NON-AB = non-abstinent smokers; cig. = cigarette; within-S = within-subjects variable; between-S = between subjects variable; Se = session; Pos. = positive; Neg. = negative; significant effects reflect analyses in which the smoking Stroop effect is the dependent variable; * = smoking Stroop effect significantly different from zero; [#] = smoking Stroop effects are significantly different from zero; ≈ reflects estimates of smoking Stroop effects from figure or other data from published paper; Cards = neutral, smoking words presented on cards; Blocked = computerized presentation of neutral, smoking words in separate blocks; Mixed = computerized presentation of neutral, smoking words in a mixed randomized sequence; VR = verbal responses were used; MR = manual (button-press) responses were used.

underlying Stroop interference have remained unclear (Mogg & Bradley, 1998). For example, in the smoking Stroop task, smokers may be poor at naming the colors of smoking-related words because they experience conditioned responses to those cues. This may result in changes in affective and physical state that could compromise color-naming performance (see Mogg & Bradley, 1998, pp. 821–822). In addition, the smoking Stroop task cannot measure the allocation of visuo-spatial attention as the task-relevant and smoking material is generally presented together in a single integrated stimulus (e.g., a colored word).

Visual-Probe Task

Task Overview

Researchers have used a second task—the visual-probe task—to derive a more direct measure of the spatial allocation of visual attention (Mogg & Bradley, 1998). On each trial, a picture pair is briefly presented on a computer screen, with one picture on the left of the screen and the other on the right. On critical trials, one picture is smoking-related and the other is neutral. When the pictures disappear, a visual probe (e.g., a dot) is presented in the position formerly occupied by one of the pictures. In some studies, participants are required to indicate the location of the visual probe (left vs. right) as quickly and as accurately as possible. In others, they are required to indicate its identity (e.g., " : " vs. " . . "). Typically, individuals are faster to respond to probes that replace motivationally salient stimuli than neutral stimuli (the "vigilance" effect). This is consistent with a shift in attention toward these stimuli. A review of visual-probe studies is presented in Table 21.2.

Association with smoking status. With a presentation duration of 500 ms, the findings have been mixed. Two studies have reported significant differences in vigilance between smokers and nonsmokers (Ehrman et al., 2002, Exps. 1, 2), and one study reported a marginally significant difference (Hogarth, Mogg, et al., 2003, Exp. 2). Three studies, however, did not find significant differences between smokers as a whole and nonsmokers at this presentation duration (Bradley et al., 2003, Exps. 1, 2; Hogarth, Mogg, et al., 2003, Exp. 1). With a presentation duration of 2,000 ms, three studies have all reported significant differences between smokers and nonsmokers (Bradley et al., 2004; Bradley et al., 2003, Exp. 2; Field et al., 2004). One study reported a between-group difference in vigilance effects for a presentation duration of 200 ms (Bradley et al., 2004). The one study that compared vigilance effects of never-smokers and ex-smokers did not find a significant difference (Ehrman et al., 2002, Exp. 2).

Associations with CSD. No studies have reported a positive association between CSD and attentional bias on the visual-probe task. Indeed, three studies reported a significant negative association (Hogarth, Mogg, Bradley, et al., 2003, Exps. 1, 2; Waters, Shiffman, Bradley, et al., 2003).

Associations with clinical outcome. The one study that assessed the prospective relations between vigilance effects and cessation outcomes reported no significant associations (Waters, Shiffman, Bradley, et al., 2003).

Associations with self-reported craving. One study reported that there were no significant correlations between self-reported craving and vigilance on the visual-probe task (Mogg & Bradley, 2002). Another study (Waters, Shiffman, Bradley, et al., 2003) reported a modest but significant positive correlation between urge measured before task completion and the vigilance effect on the first half of the task. With a presentation duration of 2,000 ms, Mogg et al. (2003)

Table 21.2 Summary of Published Studies Using the Visual-Probe Task

Study	Participants	Mean Age	Presentation duration	Task	Independent variables	Vigilance effects	Significant effects	Correlational analyses
Mogg & Bradley (2002)	27 Smokers, complete AB, NON-AB sessions	33	500 ms	Location	Abstinence (within-S)	AB = 7 ms[#] NON-AB = 8 ms[#]		No correlation between vigilance and CSD, urge
Ehrman et al. (2002, Exp. 1)	7 Smokers 23 Nonsmokers	27 35	500 ms	Location	Smoking Status (Smokers vs. Nonsmokers)	Smokers = 23 ms* Nonsmokers = 7 ms*	Main Effect Smoking Status	
Ehrman et al. (2002, Exp. 2)	67 Smokers 16 EX 25 NEVER	37 37 23	500 ms	Location	Smoking Status (Smokers vs. EX vs. NEVER)	Smokers = 12 ms* EX = 9 ms* NEVER = 1 ms	Main Effect Smoking Status	
Bradley et al. (2003, Exp. 1)	9 Smokers HRQA+ 11 Smokers HRQA– 10 Nonsmokers	22 21	500 ms	Location	Group Status (HRQA+ vs. HRQA– vs. Nonsmokers)	HRQA+ Smokers = 13 ms* HRQA– Smokers = –3 ms Nonsmokers = –1 ms	Main Effect Group Status	
Bradley et al. (2003, Exp. 2)	10 Smokers HRQA+ 15 Smokers HRQA– 20 Nonsmokers	21 21	500 ms 2,000 ms	Location	Group Status (HRQA+ vs. HRQA– vs. Nonsmokers)	500 ms: HRQA+ = 34 ms* HRQA– = 1 ms Nonsmokers = 9 ms 2,000 ms: Smokers = 11 ms* Nonsmokers ≈ –12 ms	500 ms: Main Effect Group Status 2,000 ms: Main Effect Smoking Status	
Hogarth, Mogg, Bradley, et al. (2003, Exp. 1)	4 HEAVY (20 + cigs/day) 15 LIGHT (< 20 cigs/day) 10 Nonsmokers	24 21	500 ms	Location	Group Status (HEAVY vs. LIGHT vs. Nonsmokers)	HEAVY ≈ –3 ms LIGHT ≈ 15 ms* Nonsmokers = –1 ms	Main Effect Heaviness of Smoking	

(Continued)

Table 21.2 (Continued)

Study	Participants	Mean Age	Presentation duration	Task	Independent variables	Vigilance effects	Significant effects	Correlational analyses
Hogarth, Mogg, Bradley, et al. (2003, Exp. 2)	11 HEAVY (20 + cigs/day) 25 LIGHT (< 20 cigs/day) 24 Nonsmokers	22 22 22	500 ms	Location	Group Status (HEAVY vs. LIGHT – vs. Nonsmokers)	HEAVY ≈ 2 ms LIGHT ≈ 10 ms* Nonsmokers ≈ – 1 ms	Main Effect Heaviness of Smoking	
Waters, Shiffman, Bradley, et al. (2003, Exp. 1)	141 Smokers	38	500 ms	Location	Association With Relapse, Heaviness of Smoking	Smokers = 3 ms*		Vigilance does not predict 1-week lapse, time-to-first-lapse. Neg. correlation between CSD and vigilance ($r = -.21$)
Hogarth, Dickinson, et al. (2003)	28 Smokers	22	500 ms	Location	Stimulus that signals availability of smoking (S +) vs. signal that signals unavailability (S –)	Smokers = vigilance to S + ≈ 18 ms* in final test block		Vigilance to S + correlated with craving
Mogg et al. (2003)	20 Smokers 23 Nonsmokers	23 24	2,000 ms	Identity	Group Status (Smokers vs. Nonsmokers)	Smokers = 11 ms* Nonsmokers = – 5 ms	Main Effect Smoking Status	Correlation between craving and duration of initial fixation in smokers
Field et al. (2004)	23 Smokers, complete AB, NON-AB sessions	22	2,000 ms	Identity	Abstinence (within-S)	AB = 12 ms[#] NON-AB = 14 ms[#]		

Study	Participants	Mean Age	Presentation duration	Task	Independent variables	Vigilance effects	Significant effects	Correlational analyses
Bradley et al. (2004)	20 Smokers 23 Nonsmokers	24	17 ms (Sub.); 200 ms, 2,000 ms (Supra.)	Identity	Exposure (Supra. vs. Sub.) Smoking Status (Smokers vs. Nonsmokers)	Sub.: Smokers = 6 ms Nonsmokers = 3 ms Supra. (average 200, 2,000): Smokers = 18 ms* Nonsmokers = 0 ms	Supra.: Main Effect Smoking Status	

NOTE: Vigilance effects reflect faster responses to probes replacing smoking pictures. Larger (more positive) vigilance effects reflect greater attentional bias. Waters, Shiffman, Bradley, et al. (2003) administered the visual-probe task to smokers attending a research smoking cessation clinic roughly 2 weeks before their scheduled quit day. Participants in Bradley et al. (2004) completed a subliminal version. The pair of pictures was presented for 17 ms, followed by a pair of masks (jumbled pictures) for 68 ms (in the positions that had been occupied by the pictures). A probe (arrow pointing up or down) was then immediately presented in the position of one of the masks. The task was to indicate the identity of the probe. Participants subsequently completed an awareness check.

Key: Supra. = Supraliminal; Sub. = Subliminal; NEVER = never-smokers; EX = ex-smokers; AB = abstinent smokers; NON-AB = non-abstinent smokers; within-S = within-subjects variable; between-S = between subjects variable; HRQA+ = smokers with a history of multiple quit attempts; HRQA– = smokers with one or no previous quit attempts; * = vigilance effect significantly different from zero. # = mean of related vigilance effects are significantly different from zero; ≈ reflects estimates of vigilance effects from figure or other data from published paper; Location = participants indicate whether the probe appears on the left or right; Identity = participants indicate the identity of the probe. CSD = cigarettes smoked per day found a significant correlation between initial fixation durations and craving.

Effects of abstinence and perceived availability. No studies have documented significant effects of abstinence on vigilance (Field et al., 2004; Mogg & Bradley, 2002).

Other effects. Mogg et al. (2003) monitored the eye movements of participants as they performed the visual-probe task. Smokers had significantly longer initial fixation durations on smoking-related versus control pictures (409 ms vs. 369 ms, respectively), whereas nonsmokers did not (409 ms vs. 428 ms). Within smokers, longer initial fixation durations were associated with a greater urge to smoke. Field et al. (2004) reported that participants looked at the smoking pictures for 260 ms longer than the neutral pictures in the abstinent (AB) session, and 172 ms longer in the nonabstinent (NON-AB) session. The effect of abstinence was significant.

Hogarth, Dickinson, et al. (2003) conducted the only study in which a previously neutral stimulus—when paired with tobacco smoking—acquires the ability to attract attention. Smokers received discriminative training wherein an instrumental key-press response was followed by tobacco smoking when one visual discriminative stimulus was present (S +) but not when another stimulus was present (S –). In a subsequent test phase, S + and S – were presented in a visual-probe task. Participants showed significant vigilance to S + in the final test block. Vigilance to S + on the final test block was significantly correlated with the number of times S + had been paired with tobacco smoke reinforcement in training, and with craving.

Dual-Task Paradigm

Task Overview

Dual-task paradigms have been used by cognitive psychologists to identify the degree to which performance on a primary task draws on limited capacity processing resources. Participants are asked to perform one task (e.g., hold a cigarette or a neutral object) while also performing a second task (e.g., pressing a button as quickly as possible whenever an auditory tone is presented). Performance decrements on the second task (e.g., slower responses [RTs] to auditory tones) index the amount of cognitive resources allocated to the first task.

There are some important differences between the dual-task paradigm and the Stroop task. First, the dual-task paradigm utilizes real-world smoking cues (e.g., a cigarette) that may also be lit (thereby stimulating the olfactory system). In contrast, the smoking and neutral stimuli in the Stroop task are abstract linguistic representations of these cues. Second, in the Stroop task, the participant is explicitly instructed to concentrate on the color, and to try to ignore the words. The idea is that participants will differ in how much attention is involuntarily allocated to the smoking words (an automatic process). In the dual-task paradigm, participants are explicitly instructed to attend to the cigarette or neutral cues. Thus, participants may differ in how much attention they voluntarily chose to allocate to the smoking cue (a controlled process), in addition to differences in the involuntary allocation of attention. For an overview of dual-task studies, see Table 21.3.

Association with smoking status. When the primary task was to hold a cigarette, Baxter and Hinson (2001) reported that experienced smokers were significantly slower to respond to auditory beeps (vs. the baseline condition). Novice smokers, however, were also (nonsignificantly) slower.

Associations with CSD. When the primary task is to hold a cigarette, two studies have reported no association between heaviness of smoking and cue effects (Sayette et al., 2001; Waters, Shiffman, et al., 2004).

Table 21.3 Summary of Published Studies Using the Dual-Task Paradigm

Study	Participants	Mean Age	First task	Second task	Independent variables	Cue effect	Significant effects	Correlational analyses
Sayette & Hufford (1994, Exp. 1)	40 Smokers, completed AB, NON-AB sessions	21	Hold and attend to (1) cig., (2) roll of tape	RT	Cue Type (cig. vs. tape) Abstinence (within-S)	AB = 59 ms[#] NON-AB = 47 ms[#]		Urge correlated with RTs in AB, cig.-cue session
Sayette & Hufford (1994, Exp. 2)	31 Smokers, complete AB, NON-AB sessions	22	Hold and attend to (1) cig., (2) roll of tape	RT		AB = 44 ms[#] NCN-AB = 12 ms[#]		Urge correlated with RTs in AB, cig.-cue session
Juliano & Brandon (1998)	132 Smokers	33	RT	Passive Exposure to Smoking, Neutral stimuli (e.g., stapler)	Cue Type (cig. vs. neutral, between-S) Availability (Expect-YES vs. Expect-NO, between-S)	Expect-YES, Smoking = 2 ms; Expect-YES, Neutral = 0 ms; Expect-NO, Smoking = 35 ms*; Expect-NO, Neutral = – 6 ms	Availability by Cue Type interaction	Urge correlated with RTs in Expect-YES, cig.-cue participants
Sayette et al. (2001)	67 HEAVY(21 + cigs/day) 60 LIGHT (< 6 cigs/day)	25 24	Hold and attend to (1) cig., (2) roll of tape	RT	Cue Type (cig. vs. neutral, within-S) Abstinence (7-hr vs. NON-AB, between-S) Heaviness of Smoking	Smokers (averaged over all conditions) = 44 ms*		Urge correlated with RTs in AB, HEAVY condition
Baxter & Hinson (2001, Exp. 1)	55 EXPERIENCED Smokers; 12 NOVICE Smokers (< 100 cigs. in lifetime)	U/S	(1) "hold" a cig., (2) "smoke" a cig., (3) "pseudo-smoke," (4) baseline (no task)	RT	Cigarette Task, Smoking History	EXPERIENCED ≈ 5 ms slower on "smoke" vs. baseline; NOVICE ≈ 100 ms* slower on "smoke" vs. baseline	Group by Cig. Task interaction	

(Continued)

Table 21.3 (Continued)

Study	Participants	Mean Age	First task	Second task	Independent variables	Cue effect	Significant effects	Correlational analyses
Baxter & Hinson (2001, Exp. 2)	61 EXPERIENCED Smokers 16 NOVICE Smokers (< 100 cigs. in lifetime)	U/S	(1) "hold" a cig., (2) "smoke" a cig., (3) "pseudo-smoke," (4) baseline (no task)	RT	Cigarette Task, Smoking History	EXPERIENCED ≈ 5 ms faster on "smoke" vs. baseline; NOVICE ≈ 80 ms* slower on "smoke" vs. baseline	Group by Cig. Task Interaction	
Waters, Shiffman, Sayette, et al. (2004)	158 smokers	39	Hold and attend to a cig.	RT	Nicotine Replacement (NICOTINE vs. PLACEBO) Association With Relapse	NICOTINE = 35 ms* PLACEBO = 28 ms*		RTs did not predict cessation outcomes

NOTE: Cue effects reflect differences in RTs to auditory beeps during exposure to smoking versus control cues. (In Juliano & Brandon [1998] and Waters et al. [2004], cue effects reflect changes in RT from a pre-cue baseline.) Larger (more positive) cue effects reflect greater attentional bias. Juliano and Brandon (1998) randomly assigned 3-hour AB smokers to a condition in which they expected to smoke sometime within the next 20 minutes (Expect-YES) versus a condition in which they did not expect to smoke for the next 3 hours (Expect-NO). The primary task was to press a button as quickly as possible to a series of tones. During the exposure phase, half the participants were exposed to smoking stimuli, and the other half were exposed to neutral stimuli (a stapler, pen, and pencil). Unlike other studies, participants were not instructed to hold or to attend to the cues in this study.

Key: AB = abstinent smokers; NON-AB = non-abstinent smokers; Significant effects reflect analyses in which the cue effect is the dependent variable; * = cue effect significantly different from zero; ≈ = reflects estimate of cue effects from figure or other data in published paper. # = mean of related cue effects significantly different from zero;

Associations with clinical outcome. The one study that assessed the prospective relations between cue effects and cessation outcomes reported no significant associations (Waters, Shiffman, et al., 2004).

Associations with self-reported craving. There was a significant correlation between RTs and craving in the conditions where urge to smoke was strongest (Juliano & Brandon, 1998; Sayette & Hufford, 1994, Exps. 1, 2; Sayette et al., 2001).

Effects of deprivation and perceived availability. No studies have documented significant effects of abstinence on cue effects (Sayette & Hufford, 1994; Sayette et al., 2001; Sayette & Hufford, Exp. 2, did, however, report a marginal effect). The one study that manipulated availability reported that participants who did not expect to smoke soon (Expect-NO participants) exhibited cue effects (Juliano & Brandon, 1998).

Other effects. When the primary task was to smoke a cigarette, Baxter and Hinson (2001) reported that novice smokers were slower to respond to auditory beeps (vs. the baseline condition). In contrast, the response times of experienced smokers were not slower (vs. baseline condition). Although it is possible that nicotine's effects on cognitive performance may play a role, Baxter and Hinson interpreted the results as indicating that smoking is automatized in experienced smokers and therefore does not require attentional resources. In novice smokers, the act of smoking requires attentional resources. Both groups were slower to respond to the beeps when the primary task was to pseudo-smoke the cigarette.

Correlations Between Attentional Bias Measures

Mogg and Bradley (2002) reported that there were no significant correlations between vigilance on the visual-probe task and smoking Stroop effects.

Subliminal Attentional Bias Studies

No studies have reported significant effects of smoking status or abstinence on attentional bias measures from subliminal tasks (Bradley et al., 2004; Mogg & Bradley, 2002; Munafo et al., 2003).

Discussion of Attentional Bias Literature

Most studies have shown that smokers, but not nonsmokers, exhibit robust attentional bias (Tables 21.1 and 21.2). Perhaps the two most surprising findings to emerge from these studies are that (1) abstinence appears to have little impact on attentional bias, and (2) attentional bias does not appear to be strongly associated with heaviness of smoking. On the latter point, only one study with a relatively small sample size has reported a positive association between attentional bias and heaviness of smoking in adult smokers. This suggests that currently used measures of attentional bias may not be strongly tied to tobacco dependence. On the former point, it is possible that abstinent participants recognize that they are distracted by the smoking words during the modified Stroop task, and they therefore increase the amount of effortful processing or engage in other strategic processing to overcome the processing difficulties. This "strategic override" explanation is often cited when attentional biases are unexpectedly attenuated (Mogg & Bradley, 1998). The ability to override attentional biases for high-priority stimuli has been noted by Harris and Pashler (2004). They reported that participants are distracted by their own name, but only on the first occasion that it appeared. The same was true for emotional stimuli. It is also possible that the reaction time measures are not sufficiently sensitive to detect an effect of abstinence. In contrast, as noted above, eye-tracking data did reveal significant abstinence-related differences in overt attention to the smoking pictures (Field et al., 2004).

IMPLICIT ATTITUDES

A number of measures, including the Implicit Association Test (IAT) and the priming task, purport to assess automatic affective processes.

Implicit Association Test

Task Overview

The IAT is a widely used task for investigating associations in memory. The IAT consists of two tasks. In Task 1, participants are asked to respond rapidly with a specific key press to items representing two concepts (e.g., smoking + positive), and with a different key press to items from another two concepts (e.g., not smoking + negative). In Task 2, the assignments for half of each pair are switched (such that not smoking + positive share a response, likewise smoking + negative). The central idea behind the IAT is that it is easier to map two concepts onto a single response when those concepts are more strongly associated in memory than when the concepts are unrelated or dissimilar. The critical measure (the IAT effect) is the difference in response times on Task 1 compared with Task 2.

The IAT effect is an index of the relative strength of mental associations. In the example above (termed a valence IAT), it indicates whether mental associations are stronger between smoking and positive, and not smoking and negative, than between not smoking and positive, and smoking and negative. This IAT effect is described as an implicit attitude. When me and not me concepts are used (termed a self-identification IAT), the IAT effect is an implicit measure of

self-identification. A review of IAT literature is available in Table 21.4.

Associations with smoking status. There is evidence that smokers exhibit larger (i.e., less negative) IAT effects on both the valence IAT (Chassin et al., 2002; Sherman et al., 2003, Exp. 2; Swanson et al., 2001, Exp. 3) and the self-identification IAT (Swanson et al., 2001, Exps. 2, 3). The former effect may be dependent on the contrast category for smoking (Swanson et al., Exps. 1, 2).

Associations with CSD. There is evidence that IAT effects are associated with heaviness of smoking (Sherman et al. 2003, Exp. 2).

Associations with clinical outcomes and self-reported craving. No studies have examined associations between IAT effects and cessation outcomes or craving.

Effects of abstinence and perceived availability. One study found that abstinence did not significantly influence IAT effects (Sherman et al., 2003, Exp. 2).

Other effects. Sherman et al. (2003, Exp. 1) examined IAT effects as a function of smoking stimuli, which were (1) pictures highlighting the sensory aspects of smoking (e.g., a cigarette burning in an ashtray), or (2) pictures of cigarette packages and cartons, which highlight the costs of smoking (because of the warnings on those packets). There was no effect of stimulus type.

Stimulus Response Compatibility Task

The Stimulus Response Compatibility Task (SRC) is an alternative implicit measure of the motivational or affective valence of stimuli. In the SRC task, participants perform two tasks. In Assignment 1 (A1), participants are asked to move a mannequin

Table 21.4 Summary of Published Studies Using the Implicit Association Test (IAT)

Study	Participants	Mean Age	First dimension	Second dimension	Independent variables	IAT effect	Significant effects	Correlational analyses
Swanson et al. (2001, Exp. 1)	38 Smokers 46 Nonsmokers	U/S	Smoking-Exercise or Sweets	Pleasant-Unpleasant	Smoking Status (Smoker vs. Nonsmoker)	Smokers = − 300 ms* Nonsmokers = − 354 ms*		
Swanson et al. (2001, Exp. 2)	37 Smokers 59 Nonsmokers	U/S	Smoking-Stealing	(1) Pleasant-Unpleasant (2) Me-Not Me	Smoking Status (Smoker vs. Nonsmoker)	(1) Valence: Smokers = 173 ms* Nonsmokers = 137 ms* (2) Self-Identification: Smokers = 140 ms* Nonsmokers = 93 ms*	(2) Self-Identification: Main Effect Smoking Status	
Swanson et al. (2001, Exp. 3)	35 Smokers 41 Nonsmokers	U/S	Smoking-Not Smoking	(1) Pleasant-Unpleasant (2) Me-Not Me	Smoking Status (Smoker vs. Nonsmoker)	(1) Valence: Smokers = − 69 ms Nonsmokers = − 245 ms* (2) Self-Identification: Smokers = 125 ms* Nonsmokers = − 20 ms	(1) Valence: Main Effect Smoking Status (2) Self-Identification: Main Effect Smoking Status	
Chassin et al. (2002)	446 Adolescents, Parents	13 35	Smoking-Neutral Shapes	Good-Bad	Smoking Status Children's Smoking	Smoking Mothers = − 227 ms* Ex-Smoking Mothers = − 293 ms* Nonsmoking Mothers = − 299 ms* Smoking Fathers = − 175 ms* Ex-Smoking Fathers ≈ − 326 ms* Nonsmoking Fathers ≈ − 274 ms*	Mothers Main Effect Smoking Status; Mother × Father Smoking Status Interaction	Mothers' IAT effects predict children's ever smoking[a]

(Continued)

Table 21.4 (Continued)

Study	Participants	Mean Age	First dimension	Second dimension	Independent variables	IAT effect	Significant effects	Correlational analyses
Sherman et al. (2003, Exp. 1)	61 Smokers	19	Smoking-Babies/Cuddly Animals/Insects	Good-Bad	Stimulus Type (Sensory vs. Packaging Pictures)	Sensory Pictures = 13 ms Packaging Pictures = −11 ms		IAT effects not correlated with priming effects
Sherman et al. (2003, Exp. 2)	63 HEAVY (15 + cigs/day) 93 LIGHT (<15 cigs/day) 79 Nonsmokers	20	Smoking-Babies/Cuddly Animals/Insects (Sensory stimuli)	Good-Bad	Smoking Status (Smoker vs. Nonsmoker) Abstinence (between-S)	HEAVY, AB = 7 ms HEAVY, NON-AB = −22 ms LIGHT, AB = −45 ms LIGHT, NON-AB = −55 ms Nonsmokers = −104 ms*	Main Effect Heaviness of Smoking	IAT effects not correlated with priming effects

NOTE: IAT effect reflects difference in response times on trials when smoking is paired with good/pleasant/me versus trials where smoking is paired with bad/unpleasant/not me. Larger (more positive) IAT effects reflect more positive implicit attitudes (Valence IAT), or stronger implicit self-identification with smoking (Self-Identification IAT). In Swanson et al. (2001), Exp. 3, picture stimuli were used to capture the category of smoking (e.g., a man holding a cigarette), and the contrast category "nonsmoking" (same picture but with the smoking stimuli removed).

Key: AB = abstinent smokers; NON-AB = non-abstinent smokers; U/S = undergraduate students; Significant effects reflect analyses in which the IAT effect is the dependent variable; * = IAT effect significantly different from zero.

[a]When controlling for child age, family structure, parental education, and maternal smoking, paternal smoking and their interaction. Neither fathers' nor childrens' implicit attitudes significantly predicted children's smoking.

figure toward a smoking picture or away from a neutral picture. In Assignment 2 (A2), they are asked to move a mannequin figure away from a smoking picture or toward a neutral picture. The idea behind the SRC is that it is easier to categorize positive valenced stimuli if the appropriate categorization is an approach movement, whereas it is easier to categorize negatively valenced stimuli if the appropriate categorization is an avoidance movement. The critical measure (the SRC effect) is the difference in response times on A1 compared with A2. If smokers evaluate smoking-related pictures positively, they should be faster on A1 than A2. If so, they would exhibit a positive SRC effect. Conversely, if they evaluate smoking-related pictures negatively, they should be faster on A2 than A1. If so, they exhibit a negative SRC effect.

Two studies have used the SRC task. Mogg et al. (2003) administered the SRC task to smokers ($n = 20$) and nonsmokers ($n = 23$). On each trial, a picture (smoking or neutral) was presented in the center of the screen. A mannequin figure was presented above or below the picture. Participants made responses by pressing up and down buttons on the keyboard. These responses moved the mannequin up and down on the computer screen. The mannequin disappeared as soon as it reached the edge of the picture or screen, signaling the end of the response. Smokers and nonsmokers were both faster to respond on A1 than A2 (SRC effects = 153 ms, 47 ms for smokers, nonsmokers, respectively). The SRC effect of the smokers, however, was significantly larger than that of the nonsmokers. Bradley et al. (2004) administered the SRC task to nondeprived smokers ($n = 20$) and nonsmokers ($n = 20$). Smokers, but not nonsmokers, were faster to respond on A1 than A2 (SRC effect = 105 ms, 32 ms for smokers, nonsmokers,

respectively). The SRC effect of the smokers was significantly larger than that of the nonsmokers.

Priming Task

Priming tasks have been extensively used to assess implicit attitudes in the social psychology literature (Fazio & Olson, 2003). Only two experiments have used a priming task in tobacco addiction (Sherman et al., 2003, Exps. 1, 2). In Experiment 1, participants first completed a baseline phase in which a series of adjectives (e.g., fabulous, rotten) were shown on the screen. Their task was to categorize the adjectives as good or bad by pressing either a "GOOD" or "BAD" key on a response box as quickly and accurately as possible. In the subsequent priming phase, participants saw a picture (the "prime") for 315 ms, followed by an inter-stimulus interval of 135 ms, followed by a positive or negative adjective. The primes were smoking pictures (sensory vs. packaging stimuli as discussed earlier). Differences in response times on adjectives were computed between the primed and baseline conditions. This was done for both positive and negative adjectives. Priming scores were computed to indicate the degree to which the smoking primes facilitated responding on positive adjectives as opposed to negative adjectives. Higher (more positive) priming scores reflect relatively greater facilitation in responding to positive adjectives than negative adjectives (compared to their baselines). There was a significant main effect of prime type. Priming scores were positive to the sensory stimuli (priming = 27 ms) and negative to the packaging stimuli (priming = − 43 ms).

In Experiment 2, there was a significant interaction between heaviness of smoking (light vs. heavy) and abstinence (4 hours deprived vs. just smoked). The priming scores of light smokers were more positive in the NON-AB condition (priming = – 7 ms) versus the AB condition (priming = – 25 ms). In contrast, the priming scores of heavy smokers were more positive in the AB condition (priming = 7 ms) versus the NON-AB condition (priming = – 54 ms).

Correlations Between Implicit Attitude Measures

Sherman et al. (2003) reported that the priming and IAT effects were only weakly correlated both in Experiment 1 (rs ranged from – .11 to .11) and Experiment 2 (r = .04).

Discussion of Implicit Attitude Literature

There is good evidence that the measures derived from the IAT and SRC are associated with smoking status. For the IAT, there is also evidence that the implicit attitudes are associated with heaviness of smoking. Indeed, the evidence for this association appears to be stronger than that for the attentional bias tasks, although no study has directly compared the size of the associations. To the extent that the IAT measures automatic affective processes (e.g., implicit evaluations of the "goodness" or "badness" of smoking-related stimuli), it appears that smoking dependence is associated with an increasingly positive implicit (or less negative) evaluation of these stimuli.

It is puzzling that smokers exhibit generally negative implicit evaluations on the IAT but generally positive implicit evaluations on the SRC. The IAT may be more sensitive to cultural norms, and these norms may influence participants' responses on the IAT (Rudman, 2004). It is also possible that the SRC engages different psychological mechanisms, such as those relating to approach behavior. Given that no study has directly compared performance on the IAT

and SRC, however, it is difficult to draw strong conclusions.

IMPLICIT EXPECTANCIES

Expectancy Accessibility Task

Task Overview

Response times to endorse smoking outcome expectancies are measured. Two individuals may both endorse the same outcome expectancy (e.g., Smoking makes me . . . RELAXED), but they may differ in the time taken to endorse these outcomes. The response times may contain information about the accessibility of cognitive representations that may not be possible to assess using self-report measures.

Review of Expectancy Accessibility Tasks

Litz et al. (1987) administered an accessibility task to never-smokers (n = 29) and smokers (n = 24). Participants were required to make speeded endorsements to statements relating to (1) cigarette smoking, (2) automobile driving, and (3) skydiving. Targets were positive ("relaxing") and negative ("unhealthy") outcome expectations. Smokers and never-smokers did not differ in the number of endorsements or latencies of endorsements in the automobile driving and skydiving conditions. Smokers, however, endorsed more positive targets than never-smokers, and they also made these endorsements more quickly. Smokers and nonsmokers did not differ in the number of endorsements of negative targets, or the speed of those endorsements.

Fallon (1998) administered an accessibility task to never-smokers (n = 18, mean age = 31), long-term ex-smokers (n = 18, who had quit for more than 6 months, mean age = 34), recent ex-smokers (n = 18, who had quit within the last 6 months, mean age = 31), and current smokers (*n* = 18, mean age = 22). The groups did not differ in the number of endorsements or latencies of endorsements in the automobile driving and skydiving conditions. In the cigarette smoking condition, however, smokers endorsed more positive targets than long-term ex-smokers and never-smokers. Smokers were also quicker to endorse positive targets than never-smokers. Never-smokers endorsed more negative targets than smokers and recent ex-smokers.

Palfai (2002) administered the Expectancy Accessibility task to 64 smokers (mean age = 23), who were also hazardous drinkers. Participants were randomly assigned to an AB condition (no smoking within 6 hours of the study) or a NON-AB condition. Participants responded to positive outcome expectancies preceded by "Smoking makes me" or "Television makes me" (control condition). Expectancy accessibility scores were calculated as the time to endorse control expectancies minus time to endorse smoking expectancies. Expectancy accessibility scores were not significantly moderated by abstinence. The scores, however, were positively associated with (1) CSD (and nicotine dependence) and (2) cue-elicited urges to smoke.

Memory Association Studies

Task Overview

Participants are instructed to list all the positive and negative characteristics associated with smoking that come to mind. Generally, participants are given a brief period (< 5 min) to write down the characteristics.

Review of Memory Association Studies

Sayette and Hufford (1997) examined the effect of a smoking-urge manipulation. Smokers (N = 71, mean age = 21) were given 90 seconds to list (1) all the positive

characteristics of smoking that they could think of, and (2) all the negative characteristics of smoking that they could think of. The task was completed twice. Participants generated more positive characteristics on the "high-urge" session (participants were tested just after exposure to a cigarette cue while in a state of deprivation) versus a "low-urge" session (tested after exposure to a neutral cue while nondeprived). The number of negative characteristics generated was not significantly influenced by urge condition. Urge ratings were marginally correlated with the number of positive characteristics generated.

Leung and McCusker (1999) assessed a group of smokers (*n* = 20, mean age = 22) and nonsmokers (*n* = 58, mean age = 21). Participants were asked to write down as many adjectives as possible that were associated with (1) cigarette smoking, and (2) car driving. Smokers and nonsmokers did not differ in the number of positive and negative words they generated in the control condition, or the number of negative words generated in the smoking condition. Smokers, however, did generate more positive words than the nonsmokers in the smoking condition. Moreover, the ratio of positive to negative words generated by the smokers changed over time from 0.59 in the first half of the task to 0.23 in the second half. Among the nonsmokers, the ratio remained stable (0.14 to 0.22). Thus, smoking generally has negative rather than positive associations in both smokers and nonsmokers. Smokers, however, do have more positive associations with smoking than nonsmokers, and the positive associations are generated quickly by the smokers.

Sayette et al. (2001) administered the task to heavy smokers (*n* = 67, 21 + cigs/day) and light smokers (*n* = 60, < 6 cigs/day). There were no main effects of heaviness of smoking or abstinence. There was, however, a marginally significant heaviness of smoking by abstinence interaction. Abstinence increased generation of positive characteristics for heavy smokers, but tended to decrease it for light smokers.

Summary of Implicit Expectancy Studies

Associations With Smoking Status

There is good evidence that smokers endorse more positive outcomes than non-smokers, and that they do so more rapidly (Fallon, 1998; Litz et al., 1987). One study found that never-smokers endorsed more negative outcomes than smokers and recent ex-smokers. On the memory association task, one study showed that smokers generate more positive (but not negative) characteristics than nonsmokers (Leung & McCusker, 1999).

Associations With CSD

One study showed that expectancy accessibility is associated with CSD (Palfai, 2002). Another study showed that the generation of positive and negative associations is not significantly associated with heaviness of smoking (Sayette et al., 2001).

Effects of Deprivation and Perceived Availability

Abstinence did not significantly influence expectancy accessibility scores (Palfai, 2002) or the generation of positive or negative characteristics on the memory association test (Sayette et al., 2001).

Associations With Clinical Outcome

To the best of our knowledge, no published study has examined the relations between implicit expectancies and clinical outcomes.

Associations With Self-Reported Craving

One study showed that expectancy accessibility scores were associated with cue-provoked craving (Palfai, 2002). The one study that manipulated urge state as an independent variable (through a combination of deprivation and cue exposure) showed that urge condition was significantly associated with the generation of positive, but not negative, characteristics (Sayette & Hufford, 1997).

Probability Judgment Tasks

Task Overview

Participants are asked to estimate the probability that certain smoking outcomes would occur for them. While relying on self-report, these latter measures are nonetheless considered to be implicit measures of craving, because participants presumably are unaware when they perform these tasks that it is their urges that are being measured. Judging the probability of smoking outcomes is considered to be an implicit measure of craving in the same way, for instance, that judging the loudness of background noise is used as an implicit measure of affective valence (see Sayette, Martin, Hull, et al., 2003).

Review of Probability Judgment Tasks

Sayette et al. (2001) required AB and NON-AB smokers to estimate the probability of experiencing positive (e.g., "I enjoy the taste sensations while smoking.") and negative (e.g., "Smoking is taking years off my life.") outcomes using items selected from the Smoking Consequences Questionnaire (Copeland et al., 1995). There was a marginally significant effect of abstinence. In a second study, smokers experiencing a high urge (using methods described earlier) judged positive consequences to be significantly more probable, relative to negative ones, than did NON-AB smokers (Sayette et al., 2005). A limitation of this study is that it did not include a control condition (e.g., probability judgments for a nonsmoking activity).

Correlations Between Implicit Measures

No studies have examined correlations between the expectancy accessibility and memory association tasks.

Discussion of Implicit Expectancy Literature

Clearly, there are too few published studies to draw strong conclusions. The expectancy accessibility task appears to be promising in that the implicit expectancies are associated with heaviness of smoking and urge ratings during cue reactivity. An important limitation of the tasks presented in this section, however, should be noted. Although these tasks are used to assess implicit effects, their status as implicit measures is currently uncertain. For example, the memory association tasks described in this section (e.g., listing positive and negative characteristics of smoking) have not been validated as measures of implicit cognition in any literature. Similarly, the expectancy accessibility task has not been examined in basic memory research. In particular, both the memory association task and the expectancy accessibility tasks may encourage conscious recollection or self-reflection or other explicit memory processes. Despite these important caveats, we elected to include these studies because (1) they are often used to imply implicit effects, and (2) in some cases, the "implicit" measure predicts key external variables when controlling for self-report expectancies (e.g., Palfai, 2002). Further research is required to validate their status.

OTHER IMPLICIT MEASURES

Facial Coding Studies

Sayette and Hufford (1995) used the Facial Action Coding System (FACS) to code facial expressions to smoking cues related to affective experience (termed positive Action Units (AU +) and negative Action Units [AU −]). Smokers ($N = 40$, mean age = 21) were randomly assigned to an AB condition or a NON-AB condition. AUs were assessed during a 4-second period after the participant initially observed a cigarette, and during the interval between an instruction to put down the cigarette and the time it was extinguished. The procedure was also completed using a neutral cue (roll of tape). Across both periods, more participants exhibited an AU to the cigarette cue (69 percent) than to the tape (39 percent). AB smokers showed a marginally greater probability of exhibiting an AU (82 percent) than nondeprived smokers (55 percent). AUs were longer in duration during cigarette exposure than during control exposure. During the initial observation period, participants were significantly more likely to reveal AU + than AU −. More AB smokers than NON-AB smokers exhibited AU + during this period (53 percent vs. 35 percent, respectively). This difference, however, was not statistically significant. During the later observation period, participants were significantly more likely to reveal AU − than AU +.

Sayette, Wertz, Martin, et al. (2003) investigated the effects of abstinence and perceived opportunity to smoke on facial expressions. In Experiment 1 ($N = 253$, mean age = 25), AB smokers were more likely to exhibit AU + to the cigarette than NON-AB smokers (there was no effect of abstinence on AU + to the control cue). There was also a significant opportunity by time interaction. Participants who were told they could smoke "soon" (but not immediately) became less likely to exhibit AU +, and more likely to exhibit AU −, over time (relative to participants who were told they could not smoke during the study). In Experiment 2, after lighting a cigarette, AB smokers ($n = 57$, mean age = 20) were instructed that they could smoke in (1) 15 seconds, (2) 30 seconds, or (3) 60 seconds.

Participants in the 15-second group were more likely to exhibit an AU + than those in the 60-second group. Nearly 75 percent of the 15-second participants exhibited AU +, compared with 33 percent of the 60-second participants. Taken together, the data reported by Sayette, Wertz, Martin, et al. (2003) suggest that laboratory manipulations of cigarette availability may require minimal delay in order to elicit positive affect.

Startle-Probe Studies

Geier et al. (2000), in Experiment 1, reported that smoking cues influenced startle responses in smokers ($N = 54$) in a way that was similar to that of pleasant control pictures (i.e., reduced startles). The effects were not significantly moderated by abstinence, expectancy to smoke, or acute smoking. In Experiment 2, Geier et al. reported that smoking cues influenced startle responses of never-smokers ($N = 18$) in a way that was most similar to unpleasant pictures (i.e., increased startles). Taken together, the two experiments suggest that smoking status moderates startle responses to smoking pictures. However, Orain-Pelissolo et al. (2004) reported that smoking status (smokers vs. nonsmokers) did not significantly moderate startle responses on smoking and neutral pictures (no group by picture type interaction). In sum, the effects of smoking status on startle responses to neutral and smoking pictures remains unclear.

Other Studies

Using a Gernsbacher suppression task, Zwann and Truitt (2000) reported that smokers, but not nonsmokers, had difficulty in suppressing task-irrelevant smoking-related (but not neutral) information. Jarvik et al. (1995) found that AB smokers showed enhanced lexical access for smoking-related words (vs. neutral words) compared to NON-AB smokers.

GENERAL DISCUSSION

The relative dearth of papers makes it difficult to draw strong conclusions. Thus, we summarize our thoughts on themes that cut across the tasks presented.

Clinical Relevance of Implicit Measures

We continue to believe that the implicit measures can play a valuable role in evaluating the effects of smoking-cessation interventions. One study reported an association between attentional bias and cessation outcomes (Waters, Shiffman, Sayette, et al., 2003), even after controlling for urge. Attentional bias was a better predictor of outcome than other dependence-relevant measures. Attentional bias may therefore tap an important process mediating smoking relapse. Thus, a treatment that attenuates both attentional bias and craving might do better than a treatment that reduces only craving. Nonetheless, there were also some null associations between implicit measures and clinical outcomes (e.g., Waters, Shiffman, Bradley, et al., 2003). Thus, the clinical relevance of implicit measures in tobacco dependence remains uncertain.

Association Between Implicit Measures and Tobacco Dependence

Although most published studies in the literature have shown that implicit measures are associated with smoking status, there is only modest evidence that the implicit measures are related to tobacco dependence. In particular, attentional bias may not be as strongly tied to tobacco dependence as researchers might have hoped (though see the previous section, Clinical Relevance of Implicit Measures). The IAT and expectancy accessibility task have, however, shown promising associations with heaviness of smoking.

Lack of Effect of Acute Abstinence on Implicit Measures

Acute nicotine deprivation has large effects on self-reported craving and affect, as well as a range of other physiological, subjective, and performance measures. Yet it is striking that acute nicotine deprivation does not appear to have robust effects on implicit reaction time measures (modified Stroop task, visual-probe task, dual-task paradigm, IAT, expectancy accessibility task), the memory association task, or even psychophysiological responses (startles).

It is possible that the effects of deprivation on the reaction time measures are obscured by controlled processes (see earlier discussion on attentional bias). Effects of deprivation may be better revealed on measures that more cleanly tap automatic processes. Field et al. (2004) did indeed detect significant effects of abstinence on eye movement data (more time spent looking at the cigarette stimuli in abstinence), and Sherman et al. (2003) reported significant effects of deprivation on priming in heavy smokers (more positive priming effects in abstinence). In addition, Sayette, Wertz, Martin, et al. (2003) also detected significant effects on facial expressions (more AU + on the cigarette in abstinence). Speculatively, the effects of abstinence might be better revealed by measures that provide less opportunity for interference from controlled processing (e.g., automatized eye and facial movements). Finally, Powell et al. (2002) reported that abstinence did have robust effects on attentional bias to positively and negatively valenced stimuli. Abstinence may reduce motivational responses to nonsmoking-related reinforcers, rather than potentiate responses to smoking-related information. Further research should investigate this possibility.

Methodologically, if researchers are primarily interested in the effects of self-reported craving (rather than abstinence) on implicit measures, then a manipulation that combines abstinence with cigarette exposure may yield a more powerful manipulation of craving than a simple abstinence manipulation (Sayette & Hufford, 1997; Sayette et al., 2005). Future research can ascertain if a powerful craving manipulation influences implicit measures.

Measurement Issues

The application of psychometric principles is routine in many areas of psychology (e.g., clinical rating scales). There is, however, little discussion of psychometric issues in the implicit cognition and tobacco literature. The critical measure on most implicit tasks is a difference in reaction times between two conditions. Cognitive difference scores tend to show modest reliability (e.g., Parrott, 1991). For example, Fan et al. (2001) have developed an Attention Network Test that provides a separate measure for three attention networks. They reported that the reliability correlations for alerting and orienting networks were moderate to poor (.36 and .41, respectively; the reliability of the conflict network was good at .81). Kindt et al. (1996) showed that the modified Stroop task had poor test-retest reliability. Moreover, the card and computer formats of the tasks exhibited no convergent validity. A number of other studies have documented divergent effects with different formats of the Stroop task (cited in Waters et al., 2005). Kindt et al. (p. 660) conclude that "cognitive paradigms are not applicable to emotional research without psychometric data."

Given this context, it seems important that researchers should estimate and document the reliabilities of the implicit tasks. We do note that the IAT (which evolved from the social psychology literature) has generally exhibited very robust internal and test-retest reliability (Cunningham et al.,

2001). In our review, we report that the IAT exhibited robust associations with external variables, such as smoking status and heaviness of smoking. It is tempting to conclude that the construct assessed by the IAT is more germane to tobacco dependence than that assessed by attentional bias tasks. The better reliability of the IAT, however, may in part underlie its superior performance.

Lack of Association Between Implicit Measures

Correlations between implicit measures purporting to assess a similar construct have generally been nonsignificant in this literature (Mogg & Bradley, 2002; Sherman et al., 2003). This is consistent with what is known in the implicit attitude literature (Fazio & Olson, 2003), as well as the implicit memory and self-esteem literatures (Bosson et al., 2000; Buchner & Wippich, 2000). It is tempting to interpret the lack of association as demonstrating that the different implicit tasks measure different constructs. The lack of association may also, however, reflect the measurement error associated with the implicit measures (see above). Cunningham et al. (2001) used latent variable analysis and reported that association between implicit attitude measures improved substantially when separating measurement error from estimates of stability. This latent variable approach might be useful in examining the associations between implicit measures in tobacco addiction. However, even when accounting for measurement error, it may prove more difficult to find associations between implicit measures than between explicit measures. Simple self-perceptions are likely to underlie correlations between explicit, but not implicit, measures. Finally, researchers might also examine variables that moderate the associations between implicit measures. For example, Sayette, Martin, et al. (2003) reported that nicotine abstinence significantly moderated the correlations between disparate craving-related measures (the measures were more strongly intercorrelated when participants were abstinent vs. nonabstinent).

Repeated Measurement

It would be optimal to administer the implicit measures at multiple time-points within a clinical trial. The effects of repeated measurements on many of the measures, however, is not known. We do note that implicit measures are sometimes not stable even during a single test. Waters, Shiffman, Sayette, et al. (2003) reported that the smoking Stroop effect was maximal when the smoking words first appeared, and then declined (see also Harris & Pashler, 2004). Responses to smoking stimuli may be different when those stimuli first, unexpectedly, appear. Future research should examine the effects of expectedness and time.

Final Thoughts

Researchers use implicit measures in the belief that these measures may reveal dependence-relevant processes that cannot be obtained from self-report. As yet, however, there is only modest evidence that the implicit measures are related to those variables that are of most interest to tobacco researchers—acute deprivation, dependence, and cessation. This does not mean that the implicit measures do not hold a lot of promise. For example, a number of studies have reported that attentional bias to tobacco stimuli is associated with self-reported craving (Tables 21.1, 21.2, and 21.3; see also Field et al., Chapter 11), and, as noted earlier, there is preliminary evidence of an association with cessation outcomes. In sum, research on implicit cognition and tobacco addiction is in its infancy, and much more work is required to evaluate the utility of this research approach.

REFERENCES

Baker, T. B., Piper, M. E., McCarthy, D. E., Majeskie, M. R., & Fiore, M. C. (2004). Addiction motivation reformulated: An affective processing model of negative reinforcement. *Psychological Review, 111*, 33–51.

Baxter, B. W., & Hinson, R. E. (2001). Is smoking automatic? Demands of smoking behavior on attentional resources. *Journal of Abnormal Psychology, 110*, 59–66.

Bosson, J. K., Swann, W. B., & Pennebaker, J. W. (2000). Stalking the perfect measure of implicit self-esteem: The blind men and the elephant revisited? *Journal of Personality and Social Psychology, 79*, 631–643.

Bradley, B. P., Field, M., Mogg, K., & De Houwer, J. (2004). Attentional and evaluative biases for smoking cues in nicotine dependence: Component processes of biases in visual orienting. *Behavioral Pharmacology, 15*, 29–36.

Bradley, B. P., Mogg, K., Wright, T., & Field, M. (2003). Attentional bias in drug dependence: Vigilance for cigarette-related cues in smokers. *Psychology of Addictive Behaviors, 17*, 66–72.

Buchner, A., & Wippich, W. (2000). On the reliability of implicit and explicit memory measures. *Cognitive Psychology, 40*, 227–259.

Cepeda-Benito, A., & Tiffany, S. T. (1996). The use of a dual-task procedure for the assessment of cognitive effort associated with cigarette craving. *Psychopharmacology, 127*, 155–163.

Chassin, L., Presson, C., Rose, J., & Sherman, S. J. (2002). Parental smoking cessation and adolescent risk for smoking: Potential mediating mechanisms. *Journal of Pediatric Psychology, 27*, 485–496.

Copeland, A. L., Brandon, T. H., & Quinn, E. P. (1995). The Smoking Consequences Questionnaire-Adult: Measurement of smoking outcome expectancies of experienced smokers. *Psychological Assessment, 7*, 484–494.

Cunningham, W. A., Preacher, K. J., & Banaji, M. R. (2001). Implicit attitude measures: Consistency, stability, and convergent validity. *Psychological Science, 12*, 163–170.

Ehrman, R. N., Robbins, S. J., Bromwell, M. A., Lankford, M. E., Monterosso, J. R., & O'Brien, C. P. (2002). Comparing attentional bias to smoking cues in current smokers, former smokers, and non-smokers using a dot-probe task. *Drug and Alcohol Dependence, 67*, 185–191.

Fallon, B. M. (1998). To smoke or not to smoke: The role of schematic information processing. *Cognitive Therapy and Research, 22*, 517–530.

Fan, J., Wu, Y., Fossella, J. A., & Posner, M. I. (2001). Assessing the heritability of attentional networks. *BMC Neuroscience, 2*, 14.

Fazio, R. H., & Olson, M. A. (2003). Implicit measures in social cognition research: Their meaning and use. *Annual Review of Psychology, 54*, 297–327.

Field, M., Mogg, K., & Bradley, B. P. (2004). Eye movements to smoking-related cues: Effects of nicotine deprivation. *Psychopharmacology, 173*, 116–123.

Garvey, A. J., Bliss, R. E., Hitchcock, J. L., Heinold, J. W., & Rosner, B. (1992). Predictors of smoking relapse among self-quitters: A report from the normative aging study. *Addictive Behaviors, 17*, 367–377.

Geier, A., Mucha, R. F., & Pauli, P. (2000). Appetitive nature of drug cues confirmed with physiological measures in a model using pictures of smoking. *Psychopharmacology, 150*, 283–291.

Gross, T., Jarvik, M., & Rosenblatt, M. (1993). Nicotine abstinence produces content-specific Stroop interference. *Psychopharmacology, 110*, 333–336.

Harris, C. R., & Pashler, H. E. (2004). Attention and the processing of emotional words and names. *Psychological Science, 15,* 171–178.

Heishman, S. J., Taylor, R. C., & Henningfield, J. E. (1994). Nicotine and smoking: A review of effects on human performance. *Experimental & Clinical Psychopharmacology, 2,* 345–395.

Hogarth, L. C., Dickinson, A., & Duka, T. (2003). Discriminative stimuli that control instrumental tobacco-seeking by human smokers also command selective attention. *Psychopharmacology, 168,* 435–445.

Hogarth, L. C., Mogg, K., Bradley, B. P., Duka, T., & Dickinson, A. (2003). Attentional orienting towards smoking-related stimuli. *Behavioral Pharmacology, 14,* 153–160.

Hughes, J. R., Gulliver, S. B., Fenwick, J. W., Valliere, W., Cruser, K., Pepper, S., et al. (1992). Smoking cessation among self-quitters. *Health Psychology, 11,* 331–334.

Jarvik, M. E., Gross, T. M., Rosenblatt, M. R., & Stein, R. E. (1995). Enhanced processing of smoking stimuli during smoking abstinence. *Psychopharmacology, 118,* 136–141.

Johnsen, B. H., Thayer, J. F., Laberg, J. C., & Ashjornsen, A. E. (1997). Attentional bias in active smokers, abstinent smokers, and nonsmokers. *Addictive Behaviors, 22,* 813–817.

Jorenby, D. E., Leischow, S. J., Nides, M. A., Rennard, S. I., Johnston, J. A., Hughes, A. R., et al. (1999). A controlled trial of sustained-release bupropion, a nicotine patch, or both for smoking cessation. *New England Journal of Medicine, 340,* 685–691.

Juliano, L. M., & Brandon, T. H. (1998). Reactivity to instructed smoking availability and environmental cues: Evidence with urge and reaction time. *Experimental & Clinical Psychopharmacology, 6,* 45–53.

Kindt, M., Bierman, D., & Brosschot, J. F. (1996). Stroop versus Stroop: Comparison of a card format and a single-trial format of the standard color-word Stroop task and the emotional Stroop task. *Personality and Individual Differences, 21,* 653–661.

Leung, K. S., & McCusker, C. G. (1999). Accessibility and availability of smoking-related associations in smokers. *Addiction Research, 7,* 213–226.

Litz, B. T., Payne, T. J., & Colletti, G. (1987). Schematic processing of smoking information by smokers and never-smokers. *Cognitive Therapy and Research, 11*(3), 301–313.

Mogg, K., & Bradley, B. P. (1998). A cognitive-motivational analysis of anxiety. *Behaviour Research and Therapy, 36,* 809–848.

Mogg, K., & Bradley, B. P. (2002). Selective processing of smoking-related cues in smokers: Manipulation of deprivation level and comparison of three measures of attentional bias. *Journal of Psychopharmacology, 16,* 385–392.

Mogg, K., Bradley, B. P., Field, M., & De Houwer, J. (2003). Eye movements to smoking-related pictures in smokers: Relationship between attentional biases and implicit and explicit measures of stimulus valence. *Addiction, 98,* 825–836.

Munafo, M., Mogg, K., Roberts, S., Bradley, B. P., & Murphy, M. (2003). Selective processing of smoking-related cues in current smokers, ex-smokers and never-smokers on the modified Stroop task. *Journal of Psychopharmacology, 17,* 310–316.

Orain-Pelissolo, S., Grillon, C., Perez-Diaz, F., & Jouvent, R. (2004). Lack of startle modulation by smoking cues in smokers. *Psychopharmacology, 173,* 160–166.

Palfai, T. P. (2002). Positive outcome expectancies and smoking behavior: The role of expectancy accessibility. *Cognitive Research and Therapy, 26,* 317–333.

Parrott, A. W. (1991). Performance tests in human psychopharmacology (1): Test reliability and standardization. *Human Psychopharmacology, 6,* 1–9.

Patten, C. A., & Martin, J. E. (1996). Does nicotine withdrawal affect smoking cessation? Clinical and theoretical issues. *Annals of Behavioral Medicine, 18,* 190–200.

Powell, J., Dawkins, L., & Davis, R. E. (2002). Smoking, reward responsiveness, and response inhibition: Tests of an incentive motivational model. *Biological Psychiatry, 51,* 151–163.

Powell, J., Tait, S., & Lessiter, J. (2002). Cigarette smoking and attention to signals of reward and threat in the Stroop paradigm. *Addiction, 97,* 1163–1170.

Robinson, T. E., & Berridge, K. C. (1993). The neural basis of craving: An incentive-sensitization theory of addiction. *Brain Research Review, 18,* 247–291.

Rudman, L. A. (2004). Sources of implicit attitudes. *Current Directions in Psychological Science, 13,* 79–82.

Rusted, J. M., Caulfield, D., King, L., & Goode, A. (2000). Moving out of the laboratory: Does nicotine improve everyday attention? *Behavioural Pharmacology, 11,* 621–629.

Sayette, M. A., & Hufford, M. R. (1994). Effects of cue exposure and deprivation on cognitive resources in smokers. *Journal of Abnormal Psychology, 103,* 812–818.

Sayette, M. A., & Hufford, M. R. (1995). Urge and affect: A facial coding analysis of smokers. *Experimental & Clinical Psychopharmacology, 3,* 417–423.

Sayette, M. A., & Hufford, M. R. (1997). Effects of smoking urge on generation of smoking-related information. *Journal of Applied Social Psychology, 27,* 1395–1405.

Sayette, M. A., Loewenstein, G., Kirchner, T. R., & Travis, T. (2005). Effects of smoking urge on temporal cognition. *Psychology of Addictive Behaviors, 19,* 88–93.

Sayette, M. A., Martin, C. S., Hull, J. G., Wertz, J. M., & Perrott, M. A. (2003). The effects of nicotine deprivation on craving response covariation in smokers. *Journal of Abnormal Psychology, 112,* 110–118.

Sayette, M. A., Martin, C. S., Wertz, J. M., Shiffman, S., & Perrott, M. A. (2001). A multidimensional analysis of cue-elicited craving in heavy smokers and tobacco chippers. *Addiction, 96,* 1419–1432.

Sayette, M. A., Shiffman, S., Tiffany, S. T., Niaura, R. S., Martin, C. S., & Shadel, W. G. (2000). The measurement of drug craving. *Addiction, 95,* S189–S210.

Sayette, M. A., Wertz, J. M., Martin, C. S., Cohn, J. F., Perrott, M. A., & Hobel, J. (2003). Effects of smoking opportunity on cue-elicited urge: A facial coding analysis. *Experimental & Clinical Psychopharmacology, 11,* 218–227.

Schneider, W., & Shiffrin, R. M. (1977). Controlled and automatic human information processing: I. Detection, search, and attention. *Psychological Review, 84*(1), 1–66.

Sherman, S. J., Rose, J. S., & Koch, K. (2003). Implicit and explicit attitudes toward cigarette smoking: The effects of context and motivation. *Journal of Social & Clinical Psychology, 22,* 13–39.

Sherwood, N. (1993). Effects of nicotine on human psychomotor performance. *Human Psychopharmacology: Clinical and Experimental, 8:* 155–184.

Shiffman, S., Engberg, J., Paty, J. A., Perz, W. G., Gnys, M., Kassel, J. D., et al. (1997). A day at a time: Predicting smoking lapse from daily urge. *Journal of Abnormal Psychology, 106*(1), 104–116.

Shiffman, S., Gwaltney, C. J., Balabanis, M. H., Liu, K. S., Paty, J. A., Kassel, J. D., et al. (2002) Immediate antecedents of cigarette smoking: An analysis from ecological momentary assessment. *Journal of Abnormal Psychology, 111*(4), 531–545.

Shiffman, S., Paty, J. A., Gnys, M., Kassel, J. A., & Hickcox, M. (1996). First lapses to smoking: Within-subjects analysis of real-time reports. *Journal of Consulting and Clinical Psychology, 64*(2), 366–379.

Shiffman, S., & Waters, A. J. (2004). Negative affect and smoking lapses: A prospective analysis. *Journal of Consulting and Clinical Psychology, 7*, 192–201.

Silagy, C., Mant, D., Fowler, G., & Lancaster, T. (2000). Nicotine replacement therapy for smoking cessation. *Cochrane Database System Review, 2*, CD000146. Oxford, UK: Update Software Ltd.

Stacy, A. W. (1997). Memory activation and expectancy as prospective predictors of alcohol and marijuana use. *Journal of Abnormal Psychology, 106*, 61–73.

Stewart, J., de Wit, H., & Eikelbloom, R. (1984). Role of unconditioned and conditioned drug effects in self-administration of opiates and stimulants. *Psychological Review, 91*, 251–268.

Swanson, J. E., Rudman, L. A., & Greenwald, A. G. (2001). Using the Implicit Association Test to investigate attitude-behaviour consistency for stigmatized behaviour. *Cognition & Emotion, 15*, 207–230.

Tiffany, S. T. (1990). A cognitive model of drug urges and drug-use behavior: Role of automatic and nonautomatic processes. *Psychological Review, 97*, 147–168.

Toates, F. (1986). Motivational systems. Cambridge, UK: Cambridge University Press.

U.S. Department of Health and Human Services. (1990). The health benefits of smoking cessation. A report to the Surgeon General. Washington, DC: Government Printing Office.

Waters, A. J., & Feyerabend, C. (2000). Determinants and effects of attentional bias in smokers. *Psychology of Addictive Behaviors, 14*(2), 111–120.

Waters, A. J., Sayette, M., Franken, I., & Schwartz, J. (2005). Generalizability of carry-over effects in the emotional Stroop task. *Behavior Research and Therapy, 43*, 715–732.

Waters, A. J., Sayette, M., & Wertz, J. (2003). Carry-over effects can modulate emotional Stroop effects. *Cognition & Emotion, 17*, 501–509.

Waters, A. J., Shiffman, S., Bradley, B. P., & Mogg, K. (2003). Attentional shifts to smoking cues in smokers. *Addiction, 98*, 1409–1417.

Waters, A. J., Shiffman, S., Sayette, M. A., Paty, J. A., Gwaltney, C. G., & Balabanis, M. H. (2003). Attentional bias predicts outcome in smoking cessation. *Health Psychology, 22*, 378–387.

Waters, A. J, Shiffman, S., Sayette, M. A., Paty, J. A., Gwaltney, C., & Balabanis, M. (2004). Cue provoked craving and nicotine replacement therapy in smoking cessation. *Journal of Consulting and Clinical Psychology, 72*, 1136–1143.

Wertz, J. M., & Sayette, M. A. (2001). Effects of smoking opportunity on attentional bias in smokers. *Psychology of Addictive Behaviors, 15*, 268–271.

Zack, M., Belsito, L., Scher, R., Eissenberg, T., & Corrigall, W. A. (2001). Effects of abstinence and smoking on information processing in adolescent smokers. *Psychopharmacology, 153*, 249–257.

Zwann, R. A., Stanfield, R. A., & Madden, C. J. (2000). How persistent is the effect of smoking urges on cognitive performance? *Experimental & Clinical Psychopharmacology, 8*, 518–523.

Zwann, R. A., & Truitt, T. P. (2000). Inhibition of smoking-related information in smokers and nonsmokers. *Experimental & Clinical Psychopharmacology, 8*, 192–197.

CHAPTER 22

To Drink or Not to Drink: The Role of Automatic and Controlled Cognitive Processes in the Etiology of Alcohol-Related Problems

REINOUT W. WIERS, KATRIJN HOUBEN, FREN T. Y. SMULDERS, PATRICIA J. CONROD, AND BARRY T. JONES

Abstract: Explicit measures revealed three basic types of alcohol-related cognitions: positive reinforcement, negative reinforcement (relief), and negative expectancies. Using the same typology, we review studies assessing alcohol-related cognitions with implicit measures. Most research focused on automatic appetitive responses (positive reinforcement). The common model is that an automatic appetitive response tendency can be inhibited by more controlled inhibitory processes. In addition, there is scattered evidence indicating a role for automatic aversive responses to alcohol. Negative reinforcement appears to be more difficult to assess with tests involving single associations. It is argued that the reason is that for negative reinforcement two associations are needed (negative affect < > alcohol < > positive affect). Findings are integrated into a model from which suggestions for interventions are given.

Studies investigating alcohol-related cognitions with explicit measures have identified three basic types of alcohol-related cognitions: positive reinforcement (e.g., fun), negative reinforcement (relief from negative affect), and negative expectancies (negative outcomes of drinking). The first two variables have been documented as positive predictors of prospective drinking, and the last as a negative predictor of

AUTHOR'S NOTE: The first author is funded by "VIDI" grant 452.02.005, from the Dutch National Science Foundation (N.W.O.). The authors wish to thank Brian Ostafin, Tibor Palfai, Sherry Stewart, Werner Stritzke, Andrew Waters, and Martin Zack for helpful comments on the manuscript.

prospective drinking that could be related to motivation to cut down drinking (e.g., If I continue drinking like this, I'll lose my job). In this chapter, we will review the recent literature using implicit or indirect measures (see De Houwer, Chapter 2) to assess alcohol-related cognitions using this typology. Central questions are:

1. Are the same three types of cognitions found in research using implicit measures?

2. Do implicit and explicit cognitions predict unique variance in drinking behavior and/or unique aspects of drinking behavior?

3. Do implicit and explicit alcohol-related cognitions relate to different or to the same underlying processes?

4. How do individual differences in personality relate to the development of implicit and explicit alcohol-related cognitions?

A model is presented that integrates the findings, followed by implications for interventions. First, we discuss some issues that emerged from alcohol research using explicit measures, relevant for the discussion of the findings with more implicit measures.

EXPLICIT ALCOHOL-RELATED COGNITIONS

The explicit assessment of alcohol-related cognitions has been undertaken from a variety of different theoretical frameworks. Most dominant has been the expectancy framework, proposed by Goldman and colleagues (e.g., Brown et al., 1980; Goldman et al., 1999). Other influential frameworks have been social learning theory (Bandura, 1977), cognitive behavioral therapy (e.g., Beck et al., 1993; Marlatt & Gordon, 1985), the theories of reasoned action and planned behavior (Ajzen, 1988; Fishbein & Ajzen, 1975), and motivational theories (Cooper et al., 1995; Cox & Klinger, 1988). Despite differences in the exact definitions of alcohol-related cognitions in these frameworks, some general issues emerged.

The first general issue concerns whether assessment should be unipolar or bipolar. In the attitude literature, *bipolar* assessment is common. An example is:

(E1.) Drinking alcohol is:
good ——————————— bad.

The underlying assumption of bipolar assessment is that the endpoints are opposites (correlated − 1), which, in case of attitudes, could reflect a natural tendency to classify something as either positive or as negative and not both at the same time (e.g., Russell & Carroll, 1999). This view has been challenged, because people have been found to be ambivalent about some attitude objects, with alcohol being a prime example (e.g., Conner & Sparks, 2002; note that ambivalence is at the heart of some addiction theories, e.g., Orford, 2001). In expectancy research, *unipolar* measures were found to better predict alcohol use than bipolar measures (Leigh, 1989). It has become standard practice to use *unipolar* response scales including both positive and negative expectancies (Fromme et al., 1993; Leigh & Stacy, 1993; Wiers et al., 1997). An example item:

(E2.) After a few drinks I feel good
disagree ——————————— agree.

It should be noted that a bipolar view on emotional valence and the finding that alcohol-related cognitions are best measured in a unipolar way are not necessarily incompatible: The time frame of negative and positive expectancies is different, with negative expectancies referring to more distal events (Dunn & Earleywine, 2001; Goldman et al.,

1999; Jones & McMahon, 1994), and higher dosages of alcohol (Fromme et al., 1993; Wiers et al., 1997). Hence, even though the uni- or bipolar nature of affect remains controversial (Cacioppo & Berntson, 1994; Russell & Carroll, 1999), it is clear that people hold both positive and negative alcohol-related cognitions, with the positive cognitions usually relating to immediate and negative cognitions to later outcomes.

The second issue concerns how many specific factors or dimensions are needed to represent alcohol-related cognitions. In the attitude literature, typically only positive and negative cognitions are assessed, whereas in the expectancy and motivation literature more specific factors have been proposed (e.g., Brown et al., 1980; Cooper, 1994). For positive expectancies, Leigh and Stacy (1993) and Goldman et al. (1997) showed that specific first-order expectancy factors (e.g., sexual and social enhancement) increased the prediction of alcohol use above the general higher-order factor(s). This suggests that it is useful to assess alcohol-related cognitions in more detail than general positive and negative factors only.

An important distinction in the expectancy and motivation literature concerns positive versus negative reinforcement, where the difference involves the emotional antecedent of drinking: positive or negative mood, respectively (e.g., Cooper, 1994). The literature on negative reinforcement motivations has indicated that negative reinforcement (or coping) motivations are strong positive predictors of alcohol problems (e.g., Cooper et al., 1995; Stewart et al., 2002). These findings may reflect the "clinical wisdom" that alcohol use often becomes problematic once individuals begin to drink to escape problems, which results in more negative affect in the long run (Sher, 1991).

With respect to the third type of alcohol cognitions, negative expectancies are usually found to be negatively correlated with current drinking in cross-sectional research in social drinkers (e.g., Goldman et al., 1999; Wiers et al., 1997). Jones and McMahon (1994) have found that negative expectancies predict success of abstinence of alcoholics in treatment. From this perspective, negative expectancies develop with negative experiences and should be *positively* correlated with (negative) prior drinking experience. Still, they should negatively predict (future) drinking and should be related to motivation to change behavior (Jones & McMahon, 1998). Recently, it has been shown that it is useful to assess motivations for refraining from drinking next to motivations to use alcohol (like negative expectancies, McEvoy et al., 2004). Finally, it may be useful to assess motivation for alternative behaviors from drinking (see Cox et al., Chapter 17).

In expectancy research, Goldman and colleagues have investigated the underlying memory structure of expectancies using multidimensional scaling (MDS; Goldman et al., 1999; Rather et al., 1992). A two-dimensional structure was selected reflecting two orthogonal dimensions: valence (positive vs. negative) and arousal (arousal vs. sedation). Goldman et al. (1999) observed that these dimensions also underlie affective processing, and that many expectancies can be regarded as anticipated changes in affect. Mapping of subgroups of drinkers into the two-dimensional, valence-arousal space, showed that all drinkers were on the positive side, and that the more people drink, the higher they score on the arousal dimension (Goldman et al., 1999). In a recent paper, Goldman and Darkes (2004) argued that specific expectancy factors can all be conceptualized as unique positions in the two-dimensional, valence-arousal space. A problem with this notion is the location of negative reinforcement as positive sedation, which is associated with *light* rather than with *heavy* drinking, whereas negative reinforcement motives are predictors of problem drinking. In conclusion, more factors or dimensions are needed than valence alone to represent alcohol-related cognitions, but the exact number of factors needed is an issue of debate.

Third, a general concern about the explicit assessment of alcohol-related cognitions and the prediction of drinking concerns criterion contamination (Stewart & Devine, 2000; cf. Darkes et al., 1998). When people drink a lot, they are likely to respond positively to general items like "I drink because it's fun" (Cooper, 1994). This may assess self-justifications rather than specific alcohol cognitions. In line with this concern, the predictive power of explicit alcohol cognitions decreases markedly after controlling for previous use (e.g., Jones et al., 2001; Sher et al., 1996).

In summary, there is broad agreement that there are three types of explicit alcohol-related cognitions: positive and negative reinforcement and negative cognitions, and they have been related to the two-dimensional structure of emotions (valence and arousal). This typology is used to review the literature on implicit alcohol-related cognitions.

IMPLICIT ALCOHOL-RELATED COGNITIONS

Implicit Cognition, Positive Reinforcement, and Incentive Salience

Most research using implicit measures to study alcohol-related cognitions also focused on positive reinforcement: attentional bias for alcohol-related cues (e.g., Bruce & Jones, Chapter 10; Jones et al., 2002), memory associations of alcohol with positive outcomes (e.g., Stacy, 1997; Stacy et al., Chapter 6), with positive reinforcement (e.g., Kramer & Goldman, 2003), with positive arousal (e.g., Wiers, Van Woerden, et al., 2002), and with approach action tendencies (e.g., Palfai

& Ostafin, 2003a). Findings have generally been linked to neurobiological models emphasizing incentive motivation or positive reinforcement accounts of the development and maintenance of addictive behaviors (e.g., Robinson & Berridge, 1993, 2003; Stewart et al., 1984; Wise & Bozarth, 1987). Findings regarding an attentional bias for alcohol are reviewed in other chapters (Bruce & Jones, Chapter 10; Field et al., Chapter 11); here we focus on findings regarding implicit alcohol associations.

Stacy and colleagues propose that alcohol-related associations represented in memory (e.g., positive affective outcomes related to alcohol use) can elicit a relatively automatic influence over alcohol and drug use. In a series of studies, using a variety of tests (see Stacy et al., Chapter 6), they found that the number of alcohol-related responses was predictive of higher levels of alcohol use, and this finding replicated across different measures, different populations, and different drugs of abuse (e.g., Ames & Stacy, 1998; Stacy, 1995). Importantly, Stacy (1997) demonstrated that memory associations were the strongest predictor of prospective drinking, which remained the case after controlling for earlier use, explicit measures, and personality and background variables. Hence, this line of research has demonstrated that first associations represent unique information not captured by explicit measures. In view of the research on explicit cognitions, it is noteworthy that almost all studies in this line of research have focused on *global* positive associations without differentiating more specific outcomes (e.g., positive vs. negative reinforcement). A reason may be statistical power: Many participants are already needed for global positive outcomes and many more might be needed to discern specific positive outcomes.

Recently, a variety of reaction-time paradigms have been used to assess alcohol-related cognitions, and this has been done in more dimensions than global positive only. In our own research, we have used adapted versions of the Implicit Association Test (IAT; Greenwald et al., 1998; also see Houben et al., Chapter 7) to assess alcohol associations in the two affective dimensions that were found in MDS alcohol and emotion research: valence and arousal. In a series of studies, we found that heavy drinkers associated alcoholic drinks more strongly with arousal than with sedation (as compared with sodas, Wiers, Ganushchack, et al., 2003; Wiers, Van de Luitgaarden, et al., 2005; Wiers, Van Woerden, et al., 2002). Alcohol-arousal associations were also found in alcoholics (De Houwer et al., 2004), and light drinkers were not found to hold implicit alcohol-arousal associations (Wiers, Van Woerden, et al., 2002). On the valence dimension, all of these studies found stronger negative than positive associations for alcohol as compared with soda both for light and for heavy drinkers (in contrast with explicit positive expectancies in earlier and in the same studies). To the extent that these negative associations are "real" and not an artifact of the IAT procedure (see Houben et al., Chapter 7), we argued that this pattern of results resembles the dissociation between "wanting" and "liking" proposed by Robinson and Berridge (1993, 2003). On the basis of animal research, they distinguish between two neural processes underlying natural rewards and drug responses: "wanting" and "liking," with "liking" being an important factor in early use, and "wanting" taking over once sensitization has developed. Sensitization refers to increased psychomotor activation directly and increased incentive motivation after repeated use. Importantly, "wanting" (the activation of incentive-salience) can occur in the absence of "liking." This dissociation may reflect an important feature of addiction; that compulsive use may continue in the presence of negative effects for the individual and in the absence of pleasure

(Berridge & Robinson, Chapter 31; Robinson & Berridge, 1993, 2003).

We argued that the implicit arousal associations could be related either to the motivation to approach alcohol (an appetitive response, triggered by alcohol-related stimuli), or could represent a sensitized psychomotor stimulant reaction after drinking alcohol. In two recent studies, we tested these hypotheses. In the first, we found support for the first hypothesis: Implicit arousal associations (assessed with two different tests) predicted individual differences in subjective cue-induced craving assessed 6 weeks later, after controlling for background variables, habitual drinking, and memory associations assessed at the time of the cue-induced craving manipulation (Wiers, Granzier, et al., 2005). In the second study (Van den Wildenberg et al., 2004), we tested whether implicit arousal associations in heavy drinkers were correlated with heart-rate increase following rapid consumption of approximately five alcoholic drinks (a measure of sensitivity to the stimulant properties of alcohol; Conrod et al., 2001), but this was not confirmed. A caveat was the low proportion of participants with a positive family history of alcoholism, for whom the heart-rate increase is strongest (Conrod et al., 2001).

Palfai and Ostafin (2003a; Ostafin et al., 2003) assessed the automatic activation of approach versus avoidance tendencies for alcohol in hazardous drinkers. This is a somewhat different approach, because it does not focus on the appraisal side of the emotion process, but on action tendencies (e.g., Frijda, 1986). Emotionally relevant cues can automatically trigger an action tendency, either toward the cue (approach) or away from the cue (avoidance). In one study, an adapted version of the IAT was used (Palfai & Ostafin, 2003a). Categories used were alcohol versus electricity (irrelevant contrast) combined with approach versus avoidance. Alcohol-approach associations correlated with the frequency of binge drinking and with the number of drinks per occasion. After the assessment of the IAT and questionnaire, participants were subjected to a cue-exposure procedure. IAT approach associations were correlated with urge to drink after exposure to alcohol, but not to urge to drink at baseline. Further, after controlling for baseline responses, it was found that those who scored higher on the approach IAT, exhibited stronger urge and arousal reactivity (no reactivity for valence). These findings suggest that the approach associations in this study are closely related to the arousal associations in our own work. In a recent study (Wiers, Both, et al., 2005), we assessed both valence and arousal associations and approach-avoidance associations and found that approach avoidance associations were positively correlated with positive valence and with arousal (in the absence of a correlation between valence and arousal). This suggests that approach associations are related to positive arousal associations.

The research on implicit alcohol associations presented so far has used bipolar attribute dimensions, which is at odds with the findings in the explicit literature that suggest that unipolar assessment is superior in the assessment of alcohol-related explicit cognitions (Leigh, 1989), but consistent with a bipolar view on instantaneous affect (e.g., Russell & Carroll, 1999). Given biological research that has indicated the presence of separate neural systems for approach and avoidance (e.g., Gray, 1990; Lang, 1995), it may be useful to assess implicit alcohol associations in a unipolar manner too. This has been done in a number of recent studies. Jajodia and Earleywine (2003) separately assessed positive and negative associations (against different neutral categories) using an adapted IAT and found both positive and negative associations for alcohol. Positive but not negative associations predicted unique

variance in alcohol use, but this finding has to be qualified for two reasons: Positive associations were always assessed first (and IAT effects get smaller with practice; see Wiers, Van de Luitgaarden, et al., 2005) and in the regression analysis positive associations were entered first. Houben and Wiers (2004) assessed positive, negative, arousal, and sedation associations in a series of (counterbalanced) unipolar IATs. We found the strongest effects for negative associations (effect size, $d > 1$), large effects for both positive and arousal associations (d around .8), and smaller but significant sedation associations (d around .5). Note that these findings are in line with the findings with the bipolar IATs (negative stronger than positive and arousal stronger than sedation). Interestingly, only arousal associations were significantly correlated with alcohol use and problems. These first results using unipolar IATs are promising, but it should be noted that choice of the opposing contrast category is difficult and may influence results (see De Houwer, 2002; Houben et al., Chapter 7). Using a (unipolar) primed Stroop task, Kramer and Goldman (2003) found significant positive-arousal associations in heavy drinkers and significant sedation associations in light drinkers. Ostafin et al. (2003) used a priming task to assess (unipolar) approach and avoidance tendencies. Hazardous drinkers classified target words with respect to approach or avoidance, and the targets were preceded by briefly-shown alcohol-related or neutral primes. The results on both dimensions (difference between neutral and alcohol primed approach and avoidance words) ranged from very positive to very negative (– 340 ms to 480 ms), which may indicate stronger approach tendencies in some individuals and stronger avoidance tendencies in others. Weak avoidance and not strong approach motivations predicted binge drinking and alcohol-related problems. The authors note, however, that the negative finding for approach motivations is qualified by the low reliability of the priming procedure. Hence, unipolar implicit assessment of alcohol-related cognitions shows promise. Different associations, including emotional dimensions (valence, arousal), outcomes of drinking, and action tendencies (approach vs. avoidance) can be assessed. The latter could be assessed more directly (actual movement toward or away from the stimulus; cf. Mogg et al., 2003).

Some studies investigated the effects of a priming dose of alcohol on implicit alcohol cognitions. Palfai and Ostafin (2003b) assessed primed positive and negative associations for alcohol as compared with neutral targets. Participants performed the task twice, before and after a priming dose of alcohol or placebo. It was found that the consumption of alcohol as compared with placebo made the positive associations with alcohol particularly salient. Similarly, consumption of a moderate dose of alcohol has been found to increase the activation of an alcohol-memory bias, assessed as the number of alcohol-related associations to ambiguous words (Glautier & Spencer, 1999; Havermans et al., 2004). Further, after an alcoholic sip-prime, alcohol-related words of positive affect were found to be more accessible in social drinkers (e.g., Jones & Schulze, 2000). Hence, drinking a low dose of alcohol enhances the accessibility in memory of positive reinforcement associations and approach tendencies (see Fillmore & Vogel-Sprott, Chapter 20; de Jong et al., Chapter 27).

In summary, researchers using a variety of techniques have found that in heavy drinkers, alcohol-related cues automatically grab and hold attention (Bruce & Jones, Chapter 10; Field et al., Chapter 11), and that they are automatically associated with (positive) arousal and approach action tendencies. These findings have been related to biological theories that focus on positive reinforcement and incentive motivation. In line with this, it has been found that alcohol-related cues and priming dosages make the implicit alcohol-related cognitions more salient, and that implicit alcohol associations predict cue-induced craving.

Implicit Negative Associations?

As reviewed above, there is accumulating evidence that with increasing alcohol use, people develop stronger appetitive reactions to alcohol including automatic approach tendencies. It is also evident that most people reduce alcohol consumption in their twenties, often without professional help even after high levels of consumption (e.g., Sher & Gotham, 1999). The question is what restrains their drinking. One factor concerns reduced opportunities to drink and increased responsibilities, but there is also evidence that alcohol-related cognitions play a role. When a person increasingly experiences problems related to drinking, this will be a motivator to change behavior (Jones & McMahon, 1998; Orford, 2001). From this perspective, the problem drinker is torn between two forces: an automatic approach reaction triggered by alcohol-related cues and a more controlled inhibitory response that is motivated by more distal negative outcomes (Stacy et al., 2004; Tiffany, 1990; Wiers, de Jong, et al., 2004; Wiers, Van Woerden, et al., 2002).

An additional possibility is that at least in some individuals, with repeated negative experiences, *automatic negative associations* develop that give rise to an automatic avoidance response. Note that an attentional bias for alcohol-related stimuli has generally been interpreted as a marker of an appetitive response, but could also be related to an automatic avoidance reaction, similar to findings in anxiety research (e.g., Stormark et al., 1997; see also de Jong et al., Chapter 27 and Field et al., Chapter 11).

Two studies examined associative memory responses to negative next to positive alcohol-related outcomes (Gadon et al., 2004; Leigh & Stacy, 1998). Leigh and Stacy found that previous alcohol use predicted undergraduates' associative memory responses to both positive and negative outcomes of drinking. In a series of studies, Gadon et al. (2004) developed an association instrument including frequent and infrequent positive and negative alcohol-related outcomes as well as nonalcohol-related outcomes. They found that undergraduate students' alcohol responses to highly frequent positive and negative outcomes correlated with their alcohol use. A subsequent study using the same methodology in older adults replicated this finding. In the latter sample, negative low-frequency, alcohol-related outcomes and even negative outcomes unrelated to alcohol generated more alcohol responses. This finding suggests that maturing out of heavy use might be related to increased accessibility of negative alcohol associations with age.

Some of the findings with reaction-time measures discussed in the previous section can also be interpreted as suggestive evidence for the existence of automatic negative or avoidance associations. The first concerns the replicated finding of strong negative associations in heavy drinkers in valence IATs (De Houwer et al., 2004; Houben & Wiers, 2004; Wiers, Ganushchack, et al., 2003; Wiers, Granzier, et al., 2003; Wiers, Van de Luitgaarden, et al., 2005; Wiers, Van Woerden, et al., 2002). Even though the finding is reliable, it should be noted that heavy drinkers do not hold stronger negative associations than light drinkers (if anything they tend to be somewhat less negative; cf. Waters & Sayette, Chapter 21). Further, we found that negative associations did not correlate with alcohol-related problems, while arousal associations did (Houben & Wiers, 2004; Wiers, Van de Luitgaarden, et al., 2005). Findings with a different reaction-time test to assess associations (the Extrinsic Affective Simon

Task, or EAST; De Houwer, 2003) showed that alcohol was associated as strongly with negative as with positive valence in heavy drinkers (no significant difference; De Houwer et al., 2004; Wiers, Ganushchack, et al., 2003). Because the EASTs used were bipolar, however, it remains possible that heavy drinkers hold both positive and negative associations. The findings regarding the large variance in automatic approach versus avoidance associations (Palfai & Ostafin, 2003a; Ostafin et al., 2003) also leave the possibility open that automatic avoidance associations may develop, either in some individuals or within one individual next to automatic approach associations (which would lead to "implicit ambivalence").

Is there other evidence in favor of automatic avoidance reactions? Before the current interest in implicit cognition and addiction, there was a research tradition on *aversion conditioning*, with the first experiments dating back to the 1920s (Nathan, 1985). The clinical literature can be summarized as "success and failure" (Nathan, 1985): success primarily for chemical aversion therapy (which is a biologically more related to negative response than shocks; Garcia, 1989), with higher one-year abstinence levels than usual in alcohol treatment. Failure concerns the lack of controlled studies, and the fact that most studies were performed in private clinics with high-SES (social economic status) alcoholics with good motivation for change (Nathan, 1985; Wilson, 1987, 1991). Some findings in this line of research are interesting for the present topic (automatic aversive reactions to alcohol).

A series of studies by Baker and Cannon (Baker & Cannon, 1979; Cannon et al., 1986) demonstrated that aversion therapy resulted in specific changes in subjective, behavioral, and physiological responses specific to alcohol (compared with sodas) that were consistent with acquired aversion (e.g., more negative flavor rating, overt signs of disgust, and accelerated cardiac response). The latter variable predicted the latency to the first drink (Cannon et al., 1986). Elkins (1991), following Garcia (1989), notes that taste aversion conditioning should be seen as different from classical conditioning, which subserves the learning of cognitive expectancies, and that "neither conscious mediation nor intentionality are necessary for CA [consummatory aversion] formation" (Elkins, 1991, p. 393). In his reply, Wilson (1991) agrees with Elkins (1991) that taste aversion is a form of *Evaluative Conditioning* (EC) that should be seen as an automatic process different from classical conditioning. A recent review concluded that EC is indeed a different process than classical conditioning (De Houwer et al., 2001): EC is resistant to extinction, less influenced by statistical contingency, does not require conscious awareness of the co-occurrence of neutral and emotional events, and is not modulated by occasion setting (context effects).

A final line of research relevant for the discussion of automatic approach versus aversion tendencies is research on cue reactivity, in which a variety of physiological measures have been assessed. A meta-analysis by Carter and Tiffany (1999) concluded that physiological responses were generally more in line with incentive models (approach tendencies). It may be questioned, however, to what extent the physiological data unequivocally support incentive models: One interpretation of the results (Glautier, 1999) is that emotionally relevant cues give rise to autonomic arousal (increased heart rate and skin conductance) and that this can lead either to an appetitive or to an aversive response (or perhaps both, in case of "implicit ambivalence"). This might be an explanation for the diversity of the findings. Further, a number of methodological issues need to be addressed in this area of research including a standardization of procedures (Stritzke et al., 2004), because subtle variations may dramatically change the

effects (e.g., holding vs. sipping alcohol generates opposite response patterns; Glautier et al., 1992). Grüsser and colleagues (2002) used the affective modulation of the startle response as a measure of affective valence (Lang, 1995) in response to aversive, neutral, appetitive, and alcohol-related pictures. These responses were compared with subjective measures of arousal, valence, and craving in detoxified alcoholics, social drinkers, and rarely-consuming controls (Grüsser et al., 2002). Abstinent alcoholics subjectively perceived the alcohol stimuli as more aversive than the social drinkers and the controls, and alcoholics and social drinkers experienced more arousal than the controls when alcohol-related stimuli were presented. Interestingly, in alcoholics, the startle data in response to alcohol stimuli were similar to the response to appetitive stimuli. Hence, the alcoholics *subjectively* report an *aversive* reaction to alcohol, but showed an *automatic appetitive* reaction to alcohol-related stimuli, reminiscent of the wanting versus liking dissociation proposed by Robinson and Berridge (2003). In a recent study, the mean affective startle response in a new sample of detoxified alcoholics again showed a mean positive value (Smolka et al., 2004). Interestingly, the individual startle responses showed a wide range of responses, indicating that for some the alcohol-related pictures were very aversive, whereas for others they were "better than sex" (strong appetitive response even compared with natural incentives). In summary, there is scattered evidence that indicates that at least in some people, alcohol cues can elicit an automatic aversive reaction, which is something else than an inhibition of an appetitive action tendency.

Different Underlying Processes?

In several studies and reviews of implicit cognition in substance use and misuse, it has been suggested that implicit measures may better tap into neurobiological processes involved in the etiology and maintenance of the addiction than explicit measures (e.g., Stacy, 1997; Stacy et al., 2004; Wiers et al., 2004; Wiers, Stacy, et al., 2002; Wiers, Van Woerden, et al., 2002). There are three lines of indirect evidence to support this notion.

First, several studies have shown that implicit associations predict unique variance in alcohol use after co-varying explicit measures (Jajodia & Earleywine, 2003; Kramer & Goldman, 2003; Stacy, 1997; Wiers, Van Woerden, et al., 2002). The fact that a different assessment method predicts unique variance, however, does not necessarily indicate that different processes are involved (method variance is a likely alternative). In social cognition research, it has been found that implicit measures predict different aspects of behavior than explicit measures (more spontaneous behavior; see Dovidio et al., 2001); and the same has recently been found in other areas of research, such as personality (Asendorpf et al., 2002) and psychopathology research (Huijding & De Jong, in press; Teachman & Woody, 2003). For example, Huijding and De Jong (in press) found that spider-related affective associations (assessed with the EAST), best predicted automatic fear responses, whereas explicit fear ratings best predicted strategic avoidance behavior. In alcohol research, there are some first indications that implicit measures predict spontaneous reactions to alcohol such as cue-induced craving (Palfai & Ostafin, 2003a; Wiers, Granzier, et al., 2005), but more research is needed on the associations between implicit and explicit cognitions and different aspects of drinking behavior.

Second, neurobiological research demonstrated that subcortical circuits involved in emotion and motivation that are important in addiction are not directly accessible for introspection (Bechara et al., 2003; Berridge, 2001; Robinson & Berridge, 2003; White, 1996). Implicit measures have been shown to correlate highly with activation of these structures in fMRI studies (e.g., Phelps et al., 2000). Subliminally presented pictures activate these structures in the absence of awareness (Cunningham et al., 2004). Recent research by Berridge and colleagues and by Dickinson and colleagues has demonstrated that conditioned incentive salience (underlying "wanting") can be dissociated from expected outcomes (for a review, see Berridge, 2001). Several independent studies have shown that one system can be manipulated, without affecting the other. For example, blocking the mesolimbic dopamine system blocks the incentive salience attribution but leaves the cognitive expectations unchanged, whereas prefrontal and insular lesions affect the cognitive expectations but not incentive salience (see Berridge, 2001). Again, this second line of evidence is indirect, because no direct dissociations between brain mechanisms underlying implicit versus explicit assessment of alcohol-related cognitions have been demonstrated in humans.

Third, dual-process models have been proposed in (social) cognition research (e.g., Deutsch & Strack, Chapter 4; Evans & Coventry, Chapter 3; Strack & Deutsch, 2004). Common to these models is the presence of two different learning mechanisms, one fast and associative and one slower mechanism with limited capacity. Strack and Deutsch (2004) review evidence that associations are bidirectional in the fast system, whereas they are unidirectional in the slow system (e.g., expected outcomes). As noted above, different processes are likely to underlie EC and expectancy learning (De Houwer et al., 2001).

Taken together, there is indirect evidence from different lines of research that suggests that implicit measures at least partly tap into more automatic processes than explicit measures, but this should not be seen as an absolute difference (due to "leakages" between underlying processes, Berridge, 2001; Strack

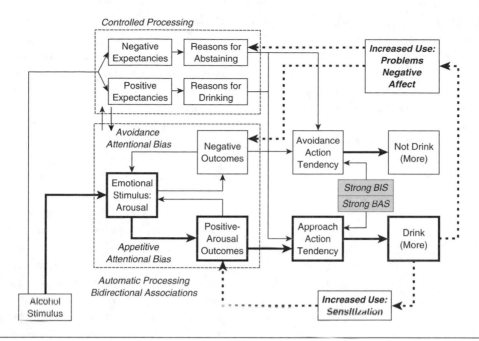

Figure 22.1 A model is depicted that attempts to integrate the findings on automatic and controlled processing in alcohol use and abuse. Thick lines develop with the development of alcohol abuse. Dashed lines are feedback loops. The upper part of the figure refers to controlled processing, with unidirectional representations. As a result of a variety of learning mechanisms (social learning, Pavlovian conditioning, expectancy learning), positive and negative expectancies develop that motivate drinking and abstaining, respectively. Meanwhile, memory associations can be formed through the mechanism of evaluative conditioning. These associations are bidirectional. As the double arrows between the two systems indicate, expectancies and associations can mutually influence each other (see Deutsch & Strack, Chapter 4). Once an individual begins to drink regularly, neural sensitization develops which will promote automatic reactions to alcohol, such as an appetitive attentional bias for alcohol, positive arousal associations and automatically triggered approach action tendencies (bold arrows). With increased use, an individual will also experience negative effects as a result of alcohol. These experiences could lead to automatic negative associations that trigger automatic avoidance action tendencies (conditioned aversion) and in negative expectancies and reasons for abstaining. These motivations could be used to abstain from drinking or to inhibit urges to drink. (approach action tendencies). Negative reinforcement exists as a positive expectancy and reason to drink. At the automatic level a negative mood may be associated with alcohol, which in turn could activate arousal associations and approach tendencies. Finally, note that an "alcohol stimulus" can be multifaceted, with sensory elements cueing appetitive responses while other elements (e.g., health warnings) may cue avoidance responses (cf. Sherman et al., 2003).

& Deutsch, 2004; and because measurement procedures are not entirely implicit or explicit, see De Houwer, Chapter 2). The three processes discussed so far are represented in Figure 22.1.

Implicit Negative Reinforcement?

The final issue in this section concerns the implicit assessment of negative reinforcement cognitions. The reason why this topic is discussed here, and not earlier, is that we propose an interpretation of the results, based on the model in Figure 22.1. It is clear that at least a subgroup of problem drinkers explicitly report to drink for reasons of negative reinforcement (stress reduction, relief from *Negative Affect,* NA). It is less clear to what extent these beliefs reflect actual affective changes (Greeley & Oei, 1999). Further, several variables moderate the perceived anxiolytic effects of alcohol, such as the timing of drinking (Sayette, 1999) and a family history of alcoholism (Sher, 1987).

One important difference between the positive reinforcement and negative alcohol-related cognitions on the one hand and the negative reinforcement cognitions on the other hand, is that an extra premise has to be added:

(I: Positive Reinforcement): Alcohol > Feel good (Positive Arousal, Appetitive Response)

(II: Negative Expectancies): Alcohol > Feel bad (Negative, Sedation, Aversive Response)

(IIIa: Negative Reinforcement): Stress / NA > Alcohol > Feel good (better).

Further, as explained in the previous section, there is evidence for a fast, automatic processing mode for affective stimuli, based on relatively simple associations, in contrast to the more cognitive resources demanding explicit expectancies (Berridge, 2001; De Houwer et al., 2001). An important difference between associations and beliefs or expectancies is that expectancies and beliefs are unidirectional, whereas associations are typically bidirectional (De Houwer, 2002; Strack & Deutsch, 2004; note, however, that the strength of the associations can be asymmetric; see McEvoy & Nelson, Chapter 5, Stacy et al., Chapter 6). When one translates negative reinforcement expectancies into bidirectional associations, one gets:

(IIIb): Feel bad (Stress / NA) < > Alcohol use < > Feel good

This comes down to two associations: The first is equivalent to negative alcohol associations, the second to positive reinforcement associations. The suggestion is then that implicit (association) measures of negative reinforcement assess *associations from alcohol with negative affect and with positive affect.* Is this idea supported by research?

Two research groups have studied implicit negative reinforcement. These studies are discussed in more detail in Birch et al. (Chapter 18). Zack and colleagues used semantic priming tasks in which participants make a lexical decision (word/nonword) for a target (Zack et al., 1999). It was investigated to what extent a prime facilitates this process. They tested problem drinkers that were either high or low on psychiatric distress. In high but not in low psychiatric distress drinkers, they found that NA words facilitated alcohol words (NA > alcohol), and they also found the opposite facilitation (alcohol > NA), in line with the interpretation presented above.

Stewart and colleagues selected students as scoring either high on explicit negative reinforcement motives ("coping drinkers") or on positive reinforcement motives ("enhancement drinkers"). In a first study (Stewart et al., 2002), a primed Stroop task was used to investigate the effects of mood primes on the response time to alcohol or neutral words. As expected, in enhancement drinkers, positive mood cues primed alcohol words and negative mood words primed alcohol in coping drinkers. Interestingly, in coping drinkers, positive mood words also primed alcohol words. One interpretation of this finding is in line with the double bidirectional association of implicit negative reinforcement represented above (see Figure 22.1): A negative mood could activate the concept alcohol, and alcohol in turn could activate positive reinforcement associations.

Taken together, these studies generally found that in a subgroup of "coping drinkers" (selected with explicit measures)

negative affect words automatically trigger alcohol-related concepts, which is related to their explicit reports of drinking to reduce stress or NA. The full negative reinforcement expectancies, however, cannot be "translated" into a single association, because the antecedent is a crucial part. Since associations are bidirectional, one would expect not only a NA > alcohol association, but also the reverse association (alcohol > NA). Results in this area appear to be generally in line with the notion. This does not mean that implicit negative reinforcement does not exist (see also Baker et al., 2004; Curtin et al., Chapter 16), but rather that they may be difficult to assess with explicit or implicit measures using single adjectives (cf. the discussion of MDS expectancy research above). More research is needed in this area, also in relation to the actual biological effects in "coping drinkers": Do coping drinkers really medicate their negative mood and reduce their stress or not, and how is this related to physiological and implicit arousal responses? From the current perspective, the second of the two bidirectional associations involved in negative reinforcement (NA < > alcohol < > positive mood) could be equal to the positive reinforcement association, with the difference being the cue (NA or not). In line with this idea, we recently found a significant positive correlation between implicit alcohol arousal associations and explicit negative reinforcement expectancies in heavy drinkers (Wiers, Van de Luitgaarden, et al., 2005). Further, there is some evidence that stress and alcohol both trigger the mesolimbic dopaminergic system; perhaps stress can trigger a sensitized alcohol response (Saal et al., 2003).

INDIVIDUAL DIFFERENCES AND THE ETIOLOGY OF ALCOHOL USE AND PROBLEMS

As noted above, a common view concerning the etiology and maintenance of alcohol use and abuse (and other addictive behaviors) is that there are two important cognitive processes at work: automatic appetitive action tendencies and controlled inhibitory processes. From this perspective, individual differences can be related to either one of these processes: People may differ in their appetitive action tendencies (and there is evidence for genetic differences in sensitization, Robinson & Berridge, 2003) and individuals may differ in the ability to inhibit these action tendencies (Bechara et al., Chapter 15; Finn et al., 1994; Ostafin et al., 2003; Stacy et al., 2004). From the present perspective, there may also be individual differences in the third process involved: the development of automatic aversion with alcohol (and a genetic factor in the development of alcohol aversion has been reported; Elkins, 1986).

Recent genetic research suggests that individual differences in the susceptibility to addictive behaviors are partly substance specific and partly general (Goldman & Bergen, 1998). With respect to the general risk factor, personality factors are a likely candidate and indeed both internalizing and externalizing behavior at age three prospectively predicted later alcoholism in boys (e.g., Caspi et al., 1996). The predictive power of externalizing behavior is relatively straightforward: This trait has been linked to a strong Behavioral Activation System (BAS), reward sensitivity, sensation seeking, behavioral undercontrol and to a weak Behavioral Inhibition System (BIS; e.g., Finn et al., 1994; Gray, 1990). Externalizing children are likely to start experimenting with alcohol early, to experience the reinforcing effects of alcohol strongly, and to lack strong inhibitory control on the urge to use. Moreover, acute and chronic alcohol and drug use significantly interfere with inhibitory control (e.g., Fillmore & Vogel-Sprott, Chapter 20; Peterson et al., 1992).

The predictive power of internalizing personality characteristics is less straightforward and might involve different mechanisms. (Note that in Gray's [1990] theory BAS and BIS represent two dimensions, hence an individual may be high on BIS and on BAS, in line with the ambivalence model on alcohol motivation where an individual can differ both on approach *and* on avoidance tendencies; Breiner et al., 1999; see also Figure 22.1.) Once internalizing individuals initiate drinking (usually late), perceived negative reinforcement may promote an escalation of use (Conrod et al., 1998). Indeed, individual differences in anxiety sensitivity (fear of anxiety-related sensations) are associated with sensitivity to the negatively reinforcing effect of alcohol on stress responses (not expectancy mediated; see MacDonald et al., 2001).

In the development of alcohol-related cognitions, there is a crucial step: the initiation of drinking. Before this, alcohol-related cognitions are socially learned, whereas after this, genetic influences related to individual differences in the reaction to alcohol influence their further development (Wiers et al., 1998). Research using questionnaires (e.g., Fossey, 1994; Wiers et al., 1998, 2000) and first associates (Dunn & Goldman, 2000) has shown that children report predominantly negative expectancies before they begin drinking alcohol themselves. These negative expectancies may inhibit the onset of drinking (cf. Caffray & Schneider, 2000). Cross-sectional studies suggest that positive expectancies develop with age, which does not imply that negative expectancies diminish but rather that positive expectancies "catch up" (Cameron et al., 2003). Once drinking begins, children score higher on positive and arousal expectancies (Dunn & Goldman, 1998, 2000), and this is more strongly the case for children of alcoholics (Wiers et al., 1998). In a recent study, Thush & Wiers (2005) tested 100 adolescents using the Single Target variety of the IAT (ST-IAT; see Houben et al., Chapter 7) and found that

arousal associations and negative explicit expectancies predicted alcohol use at a one-year follow-up. This finding suggests a causal role for (implicit) arousal associations in the early development of drinking.

Finally, personality characteristics have been related to individual differences in risk for addiction (Cloninger, 1987; Cox, 1987; Finn et al., 1994; Sher, 1991) and there is emerging evidence that personality risk factors are related to individual differences in the development of explicit alcohol-related cognitions, such as expectancies (Darkes et al., 2004) and motives (e.g., Stewart & Devine, 2000). Explicit cognitions have been shown to partially mediate the association between personality and alcohol use (Darkes et al., 2004; Finn et al., 2000; Sher et al., 1991). Obviously, the caveat noted above (criterion contamination) is also relevant here (cf. Darkes et al., 1998). As yet, few studies have investigated the association between personality and implicit alcohol-related cognitions. Notable exceptions are the studies on implicit cognition and negative reinforcement by Stewart and colleagues and by Zack and colleagues (see section entitled "Implicit Negative Reinforcement?" and Birch et al., Chapter 18). Further, Palfai and Ostafin (2003a) found that BAS scores correlated with implicit approach associations on the IAT, and Ostafin et al. (2003) found that more impulsive individuals had weaker primed associations between alcohol cues and avoidance words. Ames et al. (2005) found that the relationship between sensation-seeking and alcohol use and problems was mediated by implicit alcohol associations in high-risk adolescents.

In summary, individual differences in personality predict individual differences in alcohol use and abuse. There is preliminary evidence that part of this relationship is mediated by alcohol-related cognitions, but this conclusion is primarily based on research using explicit assessment strategies and on cross-sectional data. There clearly is a need for longitudinal studies on the development of implicit and explicit alcohol-related cognitions in relation to personality and the development of alcohol use.

CONCLUSION AND IMPLICATIONS FOR INTERVENTIONS

Individuals may differ in automatic and more controlled cognitive processes that can both influence drinking behavior. In heavy drinkers, automatic appetitive reactions triggered by alcohol cues (or by negative affect in "coping drinkers") play an important role in their drinking behavior. From the present perspective, restraint can come from two different mechanisms: an automatic mechanism that is triggered by aversion, and a more controlled effortful mechanism that inhibits an approach tendency. Interventions may target these different mechanisms. In addition, the automatization of alternative behaviors is important (Gollwitzer, 1999; see also Cox et al., Chapter 17; Prestwich et al., Chapter 29).

In *treatment*, it appears useful to try to decrease the automatic appetitive response (e.g., medication such as Naltrexone or cue-exposure; see Wiers et al., 2004). An alternative, which has a long history but has largely gone out of favor today, is to try to stimulate an automatic avoidance reaction (aversive conditioning), but therapeutic usefulness is unclear (Wilson, 1987, 1991). Perhaps an alternative could be to use less aversive methods involving reconditioning (see De Houwer

et al., 2001; Hermans & Van Gucht, Chapter 32). Some of the implicit assessment techniques could be transformed to change automatic affective and cognitive processes in alcohol abuse (see de Jong et al., Chapter 27; Wiers et al., 2004). In addition, the more controlled inhibition mechanism may be enhanced, by making negative (long-term) expectancies more salient, by increasing motivation to change, and perhaps by automatizing restraint (see Palfai, Chapter 26). In prevention, it seems useful to try to prevent the automatic processes from taking over (see Krank & Goldstein, Chapter 28). This could be done by stimulating the more controlled inhibitory processes, and in heavier drinkers by debunking explicit positive expectancies (e.g., through an expectancy challenge; Darkes & Goldman, 1993; Wiers, Van de Luitgaarden, et al., 2005; Wiers, Wood, et al., 2003) and by motivational techniques (e.g., Cox et al., Chapter 17; Marlatt et al., 1998). Cognitive behavioral strategies also target implicit and explicit beliefs by explicitly challenging problematic alcohol-related beliefs, and by implicitly challenging such beliefs by building up self-efficacy around alternative coping behaviors. Whether interventions are actually achieving the cognitive effects that they are targeting is a topic of debate (see Stewart & Conrod, in press), but will be greatly facilitated by the refinement of methods to assess alcohol cognitions. We hope this review and tentative model will stimulate further research on automatic and controlled processes in (alcohol) addiction and their applications to interventions.

REFERENCES

Ajzen, I. (1988). *Attitudes, personality and behavior*. Milton Keynes, UK: Open University Press.

Ames, S. L., & Stacy, A. W. (1998). Implicit cognition in the prediction of substance use among drug offenders. *Psychology of Addictive Behaviors, 12*, 272–281.

Ames, S. L., Sussman, S., Dent, C., & Stacy, A. W. (2005). Implicit cognition and dissociative experiences as predictors of adolescent substance use. *The American Journal of Drug and Alcohol Abuse, 31*(1), 29–162.

Asendorpf, J. B., Banse, R., & Mücke, D. (2002). Double dissociation between implicit and explicit personality self-concept: The case of shy behavior. *Journal of Personality and Social Psychology, 83*, 380–393.

Baker, T. B., & Cannon, D. S. (1979). Taste aversion therapy with alcoholics: Techniques and evidence of a conditioned response. *Behaviour Research and Therapy, 17*(3), 229–242.

Baker, T. B., Piper, M. E., McCarthy, D. E., Majeskie, M. R., & Fiore, M. C. (2004). Addiction motivation reformulated: An affective processing model of negative reinforcement. *Psychological Review, 111*(1), 33–51.

Bandura, A. (1977). *Social learning theory.* Englewood Cliffs, NJ: Prentice Hall.

Bechara, A., Damasio, A. R., & Damasio, H. (2003). The role of the amygdale in decision-making. *Annals of the New York Academy of Science, 958*, 356–369.

Beck, A. T., Wright, F. D., Newman, C. F., & Liese, B. S. (1993). *Cognitive therapy of substance abuse.* New York: Guilford.

Berridge, K. C. (2001). Reward learning: Reinforcement, incentives and expectations. *Psychology of Learning and Motivation, 40*, 223–278.

Breiner, M. J., Stritzke, W. G. K., & Lang, A. R. (1999). Approaching avoidance. A step essential to the understanding of craving. *Alcohol Research & Health, 23*, 197–206.

Brown, S. A., Goldman, M. S., Inn, A., & Anderson, L. (1980). Expectations of reinforcement from alcohol: Their domain and relation to drinking patterns. *Journal of Consulting and Clinical Psychology, 48*, 419–426.

Cacioppo, J. T., & Berntson, G. G. (1994). Relationship between attitudes and evaluative space: A critical review, with emphasis on the separability of positive and negative substrates. *Psychological Bulletin, 115*, 401–423.

Caffray, C. M., & Schneider, S. L. (2000). Why do they do it? Affective motivators in adolescents' decisions to participate in risk behaviours. *Cognition & Emotion, 14*, 543–576.

Cameron, C. A., Stritzke, W. G. K., & Durkin, K. (2003). Alcohol expectancies in late childhood: An ambivalence perspective on transitions toward alcohol use. *Journal of Child Psychology and Psychiatry, 44*, 687–698.

Cannon, D. S., Baker, T. B., Gino, A., & Nathan, P. E. (1986). Alcohol-aversion therapy: Relation between strength of aversion and abstinence. *Journal of Consulting and Clinical Psychology, 54*, 825–830.

Carter, B. L., & Tiffany, S. T. (1999). Meta-analysis of cue-reactivity in addiction research. *Addiction, 94*, 327–340.

Caspi, A., Moffitt, T. E., Newman, D. L., & Silva, P. A. (1996). Behavioral observations at age 3 years predict adult psychiatric disorders. Longitudinal evidence from a birth cohort. *Archives of General Psychiatry, 53*(11), 1033–1039.

Cloninger, C. R. (1987). Neurogenetic adaptive mechanisms in alcoholism. *Science, 236*, 410–416.

Conner, M., & Sparks, P. (2002). Ambivalence and attitudes. *European Review of Social Psychology, 12*, 37–70.

Conrod, P. J., Peterson, J. B., & Pihl, R. O. (2001). Reliability and validity of alcohol-induced heart rate increase as a measure of sensitivity to the stimulant properties of alcohol. *Psychopharmacology, 157*, 20–30.

Conrod, P. J., Pihl, R. O., & Vassileva, J. (1998). Differential sensitivity to alcohol reinforcement in groups of men at risk for distinct alcoholism subtypes. *Alcoholism: Clinical and Experimental Research, 22,* 585–597.

Cooper, M. L. (1994). Motivations for alcohol use among adolescents: Development and validation of a four-factor model. *Psychological Assessment, 6(2),* 117–128.

Cooper, M. L., Frone, M. R., Russell, M., & Mudar, P. (1995). Drinking to regulate positive and negative emotions: A motivational model of alcohol use. *Journal of Personality and Social Psychology, 69,* 990–1005.

Cox, W. M. (1987). Personality theory and research. In H. T. Blane & K. E. Leonard (Eds.), *Psychological theories of drinking and alcoholism* (pp. 55–89). New York: Guilford.

Cox, W. M., & Klinger, E. (1988). A motivational model of alcohol use. *Journal of Abnormal Psychology, 97,* 168–180.

Cunningham, W. A., Johnson, M. K., Raye, C. L., Gatenby, J. C., Gore, J. C., & Banaji, M. R. (2004). Separable neural components in the processing of black and white faces. *Psychological Science, 15,* 806–813.

Darkes, J., & Goldman, M. S. (1993). Expectancy challenge and drinking reduction: Experimental evidence for a mediational process. *Journal of Consulting and Clinical Psychology, 61,* 344–353.

Darkes, J., Greenbaum, P. E., & Goldman, M. S. (1998). Sensation-seeking disinhibition and alcohol use: Exploring issues of criterion contamination. *Psychological Assessment, 10,* 71–76.

Darkes, J., Greenbaum, P. E., & Goldman, M. S. (2004). Alcohol expectancy mediation of biopsychosocial risk: Complex patterns of mediation. *Experimental & Clinical Psychopharmacology, 12,* 27–38.

De Houwer, J. (2002). The Implicit Association Test as a tool for studying dysfunctional associations in psychopathology: Strengths and limitations. *Journal of Behaviour Therapy and Experimental Psychiatry, 33,* 115–133.

De Houwer, J. (2003). The extrinsic affective Simon task. *Experimental Psychology, 50,* 77–85.

De Houwer, J., Crombez, G., Koster, E. H. W., & De Beul, N. (2004). Implicit alcohol-related cognitions in clinical samples of heavy drinkers. *Journal of Behaviour Therapy and Experimental Psychiatry, 35,* 275–286.

De Houwer, J., Thomas, S., & Baeyens, F. (2001). Associative learning of likes and dislikes: A review of 25 years of research on human evaluative conditioning. *Psychological Bulletin, 127,* 853–869.

Dovidio, J. F., Kawakami, K., & Beach, K. R. (2001). Implicit and explicit attitudes: Examination of the relations between measures of intergroup bias. In R. Brown & S. Gaertner (Eds.), *Blackwell handbook of social psychology: Intergroup processes* (pp. 175–197). Oxford, UK: Blackwell Publishing.

Dunn, M. E., & Earleywine, M. (2001). Activation of alcohol expectancies in memory in relation to limb of the blood alcohol curve. *Psychology of Addictive Behaviors, 15,* 18–24.

Dunn, M. E., & Goldman, M. S. (1998). Age and drinking-related differences in the memory organization of alcohol expectancies in 3rd, 6th, 9th, and 12th grade children. *Journal of Consulting and Clinical Psychology, 66,* 579–585.

Dunn, M. E., & Goldman, M. S. (2000). Validation of multidimensional scaling-based modeling of alcohol expectancies in memory: Age and drinking-related differences in expectancies of children assessed as first associates. *Alcoholism: Clinical and Experimental Research, 24,* 1639–1646.

Elkins, R. L. (1986). Separation of taste-aversion-prone and taste-aversion-resistant rats through selective breeding: Implications for individual differences in conditionability and aversion-therapy alcoholism treatment. *Behavioral Neuroscience, 100*(1), 121–124.

Elkins, R. L. (1991). An appraisal of chemical aversion (emetic therapy) approaches to alcoholism treatment. *Behaviour Research and Therapy, 29*(5), 387–413.

Finn, P. R., Kessler, D. N., & Hussong, A. M. (1994). Risk for alcoholism and classical conditioning to signals for punishment: Evidence for a weak behavioral inhibition system? *Journal of Abnormal Psychology, 103,* 293–301.

Finn, P. R., Sharkansky, E. J., Brandt, K. M., & Turcotte, N. (2000). The effects of familial risk, personality, and expectancies on alcohol use and abuse. *Journal of Abnormal Psychology, 109*(1), 122–133.

Fishbein, M., & Ajzen, I. (1975). *Belief, attitude, intention and behavior: An introduction to theory and research.* Reading, MA: Addison-Wesley.

Fossey, E. (1994). *Growing up with alcohol.* London: Routledge.

Frijda, N. H. (1986). *The emotions.* Cambridge, UK: Cambridge University Press.

Fromme, K., Stroot, E., & Kaplan, D. (1993). Comprehensive effects of alcohol: Development and psychometric assessment of a new expectancy questionnaire. *Psychological Assessment, 5,* 19–26.

Gadon, L., Bruce, G., McConnochie, F., & Jones, B. T. (2004). Negative alcohol consumption outcome associations in young and mature adult social drinkers: A route to drinking restraint? *Addictive Behaviors, 29,* 1373–1387.

Garcia, J. (1989). Food for Tolman: Cognition and cathexis in concert. In T. Archer & L. Nilsson (Eds.), *Aversion, avoidance and anxiety: Perspectives on aversively motivated behavior* (pp. 45–85). Hillsdale, NJ: Lawrence Erlbaum.

Glautier, S. (1999). Do responses to drug-related cues index appetitive or aversive states? *Addiction, 94,* 346–347.

Glautier, S., Drummond, D. C., & Remington, B. (1992). Different drink cues elicit different psychophysiological responses in non-dependent drinkers. *Psychopharmacology, 106,* 550–554.

Glautier, S., & Spencer, K. (1999). Activation of alcohol-related associative networks by recent alcohol consumption and alcohol-related cues. *Addiction, 94,* 1033–1041.

Goldman D., & Bergen, A. (1998). General and specific inheritance of substance abuse and alcoholism. *Archives of General Psychiatry, 55,* 964–965.

Goldman, M. S., & Darkes, J. (2004). Alcohol expectancy multiaxial assessment: A memory network-based approach. *Psychological Assessment, 16,* 4–15.

Goldman, M. S., Del Boca, F. K., & Darkes, J. (1999). Alcohol expectancy theory: The application of cognitive neuroscience. In K. E. Leonard & H. T. Blane (Eds.), *Psychological theories of drinking and alcoholism* (2nd ed., pp. 203–246). New York: Guilford.

Goldman, M. S., Greenbaum, P. E., & Darkes, J. (1997). A confirmatory test of hierarchical expectancy structure and predictive power discriminant validation of the alcohol expectancy questionnaire. *Psychological Assessment, 9,* 145–157.

Gollwitzer, P. M. (1999). Implementation intentions. Strong effects of simple plans. *American Psychologist, 54,* 493–503.

Gray, J. A. (1990). Brain systems that mediate both emotion and cognition. *Cognition & Emotion, 4,* 269–288.

Greeley, J., & Oei, T. (1999). Alcohol and tension reduction. In K. E. Leonard & H. T. Blane (Eds.), *Psychological theories of drinking and alcoholism* (2nd ed., pp. 14–53). New York: Guilford.

Greenwald, A. G., McGhee, D. E., & Schwartz, J. L. K. (1998). Measuring individual differences in implicit cognition: the Implicit Association Test. *Journal of Personality and Social Psychology, 74,* 1464–1480.

Grüsser, S. M., Heinz, A., Raabe, A., Wessa, M., Podschus, J., & Flor, H. (2002). Stimulus-induced craving and startle potentiation in abstinent alcoholics and controls. *European Psychiatry, 17,* 188–193.

Havermans, R. C., Vancleef, L., Bylois, E., Wiers, R. W., & Jansen, A. (2004). Context dependent access to alcohol-related concepts stored in memory. *Alcohol Research, 9,* 219-222.

Houben, K., & Wiers, R. W. (2004, June). *Implicit alcohol associations: Influence of target category labels and contrast categories in a unipolar IAT.* Paper presented at the 27th Annual Scientific Meeting of the Research Society on Alcoholism, Vancouver, BC.

Huijding, J., & de Jong, P. J. (in press). Specific predictive power of automatic spider-related affective associations for controllable and uncontrollable fear responses toward spiders. *Behaviour Research and Therapy.*

Jajodia, A., & Earleywine, M. (2003). Measuring alcohol expectancies with the Implicit Association Test. *Psychology of Addictive Behaviors, 17,* 126–133.

Jones, B. C., Jones, B. T., Blundell, L., & Bruce, G. (2002). Social users of alcohol and cannabis who detect substance-related changes in a change blindness paradigm report higher levels of use than those detecting substance-neutral changes. *Phychopharmacology, 165,* 93–96.

Jones, B. T., Corbin, W., & Fromme, K. (2001). A review of expectancy theory and alcohol consumption. *Addiction, 91,* 57–72.

Jones, B. T., & McMahon, J. (1994). Negative and positive alcohol expectancies as predictors of abstinence after discharge from a residential treatment programme: A one- and three-month follow-up study in males. *Journal of Studies on Alcohol, 55,* 543–548.

Jones, B. T., & McMahon, J. (1998). Alcohol motivations as outcome expectancies. In W. R. Miller & N. Heather (Eds.), *Treating addictive behaviors* (2nd ed., pp. 75–91). New York: Plenum.

Jones, B. T., & Schulze, D. (2000). Alcohol-related words of positive affect are more accessible in social drinkers' memory than are other words when sip-primed by alcohol. *Addiction Research, 8,* 221–232.

Kramer, D. A., & Goldman, M. S. (2003). Using a modified Stroop task to implicitly discern the cognitive organization of alcohol expectancies. *Journal of Abnormal Psychology, 112,* 171–175.

Lang, P. J. (1995). The emotion probe. Studies of motivation on alcohol. *American Psychologist, 50,* 372–385.

Leigh, B. C. (1989). In search of the seven dwarves: Issues of measurement and meaning in alcohol expectancy research. *Psychological Bulletin, 105,* 361–373.

Leigh, B. C., & Stacy, A. W. (1993). Alcohol outcome expectancies: Scale construction and predictive utility in higher order confirmatory factor models. *Psychological Assessment, 5,* 216–229.

Leigh, B. C., & Stacy, A. W. (1998). Individual differences in memory associations involving the positive and negative outcomes of alcohol use. *Psychology of Addictive Behaviors, 12,* 39–46.

MacDonald, A. B., Stewart, S. H., Hutson, R., Rhyno, E., & Lee Loughlin, H. (2001). The roles of alcohol and alcohol expectancy in the dampening of responses to hyperventilation among high anxiety sensitive young adults. *Addictive Behaviors, 26,* 841–867.

Marlatt, G. A., Baer, J. S., Kivlahan, D. R., Dimeff, L. A., Larimer, M. E., Quigley, L. A., et al. (1998). Screening and brief intervention for high-risk college student drinkers: Results from a 2-year follow-up assessment. *Journal of Consulting and Clinical Psychology, 66,* 604–615.

Marlatt, G. A., & Gordon, J. R. (1985). *Relapse prevention: Maintenance strategies in the treatment of addictive behaviors.* New York: Guilford.

McEvoy, P. M., Stritzke, W. G. K., French, D. J., Lang, A. R., & Ketterman, R. L. (2004). Comparison of three models of alcohol craving in young adults: A cross validation. *Addiction, 99,* 482–497.

Mogg, K., Bradley, B. P., Field, M., & De Houwer, J. (2003). Eye movements to smoking-related pictures in smokers: Relationship between attentional biases and implicit and explicit measures of stimulus valence. *Addiction, 98,* 825–836.

Nathan, P. E. (1985). Aversion therapy in the treatment of alcoholism: Success and failure. *Annals of the New York Academy of Sciences, 443,* 357–364.

Orford, J. (2001). Addiction as excessive appetite. *Addiction, 96,* 15–31.

Ostafin, B. D., Palfai, T. P., & Wechsler, C. E. (2003). The accessibility of motivational tendencies toward alcohol: Approach, avoidance, and disinhibited drinking. *Experimental & Clinical Psychopharmacology, 11,* 294–301.

Palfai, T. P., & Ostafin, B. D. (2003a). Alcohol-related motivational tendencies in hazardous drinkers: Assessing implicit response tendencies using the modified IAT. *Behaviour Research and Therapy, 41,* 1149–1162.

Palfai, T. P., & Ostafin, B. D. (2003b). The influence of alcohol on the activation of outcome expectancies: The role of evaluative expectancy activation in drinking behavior. *Journal of Studies on Alcohol, 64,* 111–119.

Peterson, J. B., Finn, P. R., & Pihl, R. O. (1992). Cognitive dysfunction and the inherited predisposition to alcoholism. *Journal of Studies on Alcohol, 53,* 154–160.

Phelps, E. A., O'Connor, K. J., Cunningham, W. A., Funayama, E. S., Gatenby, J. C., & Gore, J. G. (2000). Performance on indirect measures of race evaluation predicts amygdala activation. *Journal of Cognitive Neuroscience, 12,* 729–738.

Rather, B. C., Goldman, M. S., Roehrich, L., & Brannick, M. (1992). Empirical modeling of an alcohol expectancy memory network using multidimensional scaling. *Journal of Abnormal Psychology, 101,* 174–183.

Robinson, T. E., & Berridge, K. C. (1993). The neural basis of drug craving: An incentive-sensitization theory of addiction. *Brain Research Reviews, 18,* 247–291.

Robinson, T. E., & Berridge, K. C. (2003). Addiction. *Annual Review of Psychology, 54,* 25–53.

Russell, J. A., & Carroll, J. M. (1999). On the bipolarity of positive and negative affect. *Psychological Bulletin, 125,* 3–30.

Saal, D., Dong, Y., Bonci, A., & Malenka, R. (2003). Drugs of abuse and stress trigger a common synaptic adaptation in dopamine neurons. *Neuron, 37,* 577–582.

Sayette, M. A. (1999). Cognitive theory and research. In K .E. Leonard & H. T. Blane (Eds.), *Psychological theories of drinking and alcoholism* (2nd ed., pp. 247–291). New York: Guilford.

Sher, K. J. (1987). Stress response dampening. In H. T. Blane & K. E. Leonard (Eds.), *Psychological theories of drinking and alcoholism* (pp. 227–271). New York: Guilford.

Sher, K. J. (1991). *Children of alcoholics, a critical appraisal of theory and research.* Chicago: University of Chicago Press.

Sher, K. J., & Gotham, H. J. (1999). Pathological alcohol involvement: A developmental disorder of young adulthood. *Development and Psychopathology, 11,* 933–956.

Sher, K. J., Walitzer, K. S., Wood, P. K., & Brent, E. E. (1991). Characteristics of children of alcoholics: Putative risk factors, substance use and abuse, and psychopathology. *Journal of Abnormal Psychology, 100*(4), 427–448.

Sher, K. J., Wood, M. D., Wood, P. K., & Raskin, G. (1996). Alcohol outcome expectancies and alcohol use: A latent variable cross-lagged panel study. *Journal of Abnormal Psychology, 105,* 561–574.

Sherman, S. J., Rose, J. S., Koch, K., Presson, C. C., & Chassin, L. (2003). Implicit and explicit attitudes toward cigarette smoking: The effects of context and motivation. *Journal of Social & Clinical Psychology, 22,* 13–39.

Smolka, M. N., Klein, S., Lemenager, T., Georgi, A., Nikitopoulos, J., Flor, H., et al. (2004, June). Emotional valence of alcohol-related stimuli and cue-induced bold activation. Paper presented at the 27th Annual Scientific Meeting of the Research Society on Alcoholism, Vancouver, BC.

Stacy, A. W. (1995). Memory association and ambiguous cues in models of alcohol and marijuana use. *Experimental & Clinical Psychopharmacology, 3,* 183–194.

Stacy, A. W. (1997). Memory activation and expectancy as prospective predictors of alcohol and marijuana use. *Journal of Abnormal Psychology, 106,* 61–73.

Stacy, A. W., Ames, S. L., & Knowlton, B. (2004). Neurologically plausible distinctions in cognition and habit relevant to drug abuse prevention. *Substance Use & Misuse, 39,* 1571–1623.

Stewart, J., De Wit, H., & Eikelboom, R. (1984). The role of unconditioned and conditioned drug effects in the self-administration of opiates and stimulants. *Psychological Review, 91,* 251–268.

Stewart, S. H., & Conrod, P. J. (in press). Introduction to the special issue on state-of-the-art in cognitive-behavioral interventions for substance use disorders. *Journal of Cognitive Psychotherapy.*

Stewart, S. H., & Devine, H. (2000). Relations between personality and drinking motives in young people. *Personality and Individual Differences, 29*(3), 495–511.

Stewart, S. H., Hall, E., Wilkie, H., & Birch, C. (2002). Affective priming of alcohol schema in coping and enhancement motivated drinkers. *Cognitive Behaviour Therapy, 31,* 68–80.

Stormark, K. M., Field, N. P., Hughdahl, K., & Horowitz, M. (1997). Selective processing of visual alcohol cues in abstinent alcoholics: An approach-avoidance conflict. *Addictive Behaviors, 22,* 509–519.

Strack, F., & Deutsch, R. (2004). Reflective and impulsive determinants of social behavior. *Personality and Social Psychology Review, 3,* 220–247.

Stritzke, W. G. K., Breiner, M. J., Curtin, J. J., & Lang, A. (2004). Assessment of substance cue reactivity: Advances in reliability, specificity and validity. *Psychology of Addictive Behaviors, 18,* 148–159.

Teachman, B. A., & Woody, S. R. (2003). Automatic processing in spider phobia: Implicit fear associations over the course of treatment. *Journal of Abnormal Psychology, 112,* 100–109.

Thush, C., & Wiers, R. W. (2005). *Explicit and implicit alcohol-related cognitions and the prediction of current and future drinking in adolescents.* Manuscript submitted for publication.

Tiffany, S. T. (1990). A cognitive model of drug urges and drug-use behavior: Role of automatic and nonautomatic processes. *Psychological Review, 97,* 147–168.

Van den Wildenberg, E., Beckers, M., Van Lambaart, F., & Wiers, R. W. (2004). Is the strength of implicit alcohol associations correlated with heart rate acceleration after alcohol consumption? Paper presented at the 27th Annual Scientific Meeting of the Research Society on Alcoholism, Vancouver, BC.

White, N. M. (1996). Addictive drugs as reinforcers: Multiple partial actions on memory systems. *Addiction, 91,* 921–949.

Wiers, R. W., Both, S., Franken, I., Iedema, T., & Kloosterman, M. (2005c). Unpublished data.

Wiers, R. W., De Jong, P. J., Havermans, R., & Jelicic, M. (2004). How to change implicit drug-related cognitions in prevention: A transdisciplinary integration of findings from experimental psychopathology, social cognition, memory and learning psychology. *Substance Use & Misuse, 39,* 1625–1684.

Wiers, R. W., Ganushchack, L., Van de Ende, N., Smulders, F. T. Y., & De Jong, P. J. (2003, May/June). Comparing implicit alcohol associations across different rt-measures: The implicit association test (IAT) versus varieties of the extrinsic affective simon task (EAST). Paper presented at the 15th Annual Convention of the American Psychological Society, Atlanta, GA.

Wiers, R. W., Granzier, J., & Havermans, R. (2005). Context effects on implicit and explicit alcohol-related cognitions. In M. Krank, A. Wall, S. H. Stewart, R. W. Wiers, & M. S. Goldman (Eds.), Context effects on alcohol cognitions. *Alcoholism: Clinical and Experimental Research, 29,* 196–206.

Wiers, R. W., Gunning, W. B., & Sergeant, J. A. (1998). Do young children of alcoholics hold more positive or negative alcohol-related expectancies than controls? *Alcoholism: Clinical and Experimental Research, 22,* 1855–1863.

Wiers, R. W., Hoogeveen, K. J., Sergeant, J. A., & Gunning, W. B. (1997). High and low dose expectancies and the differential associations with drinking in male and female adolescents and young adults. *Addiction, 92,* 871–888.

Wiers, R. W., Sergeant, J. A., & Gunning, W. B. (2000). The assessment of alcohol expectancies in school children: Measurement or modification? *Addiction, 95,* 737–746.

Wiers, R. W., Stacy, A. W., Ames, S. L., Noll, J. A., Sayette, M. A., Zack, M., et al. (2002). Implicit and explicit alcohol-related cognitions. *Alcoholism: Clinical and Experimental Research, 26,* 129–137.

Wiers, R. W., Van de Luitgaarden, J., Van den Wildenberg, E., & Smulders, F. T. Y. (2005). Challenging implicit and explicit alcohol-related cognitions in young heavy drinkers. *Addiction, 100,* 806–819.

Wiers, R. W., Van Woerden, N., Smulders, F. T. Y., & de Jong, P. J. (2002). Implicit and explicit alcohol-related cognitions in heavy and light drinkers. *Journal of Abnormal Psychology, 111,* 648–658.

Wiers, R. W., Wood, M. D., Darkes, J., Corbin, W. R., Jones, B. T., & Sher, K. J. (2003). Changing expectancies: Cognitive mechanisms and context effects. *Alcoholism: Clinical and Experimental Research, 27,* 186–197.

Wilson, G. T. (1987). Chemical aversion conditioning as a treatment for alcoholism: A re-analysis. *Behaviour Research and Therapy, 25*(6), 503–516.

Wilson, G. T. (1991). Chemical aversion conditioning in the treatment of alcoholism: Further comments. *Behaviour Research and Therapy, 29*(5), 415–419.

Wise, R., & Bozarth, M. (1987). A psychomotor stimulant theory of addiction. *Psychological Review, 94,* 469–492.

Zack, M., Toneatto, T., & MacLeod, C. M. (1999). Implicit activation of alcohol concepts by negative affective cues distinguishes between problem drinkers with high and low psychiatric distress. *Journal of Abnormal Psychology, 108,* 518–531.

CHAPTER 23

Implicit Cognition
and Drugs of Abuse

SUSAN L. AMES, INGMAR H. A. FRANKEN, AND KATE CORONGES

Abstract: This chapter focuses on a review of paradigms used in the study of drug-related spontaneously activated cognitions. The assessment methods reviewed in this chapter have roots in associative learning principles, with associative strength being a key determinant of information processing expressed as attentional and memory biases. Findings from word association methods as well as associative assessments that utilize reaction-time paradigms (e.g., semantic priming, Implicit Association Test (IAT), modified Stroop, visual dot-probe, and flicker paradigms) to evaluate relatively automatic drug-related cognitions are presented. Many of these paradigms are applicable to prevention programs interested in evaluating change in spontaneously activated drug-related cognitions in response to an intervention.

INTRODUCTION

An implicit cognition approach to drug use emphasizes the influence of spontaneously activated cognitive processes on behavioral biases through means that circumvent conscious deliberation. Assessments of implicit processes have the potential to tap into drug-related memories of events and feelings that are automatically or spontaneously activated but cannot be assessed through direct questioning of individuals. Implicit cognitive processes are relatively nonreflective processes revealed when an individual applies previously acquired knowledge without awareness on indirect measures of behavior. That is, previous experiences implicitly affect or

direct subsequent responses or reactivity to circumstances or stimuli. William James (1890) frequently referred to the observed influence of prior experience on subsequent performance with diminished conscious awareness. According to James, "Any sequence of mental action which has been frequently repeated tends to perpetuate itself; so that we find ourselves automatically prompted to think, feel, or do what we have been before accustomed to think, feel, or do, under like circumstances, without any consciously formed purpose, or anticipation of results" (James, 1890, p. 24).

For decades, the literature in basic memory research has provided evidence that some aspects of memory can be expressed by

AUTHORS' NOTE: This chapter was supported by a grant from the National Institute on Drug Abuse, DA16094.

facilitated performance on tasks requiring little or no conscious recollection of past experience (see Roediger, 1990; Schacter & Graf, 1986). Researchers exploring implicit memory in amnesic and normal populations using paradigms that tap unconscious priming effects of previously presented stimuli have shown that memory deficits affect responses on assessments of implicit processes differently than they affect responses on explicit tasks (e.g., Levy et al., 2004; Schacter, 1985, 1987; Schacter & Graf, 1986; Shimamura & Squire, 1984). This work and more recent research on impaired memory function and imaging of brain activation has helped define the influence of implicit processes on behavior and provided evidence for the neural basis of distinct memory systems (e.g., Gabrieli, 1998; Knowlton et al., 1996; Rolls, 2000; White, 1996). These findings converge on the significant influence of nonconsciously mediated or implicit cognitive processes on behavior (see Stacy, Ames, & Knowlton, 2004).

ASSESSING AUTOMATIC OR SPONTANEOUS COGNITIVE PROCESSES

Several paradigms described in the memory and social cognition literatures have been adapted to evaluate implicit cognitive processes in drug use (see Table 23.1). Unlike explicit cognitive methods and retrospective self-report strategies, these types of measures circumvent the influence of self-perceptions of behavior (see Feldman & Lynch, 1988; Nisbett & Wilson, 1977). This chapter reviews the current methods used in assessing automatic or spontaneous drug-related cognitions, and the influence of these implicit cognitions on attentional and behavioral biases. Many of these assessment methods are rooted in associative learning principles (see Yin & Knowlton, Chapter 12), with

associative strength being a key determinant of information processing expressed as attentional and memory biases. In the next sections, research findings (and relevant theory) of paradigms used in the study of spontaneously activated cognitions that influence drug-use behavior are reviewed.

Associative Memory Assessments

Word and Picture Association Tasks

An assessment approach to drug use, advanced by Stacy and colleagues, taps individual differences in memory associations established and strengthened through repetitive experiences with drugs (Stacy, 1995, 1997; Stacy et al., 1996). Stacy proposes that behavior at any moment is governed by the current pattern of activation in memory, and activation is often primarily an implicit or relatively spontaneous process (Stacy, 1997). Through repeated drug use, various cues and outcomes associated with drug use come to automatically activate thoughts about drug experiences. Anything processed during a drug-use episode (e.g., perceived affective outcomes, drug stimuli, or environmental cues) may come to elicit a conceptually related response based on associations in memory. Whether a drug-consistent cognitive state is easily activated in a variety of situations is determined by the strength of associations in memory. Simultaneous activation of competing concepts is improbable when a drug-consistent activation pattern has been elicited.

The types of measures used by Stacy and colleagues in evaluating associative links between cues or outcomes and drug use include cue-behavior association tasks (e.g., ambiguous cues such as "*bud*"), controlled association test of outcome-behavior associations (e.g., cue phrases such as "*feeling good*"; Ames & Stacy, 1998; Stacy, 1995, 1997; Stacy et al., 1996; Stacy et al., 1994;

Stacy & Newcomb, 1998), picture association tasks consisting of high-risk cues (Ames et al., 2005), and phrase and event completion tasks (Stacy et al., in press). On all tasks, participants are instructed to respond to the cue word, phrase, or picture with the first response that comes to mind. All tasks are time limited and require the generation of a discrete response to each stimulus word or phrase. The associative links revealed on these types of tasks likely tap into spontaneously activated cognitions, providing information about associative memory processes underlying drug (ab)use and memories that operate in parallel across verbal and motivational substrates (see Stacy et al., 1996).

Stacy and colleagues have demonstrated the utility of associative memory tasks in predicting substance use in college students cross-sectionally (Stacy, 1995; Stacy et al., 1994) and prospectively (Stacy, 1997), and in predicting substance use in community samples cross-sectionally (Stacy & Newcomb, 1998). Variations of these associative memory tasks have also been shown to be predictive of drug use among high-risk adolescent samples (Ames et al., 2005; Stacy et al., 1996), and among drug offenders (Ames & Stacy, 1998; Ames et al., 2002). Associative memory assessments were the best predictors of alcohol and marijuana use, while controlling for gender, ethnicity, and acculturation in studies of at-risk youth (Stacy et al., 1996) and adult drug offenders (Ames & Stacy, 1998). In another study among adult drug offenders, Ames et al. (2002) evaluated the mediating role of associative memory in the prediction of marijuana use, examining relationships among sensation seeking, memory association, marijuana use, and driving under the influence of marijuana and other drugs (DUI). The latent variable models revealed that associative memory independently predicted marijuana use and mediated the predictive effects of sensation-seeking on drug use. Individuals higher in sensation-seeking

were more likely to generate associates of marijuana use in response to the associative memory tasks. Additionally, memory associations had a significant indirect effect on DUI, mediated through marijuana use. Findings were similar in a study of high-risk youth, which examined the relative contributions of dissociative experiences, memory associations, and sensation-seeking in structural models of drug use and problem experiences (Ames et al., 2005).

In a prospective study of substance use among 340 college students, Stacy (1997) evaluated the predictive effects of associative memory measures and explicit cognitions as measured by outcome expectancies, while controlling for potential confounding predictors and prior substance use. Latent variable models revealed assessments of associative memory to be better predictors of subsequent alcohol and marijuana use than outcome expectancies, sensation-seeking, acculturation, and gender. Outcome expectancies and sensation-seeking were also predictive of alcohol use, but not marijuana use, in this study. These findings provide evidence of the influence of different aspects of cognition involved in drug-use motivation: an implicit cognition component represented by the spontaneous activation of drug-related cognitions, and a more deliberate or explicit cognitive process represented by outcome expectancies (Stacy, 1997). This work demonstrates the prospective prediction by implicit measures over and above what is learned from self-report measures of behavior.

Taken together, the studies reviewed here provide evidence that associative memory measures tap into relatively spontaneous drug-related cognitions and provide information about individual differences in associative memory that correlate with and predict behavior. The associative memory assessments reviewed in this section are consistent with the concept of immediately accessed thoughts; that is, the time limits and instructions to respond quickly to task items should mitigate extensive post-access processing. Nevertheless, it is possible that individuals may block or "filter" associates in these types of tasks (see Jacoby & Kelley, 1991).

Other researchers have used similar assessments to evaluate associates of a variety of behaviors. Benthin et al. (1995) used a word association task to examine cognitive and affective associates of some health-threatening (e.g., marijuana use, drinking beer) and health-enhancing behaviors (e.g., exercise, condom use) among a sample of adolescents. When adolescents were asked to think for a moment about a specific behavior and then write the first five thoughts that came to mind while thinking about that behavior, they generated many similar positive associates to health-threatening behaviors (e.g., having fun), while generating few common positive associates of health-enhancing behaviors. In general, participants generated more negative than positive associates to cues relating to alcohol, tobacco, and marijuana use. For example, 63 percent of words elicited by the cued behavior "smoking marijuana" were negative. But, adolescents who reportedly engaged in marijuana use produced a higher percent of positive outcomes (e.g., relaxation) than those who reported never having used marijuana. In a similar study, Leeming et al. (2002) adapted the methods used by Benthin et al. (1995) to generate associates of alcohol, tobacco, inhalants, ecstasy, and heroin use among a group of young adolescents. In content analyses of the distribution of spontaneously generated responses, they also found that 63 percent of all responses generated were negative in content (e.g., health problems) and only 8 percent were positive (e.g., having a good time).

Some researchers have adapted word association methods to evaluate group differences in associative links to ambiguous drug-relevant words and found that drug users generated significantly more drug-related associates than nonusers (e.g., Green &

Galbraith, 1986; Haertzen et al., 1974), and that specific cues could be used to target associative memories reflecting various stages of addiction (Haertzen & Ross, 1980). These findings provide information about salient drug-relevant associative structures and evidence that associative memory methods can be used in a variety of situations to elicit highly accessible and strongly activated memories that help define differential involvement in a particular subculture or group (e.g., drug users vs. nondrug users). Associative links are learned and elaborated through cultural learning as well as through direct experience (see McCusker, 2001) and these influences are reflected in the likelihood of drug-related responses on associative memory tasks (see Stacy et al., 1994).

Continued Association Method

The continued association assessment method has been effectively used in basic memory research as a means of eliciting associates of stimuli to reveal how meaningful a particular cue is to a group or individual (e.g., Noble, 1952; Szalay & Deese, 1978; Underwood, 1959). This method shares the same basic rationale as other word association methods but requires that individuals provide multiple responses to the same repeated cue (e.g., *pot:* ____; *pot:* ____; *pot:* ____), thereby increasing the potential to detect more variability in drug-related cognitions and their influence on behavior. Szalay and his colleagues advocate the use of this method proposing that dominant or salient responses occur early in the method of continued associations but not necessarily only in the first position.

Szalay and colleagues have inferred subjective meaning from the distributions of responses to free associations and their behavioral implications through the use of open-ended analytic analyses (i.e., Associative Group Analysis) of the responses to theme words and pictures (Szalay, Carroll, et al., 1993; Szalay &

Deese, 1978). In studies of alcohol and other drug use, Szalay and colleagues found the continuous free association assessment approach provided response content that could differentiate dominant perceptions and attitudes of drug users from nondrug users (Szalay, Canino, et al., 1993; Szalay, Inn, et al., 1993; Szalay, Vilov, et al., 1992) and pretreatment and posttreatment drug users (Szalay, Bovasso, et al., 1992; Szalay, Carroll, et al., 1993). In this work, Szalay found that marijuana and other drug users generated more positive content (e.g., fun, relaxed) to cued themes than nonusers. Drug users also generated less negative content than nonusers, whereas nonusers generated more associates related to harmful and negative consequences of drug use (Szalay, Canino, et al., 1993; Szalay et al., 1999; Szalay, Vilov, et al., 1992). Szalay, Carroll, et al. (1993) also found drug users generated more associative responses relating to negative consequences of use (e.g., danger) following treatment. Szalay's approach is based on the assumption that vulnerability to drug (ab)use is shaped by individual differences in one's "internal world" and by an individual's dominant motivations and perceptions (Szalay et al., 1999).

Reaction-Time Paradigms

Semantic Priming and Associative Memory

Semantic priming paradigms are frequently used in basic memory research to examine the influence of associative memory structures. These types of tasks are believed to assess automatic information processing (see Schacter, 1992). In semantic priming tasks, exposure to a "prime" word or phrase should facilitate responding to associates that are semantically or conceptually related. To date, several alcohol studies have examined facilitatory effects of priming (i.e., activation of associative memory) to examine alcohol-related cognitions (e.g., Feldtkeller et al., 2001; Hill & Paytner, 1992; Weingardt

et al., 1996; Zack et al., 1999), but we found only one study that focused on priming effects in opiate-dependent individuals.

Weinstein et al. (2000) examined the effects of "contextual" priming on the processing of drug and craving-related words in opiate-dependent individuals awaiting methadone following a period of abstinence, opiate-dependent individuals actively using and/or receiving methadone, and a control group of family members. The priming task involved reading sentences describing withdrawal, craving, or neutral contexts followed by either drug-related (compatible), neutral, or nonsense words. Weinstein et al. hypothesized that participants should react faster when processing words compatible with their salient state. That is, the influence of withdrawal in abstinent methadone patients should increase attentional biases toward craving and withdrawal-related information. They found, however, that the craving and withdrawal prime sentences did not facilitate processing of information in abstinent methadone participants anymore so than in the group of opiate-dependent users. Overall, the opiate-dependent groups responded faster to drug-related words that followed withdrawal-related sentences (but not craving-related sentences) as compared to neutral words that followed neutral sentences (Weinstein et al., 2000). This study provides preliminary evidence of biases elicited by "contextual" priming of withdrawal-related information. Studies that replicate this finding in other drug-dependent populations will help in understanding context effects in automatic information processing and their influence on behavior.

Implicit Association Test (IAT) and Evaluative Bias

The Implicit Association Test (IAT) is a categorization task that measures the relative strength of pairs of associates through rate of

(Text continues on page 372)

Table 23.1 Summary of Studies Addressing Implicit Cognitive Processes and Other Drugs of Abuse

Study	Construct assessed	Methods used	Drug	Population	Findings
Ames & Stacy, 1998	Associative Memory	Cue-behavior and outcome-behavior association tasks	Marijuana	Drug offenders	Associative memory correlates with self-reports of marijuana use
Ames et al., 2005	Associative Memory	Cue-behavior, outcome-behavior, picture association tasks	Marijuana	At-risk adolescents	Associative memory correlates with drug use, mediates predictive effects of sensation-seeking
Ames et al., 2002	Associative Memory	Cue-behavior, outcome-behavior, picture association tasks	Marijuana	Drug offenders	Associative memory correlates with drug use, mediates the predictive effects of sensation-seeking
Stacy, 1995	Associative Memory	Cue-behavior, object association	Marijuana	College students	Associative memory correlates with drug use, controlling for gender and acculturation; object association independently predicts marijuana use
Stacy, 1997	Associative Memory	Cue-behavior and outcome-behavior association tasks	Marijuana	College students	Memory associations predict marijuana use prospectively, controlling for prior use, gender, expectancies, sensation-seeking, and acculturation
Stacy et al., 1996	Associative Memory	Cue-behavior and outcome-behavior association tasks	Marijuana	At-risk adolescents	Memory associations predict marijuana use, controlling for confounding variables
Benthin et al., 1995	Associative Memory	Word association (associates of specified behaviors)	Marijuana	Adolescents	More negative associates generated for drug-related cues. Adolescents reporting marijuana use produced more positive outcomes than those who never used
Green & Galbraith, 1986	Associative Memory	Word association (double-entendre words)	Various drugs	College students and drug addicts	Addicts generate significantly more drug-related associations than college students, but not more associates of aggressive behavior

Study	Construct assessed	Methods used	Drug	Population	Findings
Haertzen et al., 1974	Associative Memory	Word association	Various drugs	Opiate dependents and normal controls	Heroin addicts generate more heroin associations than associates of other drugs
Haertzen & Ross, 1980	Associative Memory	Word association	Opiates	Opiate addicts	Specific cues target associative memories reflecting various stages in the addiction process
Leeming et al., 2002	Associative Memory	Word association	Marijuana Heroin Ecstasy	Adolescents	More negative associates for drug cues were generated, only 8 percent were positive
Szalay, Bovasso, et al, 1992	Associative Memory	Continued free association	Cocaine, crack, and other drugs	Pre- and posttreatment drug addicts and nonusers	Posttreatment group associated drug cues with more negative consequences (e.g., sickness). Pretreatment group responses were more related to entertainment. Nonusers showed similar patterns of associates as posttreatment group
Szalay, Canino, et al., 1993	Associative Memory	Continued free association	Marijuana, cocaine, and crack	Drug users and nonusers	Drug users generated more response content related to fun, entertainment, and euphoric effects. Nondrug users generated more content related to harmful consequences
Szalay, Carroll, et al., 1993	Associative Memory	Continued free association and picture association	Crack and cocaine, and other drugs	Pre- and posttreatment crack, cocaine, and other drug addicts	Pretreatment generated specific drug-relevant responses, whereas posttreatment associative responses related to negative consequences
Szalay, Inn, et al., 1993	Associative Memory	Continued free association	Marijuana, crack, cocaine, and other drugs	Grade school to graduate student users and nonusers	Drug users associate drugs with positive experiences and feelings, and are more familiar with drug names, methods, and effects. Nonusers associate drugs with more negative consequences

(Continued)

Table 23.1 (Continued)

Study	Construct assessed	Methods used	Drug	Population	Findings
Szalay, Vilov, et al., 1992	Associative Memory	Continued free association	Marijuana and other drugs	College student users and nonusers	Drug users generated more response content related to drug use, and less negative content than nonusers
Weinstein et al., 2000	Associative Memory	Contextual priming	Opiates	Opiate-dependents and family members	Opiate-dependents responded faster to drug-related words following withdrawal-related sentences as compared to neutral words that followed neutral sentences
Field et al., 2004	Evaluative Bias	Implicit Association Test	Marijuana	Marijuana users and nonusers	More negative associations for marijuana-related words in nonusers; no significant differences for positive marijuana associations between users and non-users
	Attentional Bias	Visual Dot-Probe			Attentional bias toward marijuana-related words found in marijuana users with high craving levels
Franken, Kroon, et al., 2000	Attentional Bias	Probe detection (attentional cueing task)	Cocaine	Cocaine addicts	Attentional bias for drug cues found in patients with higher scores on obsessive cocaine thoughts and higher craving scores
Lubman et al., 2000	Attentional Bias	Pictorial Probe Detection	Opiates	Heroin addicts	Addicts showed an attentional bias toward pictures depicting drug-related items
Copersino et al., 2004	Attentional Bias	Word Stroop	Cocaine	Cocaine addicts and nonusers, cocaine-dependent schizophrenics, and nonusing schizophrenics	Attentional bias for cocaine cues was found in cocaine addicts only and not in cocaine-dependent schizophrenics Cocaine addicts also reported significantly more craving than cocaine-dependent schizophrenics

Study	Construct assessed	Methods used	Drug	Population	Findings
Franken et al., 2004	Attentional Bias	Word Stroop	Opiates	Heroin addicts	Addicts had an attentional bias toward heroin-related words that decreased after haloperidol
Franken, Kroon, Wiers, et al., 2000	Attentional Bias	Word Stroop	Opiates	Heroin addicts	Heroin addicts had an attentional bias toward heroin-related words
Jones et al., 2003	Attentional Bias	Flicker paradigm	Marijuana	Marijuana users	Heavier use associated with more attention for cannabis-related changes in a picture
Jones et al., 2002	Attentional Bias	Flicker paradigm	Marijuana	Marijuana users	Subjects who detected cannabis-related changes in a picture reported higher levels of use

processing. The basic assumption is that individuals react faster when categorizing strongly associated concepts that share a response key (i.e., compatible situation) and slower when categorizing concepts that are less likely to be associated and share a response key (i.e., incompatible situation; see Greenwald et al., 1998). To date, most studies that have adapted the IAT to evaluate relatively automatic associations in drug use focus on alcohol and tobacco use. Recently, Field et al. (2004) extended the use of the IAT to study evaluative associations in a sample of marijuana users and nonmarijuana users. Consistent with theories of associative memory, they expected marijuana users with relatively positive implicit cognitions toward drug use to react faster in categorizing stimuli highly associated in memory (e.g., marijuana + positive words) than when categorizing stimuli not highly associated in memory (e.g., marijuana + negative words). Alternatively, individuals with more negative associations with marijuana should process marijuana words paired with negative words faster. Overall, Field et al. found more negative associations for marijuana-related words in the group of nonmarijuana users but no significant differences for positive marijuana associations between users and nonusers. These findings are consistent with IAT effects found in studies on alcohol (e.g., Wiers et al., 2002) and smoking (e.g., Swanson et al., 2001).

There is still opportunity to explore influences on IAT effects in addiction research. For example, measurement approaches can be modified (see Wiers et al., 2002), contextual parameters varied (see Mitchell et al., 2003; Olson & Fazio, 2004), and changes in automatic processing in response to treatment assessed (see Teachman et al., 2003).

Visual Dot-Probe and Attentional Bias

A few researchers have examined attentional biases in cocaine, cannabis, and heroin users, but most studies focusing on attentional biases in addiction research have focused on alcohol and tobacco use (see Franken, 2003, for review). In the IAT study reviewed above, Field et al. (2004) also evaluated group differences in attentional biases among marijuana users and nonusers with a visual-probe task. With this task, individuals are expected to react faster to a probe that immediately appears on a computer screen in an area that was previously attended to than to a probe that appears in an area that was not previously attended to. That is, marijuana users should react faster to a probe that replaces a marijuana-related word than to a control word because of selective attention to marijuana-associated cues. Field et al. found that marijuana users reporting high levels of craving demonstrated significant attentional bias for marijuana-related words on the visual-probe task. Marijuana users reporting low levels of craving, however, did not show an attentional bias for marijuana words. These findings are consistent with a dot-probe study by Franken, Kroon, and Hendriks (2000) in which cocaine craving among cocaine users was correlated with attentional bias. In this study, more attentional bias for drug cues in cocaine-dependent patients was associated with higher scores on obsessive cocaine thoughts and higher craving scores. In another study, Lubman et al. (2000) demonstrated attentional bias in opiate-dependent patients measured with a pictorial version of the dot-probe task. In this study, addicts were faster in reacting to probes that replaced drug pictures as compared to neutral pictures, suggesting an attentional bias for picture cues.

Stroop Tasks and Attentional Bias

Another reaction-time measure of attentional bias is the Stroop task (Williams et al., 1996). In a typical Stroop task, key concept-related words and neutral words are presented in four different colors and the subject names the color of the word as quickly as possible while ignoring word meaning. A Stroop effect suggests that activation and accessibility of concepts related to a salient state affect what stimuli an individual selectively attends to (i.e., color or word meaning). Activation occurs relatively spontaneously likely involving implicit processes in the color-naming of words related to salient concerns.

In a study among a sample of abstinent heroin users, Franken, Kroon, Wiers, et al. (2000) found an attentional bias for heroin-related words with the use of a modified Stroop. Although the Stroop paradigm captures a relatively automatic or involuntary processing of meaning, this does not imply that this process occurs completely outside awareness. A "subliminal" Stroop has been used to assist in determining whether attentional biases occur outside awareness. With this paradigm, the duration of subliminally presented Stroop words (a few milliseconds) is too short for an individual to be consciously aware of the meaning of words. In contrast to the "supraliminal" Stroop, Franken, Kroon, Wiers, et al. (2000) did not find a subliminal Stroop effect in heroin addicts. These findings provide suggestive evidence that heroin-dependent subjects experience an implicit cognitive bias for heroin-related cues but this bias does not occur completely outside awareness. Franken et al. (2004) recently replicated the finding of an attentional bias in heroin-dependent patients with the use of a supraliminal Stroop paradigm, contributing further to the evidence of an attentional bias effect. In this study, Franken et al. (2004) also found that attentional bias for heroin cues decreased in abstinent heroin-dependent patients after a single dose of the dopamine antagonist haloperidol. Similarly, with the use of a modified Stroop, Copersino et al. (2004) found an attentional processing bias for

cocaine-related cues among cocaine-dependent individuals (but not cocaine-dependent schizophrenic patients). Additionally, only among the cocaine-dependent individuals was severity of cocaine craving correlated with attentional bias.

Attentional biases measured with Stroop paradigms have been shown to be predictive of alcohol (Cox et al., 2002) and smoking (Waters, Shiffman, et al., 2003) treatment outcomes. Recently, Marissen et al. (2004) found attentional bias predicted relapse at 3-month follow-up in heroin-dependent individuals, whereas subjective craving experience and physiological cue reactivity did not predict relapse in this population. Marissen et al. found that attentional bias in abstinent heroin-dependent patients decreased following treatment but cue-exposure therapy did not reduce attentional bias to heroin-related words any more than a control therapy. Although research indicates that implicit cognitive processes such as attentional bias may tap important components of drug dependence, it is not yet clear whether these processes can be sufficiently modified by current therapeutic interventions.

Flicker Paradigm and Attentional Bias

Another measure of attentional processing of drug-related stimuli is the flicker paradigm, a change-detection task (see Jones et al., 2002). In this paradigm, two versions of visual scenes are transiently presented repeatedly on a monitor. Objects in one scene are slightly different (e.g., deleted or rotated) from the original scene, and detection of this change is assessed. Jones et al. (2002) adapted this paradigm to evaluate information processing biases in social alcohol and marijuana users with the use of two competing stimuli in one scene (i.e., changes in a substance specific stimulus and a neutral stimulus). They demonstrated that participants who detected a marijuana-related change in the visual scene reported higher levels of marijuana use than participants who detected a neutral change. In another study, Jones et al. (2003) found that heavier marijuana users detected marijuana-related changes faster (with fewer flickers) than neutral-related changes. Interestingly, these findings were obtained within a group of social users, suggesting that this paradigm is sufficiently sensitive to reveal information-processing biases in social users (see Jones et al., 2003). These studies suggest that marijuana (and alcohol) use is associated with a cognitive bias towards substance-related stimuli, but the extent to which this task taps implicit processes requires further evaluation. The very limited duration of the scenes on the screen, however (250 ms; see Jones et al., 2002), makes it likely that implicit cognitive processes are involved. It is possible that each transient exposure through a priming mechanism influences subsequent detection and this information processing is faster for drug users exposed to relevant drug-related stimuli.

IMPLICATIONS FOR PREVENTION

Many of the paradigms reviewed in this chapter are applicable to interventions interested in evaluating change in spontaneously activated drug-related cognitions in response to an intervention. To date, cognitive processes that operate automatically have not been the focus of prevention research in the field of addictions, but changing automatic associative effects could be a fundamental adjunct to interventions. As noted by DiChiara (2002), "Both cognitive, conscious (explicit/declarative), as well as associative, unconscious (implicit/procedural) mechanisms contribute to purposeful behavior" (p. 76). If we assume that behavior is not only influenced by deliberate but also automatic processes, then components of an intervention must become implicitly activated in memory to compete with pre-existing, implicit drug-related cognitions. To enhance the relative accessibility of program information, interventions may need to include components focused on establishing and strengthening new associations that become part of what is spontaneously activated in memory to affect behavior (Stacy & Ames, 2001).

CONCLUSION

Although the associative-memory and reaction-time tasks described in this chapter appear to tap relatively spontaneous cognitions toward drug use, it is difficult to rule out the possibility that these methods may be contaminated by post-access processes. Do these tasks tap overlapping or unique dimensions of implicit cognitions or some other processes? Currently, there is a need to evaluate the convergent validity of the various reaction-time and associative-memory paradigms in addiction research. In one study that evaluated convergent validity of implicit measures of self-esteem, Bosson et al. (2000) found only small correlations between the Implicit Association Test and priming tasks. In another study among smokers, Mogg & Bradley (2002) found no significant correlations among three measures of processing biases (i.e., visual-probe task, and masked and unmasked Stroop tasks). Even within a single task, different measures may tap different constructs. For example, Waters, Sayette, Franken, et al. (2005) and Waters, Sayette, and Wertz (2003) showed that two different Stroop measures could be taken from one single task. One measure (i.e., Stroop effect) reflects the influence of the emotional salience of drug-related words on attentional processes within a short time frame (i.e., within a second). Another measure (i.e., carryover effect) reflects processing of the salient word occurring more than a second after the word is removed from the screen, thereby tapping the difficulty in disengaging attention from emotionally salient stimuli (Waters, Sayette, et al., 2005). Continued research that evaluates the contribution of automatic processes in drug-use motivation will help define the varying dimensions of implicit cognition, and the value added by including implicit cognition indices and components to prevention and treatment efforts.

REFERENCES

Ames, S. L., & Stacy, A. W. (1998). Implicit cognition in the prediction of substance use among drug offenders. *Psychology of Addictive Behaviors, 12*(4), 272–281.

Ames, S. L., Sussman, S., Dent, C., & Stacy, A. W. (2005). Implicit cognition and dissociative experiences as predictors of adolescent substance use. *American Journal of Drug and Alcohol Abuse, 31*(1), 29–162.

Ames, S. L., Zogg, J. B., & Stacy, A. W. (2002). Implicit cognition, impulsive sensation seeking, marijuana use, and driving behavior among drug offenders. *Personality and Individual Differences, 33*(7), 1055–1072.

Benthin, A., Slovic, P., Moran, P., Severson, H., Mertz, C. K., & Gerrard, M. (1995). Adolescent health-threatening and health-enhancing behaviors: A study of word association and imagery. *Journal of Adolescent Health, 17,* 143–152.

Bosson, J. K., Swann, W. B., & Pennebaker, J. W. (2000). Stalking the perfect measure of implicit self-esteem: The blind men and the elephant revised. *Journal of Personality and Social Psychology, 79*(4), 631–643.

Copersino, M. L., Serper, M. R., Vadhan, N., Goldberg, B. R., Richarme, D., Chou, J. C. Y., et al. (2004). Cocaine craving and attentional bias in cocaine-dependent schizophrenic patients. *Psychiatry Research, 128,* 209–218.

Cox, W. M., Hogan, L. M., Kristian, M. R., & Race, J. H. (2002). Alcohol attentional bias as a predictor of alcohol abusers' treatment outcome. *Drug and Alcohol Dependence, 68*(3), 237–243.

DiChiara, G. (2002). Nucleus accumbens shell and core dopamine: Differential role in behavior and addiction. *Behavioural Brain Research, 137,* 75–114.

Feldman, J. M., & Lynch, J. G. (1988). Self-generated validity and other effects of measurement on belief, attitude, intention, and behavior. *Journal of Applied Psychology, 73,* 421–435.

Feldtkeller, B., Weinstein, A., Cox, W. M., & Nutt, D. (2001). Effects of contextual priming on reactions to craving and withdrawal stimuli in alcohol-dependent participants. *Experimental & Clinical Psychopharmacology, 9,* 343–351.

Field, M., Mogg, K., & Bradley, B. P. (2004). Cognitive bias and drug craving in recreational cannabis users. *Drug and Alcohol Dependence, 74,* 105–111.

Franken, I. H. A. (2003). Drug craving and addiction: Integrating psychological and neuropsychopharmacological approaches. *Progress in Neuro-Psychopharmacology & Biological Psychiatry, 27*(4), 563–579.

Franken, I. H. A., Hendriks, V. M., Stam, C. J., & van den Brink, W. (2004). A role for dopamine in the processing of drug cues in heroin dependent patients. *European Neuropsychopharmacology, 14,* 503–508.

Franken, I. H. A., Kroon, L. Y., & Hendriks, V. M. (2000). Influence of individual differences in craving and obsessive cocaine thoughts on attentional processes in cocaine abuse patients. *Addictive Behaviors, 25,* 99–102.

Franken, I. H. A., Kroon, L. Y., Wiers, R. W., & Jansen, A. (2000). Selective cognitive processing of drug cues in heroin dependence. *Journal of Psychopharmacology, 145*, 395–400.

Gabrieli, J. D. E. (1998). Cognitive neuroscience of human memory. *Annual Review of Psychology, 49*, 87–115.

Green, P. D., & Galbraith, G. G. (1986). Associative responses to double entendre drug words: A study of drug addicts and college students. *Personality and Social Psychology Bulletin, 12*(1), 31–39.

Greenwald, A. G., McGhee, D. E., & Schwartz, J. K. L. (1998). Measuring individual differences in implicit cognition: The implicit association test. *Journal of Personality and Social Psychology, 74*, 1464–1480.

Haertzen, C. A., Hooks, N. T., & Pross, M. (1974). Drug associations as a measure of habit strength for specific drugs. *Journal of Nervous and Mental Disease, 158*(3), 189–197.

Haertzen, C. A., & Ross, F. E. (1980). Effects of clean, drug relevant, and drug word stimuli upon verbal associations to stages of addiction and steps in drug-taking. *Addictive Behaviors, 5*(4), 285–298.

Hill, A. B., & Paytner, S. (1992). Alcohol dependence and semantic priming of alcohol related words. *Personality and Individual Differences, 13*(6), 745–750.

Jacoby, L. L., & Kelley, C. M. (1991). A process dissociation framework for investigating unconscious influences: Freudian slips, projective tests, subliminal perception, and signal detection theory. *Current Directions in Psychological Science, 1*, 174–179.

James, W. (1890). *Habit.* New York. Henry Holt.

Jones, B. C., Jones, B. T., Blundell, L., & Bruce, G. (2002). Social users of alcohol and cannabis who detect substance-related changes in a change blindness paradigm report higher levels of use than those detecting substance-neutral changes. *Psychopharmacology, 165*(1), 93–96.

Jones, B. T., Jones, B. C., Smith, H., & Copley, N. (2003). A flicker paradigm for inducing change blindness reveals alcohol and cannabis information processing biases in social users. *Addiction, 98*(2), 235–244.

Knowlton, B. J., Mangels, J. A., & Squire, L. R. A. (1996). Neostriatal habit learning system in humans. *Science, 273*, 1399–1402.

Leeming, D., Hanley, M., Lyttle, S. (2002). Young people's images of cigarettes, alcohol and drugs. *Drugs: Education, prevention and policy, 9*(2), 169–185.

Levy, D. A., Starck, C. E. L., & Squire, L. R. (2004). Intact conceptual priming in the absence of declarative memory. *Psychological Science, 15*(10), 680–686.

Lubman, D. I., Peters, L. A., Mogg, K., Bradley, B. P., & Deakin, J. F. W. (2000). Attentional bias for drug cues in opiate dependence. *Psychological Medicine, 30*(1), 169–175.

Marissen, M. A. E., Franken, I. H. A., Waters, A. J., Blanken, P., van den Brink, W., & Hendriks, V. M. (2004). Attentional bias predicts relapse in heroin dependence following treatment. Manuscript submitted for publication.

McCusker, C. G. (2001).Cognitive biases and addiction: An evolution in theory and method. *Addiction, 96*, 47–56.

Mitchell, J. P., Nosek, B. A., & Banaji, M. R. (2003). Contextual variations in implicit evaluation. *Journal of Experimental Psychology: General, 132*(3), 455–469.

Mogg, K., & Bradley, B. P. (2002). Selective processing of smoking-related cues in smokers: Manipulation of deprivation level and comparison of three measures of processing bias. *Journal of Psychopharmacology, 16*(4), 385–392.

Nisbett, R. E., & Wilson, T. D. (1977). Telling more than we can know: Verbal reports on mental processes. *Psychological Review, 84,* 231–259.

Noble, C. E. (1952). An analysis of meaning. *Psychological Review, 59,* 421–430.

Olson, M. A., & Fazio, R. H. (2004). Reducing the influence of extrapersonal associations on the Implicit Association Test: Personalizing the IAT. *Journal of Personality and Social Psychology, 86,* 653–667.

Roediger, H. L. (1990). Implicit memory: Retention without remembering. *American Psychologist, 45,* 1043–1056.

Rolls, E. T. (2000). Memory systems in the brain. *Annual Review of Psychology, 51,* 599–630.

Schacter, D. L. (1985). Priming of old and new knowledge in amnesic patients and normal subjects. *Annals of the New York Academy of Science, 444,* 41–53.

Schacter, D. L. (1987). Implicit expressions of memory in organic amnesia: Learning of new facts and associations. *Human Neurobiology, 6*(2), 107–118.

Schacter, D. L. (1992). Understanding implicit memory: A cognitive neuroscience approach. *American Psychologist, 47*(40), 559–569.

Schacter, D. L., & Graf, P. (1986). Preserved learning in amnesic patients: Perspectives from research on direct priming. *Journal of Clinical & Experimental Neuropsychology, 8*(6), 727–743.

Shimamura, A. P., & Squire, L. R. (1984). Paired-associate learning and priming effects in amnesia: A neuropsychological study. *Journal of Experimental Psychology: General, 113,* 556–570.

Stacy, A. W. (1995). Memory association and ambiguous cues in models of alcohol and marijuana use. *Experimental & Clinical Psychopharmacology, 3,* 183–194.

Stacy, A. W. (1997). Memory activation and expectancy as prospective predictors of alcohol and marijuana use. *Journal of Abnormal Psychology, 106*(1), 61–73.

Stacy, A. W., & Ames, S. L. (2001). Implicit cognition theory in drug use and driving under the influence interventions. In S. Sussman (Ed.), *Handbook of program development in health behavior research and practice* (pp. 107–130). Thousand Oaks, CA: Sage.

Stacy, A. W., Ames, S. L., & Knowlton, B. (2004). Neurologically plausible distinctions in cognition relevant to drug use etiology and prevention. *Substance Use and Misuse, 39,* 1571–1623.

Stacy, A. W., Ames, S. L., Sussman, S., & Dent, C. W. (1996). Implicit cognition in adolescent drug use. *Psychology of Addictive Behaviors, 10*(3), 190–203.

Stacy, A. W., Ames, S. L., Ullman, J. B, Zogg, J. B., & Leigh, B. C. (in press). Spontaneous cognition and HIV risk behavior. *Psychology of Addictive Behavior.*

Stacy, A. W., Leigh, B. C., & Weingardt, K. R. (1994). Memory accessibility and association of alcohol use and its positive outcomes. *Experimental & Clinical Psychopharmacology, 2,* 269–282.

Stacy, A. W., & Newcomb, M. D. (1998). Memory association and personality as predictors of alcohol use: Mediation and moderator effects. *Experimental & Clinical Psychopharmacology, 6*(3), 280–291.

Swanson, J. E., Rudman, L. A., & Greenwald, A. G. (2001). Using the implicit association test to investigate attitude-behaviour consistency for stigmatized behaviour. *Cognition & Emotion, 15,* 207–230.

Szalay, L. B., Bovasso, G., Vilov, S., & Williams, R. E. (1992). Assessing treatment effects through changes in perceptions and cognitive organization. *American Journal of Drug and Alcohol Abuse, 18*(4), 407–428.

Szalay, L. B., Canino, G., & Vilov, S. K. (1993). Vulnerabilities and cultural change: Drug use among Puerto Rican adolescents in the United States. *International Journal of the Addictions, 28*(4), 327–354.

Szalay, L. B., Carroll, J. F., & Tims, F. (1993). Rediscovering free associations for use in psychotherapy. *Psychotherapy, 30*(2), 344–356.

Szalay, L. B., & Deese, J. (1978) *Subjective meaning and culture. An assessment through word association.* Hillsdale, NJ: Lawrence Erlbaum.

Szalay, L. B., Inn, A., Strohl, J. B., & Wilson, L. C. (1993). Perceived harm, age, and drug use: Perceptual and motivational dispositions affecting drug use. *Journal of Drug Education, 23*(4), 333–356.

Szalay, L. B., Strohl, J. B., & Doherty, K. T. (1999). *Psychoenvironmental forces in substance abuse prevention.* New York: Kluwer Academic/Plenum.

Szalay, L. B., Vilov, S., & Strohl, J. B. (1992). Charting the psychological correlates of drug abuse. In R. R. Watson (Ed.), *Alcohol and drug abuse reviews: Vol. 4. Drug abuse treatment.* Totowa, NJ: Humana.

Teachman, B. A., Woody, S. R., & Brownell, K. D. (2003). Automatic processing in spider phobia: Implicit fear associations over the course of treatment. *Journal of Abnormal Psychology, 112*(1), 100–109.

Underwood, B. J. (1959). Verbal learning in the educative processes. *Harvard Educational Review, 29,* 107–117.

Waters, A. J., Sayette, M. A., Franken, I. H. A., & Schwartz, J. E. (2005). Carry-over effects may capture a component of attentional bias. *Behaviour Research and Therapy,* 715–732.

Waters, A. J., Sayette, M. A., & Wertz, J. M. (2003). Carry-over effects can modulate emotional Stroop effects. *Cognition & Emotion, 17*(3), 501–509.

Waters, A. J., Shiffman, S., Sayette, M. A., Paty, J. A., Gwaltney, C. J., & Balabanis, M. H. (2003). Attentional bias predicts outcome in smoking cessation. *Health Psychology, 22*(4), 378–387.

Weingardt, K., Stacy, A. W., & Leigh, B. C. (1996). Automatic activation of alcohol concepts in response to positive outcomes of alcohol use. *Alcoholism: Clinical and Experimental Research, 20,* 25–30.

Weinstein, A. V., Feldtkeller, B. T., Myles, J., Law, F., & Nutt, D. J. (2000). The processing of automatic thoughts of drug use and craving in opiate-dependent individuals. *Experimental & Clinical Psychopharmacology, 8,*(4), 549–553.

White, N. M. (1996). Addictive drugs as reinforcers: Multiple partial actions on memory systems. *Addiction, 91,* 921–949.

Wiers, R. W., van Woerden, N., Smulders, F. T. Y., & de Jong, P. J. (2002). Implicit and explicit alcohol-related cognitions in heavy and light drinkers. *Journal of Abnormal Psychology, 111,* 648–658.

Williams, J. M. G., Mathews, A., & MacLeod, C. (1996). The emotional Stroop task and psychopathology. *Psychological Bulletin, 120*(1), 3–24.

Zack, M., Toneatto, T., & MacLeod, C. M. (1999). Implicit activation of alcohol concepts by negative affective cues distinguishes between problem drinkers with high and low psychiatric distress. *Journal of Abnormal Psychology, 108,* 518–531.

CHAPTER 24

Implicit Cognition in Problem Gambling

Martin Zack and Constantine X. Poulos

Abstract: This overview describes three implicit paradigms used to assess activation of semantic networks in problem gamblers. Stroop interference to gambling stimuli discriminates between different subtypes of gamblers (slots vs. racetrack bettors) and is absent in nonproblem gamblers. Response time to alcohol words paired with gambling win versus loss words on the Implicit Association Test discriminates between problem gamblers with different propensities to drink in response to gambling wins versus losses. Reading latency to gambling words under the influence of amphetamine in a pharmacological priming paradigm called the Lexical Salience Task discriminates problem gamblers from problem drinkers and healthy controls. The findings show that trait factors, learning history, and pharmacological probes all moderate implicit gambling-related cognitions in problem gamblers.

INTRODUCTION

Stacy et al. (1994) proposed that addictive behavior is "mediated" by implicit associations in memory, which link prior associates of addictive reinforcers with future seeking and use. Hills and Dickerson (2002) summarized this argument, noting that "Stacy and colleagues question the rational view of decision making which assumes people consciously weigh pros and cons, all of which are equally accessible from memory. Instead, they invoke the spreading activation model of memory to suggest that closely associated concepts in memory such as *have fun–drink*

alcohol (or *feel good–gamble*) will be most highly accessible and will automatically come to mind to direct behavioural 'decisions'" (p. 598). Three critical ideas are expressed here: First, cognitive events often exert causal effects on addictive behavior. Second, these cognitions can be activated automatically by relevant cues. Third, cognitive activation can operate outside awareness to bias decisions and overt behavior toward addictive reinforcers and away from adaptive alternatives.

Although formally classified as an Impulse Control Disorder in the *DSM-IV* (American Psychiatric Association, 1994), considerable evidence supports the characterization of

AUTHOR'S NOTE: The authors wish to thank Ms. Tracy Woodford for her valuable assistance in the amphetamine study and Mr. Ken Seergobin for programming the computer tasks.

Funding for this research was provided by the National Center of Responsible Gaming and the Ontario Problem Gambling Research Centre.

pathological or problem gambling as a form of addiction. Like drug or alcohol addiction, problem gambling involves symptoms of tolerance, withdrawal, and strong urges or cravings, along with high rates of relapse (e.g., Castellani & Rugle, 1995). Problem gamblers are also more likely to exhibit anomalies in genes that code for dopamine receptors, much like substance abusers (Comings & Blum, 2000). Neuroimaging research also shows that acute anticipation and receipt of monetary rewards, core elements of gambling activity, activate discrete brain regions associated with the reinforcing effects of addictive drugs (Knutson et al., 2001). These kinds of evidence strongly suggest that problem gambling is a form of addiction.

In recent years, changes in policy and the advent of the Internet have led to drastic increases in the availability of gambling activities. This trend has coincided with a surge in the incidence of problem gambling, a disorder once considered rare (Volberg, 2002). The relative recency of widespread problem gambling compared to other forms of addiction, like alcoholism or drug abuse, has resulted in a lag in research on implicit cognition in problem gambling. Nevertheless, a handful of studies have been identified, which employ a range of methodologies to investigate implicit cognitive processes in problem gambling. Implicit tasks have been used to investigate a dual-process model of cognition in problem gamblers (see Evans & Coventry, Chapter 3). The present overview aims to illustrate the progression in the nature of the questions posed about problem gambling and the implicit procedures used to answer them.

THE MODIFIED STROOP TASK

Background

The modified or emotional Stroop is among the most widely used tasks for the assessment of implicit cognition in psychopathology (Williams et al., 1996). Like the original or "classic" Stroop (Stroop, 1935), the dependent measure in the modified Stroop task is latency to name the print color of a word stimulus. In the modified Stroop, slower color-naming of schema-relevant words reflects greater involuntary attention to clinically relevant words as compared with neutral words (Kahneman & Chajczyk, 1983). This bias, in turn, is presumed to reflect the activation of the corresponding concepts in memory, and provides one operational definition of the "salience" of a class of stimuli.

The modified Stroop has been successfully applied to the investigation of addiction-specific schemata. It appears to be sensitive to trait (e.g., problem vs. social drinker; Stetter et al., 1995), and state factors such as short-term cigarette abstinence versus nonabstinence (Gross et al., 1993). Interference to smoking words also predicts individual differences in nicotine dependence and the self-reported desire to smoke following overnight abstinence in adolescent smokers (Zack et al., 2001). It has been suggested that interference on the modified Stroop provides an operational definition of drug "wanting" in smokers (see Mogg & Bradley, 2002). Thus, the modified Stroop would appear to reflect incentive salience of addictive stimuli proposed by Robinson and Berridge (2001).

The modified Stroop would appear to be well suited to an initial investigation of implicit addiction-specific biases in problem gamblers. This research is discussed below.

Initial Study on Implicit Gambling-Related Cognitions Using the Modified Stroop

McCusker and Gettings (1997) used a card version of the modified Stroop task to assess interference to gambling-related words in treatment seeking (Gamblers' Anonymous) problem gamblers ($N = 15$) whose primary form of gambling was "fruit" machines (i.e., slot machines) or horse racing. The target stimuli were words related to each subtype of gambling (e.g., slots, jockey) that were compared to length- and frequency-matched drug-related (e.g., grass, needle) and neutral (e.g., egg, statue) words.

Overall, problem gamblers displayed significantly slower color-naming of gambling versus neutral or drug-related words, whereas nongambler control subjects displayed no such bias. Although drug and alcohol use data for the problem gamblers were not provided, they displayed no differences in color-naming of drug-related versus neutral words and did not differ from the spouses or controls in color-naming of drug-related words themselves. This indicates that the interference they displayed to gambling words was not a general response to addiction-related stimuli. In addition, the interference effects for gambling words were selective for each subtype of gambling, with slots players displaying significant interference to slots-related words only, whereas racetrack players displayed interference to track-related words only. The finding of Stroop interference to gambling words has recently been replicated, using a computerized task and manual rather than vocal response latency as the dependent measure (Boyer & Dickerson, 2003). Although these authors assert that their findings support a dimensional basis for biases in implicit gambling-related cognition based on degree of impaired impulse control rather than problem gambler status, their measure of impaired control correlates with problem gambling scores on the SOGS (South Oaks Gambling Screen), suggesting that impaired impulse control is essentially a proxy variable for problem gambling in this study.

The Stroop data for problem gamblers suggest that gambling pathology has similar effects on involuntary attention as substance-based addictions. The finding that subtype of gambler predicted the specific type of gambling stimuli that elicited interference

further corroborates the role of experiential factors and implies that gambling-related cognitive schemata are not uniform. This is consistent with the high degree of heterogeneity in symptoms and gambling profiles often cited in the literature on problem gambling (Dickerson & Baron, 2000).

The heterogeneity of problem gambling would be expected to create large individual differences in the gambling schema, with corresponding limits on the range of stimuli that are reliably schema-relevant. This can cause difficulties for research by restricting the number of verbal stimuli available to investigate implicit cognition in problem gamblers.

By establishing the discriminant validity of implicit gambling-related cognitions as an index of problem gambler status or impaired control, the findings from McCusker and Gettings (1997) provide a good foundation for subsequent research. The use of the Stroop enables direct comparisons with other types of addictive disorders. At the same time, the moderating effects of problem gambling severity and state factors such as primed motivation to gamble remain important issues for further investigation.

Although the modified Stroop is internally valid and sensitive, it is not particularly suitable to the assessment of implicit cognitive associations. Such associations may explain patterns of cue-reactivity beyond increased salience per se.

For example, the word "wager" may be highly salient to a problem gambler. Antecedents (cues) and consequences (reinforcement), however, can strongly influence the motivation to wager. From a cognitive perspective, these events would be coded as associates of wagering in the gambling network. As a result, it should be possible to evaluate the role of antecedents and consequences on gambling by measuring priming and interference in response time when a gambling activity word (wager) is preceded or followed by a word whose corresponding concept is associated (e.g., lucky) or not associated (e.g., lumber) with gambling in memory.

Assessing these types of associations may be important because cue-induced cognitive associations may reflect a person's learning history and may therefore be especially sensitive to individual differences in gambling-related psychopathology. For example, a measure of implicit cognitive associations may distinguish gamblers with differing motives for gambling (e.g., coping vs. enhancement; see Chapter 18 by Birch and colleagues in this volume for additional information on these motives) and differing degrees of comorbidity (e.g., alcohol misuse). The second study (Zack et al., 2005), described below, investigates these issues.

ASSESSING GAMBLING-ALCOHOL ASSOCIATIONS WITH THE IMPLICIT ASSOCIATION TEST

The Implicit Association Test (IAT) was first developed to evaluate involuntary cognitive responses to social stimuli, such as evaluative judgments about names that typify members of an out-group (Greenwald et al., 1998). Since its inception, numerous studies have used this task to assess implicit attitudes (cf. Nosek et al., 2005). The specific strengths and applications of the IAT are detailed elsewhere in this volume (Fadardi et al., Chapter 9; Houben et al., Chapter 7).

Briefly, the task involves rapidly classifying individual words denoting various classes of target stimuli. The primary question is whether classification is facilitated or inhibited when two categories of words are mapped onto the same response key (e.g., alcohol + positive consequences). Facilitation in response time indicates that the congruently mapped categories are implicitly associated; inhibition indicates that the categories are dissociated or independent.

In the present case, the hypothesis that positive gambling outcomes are associated with alcohol predicts that response time will be faster on trials where words like "jackpot" and "beer" entail the same response (press left key) than on trials where words like "forfeit" and "beer" entail the same response (press left key). Note, the key designation itself (left/right) is unimportant; the critical issue is whether the categories that are mapped onto the same response key in a given phase are related (e.g., jackpot and beer) or unrelated (e.g., forfeit and beer).

The IAT has been used to assess implicit associations between alcohol and positive versus negative outcomes and between alcohol and arousal versus sedation effects in light and heavy drinkers (Wiers et al., 2002). In that study, IAT effects correlated with drinking behavior within a prospective design, supporting the predictive validity of this task.

As well, the IAT can reliably detect associations with fewer than 10 exemplars for the target category. This is an important consideration in the case of gambling, which (as noted above) is a category with relatively few viable exemplars.

The predictive validity of the IAT for future drinking behavior implies that this task might also be sensitive to contingent patterns of addictive behavior in individuals with different learning histories. Specifically, the IAT may reveal implicit associations between gambling outcomes and alcohol use in problem gamblers with differing patterns of gambling and drinking and differing degrees of co-morbid alcohol misuse. The ability to assess these types of associative processes is important given the high degree of co-morbidity in gambling and alcohol use disorders (Kausch, 2003).

To test this possibility, we (Zack et al., 2005) assessed responses to alcohol words paired with words denoting gambling win outcomes (e.g., jackpot) versus gambling loss outcomes (e.g., forfeit) in the IAT. Subjects ($N = 144$; 34 women) were recruited by newspaper ads from two urban Canadian populations, and all met criteria for problem gambling on the South Oaks Gambling Screen (SOGS; Lesieur & Blume, 1987). Alcohol misuse was measured by the Brief Michigan Alcohol Screening Test (BMAST; Pokorny et al., 1972). Using a cutoff score of six, roughly half the sample could be classified as problem drinkers. Following the IAT, subjects completed a scale to determine their tendency (more likely, not more likely) to drink in response to gambling wins and in response to gambling losses. In addition, they completed the Drinking Motives Questionnaire (DMQ; Cooper et al., 1992) to assess nongambling-specific drinking motives.

The primary research question was: What is the effect of gambling win/loss words on response time to alcohol words as a function of one's tendency to drink in response to a gambling win versus a loss? Previous research had shown that wins and losses represent distinct discriminative stimuli for gambling (Stewart et al., 2002), suggesting that a parallel relationship might apply with respect to these gambling outcomes and alcohol use. Such an association could help to explain patterns of comorbid gambling and alcohol misuse and might also inform interventions to weaken the linkage of these behaviors.

The study found an overall facilitatory effect of gambling wins on response time to alcohol words. The degree of facilitation was also significantly greater in subjects who said they were more likely to drink when they won at gambling. In addition, severity of alcohol misuse on the BMAST directly predicted the degree of win-based facilitation of alcohol words on the IAT. Supplemental analyses confirmed that this was not mediated by a greater self-reported tendency for problem drinkers to drink in response to wins. In contrast to the significant IAT effects related to win-based drinking, the reported tendency to drink in response to gambling losses had no effect on mean IAT responses to alcohol words. This latter finding was in contrast to the expected facilitatory effect

of gambling loss words on response time to alcohol words in the gamblers who said they were more likely to drink when they lost. This apparent inconsistency may reflect the influence of variation in problem gambling severity, as regression analyses found that SOGS scores directly predicted the degree of facilitation on loss-alcohol trials in loss-based drinkers.

Scores from the DMQ subscales revealed that drinking in response to gambling wins was most strongly correlated with drinking to enhance positive affect, whereas drinking in response to gambling losses was most strongly correlated with drinking to cope with negative affect. These intercorrelations support the validity of the gambling-specific drinking scales. Neither the enhancement nor the coping subscale of the DMQ, however, reliably predicted win-based facilitation of alcohol words on the IAT, indicating that gambling-specific drinking patterns were critical to the degree of win-alcohol facilitation.

The findings of this study are consistent with those of a previous study on negative emotional priming of alcohol concepts in problem drinkers (Zack et al., 1999; see also Birch et al., Chapter 18, for additional details). They indicate that both trait factors (in this case concurrent problem drinking and problem gambling) and situational factors (i.e., contingent gambling-drinking patterns) moderate implicit associations between gambling outcomes and alcohol use. The present findings imply that efforts to extinguish the association between winning at gambling and drinking may have a general beneficial effect on alcohol use (and its attendant effects on decision making and impulsivity) in problem gamblers. In addition, this extinction approach may be particularly useful for gamblers who already evidence clinically significant levels of alcohol misuse.

For example, exposure to alcoholic beverages (coupled with drinking response prevention) during an episode of preprogrammed win or loss trials on a slot machine may help to establish a dissociation between gambling and alcohol consumption. Ladouceur and colleagues have found that such in vivo manipulations facilitate cognitive restructuring in problem gamblers (Ladouceur et al., 2002). It should also be acknowledged, however, that, although general associations between gambling and alcohol may be amenable to such interventions, more specific (i.e., win/loss– alcohol) associations may be more resistant to extinction (Wiers et al., 2004).

PHARMACOLOGICAL PRIMING OF GAMBLING COGNITIONS: THE LEXICAL SALIENCE TASK

In experimental studies, drugs are often used to probe the neurochemical substrates of addictive behavior (Stewart & de Wit, 1987). If administration of a drug increases drug-seeking behavior, it follows that its administration should also increase activation of semantic memory networks related to the addictive reinforcer. This logic provides a framework for the next study, which we describe below.

The third study on implicit cognition in problem gambling adopted a cognitive neuroscience approach to investigate the effects of a pharmacological challenge in problem gamblers (Zack & Poulos, 2004). The between-subjects variables were gambler status (problem vs. nonproblem) and drinker status (problem vs. nonproblem), which were fully crossed, leading to a 2 × 2 factorial design. Nonproblem gamblers were individuals who gambled infrequently and scored < 4 on the SOGS. Nonproblem drinkers were individuals who drank socially and scored < 8 on the Alcohol Dependence Scale (Ross et al., 1990). The pharmacological challenge was a moderate (30 mg) oral dose of the prototypic psychomotor stimulant, d-amphetamine.

The rationale for the study was twofold: First, there is considerable debate as to whether problem gambling is better characterized as an addiction or an impulse control disorder (e.g., Blaszczynski, 1999). As noted earlier, however, a growing literature on genetic, neurochemical, and clinical similarities between problem gamblers and substance abusers indirectly supports the assertion that problem gambling is an addiction. Evidence indicating a neurochemical similarity between problem gamblers and substance abusers would corroborate the existing evidence that problem gambling is an addiction.

Second, it is unclear whether the overlap between problem gambling and substance addiction involves a generic process (e.g., compulsive seeking behavior), or a specific process (e.g., activation of a particular set of neurochemical processes and concomitant subjective effects). Evidence indicating a differential effect of amphetamine in problem gamblers versus abusers of alcohol, a drug that has different neurochemical properties than amphetamine, would support the specificity hypothesis. The specificity hypothesis is based on a wealth of evidence showing that amphetamine, at a range of doses, does not prime alcohol consumption in animals familiar with alcohol (e.g., Halladay et al., 1999; Linseman, 1990).

The choice of amphetamine as a neurochemical probe was based on early research that found that problem gamblers describe an imagined bout of gambling in terms that are strikingly similar to those used by psychostimulant abusers to describe the effects of their drug use (Hickey et al., 1986). In addition, the stereotypic profile of response to stimulants closely mirrors the highly stereotyped pattern often seen in gambling behavior. Finally, several bio-assay studies had found indirect evidence of anomalies in brain catecholamine (dopamine and norepinephrine) function in problem gamblers versus healthy individuals, using metabolite levels in cerebrospinal fluid to detect these effects (Bergh et al., 1997). Activation of the brain catecholamine systems is critically involved in the subjective and behavioral effects of psychostimulant drugs (e.g., Ventura et al., 2003), further suggesting that problem gambling may induce psychostimulant-like neurochemical effects.

The hypothesis that amphetamine would activate gambling-specific motivational responses stemmed from research on a phenomenon called cross-priming. This phenomenon involves the noncontingent delivery of a small dose of one drug to elicit seeking of another drug with similar properties. For example, animals with a history of cocaine self-administration will display cocaine-seeking behavior in response to a priming dose of another psychostimulant, amphetamine (Schenk & Partridge, 1999). In contrast, cocaine-familiar animals will not display such cross-priming in response to a nonstimulant drug like THC, the active ingredient in marijuana (Schenk & Partridge, 1999). The occurrence of cross-priming is believed to indicate that the reinforcing effects of the prime and target drugs are mediated by common neurochemical substrates (e.g., Stewart & de Wit, 1987). In the present case, evidence that amphetamine selectively activated motivation to gamble would indicate that the reinforcing effects of gambling and psychostimulant drugs are mediated by common neurochemical substrates.

As noted in earlier sections, implicit cognitive tasks provide a sensitive and internally valid means of assessing addictive motivation. This is evident in the relative salience of words denoting addictive stimuli as compared with neutral stimuli. Interference on the modified Stroop task and facilitation on the IAT task each provide an operational definition of salience. In the case of the IAT, this salience is conferred or amplified by exposure to motivationally relevant associate cues. Both the Stroop and IAT, however, engage processes that may be susceptible to

the generic effects of a pharmacological probe. For example, inhibition of a prepotent reading response will critically influence performance on the Stroop, irrespective of the semantic content of the word stimulus. Similarly, decision-making proficiency will critically influence performance on the IAT, regardless of the categories involved (Mierke & Klauer, 2003). Because psychoactive drugs can powerfully influence each of these generic processes (Servan-Schreiber et al., 1998), implicit cognitive biases induced by a drug probe on these tasks may be obscured by drug-induced ceiling or floor effects or may interact with generic effects in a manner that hampers clear interpretation. To minimize these potential problems, it is desirable to employ a task that engages the minimum number of cognitive processes to measure "accessibility" of a concept in memory (see McCusker, 2001).

The semantic priming literature has shown that rapid reading of verbal stimuli is a highly robust procedure for assessing primed access to a target concept (Neely, 1991). In that case, priming is inferred from faster reading (shorter response latencies) of target words on trials where the prime word that immediately precedes the target is conceptually related (e.g., salt) rather than unrelated (e.g., sod) to the target (e.g., pepper). Because reading is highly automatized, reading latency provides an index of target accessibility that is relatively unaffected by other executive processes (e.g., inhibition, decision-making; Owen et al., 2004).

To evaluate the effects of a pharmacological prime on accessibility of target concepts, we modified the semantic priming rapid reading task from its conventional form. The general logic was that amphetamine would serve as the prime for gambling-related cognitions in problem gamblers. Accordingly, the verbal primes that precede each target in the conventional reading task were removed in the modified task. To distinguish this task from the conventional semantic priming task, we refer to it as the Lexical Salience Task (LST). On any trial, subjects simply saw a fixation stimulus (e.g., &&&&) and responded as quickly as possible to the target word (e.g., wager). Target stimuli were degraded with asterisks (e.g., w*a*g*e*r), a procedure shown to increase priming effects (Stanovich & West, 1983), and previously employed in studies using the reading task to assess implicit addictive cognitions (Weingardt et al., 1996).

The dependent variable was time to read the target stimulus aloud, which was registered by a voice-activated response key (microphone attached to the computer). Faster reading responses (i.e., shorter response latencies) to a class of targets (e.g., gambling words) under the influence of the drug versus placebo would provide an index of pharmacological priming of the addiction schema. In the present case, the modified rapid reading task included five classes of target words, gambling, alcohol, positive affect (e.g., happy), negative affect (e.g., anxious), and neutral (e.g., window), all of which were categorized and matched on length, and frequency. Categories and items were randomized over trials. Testing occurred 90 minutes after receipt of the capsule, and drug versus placebo was counterbalanced and administered in a double blind manner on two procedurally identical test sessions.

The study found that amphetamine primed motivation to gamble. This was supported by ratings on modified visual analogue scales, in which gamblers reported a significant increase in desire to gamble and a significant decrease in confidence to refrain from gambling under amphetamine relative to placebo. Problem drinkers displayed no such change in motivation for alcohol under amphetamine.

On the LST, amphetamine produced strikingly different effects in problem gamblers than in nonproblem gamblers. In nonproblem gamblers, amphetamine led to an undifferentiated improvement in reading responses (i.e., shorter response latencies) to all five classes of words. This is consistent with the generic improvement in mental fluency expected from a psychostimulant drug (Servan-Schreiber et al., 1998). By contrast, in problem gamblers, amphetamine selectively facilitated reading responses (shorter latencies) to gambling words, and selectively inhibited reading responses (longer latencies) to neutral words. Amphetamine had no significant priming effect on response time to alcohol words in problem drinkers or comorbid problem gambler drinkers, further supporting the specificity of the cross-priming effects for gamblers.

Scores on the Multiple Affective Adjective Checklist (MAACL; Zuckerman & Lubin, 1965) increased significantly but nonspecifically, under amphetamine, and were not affected by group. In addition, neither the overall score nor the subscale scores on the MAACL correlated with scores on the desire scales or LST. Thus, affective responses to amphetamine do not appear to account for its effects on self-report or cognitive indices of motivation to gamble.

The selective facilitation of gambling words was hypothesized: Under the influence of a pharmacological prime for gambling, gambling concepts should become more accessible. The inhibition of neutral words was both unexpected and striking given amphetamine's generic facilitatory effects on mental fluency. This combined pattern of results reflects a "polarizing" effect of the drug prime on motivationally relevant versus motivationally irrelevant concepts in memory. Selective facilitation of response time to gambling words indicated that gambling concepts were more accessible under amphetamine. In terms of this logic, selective slowing of response time to neutral words indicated that neutral concepts were less accessible under amphetamine.

As we noted in our original article, activation or priming of an incentive motivational system operates to suppress other motivational systems as well as irrelevant activities and cues (Volkow et al., 2004). In Robinson and Berridge's (2001) model of addiction, incentive motivation is dysregulated by repeated exposure to addictive substances, which results in pathological "wanting" or craving. As a corollary to this model, Kostowski (2002) proposed that such pathological drug "wanting" involves concurrent pathological suppression of irrelevant activities and these combined factors mediate compulsive drug-seeking to the exclusion of normal adaptive behaviors. This general framework makes sense of the present findings. The selective facilitation of reading responses to gambling words in problem gamblers can be interpreted as targeted wanting whereas the concurrent slowing of responses to neutral words reflects a linked suppression of irrelevant stimuli. This interpretation is corroborated by the self-reported motivational effects of amphetamine discussed below.

The relevance of primed responses on the LST to gambling-related pathology was supported by correlational data. Specifically, severity of gambling problems in terms of maximum financial loss in a single gambling episode significantly predicted (faster) responses to gambling words under amphetamine, controlling for responses to gambling words under placebo (i.e., unprimed accessibility of schema-relevant concepts). Similarly, both maximum loss and scores on the diagnostic inventory for problem gambling, the SOGS (Lesieur & Blume, 1987), significantly predicted (slower) responses to neutral words under amphetamine, controlling for responses to neutral words under placebo. Finally, in addition to these trait measures, the LST was also sensitive to state measures. Specifically, self-reported desire to gamble was significantly correlated with response time to gambling words under amphetamine, controlling for response time to gambling words under placebo and for desire to gamble under placebo. The greater the reported desire to gamble under the drug,

the faster was the response time to gambling words.

Taken together, the findings from this study demonstrate an important commonality between psychostimulant drug effects and motivation to gamble. These effects are evident in terms of biases in implicit activation of gambling versus neutral concepts as well as self-reported motivation to gamble. The evidence from the LST suggests that it may provide a useful tool for exploring pharmacological priming effects in a highly sensitive, internally valid manner. Accordingly, we have since demonstrated that a low-dose of diazepam, which has similar neurochemical effects to alcohol, selectively primes reading responses to alcohol words in problem drinkers (Poulos & Zack, 2004). Thus, the LST appears to afford a simple, unambiguous measure of primed motivation to engage in addictive behavior and the concomitant salience of addictive reinforcers. Conceptually, the evidence of pharmacological priming of semantic memory networks strengthens the assertion that accessibility of addiction concepts provides an operational definition of the motivation to engage in addictive behavior. At a more practical level, the LST may have value in the assessment of putative medications designed to treat addictive behavior. Evidence that a medication modulates the response to gambling activity or psychostimulant drug primes on implicit measures like the Stroop or LST would support this possibility.

SUMMARY AND FUTURE DIRECTIONS

As noted earlier, problem gambling is a disorder characterized by a high degree of heterogeneity. Delineating subtypes or dimensions of gambling pathology will be important for effective intervention. The implicit cognitive procedures described in this chapter, along with those described in other chapters in this volume, should provide valuable tools for defining these subtypes and dimensions in a sensitive and objective way. Such tasks may also assist in defining the relationship between specific neurochemical processes and the psychological constructs (e.g., motives, expectancies) that influence problem gambling. This in turn will facilitate the development of new and better treatments for this serious disorder.

The studies reported above provide a brief but clear depiction of implicit cognitive processes in problem gambling. The evidence shows that problem gambling shares many of the same cognitive biases with respect to target reinforcers as alcoholism and drug abuse. As in the case of these more familiar addictions, implicit cognitive biases in problem gambling appear to be influenced by trait as well as state factors. The importance of learning history as a moderating factor is also evident, highlighting the value of implicit cognition as an index of individual differences

in gambling pathology. Finally, the incorporation of pharmacological primes into conventional implicit cognitive paradigms permits investigation of the role of specific neurochemical processes on addictive motivation in a manner that is both sensitive and relatively immune to distortion.

Drugs of abuse can have both acute and chronic disruptive effects on basic mental functions. Research on implicit cognition in substance abusers is inherently vulnerable to these effects. By contrast, problem gambling involves no direct exposure to pharmacological agents, yet appears to engage many of the same processes as substance addiction. As such, research on implicit cognition in problem gambling not only serves a practical goal of informing treatment and prevention of this disorder; it also provides a means of assessing the role of implicit cognitive processes in addiction where the neurotoxic effects of abused substances are not a factor.

REFERENCES

American Psychiatric Association. (1994). *Diagnostic and statistical manual of mental disorders* (4th ed.). Washington, DC: Author.

Bergh, C., Eklund, T., Sodersten, P., & Nordin, C. (1997). Altered dopamine function in pathological gambling. *Psychological Medicine, 27,* 473–475.

Blaszczynski, A. (1999). Pathological gambling: An impulse control, addictive or obsessive-compulsive disorder? *Anuario de Psicologia, 30,* 93–109.

Boyer, M., & Dickerson, M. (2003). Attentional bias and addictive behaviour: Automaticity in a gambling-specific modified Stroop task. *Addiction, 98,* 61–70.

Castellani, B., & Rugle, L. (1995). A comparison of pathological gamblers to alcoholics and cocaine misusers on impulsivity, sensation seeking, and craving. *International Journal on Addictions, 30,* 275–289.

Comings, D. E., & Blum, K. (2000). Reward deficiency syndrome: Genetic aspects of behavioral disorders. *Progress in Brain Research, 126,* 325–341.

Cooper, M. L., Russell, M., Skinner, J. B., & Windle, M. (1992). Development and validation of a three-dimensional measure of drinking motives. *Psychological Assessment, 42,* 123–132.

Dickerson, M., & Baron, E. (2000). Contemporary issues and future directions for research into pathological gambling. *Addiction, 95,* 1145–1159.

Greenwald, A. G., McGhee, D. E., & Schwartz, J. L. K. (1998). Measuring individual differences in implicit cognition: The implicit association test. *Journal of Personality and Social Psychology, 74,* 1464–1480.

Gross, T. M., Jarvik, M. E., & Rosenblatt, M. R. (1993). Nicotine abstinence produces content-specific Stroop interference. *Psychopharmacology, 110,* 333–336.

Halladay, A. K., Wagner, G. C., Hsu, T., Sekowski, A., & Fisher, H. (1999). Differential effects of monoaminergic agonists on alcohol intake in rats fed a tryptophan-enhanced diet. *Alcohol, 18,* 55–64.

Hickey, J. E., Haertzen, C. A., & Henningfield, J. E. (1986). Simulation of gambling responses on the Addiction Research Center Inventory. *Addictive Behaviors, 11,* 345–349.

Hills, A. M., & Dickerson, M. (2002). Emotion, implicit decision making and persistence at gaming. *Addiction, 97,* 598–599.

Kahneman, D., & Chajczyk, D. (1983). Tests of the automaticity of reading: Dilution of Stroop effects by color-irrelevant stimuli. *Journal of Experimental Psychology: Human Perception and Performance, 9,* 497–509.

Kausch, O. (2003). Patterns of substance abuse among treatment-seeking pathological gamblers. *Journal of Substance Abuse Treatment, 25,* 263–270.

Knuston, B., Fong, G. W., Adams, C. M., Varner, J. L., & Hommer, D. (2001). Dissociation of reward anticipation and outcome with event-related fMRI. *Neuroreport, 12,* 3683–3687.

Kostowski, W. (2002). Drug addiction as drive satisfaction ('antidrive') dysfunction. *Acta Neurobiologica Experimenta, 62,* 111–117.

Ladouceur, R., Sylvain, C., Boutin, C., & Doucet, C. (2002). *Understanding and treating the pathological gambler.* New York: Wiley.

Lesieur, H. R., & Blume, S. B. (1987). The South Oaks Gambling Screen (SOGS): A new instrument for identification of pathological gamblers. *American Journal of Psychiatry, 144,* 1184–1188.

Linseman, M. A. (1990). Effects of dopaminergic agents on alcohol consumption by rats in a limited access paradigm. *Psychopharmacology, 100,* 195–200.

McCusker, C. G. (2001). Cognitive biases and addiction: An evolution in theory and method. *Addiction, 96,* 47–56.

McCusker, C. G., & Gettings, B. (1997). Automaticity of cognitive biases in addictive behaviours: Further evidence with gamblers. *British Journal of Clinical Psychology, 36,* 543–554.

Mierke, J., & Klauer, K. C. (2003). Method-specific variance in the implicit association test. *Journal of Personality and Social Psychology, 85,* 1180–1192.

Mogg, K., & Bradley, B. P. (2002). Selective processing of smoking-related cues in smokers: Manipulation of deprivation level and comparison of three measures of processing bias. *Journal of Psychopharmacology, 16,* 385–392.

Neely, J. H. (1991). Semantic priming effects in visual word recognition: A selective review of current findings and theories. In D. Besner & G. W. Humphreys (Eds.), *Basic processes in reading: Visual word recognition* (pp. 264–337). Hillsdale, NJ: Lawrence Erlbaum.

Nosek, B. A., Greenwald, A. G., & Banaji, M. R. (2005). Understanding and Using the Implicit Association Test: II. Method variables and construct validity. *Personality and Social Psychology Bulletin, 31,* 166–180.

Owen, W. J., Borowsky, R., & Sarty, G. E. (2004). fMRI of two measures of phonological processing in visual word recognition: Ecological validity matters. *Brain and Language, 90,* 40–46.

Pokorny, A. D., Miller, B. A., & Kaplan, H. B. (1972). The brief MAST: A shortened version of the Michigan Alcoholism Screening Test. *American Journal of Psychiatry, 129,* 342–345.

Poulos, C. X., & Zack, M. (2004). Low dose diazepam primes motivation for alcohol and alcohol-related semantic networks in problem drinkers. *Behavioural Pharmacology, 15,* 503–512.

Robinson, T. E., & Berridge, K. C. (2001). Incentive sensitization and addiction. *Addiction, 96,* 103–114.

Ross, H. E., Gavin, D. R., & Skinner, H. A. (1990). Diagnostic validity of the MAST and the Alcohol Dependence Scale in the assessment of *DSM-III* alcohol disorders. *Journal of Studies on Alcohol, 51,* 506–513.

Schenk, S., & Partridge, B. (1999). Cocaine-seeking produced by experimenter-administered drug injections: Dose-effect relationships in rats. *Psychopharmacology, 147,* 285–290.

Servan-Schreiber, D., Carter, C. S., Bruno, R. M., & Cohen, J. D. (1998). Dopamine and the mechanisms of cognition: Part II. D-amphetamine effects in human subjects performing a selective attention task. *Biological Psychiatry, 43,* 723–729.

Stacy, A. W., Leigh, B. C., & Weingardt, K. R. (1994). Memory accessibility and association of alcohol use and its positive outcomes. *Experimental & Clinical Psychopharmacology, 2,* 269–282.

Stanovich, K. E., & West, R. F. (1983). On priming by a sentence context. *Journal of Experimental Psychology: General, 112,* 1–36.

Stetter, F., Ackermann, K., Bizer, A., Straube, E. R., & Mann, K. (1995). Effects of disease-related cues in alcoholic inpatients: Results of a controlled 'Alcohol Stroop' study. *Alcoholism: Clinical and Experimental Research, 19,* 593–599.

Stewart, J., & de Wit, H. (1987). Reinstatement of drug-taking behavior as a method of assessing incentive motivational properties of drugs. In M. A. Bozarth (Ed.), *Methods of assessing the reinforcing properties of abused drugs* (pp. 211–227). New York: Springer-Verlag.

Stewart, S. H., Zack, M., Klein, R., Loba, P., & Fragopoulos, F. (2002, September). *Gambling motives and drinking motives in pathological gamblers who drink when gambling.* Paper presented at the World Forum on Drugs and Dependencies: Impacts and Responses, Montreal, QC.

Stroop, J. R. (1935). Studies of interference in serial verbal reactions. *Journal of Experimental Psychology, 18,* 643–662.

Ventura, R., Cabib, S., Alcaro, A., Orsini, C., & Puglisi-Allegra, S. (2003). Norepinephrine in the prefrontal cortex is critical for amphetamine-induced reward and mesoaccumbens dopamine release. *Journal of Neuroscience, 23,* 1879–1885.

Volberg, R. A. (2002). The epidemiology of pathological gambling. *Psychiatric Annals, 32,* 171–178.

Volkow, N. D., Fowler, J. S., Wang, G.-J., & Swanson, J. M. (2004). Dopamine in drug abuse and addiction: Results from imaging studies and treatment implications. *Molecular Psychiatry, 9,* 557–569.

Weingardt, K. R., Stacy, A. W., & Leigh, B. C. (1996). Automatic activation of alcohol concepts in response to positive outcomes of alcohol use. *Alcoholism: Clinical and Experimental Research, 20,* 25–30.

Wiers, R. W., de Jong, P. J., Havermans, R., & Jelicic, M. (2004). How to change implicit drug use-related cognitions in prevention: A transdisciplinary integration of findings from experimental psychopathology, social cognition, memory, and experimental learning psychology. *Substance Use & Misuse, 39,* 1625–1684.

Wiers, R. W., Van Woerden, N., Smulders, F. T. Y., & de Jong, P. J. (2002). Implicit and explicit alcohol-related cognitions in heavy and light drinkers. *Journal of Abnormal Psychology, 111,* 648–658.

Williams, J. M., Mathews, A., & MacLeod, C. (1996). The emotional Stroop task and psychopathology. *Psychological Bulletin, 120,* 3–24.

Zack, M., Belsito, L., Scher, R., Eissenberg, T., & Corrigall, W. A. (2001). Effects of abstinence and smoking on information processing in adolescent smokers. *Psychopharmacology, 153,* 249–257.

Zack, M., & Poulos, C. X. (2004). Amphetamine primes motivation to gamble and gambling-related semantic networks in problem gamblers. *Neuropsychopharmacology, 29,* 195–207.

Zack, M., Stewart, S. H., Klein, R. M., Loba, P., & Fragopoulos, F. (2005). Contingent gambling-drinking patterns and problem drinker status moderate implicit gambling-alcohol associations in problem gamblers. *Journal of Gambling Studies: Special Issue on Co-Morbid Gambling and Alcohol Use Disorders, 21,* 325–354.

Zack, M., Toneatto, T., & MacLeod, C. M. (1999). Implicit activation of alcohol concepts by negative affective cues distinguishes between problem drinkers with high and low psychiatric distress. *Journal of Abnormal Psychology, 108,* 518–531.

Zuckerman, M., & Lubin, B. (1965). *Multiple Affect Adjective Checklist.* San Diego, CA: Educational and Industrial Testing Service.

CHAPTER 25

Implicit Cognition and Cross-Addictive Behaviors

Brian D. Ostafin and Tibor P. Palfai

Abstract: Concurrent use of alcohol and tobacco is one of the most common types of cross-addictive behaviors. This chapter proposes that implicit cognition methods can add to the understanding of why alcohol and tobacco use are associated with each other. The first section begins by reviewing the data on the co-occurrence of alcohol and smoking behavior. The second section discusses the cognitive-motivational mechanisms that have been proposed to mediate the association between alcohol and tobacco use. The third section presents theories that incorporate a role for automatic processes in substance use and research that has utilized implicit cognition methods in examining cross-addictive behaviors. Clinical implications of an implicit cognition perspective of cross-substance use are presented in the fourth section.

INTRODUCTION

Individuals who engage in one form of addictive behavior are more likely to engage in others as well (Tsuang et al., 1998). One of the best documented of these cross-addictions is between alcohol and tobacco use. Heavier users of alcohol are more likely to smoke cigarettes and heavier users of tobacco are more likely to drink alcohol (Hughes, 1993; Zacny, 1990). Such observations have led investigators to try to better understand why these behaviors tend to be associated with one another and to design intervention strategies that may be utilized to address cross-substance use. A number of mechanisms have been proposed to account for the interaction between alcohol and nicotine use. Some researchers have focused on understanding this pattern of substance use by identifying underlying individual differences such as genetic or temperament factors (Bierut et al., 2000). Others have attempted to identify the mechanisms by which the use of one substance influences the use of another (Little, 2000; Monti et al., 1995). For those who are dependent on one or both of these substances, both the presence and absence of one substance may influence behaviors associated with the other. The current chapter examines how implicit cognition methods may elucidate key mechanisms that underlie the co-occurrence of addictive behaviors by focusing on alcohol-tobacco interactions.

AUTHOR'S NOTE: We would like to thank Michael Sayette, Reinout Wiers, and an anonymous reviewer for their helpful comments on an earlier version of this chapter.

The chapter begins with a brief review of laboratory studies of alcohol-tobacco interactions. These studies have begun to clarify how cues, pharmacological properties, and access/restriction to one substance influence motivation to use another substance. In the second section, a variety of cognitive-motivational mechanisms are discussed as mediators of the association between alcohol and tobacco. Mechanisms that underlie cross-substance use include specific learned associations between alcohol and smoking cues and other contextual factors that support co-occurrent alcohol and tobacco use. Alcohol and nicotine serve a number of important affective functions for one another, including both the enhancement of reinforcing effects and the reduction of punishing effects of the second substance. Additionally, there is evidence that these substances may activate general systems to alleviate negative affect and increase appetitive responding, not only to the co-occurring substance but also to nonsubstance rewards.

The role of implicit cognition in these cognitive-motivational mechanisms is discussed in the third section. Through the use of implicit measures, it is proposed that investigators will be able to better understand the characteristics of representational structures and elucidate key cognitive-motivational processes that underlie alcohol-tobacco interactions. The utility of this approach is examined with evidence from the few studies that have utilized implicit cognition methods in examining cross-substance use. Clinical implications are discussed in the fourth and final section.

A BRIEF REVIEW OF LAB STUDIES OF ALCOHOL-TOBACCO INTERACTIONS

The concurrent use of alcohol and cigarettes is a phenomenon well-known to clinicians and researchers. Put succinctly, "smokers tend to drink and drinkers tend to smoke" (Shiffman & Balabanis, 1995, p. 19). As many as 90 percent of alcoholics smoke (National Institute on Alcohol Abuse and Alcoholism, 1998), and tend to smoke more than nonalcoholic smokers (Hughes, 1993). Likewise, smokers are more likely to drink than nonsmokers (Shiffman & Balabanis, 1995; Zacny, 1990). Additionally, alcohol or tobacco use constitutes a risk for developing a use disorder in the other substance. Tobacco dependence and alcohol-use disorders have been demonstrated to be related both in cross-sectional (Gulliver et al., 2000; John et al., 2003) and prospective (Jensen et al., 2003; Sher et al., 1996) research. Further, there is evidence that using one substance may make it more difficult to abstain from using the other substance (Hughes, 1993; Murray et al., 1995; Sobell et al., 1990).

Experimental research has begun to examine the specific nature of how one substance influences use of a second substance. Most of the research focuses on the effects of alcohol on smoking responses. For example, alcohol administration studies have found that alcohol consumed in the lab leads to increased urges to smoke (Burton & Tiffany, 1997; Rohsenow et al., 1997; Sayette et al., in press), greater smoking behavior (Griffiths et al., 1976; Mello et al., 1980; Nil et al., 1984), and more postsmoking satisfaction and reinforcement (Hughes et al., 2000; Rose et al., 2002). Alcohol cues have also been shown to affect smoking-related responses. In drinkers who smoke, presentation of alcohol-related cues such as a glass of a preferred alcoholic beverage has been shown to elicit smoking urges (Cooney et al., 2003; and see Drobes, 2002; Rohsenow et al., 1997). Additionally, evidence has suggested that attempts to control alcohol urges through suppression may increase smoking motivation as indexed by more intense smoking behavior (i.e., number of puffs on a cigarette [Palfai et al., 1997]).

There is considerably less research on the effects of smoking on alcohol-related responses (Shiffman & Balabanis, 1995). One study found that smoking administration led to increased motivation for alcohol (Perkins et al., 2000). Male participants who had consumed a preload of alcohol and who had recently smoked worked harder to obtain more alcohol than did participants who had been deprived of nicotine overnight, though this effect did not hold for females. Additional evidence suggests that smoking cues may elicit alcohol urges (Drobes, 2002) and nicotine deprivation has been demonstrated to elicit alcohol urges and to increase alcohol consumption in a taste-test drinking task (Palfai et al., 2000). Cooney and colleagues (Cooney et al., 2003) did not find an effect of nicotine deprivation on alcohol urges, but the authors note that their sample consisted of alcohol-dependent subjects who were in treatment and who may thus not view alcohol use as a viable response to regulate their negative affect.

COGNITIVE-MOTIVATIONAL MECHANISMS IN THE ASSOCIATION BETWEEN ALCOHOL AND TOBACCO USE

A number of cognitive-motivational models have been proposed by addiction researchers to account for the association between alcohol and tobacco use (Drobes, 2002; Little, 2000; Monti et al., 1995; Shiffman & Balabanis, 1995). These models can be broadly differentiated as priming and coping models. Priming models propose that the use of one substance will activate cognitive and motivational representations such that the use of the second substance becomes more likely. Monti et al. (1995) note a number of specific processes that may mediate priming effects. For example, classical conditioning may occur such that any environmental cue present during the use of a substance can come to activate the behavioral responses associated with that substance. Thus, if a person smokes right before consuming alcohol, smoking cues (in addition to other contextual cues) can come to act as conditioned stimuli that prime drinking behavior. From a neurological perspective, both alcohol and nicotine may activate a general approach motivational system (Gray, 1994; Panksepp, 1998; Wise, 1988) that would increase appetitive responses to cues of reward, including cues of the second substance. The activation of the appetitive motivational system by one substance may also increase the incentive salience of the second substance (Little, 2000; Watson & Little, 1999), further strengthening the association between the cross-substance use.

Coping models propose that a link between alcohol and smoking behavior may be functional in that each substance has negative reinforcing effects. A number of processes may mediate coping model effects (Monti et al., 1995). From a social learning perspective, because both alcohol and nicotine have negative reinforcing properties, both may be used to cope with similar stressors. Additionally, if access to one substance is restricted during stress, the second substance may become an increasingly salient negative reinforcement behavioral option (Vuchinich & Tucker, 1988). From a neuropsychological perspective, one substance can be used to offset aversive states associated with the second substance. For example, attention deficits resulting from alcohol intoxication (Koelega, 1995) may be offset by smoking-elicited increases in attention skills (e.g., sustained attention and fewer errors in a reaction-time task [Rezvani & Levin, 2001]). Neurological processes may mediate these negative reinforcement effects. Because dopamine depletion is a neurological correlate of alcohol craving (Wise, 1988), smoking may be negatively reinforcing through its ability to increase dopamine (Monti et al., 1995).

Although priming and coping models account for a variety of processes thought to underlie concurrent alcohol and smoking behavior, they are not exhaustive. For example, cross-tolerance processes may occur such that tolerance to both the reinforcing and negative effects of one substance may lead to tolerance to the second substance (Little, 2000). Tolerance to the reinforcing effects may lead to increased use of the second substance because more is needed to obtain the desired positive state. Tolerance to the negative effects may lead to increased use of the second substance because negative consequences are discounted in decisions to use. In sum, there are a number of cognitive-motivational mechanisms that may be involved in cross-substance use and addiction researchers have begun to use implicit cognition theory and methods to help understand how these mechanisms are represented in memory.

AUTOMATIC PROCESSES AND CROSS-ADDICTION

Addiction researchers have shown increasing interest in the distinction made by cognitive scientists between automatic and controlled processes (Posner & Snyder, 1975; Shiffrin & Schneider, 1977). Although the terms automatic and implicit are often used interchangeably and several definitions have been proposed for these constructs (e.g., Greenwald & Banaji, 1995; Roediger, 1990), we will use *automatic* to refer to properties of mental processes and *implicit* to refer to tasks used to measure automatic processes (also see De Houwer, Chapter 2). From this perspective, the properties of mental processes that are defined as automatic are those that are (1) unintentional, (2) efficient (i.e., effortless), (3) difficult to control, and (4) not involving awareness (of the stimulus itself, of the way a stimulus influences later thought/behavior, or of the way a stimulus is evaluated or categorized [Bargh, 1992, 1994]). Controlled processes

can be oppositely defined—as being intentional, effortful, controllable, and involving awareness. Additionally, Bargh (1994) has argued that whereas each of the four features tends to be jointly present in controlled processes, they often do not co-occur in automatic processes. That is, the presence of only one feature is sufficient to define a cognitive process as automatic.

A number of theoretical models of substance-use behavior have been proposed that incorporate automatic processes (Baker et al., 1987; Goldman et al., 1991; Leigh & Stacy, 1991; Ryan, 2002; Stacy, 1995; Stephens & Marlatt, 1987; Tiffany, 1990). These theories make the contribution of modeling the processes that may be involved in the "loss of control" experience that is central to addictive behavior (McCusker, 2001; Widiger & Smith, 1994). More recently, implicit cognition methods have begun to be successfully utilized to examine specific instances of automatic processes related to substance use. Although the majority of this research has been conducted on automatic processes involved in the use of a single substance (typically alcohol or smoking), the processes may also have important implications for understanding cross-drug use. Three areas in which automatic processes may be importantly involved in substance use include the following: (1) perception, (2) affect/evaluation, and (3) goal-directed behavior.

Automatic Processes and Perceptual Biases

Perceptual biases may be manifested as selective attention such that environmental stimuli are likely to automatically draw attention if they have been frequently processed (e.g., been involved in thought or behavior) or if they are motivationally salient; that is, if they are relevant to current goals (Barsalou, 1983; Wegner & Bargh, 1998; see also Bruce & Jones, Chapter 10; Field et al., Chapter 11). In this vein, emotion researchers have proposed that stimuli with strong affective valence (i.e., those that are relevant to an organism's goals or values) are more likely to automatically attract attention than stimuli with weak affective valence (Lang et al., 2000; and see Wentura et al., 2000).

Perceptual biases have been proposed to facilitate addictive behavior, especially in the incentive sensitization theory (Robinson & Berridge, 1993, 2001). This theory argues that with recurrent drug use, mesolimbic dopamine activity imparts incentive salience onto drug stimuli with the result that those stimuli automatically draw attention (as well as activate approach behavioral tendencies and the experience of "wanting"). Addiction researchers have found attentional biases for substance-use cues in heavy drinkers and smokers using Stroop tasks (Gross et al., 1993; Stetter et al., 1995), dichotic listening tasks (Sayette & Hufford, 1994; Stetter et al., 1994), lexical decision tasks (Jarvik et al., 1995), visual-probe tasks (Bradley et al., 2003; Mogg et al., 2003), and eye-movement tasks (Mogg et al., 2003). Of note, the attention biases found in the Mogg et al. (2003) study were strongly correlated with valence ratings of the smoking stimuli, converging with the Lang et al. (2000) proposal that affect valence predicts capacity to attract attention.

In addition to their role in the use of single substances, perceptual biases may facilitate cross-addictive behavior. Motivated states are posited in both priming (approach toward cues of reward) and coping (approach toward cues of relief) models (Baker et al., 1987). To the extent that these motivational states are activated, attention may be preconsciously biased toward the salient cues (of reward or relief), facilitating further information processing of these stimuli and use of that information in behavioral decisions (Stacy et al., 1996). Two published studies utilizing implicit cognition methods in cross-addictive behavior have examined the effects of drug motivational states on perceptual biases. Palfai et al. (2000) elicited a coping

motivational state by depriving regular smokers of nicotine for 6 hours and assessed perceptual biases toward alcohol stimuli with a lexical decision task. The results indicated that the deprivation group did not have faster latencies than the control group for recognizing the alcohol stimuli as words. Zack and Poulos (2004) elicited a priming motivational state in problem gamblers with a dose of amphetamine (versus a placebo group) and assessed perceptual biases toward gambling (alcohol, positive affect, negative affect, and neutral stimuli with a word-naming task. The results indicated that the amphetamine dose led to faster reading speed (compared to placebo) of gambling words, but not the other four word categories. These studies indicate that at least in some conditions, perceptual biases for cross-addictive stimuli may occur.

Future research could examine the motivational elements necessary to elicit perceptual biases such as (1) whether biases occur only in priming/positive reinforcement states, (2) whether source (drug-related withdrawal or priming versus other types of negative and positive affect) or intensity of motivation state matters, and (3) whether perceptual bias is specific to similar classes of drugs and behavior (as the Zack & Poulos [2004] findings of no effects on alcohol words would suggest). Additionally, as conditioned learning models of priming propose that a cue of one substance can become associated with cues of a second substance through frequent co-occurrence (Monti et al., 1995), future research may examine whether one substance can elicit perceptual bias toward the second substance in the absence of a motivation state.

Automatic Processes and Affect Representations

Attention biases toward substance-use stimuli may lead to other automatic information processing that facilitates use behavior. Implicit cognition research has indicated that affective relevance (i.e., "good and to be approached" or "bad and to be avoided") may be the first information extracted from perceptions of stimuli (Bargh et al., 1989). A variety of implicit cognition methods have been utilized to demonstrate that associative strength influences whether a stimulus will automatically activate an affective response (Fazio, 2001; Greenwald & Banaji, 1995; Musch & Klauer, 2003). Of note, perceptions of stimuli do not have to reach the threshold of awareness to automatically activate affective information, as demonstrated by subliminal affective priming (Berridge & Winkielman, 2003; Murphy & Zajonc, 1993).

Addiction theories have proposed that through experience (and vicarious learning) of the affective consequences of substance use, substance-use cues can come to activate affective representations that support approach toward and consumption of the substance (Baker et al., 1987; Cox & Klinger, 1988; Goldman et al., 1999; Stewart et al., 1984). Recent research utilizing implicit cognition methods has demonstrated automatically activated associations between substance-use cues and affect representations (affective valence, salience, and behavioral dispositions) with the IAT (Jajodia & Earleywine, 2003; Palfai & Ostafin, 2003; Wiers et al., 2002), affective priming tasks (Ostafin et al., 2003; Ostafin et al., 2001), outcome association tasks (Ames & Stacy, 1998; Stacy, 1997; Weingardt et al., 1996), and tasks utilizing symbolic approach and avoidance behavior responses (Mogg et al., 2003).

A number of cognitive-motivational mechanisms may be involved in the creation of cross-substance affective salience. From a priming model perspective, use of one substance may activate a general appetitive motivation system, increasing the incentive salience of the second substance when it is used (Watson & Little, 1999), creating a positive reinforcement association (see also research reported in Zack & Poulos, Chapter 24). A recent study found that participants who consumed alcohol displayed positive affect facial expressions (and stronger smoking urges) in a smoking-cue exposure phase than did participants who consumed placebo (Sayette et al., in press). From a coping model perspective, negative affect elicited by use (or withdrawal) of one substance may be reduced by use of the second substance (Monti et al., 1995), creating a negative reinforcement association.

The results of two implicit cognition tasks used in our research may be understood through priming and coping models of cross-substance use. First, Ostafin and Palfai (2003) assessed the strength of alcohol-approach motivation associations with an affective priming task that consisted of observing briefly presented primes of alcohol or water pictures and categorizing target words as being related to "approach" or "avoid" as quickly as possible. The results indicated that controlling for alcohol consumption, amount of smoking predicted stronger alcohol-approach associations. This finding is consistent with a priming model in that smoking that precedes alcohol use could activate an approach motivational state, making alcohol a more appetitive cue in smokers who drink. Second, Palfai et al. (2000) assessed the accessibility of alcohol expectancies with a sequential priming task that consisted of reading briefly presented primes ("Alcohol makes me" or "I am generally") and indicating as "true" or "false" whether a positive or negative expectancy word was related to the prime. The results indicated that in nicotine-deprived participants (compared to participants who smoked as usual), both positive and negative expectancies were more accessible, more positive expectancies were endorsed than negative expectancies, and expectancy accessibility partially mediated the relation between deprivation and alcohol consumption in an ad lib drinking task. These findings are consistent with a coping model in that a deprivation state may preferentially activate positive alcohol expectancies, leading to greater alcohol consumption.

Future research in this area could benefit by examining (1) what stimuli associated with one substance (e.g., interoceptive cues such as positive or negative affect resulting from use or deprivation of that substance, visual cues of the substance, etc.) are capable of eliciting cross-substance affect representations, and (2) whether the affect associations are specific to the cross-substance or are generalized to other non-substance incentives as well (Kambouropoulos & Staiger, 2001).

Automatic Processes and Goal-Directed Behavior

Automatic processes may also be implicated in substance use via the mental representations involved in goal-directed behavior. Bargh and his colleagues (Bargh, 1990; Bargh & Chartrand, 1999, 2000; Bargh & Ferguson, 2000; Wegner & Bargh, 1998) have proposed several paths by which automatic processes may influence behavior. First, as previously mentioned, goal activation can influence what environmental stimuli "jump out" for additional processing (Barsalou, 1983). Second, activation of a goal may automatically activate behavior used in the past to attain the goal. Aarts and Dijksterhuis (2000) demonstrated that when subjects were primed with the goal concept of "traveling," the behavioral concept of "cycling" was activated in a reaction-time task for habitual bicyclers but not for nonbicyclers (and that this difference did not occur with "nontraveling" goal concept primes). Third, goals can be automatically activated so that their effects (guiding perception and priming behavior) may also emerge without awareness. In two studies, Chartrand and Bargh (1996) found that the social information processing goal of "forming an impression" of a person could be primed automatically, either without awareness of the stimuli by presenting impression-related words subliminally or without awareness of how the stimuli influence later behavior by presenting a "language test" that consisted of several impression formation–related words such as "evaluate" (vs. memory-related words such as "remember"). In both cases, participants who were primed with the impression words were more likely to form an impression about a social target on a subsequent task that was ostensibly unrelated to the priming task.

There is evidence that each of these automatic processes involved in goal-directed behavior plays a role in substance use. As previously reviewed, heavy alcohol and tobacco use predicts automatic attention bias toward substance-related cues. Substance-use goal concepts have also been demonstrated to activate substance-use behavior concepts (see Curtin et al., Chapter 16). Outcome association tasks (Ames & Stacy, 1998; Stacy, 1995) that present a desirable outcome state (e.g., "having a good time") and ask participants to "write the first behavior that comes to mind" have found that substance-related behavior responses predict level of substance use. In addition, goal concepts can be automatically primed and influence substance-use behavior, as research by Goldman and his colleagues (Roehrich & Goldman, 1995; Stein et al., 2000) have demonstrated. These studies found that when participants were primed with desirable outcome states (e.g., via a Stroop task that consisted of several positive alcohol outcome words), they consumed more (placebo and alcoholic) beer in an ad lib drinking task. Like Chartrand and Bargh (1996), the outcome prime effect on behavior is defined as automatic because the experiment was set up as two different studies (the Stroop "word recognition" task and the ostensibly unrelated taste test) to prevent awareness of the relation between the two events (verified by a manipulation check).

Coping models suggest that goal concept activation may influence cross-substance use.

The social learning model discussed by Monti et al. (1995) suggests that because a variety of substances reduce negative affect, negative reinforcement goals should activate behavioral concepts associated with a number of substances. A similar logic would hold for positive reinforcement goals. No cross-substance research has examined these processes with implicit cognition methods. Future research could examine (1) whether the reinforcement goals do in fact activate cross-substance behavior concepts, (2) whether strength of activation is a function of frequency of substance use in the service of reinforcement goals, and (3) whether negative (and potentially positive) reinforcement goals can be nonconsciously activated as Baker has recently suggested (Baker et al., 2004).

CLINICAL IMPLICATIONS

Future research in the role of automatic processes in cross-substance use may have implications for assessment and treatment. Perhaps most broadly, assessing automatic processes such as substance-affect associations may help to predict likelihood of changing the addictive behavior. A number of implicit cognition theorists have noted that automatic processes may be more likely to influence behavior in situations lacking either the motivation or the opportunity (or both) to utilize conscious, controlled processes to self-regulate (Fazio & Towles-Schwen, 1999). Evidence suggests that implicit measures are better able to predict behavior under these conditions than are explicit measures (Asendorpf et al., 2002; Fazio et al., 1995). Consequently, assessing the strength of automatic processes may indicate likelihood of substance use in high-risk situations in which either opportunity or motivation for self-regulation is low (Marlatt, 1996). Related, if automatic processes preferentially influence behavior in high-risk situations, implicit measures could be used as "test-probes" to assess

whether an intervention was successful (Rachman, 1980).

Implicit cognition theory and methods may also contribute to the development of effective treatments. Given initial evidence that implicit measures may predict treatment outcome (Waters et al., 2003), it may be of use to tailor treatments that can alter automatic processes. Several such strategies have been proposed (Gabbard & Westen, 2003; Goldfried, 2003; Segal et al., 1999; Wiers et al., 2004). A commonality among a number of these strategies is that memory structures are proposed to change by incorporating information that is discrepant from them. As Foa and Kozak (1986) have noted, modification of memory structures will be most likely to occur when the memory structure is activated. Thus, it is important to determine which cues most closely resemble a "stimulus input prototype" capable of activating the memory structure. Brewin (1989) points out that this may be a challenge given that the majority of stimuli input are not represented in awareness, reducing the client's ability to self-report on important contextual features. Indeed, Baker et al. (2004) propose that a great deal of addictive behavior is elicited by nonconscious perception of stimuli associated with negative affect. Implicit cognition methods such as subliminal priming may help to provide information about the stimuli involved in eliciting single- and cross-substance use.

Implicit cognition methods may also yield information about the choice of treatment targets. It may be that focus on individual automatic processes such as substance-use behavior or expectancy associations will serve as key elements in treatment. Alternatively, a number of addiction researchers have proposed an integrated memory network to account for drug use (Baker et al., 1987; Niaura et al., 1991; Tiffany, 1990). These theories are largely derived from Lang's (1979) bioinformational network theory of emotion that proposes that an emotion state consists of integrated behavioral, physiological, and verbal expressive response elements. It may be that the activation of an approach motivation system (toward cues of reward or relief) elicits an integrated response including a number of automatic processes. Although there is debate over which response elements may be involved (Tiffany, 1990), implicit measures used by Mogg et al. (2003) and Palfai et al. (2000) suggest that such integration may occur. Moreover, if a motivational state underlies a number of automatic processes involved in substance use, then treatment emphasis may focus on deactivating that state (e.g., through emotion regulation strategies, Naltrexone, etc.).

In summary, although there is limited research utilizing implicit cognition methods to study cross-addiction, these methods hold promise for developing a greater understanding of the processes involved in such behavior. In combination with basic implicit cognition research and addiction research using these methods to study single-substance use, the few studies that have used implicit cognition methods to study cross-addiction suggest that a number of automatic processes may be involved in cross-substance use. Future research on these automatic processes may help to clarify the mechanisms involved in coping and priming models of cross-substance use and may also help in the creation of clinical interventions designed to alter these processes.

REFERENCES

Aarts, H., & Dijksterhuis, A. (2000). Habits as knowledge structures: Automaticity in goal-directed behavior. *Journal of Personality and Social Psychology, 78,* 53–63.

Ames, S. L., & Stacy, A. W. (1998). Implicit cognition in the prediction of substance use among drug offenders. *Psychology of Addictive Behaviors, 12,* 272–281.

Asendorpf, J. B., Banse, R., & Muecke, D. (2002). Double dissociation between implicit and explicit personality self-concept: The case of shy behavior. *Journal of Personality and Social Psychology, 83,* 380–393.

Baker, T. B., Morse, E., & Sherman, J. E. (1987). The motivation to use drugs: A psychobiological analysis of urges. In C. Rivers (Ed.), *The Nebraska symposium on motivation: Alcohol use and abuse* (pp. 257–323). Lincoln: University of Nebraska Press.

Baker, T. B., Piper, M. E., McCarthy, D. E., Majeskie, M. R., & Fiore, M. C. (2004). Addiction motivation reformulated: An affective processing model of negative reinforcement. *Psychological Review, 111,* 33–51.

Bargh, J. A. (1990). Auto-motives: Preconscious determinants of social interaction. In E. T. Higgins & R. M. Sorrentino (Eds.), *Handbook of motivation and cognition* (Vol. 2, pp. 93–130). New York: Guilford.

Bargh, J. A. (1992). The ecology of automaticity: Toward establishing the conditions needed to produce automatic processing effects. *American Journal of Psychology, 105,* 181–199.

Bargh, J. A. (1994). The four horsemen of automaticity: Awareness, intention, efficiency, and control in social cognition. In R. S. Wyer & T. K. Srull (Eds.), *Handbook of social cognition* (2nd ed., Vol. 1, pp. 1–40). Hillsdale, NJ: Lawrence Erlbaum.

Bargh, J. A., & Chartrand, T. L. (1999). The unbearable automaticity of being. *American Psychologist, 54,* 462–479.

Bargh, J. A., & Chartrand, T. L. (2000). The mind in the middle: A practical guide to priming and automaticity research. In H. T. Reis & C. M. Judd (Eds.), *Handbook of research methods in social and personality psychology* (pp. 253–285). New York: Cambridge University Press.

Bargh, J. A., & Ferguson, M. J. (2000). Beyond behaviorism: On the automaticity of higher mental processes. *Psychological Bulletin, 126,* 928–945.

Bargh, J. A., Litt, J., Pratto, F., & Spielman, L. A. (1989). On the preconscious evaluation of social stimuli. In A. F. Bennett & K. M. McConkey (Eds.), *Cognition in individual and social contexts* (pp. 357–370). Amsterdam, The Netherlands: Elsevier/North-Holland.

Barsalou, L. W. (1983). Ad hoc categories. *Memory & Cognition, 11,* 211–227.

Berridge, K. C., & Winkielman, P. (2003). What is an unconscious emotion? *Cognition & Emotion, 17,* 181–211.

Bierut, L. J., Schuckit, M. A., Hesselbrock, V., & Reich, T. (2000). Co-occurring risk factors for alcohol dependence and habitual smoking. *Alcohol Research & Health, 24,* 233–241.

Bradley, B. P., Mogg, K., Wright, T., & Field, M. (2003). Attentional bias in drug dependence: Vigilance for cigarette-related cues in smokers. *Psychology of Addictive Behaviors, 17,* 66–72.

Brewin, C. R. (1989). Cognitive change processes in psychotherapy. *Psychological Review, 96,* 379–394.

Burton, S. M., & Tiffany, S. T. (1997). The effect of alcohol consumption on craving to smoke. *Addiction, 92,* 15–26.

Chartrand, T. L., & Bargh, J. A. (1996). Automatic activation of impression formation and memorization goals: Nonconscious goal priming reproduces effects of explicit task instructions. *Journal of Personality and Social Psychology, 71,* 464–478.

Cooney, J. L., Cooney, N. L., Pilkey, D. T., Kranzler, H. R., & Oncken, C. A. (2003). Effects of nicotine deprivation on urges to drink and smoke in alcoholic smokers. *Addiction, 98,* 913–921.

Cox, W. M., & Klinger, E. (1988). A motivational model of alcohol use. *Journal of Abnormal Psychology, 97,* 168–180.

Drobes, D. J. (2002). Cue reactivity in alcohol and tobacco dependence. *Alcoholism: Clinical and Experimental Research, 26,* 1928–1929.

Fazio, R. H. (2001). On the automatic activation of associated evaluations: An overview. *Cognition & Emotion, 15,* 115–141.

Fazio, R. H., Jackson, J. R., Dunton, B. C., & Williams, C. J. (1995). Variability in automatic activation as an unobtrusive measure of racial attitudes: A bona fide pipeline? *Journal of Personality and Social Psychology, 69,* 1013–1027.

Fazio, R. H., & Towles-Schwen, T. (1999). The MODE model of attitude-behavior processes. In S. Chaiken & Y. Trope (Eds.), *Dual process theories in social psychology* (pp. 97–116). New York: Guilford.

Foa, E. B., & Kozak, M. J. (1986). Emotional processing of fear: Exposure to corrective information. *Psychological Bulletin, 99,* 20–35.

Gabbard, G., & Westen, D. (2003). On therapeutic action. *International Journal of Psychoanalysis, 84,* 823–841.

Goldfried, M. R. (2003). Cognitive-behavior therapy: Reflections on the evolution of a therapeutic orientation. *Cognitive Therapy and Research, 27,* 53–69.

Goldman, M. S., Brown, S. A., Christiansen, B. A., & Smith, G. T. (1991). Alcoholism and memory: Broadening the scope of alcohol-expectancy research. *Psychological Bulletin, 110,* 137–146.

Goldman, M. S., Del Boca, F. K., & Darkes, J. (1999). Alcohol expectancy theory: The application of cognitive neuroscience. In K. E. Leonard & H. T. Blane (Eds.), *Psychological theories of drinking and alcoholism* (2nd ed., pp. 203–246). New York: Guilford.

Gray, J. A. (1994). Three fundamental emotion systems. In R. J. Davidson & P. Ekman (Eds.), *The nature of emotion: Fundamental questions* (pp. 243–247). New York: Oxford University Press.

Greenwald, A. G., & Banaji, M. R. (1995). Implicit social cognition: Attitudes, self-esteem, and stereotypes. *Psychological Review, 102,* 4–27.

Griffiths, R. R., Bigelow, G. E., & Liebson, I. (1976). Facilitation of human tobacco self-administration by ethanol: A behavioral analysis. *Journal of Experimental Analysis of Behavior, 25,* 279–292.

Gross, T. M., Jarvik, M. E., & Rosenblatt, M.R. (1993). Nicotine abstinence produces context-specific Stroop interference. *Psychopharmacology, 110,* 333–336.

Gulliver, S. B., Kalman, D., Rohsenow, D. J., Colby, S. M., Eaton, C. A., & Monti, P. M. (2000). Smoking and drinking among alcoholics in treatment: Cross-sectional and longitudinal relationships. *Journal of Studies on Alcohol, 61,* 157–163.

Hughes, J. R. (1993). Treatment of smoking cessation in smokers with past alcohol/drug problems. *Journal of Substance Abuse Treatment, 10,* 181–187.

Hughes, J. R., Rose, G. L., & Callas, P. W. (2000). Nicotine is more reinforcing in smokers with a past history of alcoholism than in smokers without this history. *Alcoholism: Clinical and Experimental Research, 24,* 1633–1638.

Jajodia, A., & Earleywine, M. (2003). Measuring alcohol expectancies with the implicit association test. *Psychology of Addictive Behaviors, 17,* 126–133.

Jarvik, M. E., Gross, T. M., Rosenblatt, M. R., & Stein, R. E. (1995). Enhanced lexical processing of smoking stimuli during smoking abstinence. *Psychopharmacology, 118,* 136–141.

Jensen, M. K., Sorensen, T. I., Anderson, A. T., Thorsen, T., Tolstrup, J. S., Godtfredsen, N.S., et al. (2003). A prospective study of the association between smoking and later alcohol drinking in the general population. *Addiction, 98,* 355–363.

John, U., Meyer, C., Rumpf, H. J., & Hapke, U. (2003). Probabilities of alcohol high-risk drinking, abuse or dependence estimated on grounds of tobacco smoking and nicotine dependence. *Addiction, 98,* 805–814.

Kambouropoulos, N., & Staiger, P. K. (2001). The influence of sensitivity to reward on reactivity to alcohol-related cues. *Addiction, 96,* 1175–1185.

Koelega, H. (1995). Alcohol and vigilance performance: A review. *Psychopharmacology, 118,* 233–249.

Lang, P. J. (1979). A bio-informational theory of emotional imagery. *Psychophysiology, 16,* 495–512.

Lang, P. J., Davis, M., & Öhman, A. (2000). Fear and anxiety: Animal models and human cognitive psychophysiology. *Journal of Affective Disorders, 61,* 137–159.

Leigh, B. C., & Stacy, A. W. (1991). On the scope of alcohol expectancy research: Remaining issues of measurement and meaning. *Psychological Bulletin, 110,* 147–154.

Little, H. J. (2000). Behavioral mechanisms underlying the link between smoking and drinking. *Alcohol Research & Health, 24,* 215–224.

Marlatt, G. A. (1996). Taxonomy of high-risk situations for alcohol relapse: Evolution and development of a cognitive-behavioral model. *Addiction, 91,* S37–S49.

McCusker, C. G. (2001). Cognitive biases and addiction: An evolution in theory and method. *Addiction, 96,* 47–56.

Mello, N. K., Mendelson, J. H., Sellers, M. L., & Kuehnle, J. C. (1980). Effect of alcohol and marijuana on tobacco smoking. *Clinical Pharmacology & Therapeutics, 27,* 202–209.

Mogg, K., Bradley, B. P., Field, M., & De Houwer, J. (2003). Eye movements to smoking-related pictures in smokers: Relationship between attentional biases and implicit and explicit measures of stimulus valence. *Addiction, 98,* 825–836.

Monti, P. M., Rohsenow, D. J., Colby, S. M., & Abrams, D. B. (1995). Smoking among alcoholics during and after treatment: Implications for models, treatment strategies and policy. In J. B. Fertig & J. P. Allen (Eds.), *Alcohol and tobacco: From basic science to policy* (NIAAA Research Monograph No. 30, pp. 187–206). Washington, DC: U.S. Department of Health and Human Services.

Murphy, S. T., & Zajonc, R. B. (1993). Affect, cognition, and awareness: Affective priming with optimal and suboptimal stimulus exposures. *Journal of Personality and Social Psychology, 64,* 723–739.

Murray, R. P., Istvan, J. A., Voelker, H. T., Rigdon, M. A., & Wallace, M. D. (1995). Level of involvement with alcohol and success at smoking cessation in the Lung Health Study. *Journal of Studies on Alcohol, 56,* 74–82.

Musch, J., & Klauer, K. C. (2003). *The psychology of evaluation.* Mahwah, NJ: Lawrence Erlbaum.

National Institute on Alcohol Abuse and Alcoholism. (1998). Alcohol and tobacco. (*Alcohol Alert,* No. 39). Rockville, MD: Author.

Niaura, R., Goldstein, M., & Abrams, D. (1991). A bioinformational systems perspective on tobacco dependence. *British Journal of Addiction, 86,* 593–597.

Nil, R., Buzzi, R., & Battig, K. (1984). Effects of single doses of alcohol and caffeine on cigarette smoke puffing behavior. *Pharmacology, Biochemistry, and Behavior, 20,* 583–590.

Ostafin, B. D., & Palfai, T. P. (2003). An implicit measure of alcohol-approach associations in smokers. Unpublished raw data.

Ostafin, B. D., Palfai, T. P., & Wechsler, C. E. (2003). The accessibility of motivational tendencies toward alcohol: Approach, avoidance, and disinhibited drinking. *Experimental & Clinical Psychopharmacology, 11,* 294–301.

Ostafin, B. D., Tzilos, G., & Palfai, T. P. (2001, November). Affective salience of outcome expectancies for smoking: An implicit measure of motivation to change. Poster session presented at the annual meeting of the Association for the Advancement of Behavior Therapy, Philadelphia, PA.

Palfai, T. P., Colby, S. M., Monti, P. M., & Rohsenow, D. J. (1997). Effects of suppressing the urge to drink on smoking topography: A preliminary study. *Psychology of Addictive Behaviors, 11,* 115–123.

Palfai, T. P., Monti, P. M., Ostafin, B., & Hutchison, K. (2000). Effects of nicotine deprivation on alcohol-related information processing and drinking behavior. *Journal of Abnormal Psychology, 109,* 96–105.

Palfai, T. P., & Ostafin, B. D. (2003). Alcohol-related motivational tendencies in hazardous drinkers: Assessing implicit response tendencies using the modified IAT. *Behaviour Research and Therapy, 41,* 1149–1162.

Panksepp, J. (1998). *Affective neuroscience: The foundations of human and animal emotions.* London: Oxford University Press.

Perkins, K. A., Fonte, C., & Grobe, J. E. (2000). Sex differences in the acute effects of cigarette smoking on the reinforcing value of alcohol. *Behavioural Pharmacology, 11,* 63–70.

Posner, M. I., & Snyder, C. R. R. (1975). Attention and cognitive control. In R. L. Solso (Ed.), *Information processing and cognition: The Loyola symposium* (pp. 55–85). Hillsdale, NJ: Lawrence Erlbaum.

Rachman, S. (1980). Emotional processing. *Behaviour Research and Therapy, 18,* 51–60.

Rezvani, A. H., & Levin, E. D. (2001). Cognitive effects of nicotine. *Biological Psychiatry, 49,* 258–267.

Robinson, T. E., & Berridge, K. C. (1993). The neural basis of drug craving: An incentive-sensitization theory of addiction. *Brain Research Reviews, 18,* 247–291.

Robinson, T. E., & Berridge, K. C. (2001). Incentive-sensitization and addiction. *Addiction, 96,* 103–114.

Roediger, H. L. (1990). Implicit memory: Retention without remembering. *American Psychologist, 45,* 1043–1056.

Roehrich, L., & Goldman, M. S. (1995). Implicit priming of alcohol expectancy memory processes and subsequent drinking behavior. *Experimental & Clinical Psychopharmacology, 3,* 402–410.

Rohsenow, F. J., Monti, P. M., Colby, S. M., Gulliver, S. B., Sirota, A. D., Niaura, R. S., et al. (1997). Effects of alcohol cues on smoking urges and topography among alcoholic men. *Alcoholism: Clinical and Experimental Research, 21,* 101–107.

Rose, J. E., Brauer, L. H., Behm, F. M., Cramblett, M., Calkins, K., & Lawhon, D. (2002). Potentiation of nicotine reward by alcohol. *Alcoholism: Clinical and Experimental Research, 26,* 1930–1931.

Ryan, F. (2002). Detected, selected, and sometimes neglected: Cognitive processing of cues in addiction. *Experimental & Clinical Psychopharmacology, 10,* 67–76.

Sayette, M. A., & Hufford, M. R. (1994). Effects of cue exposure and deprivation on cognitive resources in smokers. *Journal of Abnormal Psychology, 103,* 812–818.

Sayette, M. A., Martin, C. S., Wertz, J. M., Perrott, M. A., & Peters, A. R. (in press). The effects of alcohol on cigarette craving in heavy smokers and tobacco chippers. *Psychology of Addictive Behaviors.*

Segal, Z. V., Lau, M. A., & Rokke, P. D. (1999). Cognition and emotion research and the practice of cognitive-behavioural therapy. In T. Dalgeish & M. J. Power (Eds.), *Handbook of cognition and emotion* (pp. 705–726). New York: John Wiley.

Sher, K. J., Gotham, H. J., Erickson, D. J., & Wood, P. K. (1996). A prospective, high-risk study of the relationship between tobacco dependence and alcohol use disorders. *Alcoholism: Clinical and Experimental Research, 20,* 485–492.

Shiffman, S., & Balabanis, M. (1995). Associations between alcohol and tobacco. In J. B. Fertig & J. P. Allen (Eds.), *Alcohol and tobacco: From basic science to policy* (NIAAA Research Monograph No. 30, pp. 17–36). Washington, DC: U.S. Department of Health and Human Services.

Shiffrin, R. M., & Schneider, W. (1977). Controlled and automatic human information processing: II. Perceptual learning, automatic attending, and a general theory. *Psychological Review, 84,* 127–190.

Sobell, L. C., Sobell, M. B., Kozlowski, L. T., & Toneatto, T. (1990). Alcohol or tobacco research versus alcohol and tobacco research. *British Journal of Addiction, 85,* 263–269.

Stacy, A. W. (1995). Memory association and ambiguous cues in models of alcohol and marijuana use. *Experimental & Clinical Psychopharmacology, 3,* 183–194.

Stacy, A. W. (1997). Memory activation and expectancy as prospective predictors of alcohol and marijuana use. *Journal of Abnormal Psychology, 106,* 61–73.

Stacy, A. W., Ames, S. L., Sussman, S., & Dent, C. W. (1996). Implicit cognition in adolescent drug use. *Psychology of Addictive Behaviors, 10,* 190–203.

Stein, K. D., Goldman, M. S., & Del Boca, F. K. (2000). The influence of alcohol expectancy priming and mood manipulation on subsequent alcohol consumption. *Journal of Abnormal Psychology, 109,* 106–115.

Stephens, R. S., & Marlatt, G. A. (1987). Creatures of habit: Loss of control over addictive and nonaddictive behaviors. *Drugs and Society, 1,* 85–103.

Stetter, F., Ackerman, K., Bizer, A., Straube, E. R., & Mann, K. (1995). Effects of disease-related cues in alcohol inpatients: Results of a controlled "alcohol Stroop" study. *Alcoholism: Clinical and Experimental Research, 19,* 593–599.

Stetter, F., Chaluppa, C., Ackerman, K., Straube, E. R., & Mann, K. (1994). Alcoholics' selective processing of alcohol related words and cognitive performance on a Stroop task. *European Psychiatry, 9,* 71–76.

Stewart, J., de Wit, H., & Eikelboom, R. (1984). Role of unconditioned and conditioned drug effects in the self-administration of opiates and stimulants. *Psychological Review, 91,* 251–268.

Tiffany, S. T. (1990). A cognitive model of drug urges and drug-use behavior: Role of automatic and nonautomatic processes. *Psychological Review, 97,* 147–168.

Tsuang, M. T., Lyons, M. J., Meyer, J. M., Doyle, T., Eisen, S. A., Goldberg, J., et al. (1998). Co-occurrence of abuse of different drugs in men: The role of drug-specific and shared vulnerabilities. *Archives of General Psychiatry, 55,* 967–972.

Vuchinich, R. E., & Tucker, J. A. (1988). Contributions from behavioral theories of choice to an analysis of alcohol abuse. *Journal of Abnormal Psychology, 97,* 181–195.

Waters, A. J., Shiffman, S., Sayette, M. A., Paty, J. A., Gwaltney, C. G., & Balabanis, M. H. (2003). Attentional bias predicts outcome in smoking cessation. *Health Psychology, 22,* 378–387.

Watson, W. P., & Little, H. J. (1999). Prolonged effects of chronic ethanol consumption on response to nicotine: Interaction with environmental cues. *Neuropharmacology, 38,* 587–595.

Wegner, D. M., & Bargh, J. A. (1998). Control and automaticity in social life. In D. T. Gilbert, S. T. Fiske, & G. Lindzey (Eds.), *Handbook of social psychology* (4th ed., pp. 446–496). Boston: McGraw-Hill.

Weingardt, K. R., Stacy, A. W., & Leigh, B. C. (1996). Automatic activation of alcohol concepts in response to positive outcomes of alcohol use. *Alcoholism: Clinical and Experimental Research, 20,* 25–30.

Wentura, D., Rothermund, K., & Bak, P. (2000). Automatic vigilance: The attention-grabbing power of approach and avoidance related social information. *Journal of Personality and Social Psychology, 78,* 1024–1037.

Widiger, T. A., & Smith, G. T. (1994). Substance use disorder: Abuse, dependence, and dyscontrol. *Addiction, 89,* 267–282.

Wiers, R. W., de Jong, P. J., Havermans, R., & Jelicic, M. (2004). How to change implicit drug use-related cognitions in prevention: A transdisciplinary integration of findings from experimental psychopathology, social cognition, memory, and experimental learning psychology. *Substance Use & Misuse, 39,* 1625–1684.

Wiers, R. W., Van Woerden, N., Smulders, F. T. Y, & de Jong, P. J. (2002). Implicit and explicit alcohol-related cognitions in heavy and light drinkers. *Journal of Abnormal Psychology, 111,* 648–658.

Wise, R. A. (1988). The neurobiology of craving: Implications for the understanding and treatment of addiction. *Journal of Abnormal Psychology, 97,* 118–132.

Zack, M., & Poulos, C. X. (2004). Amphetamine primes motivation to gamble and gambling-related semantic networks in problem gamblers. *Neuropsychopharmacology, 29,* 195–207.

Zacny, J. P. (1990). Behavioral aspects of alcohol-tobacco interactions. In M. Galanter (Ed.), *Recent developments in alcoholism* (Vol. 8, pp. 205–219). New York: Plenum.

Section VI

APPLYING IMPLICIT COGNITIONS TO PREVENTION AND TREATMENT

CHAPTER 26

Automatic Processes in the Self-Regulation of Addictive Behaviors

Tibor P. Palfai

S elf-regulation typically refers to the ability to control or modify inner states and behavior to attain desired outcomes (Vohs & Baumeister, 2004). This is particularly challenging when one is faced with the task of behaving in a manner that is contrary to habits or immediate preferences (Mischel et al., 1996). In such cases, one must act in opposition to a dominant response tendency to pursue more distal outcomes (Rachlin, 2000). This form of self-regulation (often called "self-control") is perhaps best exemplified in efforts to change addictive behaviors. With repeated use, a variety of internal and external cues may come to serve as triggers for well practiced, affect modulating patterns of substance-use behavior (Baker et al., 1987; Baker et al., 2004). Self-control of addictive behavior requires that the individual refrain from pursuing a valued incentive even though the pursuit of that incentive is supported by the

immediate context. How does this type of self-regulation occur and can it become automatic? The current paper examines research on automatic processes in self-regulation and discusses its potential implications for enhancing interventions for addictive behaviors.

SELF-REGULATION OF ADDICTIVE BEHAVIORS: A GOAL SYSTEMS PERSPECTIVE

One way of understanding the self-regulation of addictive behavior is in terms of goal processes (Gollwitzer & Moskowitz, 1996; Karoly, 1999; Kruglanski, 1996). Changing patterns of addictive behaviors involves the setting of new goals (e.g., reduce my alcohol use) and standards for behavior (e.g., do not have more than two alcoholic beverages on any occasion). The new health behavior goal

AUTHOR'S NOTE: Preparation of this article was supported by grant #R01 AA11534 from the National Institute on Alcohol Abuse and Alcoholism.

must be selected in relevant contexts, effectively transformed to behavior, and maintained over time. Self-regulation entails the use of a variety of cognitive, affective, and behavioral processes that allow one to maintain the pursuit of a health goal in the face of competing goals and environmental demands (Karoly, 1993). Effective self-regulation depends not only on what happens during relevant contexts (e.g., one attends a party), but also what the individual does before (e.g., developing plans of how to employ coping strategies), and after the situation is encountered (e.g., evaluation of goal efforts; Karoly, 1999). The extended nature of goal pursuit in efforts to change addictive behaviors means that these phases do not unfold in a linear fashion but rather influence one another in an ongoing manner (e.g., evaluation of success in self-regulation modifies planning for the subsequent occasion). Similarly, the relative importance of self-regulatory processes may change from initiation of an effort to change addiction-related behavior to the long-term maintenance of this change (Rothman, 2000).

In addition to establishing new goals and standards for behavior, the individual must have a means of monitoring internal and external information that signifies progress or failure with respect to these standards to decide whether to take action. Once action is determined as necessary, the individual must select a means to pursue the desired goal (e.g., using a coping skill) and implement specific actions (Karoly, 1993). Even when goals are being executed, they must be protected from other goals that may assume priority (Kuhl, 1985). Kuhl has proposed a number of action control strategies that are used to protect an intention from interference: (1) selective attention to goal-related information, (2) modulation of affect to facilitate goal pursuit, (3) enhancing the emotional or motivational basis for the goal, and (4) inhibition of counterintentional behaviors and competing goals.

Each of these components of self-regulation is facilitated through the intentional use of specific strategies that may be monitored and employed as the context demands it (Kuhl & Goschke, 1994). Most (e.g., Baumeister & Heatherton, 1996; Brown, 1998; Tiffany, 1990) have viewed the self-regulation of addictive behaviors as the product of conscious, controlled processes (Shiffrin & Schneider, 1977). Consciousness permits the flexible use of strategies to adapt to novel contexts and direct processing resources where needed (Yates, 1985).

Consider, for instance, some possible steps in the act of self-regulation for the drinker who is attempting to reduce alcohol consumption. Success in this effort is likely to depend on the intentional, deliberate use of cognitive and behavioral skills (e.g., Miller & Brown, 1991). The drinker may use a variety of self-regulatory processes including choosing to limit drinking in a given context, deciding on a standard of what is acceptable use, actively retrieving a variety of strategies to help limit consumption, focusing attention on information about progress or potential threats to this goal (e.g., an old drinking buddy enters the bar), or bolstering the importance of the self-control goal by intentionally bringing relevant information into awareness (e.g., pros of changing). Each of the steps that support the goal of self-control appears to be intentional, effortful, and consciously controlled. If cognitive resources were compromised by stress or fatigue, we might expect that he or she would have more difficulty achieving these self-regulatory objectives (Drobes et al., 1994; Muraven & Baumeister, 2000).

This view of self-control as mediated by conscious processes is one that has had a strong influence on the development of addiction treatments and interventions. There has, however, been increasing interest in understanding the potential role of nonconscious processes in self-control. Can components of self-regulation become automatic? This question is being asked with increasing regularity (Fitzsimons & Bargh, 2004; Lord & Levy, 1994; Moskowitz, 2001) as evidence suggests that goal pursuit may be initiated and maintained without intention or awareness (Bargh & Ferguson, 2000). This research raises the intriguing possibility that the self-control of addictive behavior itself may develop characteristics of automaticity, thereby changing the impact of factors that typically lead to self-regulation failure (Palfai, 2004).

AUTOMATICITY IN SELF-REGULATION

Defining Automaticity

Before addressing the issue of what it would mean to say that self-control of addictive behaviors might be automatic, it is useful to briefly elaborate on the distinctions between controlled and automatic processes. Controlled processes have historically been equated with functions of consciousness; they are intentional, consume limited resources, involve subjective awareness, and are controllable (Wegner & Bargh, 1998). Automatic processes, on the other hand, are those that do not involve consciousness. Judgments, inferences, and perception are said to occur automatically when they are not deliberately initiated by the individual, occur without awareness, unfold with few demands on limited processing capacity (i.e., efficiency), and are not modified once initiated. As Bargh (1994) has convincingly argued, however, these attributes do not always co-occur. Most of the automatic social-cognitive phenomena studied (e.g., automatic inferences, automatic evaluations, misattribution effects) involve some elements of controlled processing (Bargh, 1994). Such findings have led to the conceptualization of automaticity as a category of features that includes the absence of awareness, lack of intentionality, efficiency,

and uncontrollability. Automatic social cognition is the product of various combinations of these features (Bargh, 1994).

In What Sense Can Self-Control Be Automatic?

Given this broad conception of automaticity, the question of whether self-control may become automatic is one that pertains to the intentionality, awareness, effort, and controllability of the self-regulatory processes that mediate the pursuit of a health behavior change goal. Research suggests that each of the major self-regulation components described above (e.g., activating goals, choosing means, maintaining goal pursuit) may exhibit some or all of the characteristics of automaticity.

Automaticity in Goal Activation

Before self-regulatory processes may be initiated, the individual must have a way of activating or triggering the self-regulation goal in relevant contexts (Karoly, 1993). Bargh and colleagues (Bargh & Chartrand, 1999; Bargh & Ferguson, 2000; Bargh & Gollwitzer, 1994) have conducted a series of studies showing that goals may be automatically activated by situational cues and that they may be pursued without conscious awareness. What is most striking about these automatic effects is that they produce similar effects on emotion, cognition, and behavior as explicitly activated goals (Bargh & Chartrand, 1999). For example, priming an achievement goal with achievement-related words (e.g., success) has been shown to increase performance on a subsequent verbal task (Bargh et al., 2001). With repeated pursuit of the same goal within specific contexts, the individual develops automatic associations between cues, goals, and behaviors in memory (Bargh & Gollwitzer, 1994). This allows for goals to be triggered rapidly and without intention upon exposure to relevant cues.

Self-regulatory goals may operate in the same manner and guide supporting cognition and behavior (Fitzsimons & Bargh, 2004; Moskowitz, 2001). For example, stereotype responses may be countered by the activation of egalitarian goals (Moskowitz et al., 1999). For those who wish to treat individuals fairly regardless of race or ethnicity (so-called "chronic egalitarians"), exposure to faces of a race other than their own increases the accessibility of egalitarian goals as measured in primed lexical decision tasks (Moskowitz et al., 1999). Fishbach and colleagues (2003) have suggested that this type of automatic activation may also provide an important self-regulatory function in self-control of health behaviors such as dieting. With repeated efforts to maintain diets in the face of tempting cues, dieters may come to develop associations between the goal of dieting and variety of tempting foods. Over time, these repeated activation patterns may come to influence the development of cognitive-motivational networks such that dieting goals are automatically activated in the presence of tempting cues. In one experiment, self-regulatory success for dieting was associated with the degree to which tempting cues served to prime diet-related words. Among those who showed higher levels of commitment to dieting, greater success in the pursuit of the goal of dieting was associated with faster responses to make lexical judgments of diet-related words when they were primed by tempting cues. Moreover, these effects were observed with subliminal primes, suggesting that the activation of these goals may occur without intention or awareness (Fishbach et al., 2003).

Similar processes may operate in the self-control of addictive behaviors. The mere presentation of addiction-related cues may come to automatically activate self-regulatory goals for those who are attempting to change their addictive behavior. The ability to rapidly activate self-control goals upon exposure to addiction-related contexts may be critical for self-regulatory success as the processing of information pertinent to the goal of health behavior change may be initiated before addiction-related memory representations are activated.

Automaticity in Monitoring and Discrepancy Detection

A second key component in many self-regulatory models is information monitoring and discrepancy detection (e.g., Carver & Scheier, 1998; Powers, 1973). To pursue goals associated with behavior change, individuals must be able to monitor the environment for goal-related information and identify critical periods in which there is a discrepancy between the current state and the desired state. Although a given health behavior change goal (e.g., reduce drinking) may be represented at higher levels of the goal hierarchy, it may be instantiated through a number of specific subgoals (Bagozzi & Edwards, 1998), each with specific standards and specific types of information input. At each level of the goal hierarchy, the individual represents information relevant to a standard as well as information regarding the state of the system with respect to that standard. Addictive behavior change will likely involve both approach (e.g., talk to people who are not drinking alcohol at the party) and avoid (e.g., do not drink any spirits) subgoals that will trigger different forms of feedback monitoring (Carver & Scheier, 1998). These monitoring processes are central for action as they allow for the identification of discrepancies between a salient goal (or subgoal) and goal-related activity (Lord & Levy, 1994; Powers, 1973) that help prioritize action-related processing resources.

When the self-control goal is activated, individuals monitor information that is relevant to its pursuit. For addictive behaviors, this monitoring may include a number of targets including internal cues related to substance use, amounts consumed, opportunities for use, and cues that signal safety and alternatives to drinking. Although monitoring processes may be deliberate and intentional, the fact that there are multiple sources of information related to goals and that multiple goals are processed in parallel means that individuals must develop efficient processing systems that only demands conscious resources when necessary (Lord & Levy, 1994; Wegner, 1994).

Evidence from a number of experimental paradigms suggests that chronically and temporarily activated goals may influence cognitive processing of goal-relevant external stimuli without intention or awareness (Aarts et al., 2001; Bargh, 1982; Bargh & Pratto, 1986; Moskowitz, 2002). Similar processes may operate in the monitoring of internal stimuli. Extensive research on "current concerns," for example, has shown that important nonconscious goals may influence thoughts and images that come to mind (see Klinger & Cox, 2004). Such unintentional goal-driven effects have also been described in Wegner's research on ironic processes (Wegner, 1994) in which the initiation of specific processing goals (e.g., suppress a specific target) may initiate automatic monitoring of internal cues related to that goal (see Wegner & Erber, 1992).

Moskowitz (2001) has suggested that monitoring processes may be automatically initiated upon exposure to discrepancy-related information. In a series of experiments, Moskowitz (2002) has shown that the induction of a discrepancy between goal-related standards and behavior produces unintentional selective attention and more efficient processing of goal-related stimuli in the environment. For example, athletes who contemplated failure in their athletic endeavors showed greater subsequent Stroop interference effects to athletic-related words (Exp. 1)

compared with those who thought about successes. Similarly, those who were induced to think about times that they failed to live up to the ideal of egalitarianism showed greater interference on a subsequent response-time task on which egalitarian words were presented as distracters (Exp. 2).

This research on goals and cognitive processing suggest that key processes underlying monitoring and discrepancy detection may operate without intention and with high efficiency. For those who are attempting to change their addictive behavior, automatic monitoring of information that signals not only success in striving but also threat may be monitored without intention or awareness once self-control goals have become established and are readily activated.

Automaticity in the Activation of Means

Discrepancies between standards and output at higher levels of the goal hierarchy are resolved at lower levels (Lord & Levy, 1994). Successful attainment of a "health behavior change" goal is dependent on the operation of more concrete, lower-order subgoals and means. Once a goal has been activated, the individual must next select strategies to pursue this goal. For those attempting to change addictive behaviors, this process may entail the selection of a specific coping skill and the generation of positive coping expectancies. Processes of discrepancy resolution, however, need not be deliberate or even involve awareness (Aarts & Dijksterhuis, 2000; Moskowitz, 2001). Goal activation may automatically influence the means that are selected for goal pursuit (Aarts & Dijksterhuis, 2000; Shah & Kruglanski, 2000). Lexical decision studies have shown that the activation of goals through the presentation of goal-related stimuli (e.g., fitness) increases the accessibility of means that are used to obtain those goals (e.g., cycling; Aarts & Dijksterhuis, 2000;

Kruglanski et al., 2002). Moreover, these effects are observed even when subjects are subliminally exposed to goal cues outside of awareness. This automatic activation of means may be critical for the self-control of addictive behaviors as it may lead to more rapidly initiated coping responses in high-risk contexts. Self-control responses that are initiated earlier reduce the likelihood that appetitive motivational systems are fully activated in contexts that include temptation-related cues (Metcalf & Mischel, 1999).

Automaticity in Action-Control Processes

Once the goal has been activated and information related to the goal is being monitored, there are a number of key volitional processes that are critical to ensure that the goal is executed in the face of multiple other goals that may compete for processing resources. Although each of these strategies may be deliberate and consciously controlled, there is evidence that the critical action control strategies may be executed without intention; rather they operate through automatic inhibition and activation mechanisms (Lord & Levy, 1994). The establishment of a specific goal or intention automatically primes information that is related to the goal and suppresses information that is in competition with that goal. These automatic processes of inhibition and facilitation operate at each level of the self-regulatory hierarchy to influence attention, emotion, memory, and motor control (Dagenbach & Carr, 1994; Lord & Levy, 1994; Nigg, 2000).

Inhibiting Alternative Goal-Related Information

Successful goal-striving depends on successful interference control in which internal and external distracters are prevented from interfering with working memory (Nigg, 2000). Shah and colleagues (Shah et al.,

2002) have conducted a number of experiments that suggest that goals may be automatically shielded through inhibition processes. On a modified primed lexical decision task, for example, subjects showed slower response times (suggesting less activation) to identify goal-related words as personal attributes when preceded by subliminally presented primes of alternative goals. The magnitude of goal inhibition is stronger for goals that individuals are more committed to attaining. Indeed, the degree to which one is able to inhibit alternative goals is associated with persistence and success in goal striving (Shah et al., 2002).

Other work has also suggested that individuals who are more successful in their self-regulation efforts demonstrate stronger automatic inhibition processes (Diefendorff et al., 1998; Newman, 1998; Nigg, 2000). For example, Diefendorff et al. (1998) found that the strength of the negative priming effect (i.e., the degree to which participants were slower to respond to previously ignored items) was positively correlated with reported self-regulatory success for important health goals, including fitness, exercise, and weight management. What this and many other studies of inhibitory processes in emotion and cognition have shown is that self-regulatory success is associated with the ability to automatically inhibit information that is inconsistent with the currently pursued goal. Although this ability may be influenced by biological and other individual difference factors (Nigg, 2000), changes in the representational structures of goal systems through commitment and goal importance may also affect the ability to employ these automatic action control processes (Shah et al., 2002).

Summary: Automatic Processes in Self-Regulation

The above research suggests that most of the components that are viewed as central to effective self-control are mediated in part by automatic processes. Goal activation, monitoring, means selection, and a variety of action control processes, may operate automatically. Does this mean that the models of self-regulation that are based on controlled processes are incorrect? No, what it does suggest is that many of the elements that are considered to be important in goal-striving may develop characteristics of automaticity.

The ability to initiate and maintain processes that will support the self-regulatory goal without deliberation, with minimal effort, and without the need for conscious monitoring provides significant advantages for one who is attempting to change addictive behaviors. Not only are the self-control goals more likely to be executed, but the individual may be less susceptible to the types of internal states and external cues that are often associated with self-control failure (Baumeister & Heatherton, 1996). High-risk contexts for addictive behaviors (e.g., negative affect; fatigue) are often synonymous with those that deplete cognitive resources viewed as central for self-regulation (Muraven & Baumeister, 2000). The ability to execute self-control skills with fewer limited-processing resources makes it less likely that the pursuit of self-control goals is interrupted by high-risk cues and allows the individual to direct limited processing resources to specific elements of self-control that may represent a challenge (e.g., intensity of distracters). Thus, automaticity in self-control confers a number of advantages in the prevention of relapse to addiction.

CLINICAL IMPLICATIONS AND AREAS FOR FUTURE RESEARCH

The above studies provide a number of clues to how interventions may be developed to account for the distinct processing systems that mediate self-control and addiction and that capitalize on the advantages of making elements of self-control automatic. Interventions

may increase their effectiveness to the extent that they enhance the automaticity of self-control processes and/or change the automatic processes that support addictive behaviors.

Enhancing Automaticity of Self-Regulation Through Practice

The most direct way to increase these self-regulatory abilities is through practice (Fitzsimons & Bargh, 2004). An extensive body of research that has shown how practice may decrease the need for controlled processes to execute skills (Kanfer, 1996; Shiffrin & Dumais, 1982). Information that supports goal-directed behavior may be transformed through practice to become utilized by different levels of control. Through repeated use of skills in response to specific cues, the individual develops the ability to activate goals and means that will facilitate self-control automatically (Aarts & Dijksterhuis, 2000). Indeed, cue exposure training for alcohol that incorporates skill training (e.g., Monti et al., 1993) may derive part of its success through this method. Through repeated use of skills in the presence of alcohol-related cues (either internal or external), the individual is able to become more likely to activate relevant skills and become increasingly efficient with coping responses (e.g., using a drink refusal skill or ordering a soda). Practice may benefit not only the use of coping skills but also the use of action control skills. Repeated experience with the use of different volitional strategies to enhance motivation, modulate affect, and maintain attention may also be useful supplements to cognitive-behavioral treatment approaches.

Planning and Self-Control: The Deliberate Use of Automatic Processes

A second way that one may utilize automatic processes in the self-regulation of addictive behavior is through planning. Although planning is itself a conscious strategy, it enables the individual to prospectively engage automatic self-control processes by forming and rehearsing context-specific responses. Planning allows one to mentally simulate goal-striving processes prior to a situation that requires coping and anticipate obstacles to goal attainment. Through planning, the individual may determine characteristics of his or her environment in advance to activate self-regulation goals when needed (e.g., placing a daily calorie counter on the refrigerator).

Research on implementation intentions (Gollwitzer, 1999; Prestwich et al., Chapter 29) has shown that certain planning strategies may increase one's ability to execute goal-related behaviors automatically in relevant contexts. Implementation intentions consist of propositional statements of an intended action that are associated with specific contexts. They take the form, "When I encounter situation X, I will do Y." Associating a specific action with an anticipated cue in memory increases the likelihood that the action will be automatically activated during critical situational contexts (Gollwitzer, 1999). The specific skill is automatically activated and maintained by prespecified environmental cues even though the individual is aware that he or she is using a skill that was learned for coping. Implementation intentions may not only increase the automaticity of action initiation, but also increase the accessibility of cues for the initiation of self-control behavior and protect the behavior from distracters and alternative goals (Gollwitzer, 1999). Implementation intentions have been shown to influence a number of health behaviors (Gollwitzer & Oettingen, 1998), including improving diet (Verplanken & Faes, 1999), and reducing smoking behavior (Greene & Palfai, 2004).

Implementation intentions may be integrated with more extensive planning that utilizes temporal and situational cues. Moreover, the use of implementation intentions may be used to help the initiation of coping skills as well as for other action control processes such as motivation or affective control (Gollwitzer, 1999; Kuhl & Fuhrmann, 1998). The association of specific behavioral responses to specific situational cues, however, represents both an advantage and disadvantage for self-regulatory behavior. First, for some addictive behaviors it may be very difficult and cumbersome to generate multiple implementation intentions for the wide range of contexts in which the behavior occurs (e.g., smoking). Second, it may be difficult to plan for novel contexts in which drug-use motivation is activated. In such cases, it may be more important to incorporate higher-order scripts, action plans, or even subgoals in self-regulatory plans that are linked with more general contexts. These midlevel constructs between specific behaviors and general intentions may permit the flexibility needed to adapt to changing contexts while at the same time maintaining the specificity necessary to enhance action initiation (Abraham et al., 1998). Higher-order action identification will be more stable if the situational context shifts or is unexpected (Vallacher & Wegner, 1987). The range and limits of "strategic automaticity" (Gollwitzer, 1999) provided by implementation intentions and other planning techniques has yet to be fully explored and is one area that holds great promise in the development of interventions.

Changing the Activation of Addiction-Related Motivational Systems

In addition to increasing the automaticity of self-control systems, investigators have utilized a number of planning strategies that may be used to decrease the activation of addiction-related motivational systems. Specific planning strategies, such as stimulus control (Kanfer, 1986), scheduled smoking (Cinciripini et al., 1995), and cue exposure (Monti et al., 1993) influence motivational systems underlying addictive behavior by either changing the likelihood that these systems will be activated in subsequent contexts (e.g., stimulus control), or modifying the association between substance cues and addiction-related motivational systems. Self-management approaches to self-regulation make great use of this in the strategy of stimulus control (Kanfer, 1986) in an effort to deactivate the "hot systems" (Metcalfe & Mischel, 1999) that maintain addictive behaviors (e.g., get rid of the alcohol that you keep in the house "in case" guests come over). Scheduled smoking (Cinciripini et al., 1995) is a deliberate self-control strategy that attempts to modify typical behavioral responses to smoking-related contexts. Smokers are instructed to use cigarettes at regularly scheduled times throughout the day instead of in response to usual cues. Similarly, cue exposure training involves repeated exposure to substance-related cues with prevention of an addiction-related response in an attempt to differentially activate behavioral responses to high-risk triggers.

CHANGING THE CONTENT AND STRUCTURE OF MEMORY REPRESENTATIONS

Two of the central puzzles in treatment of addictive disorders are (1) how do verbal, conscious strategies that are used to change addictive behaviors influence automatic responses to substance-related contexts, and (2) how does this transformation take place? For example, do efforts to modify positive expectancies about the effects of alcohol through expectancy challenge procedures (Darkes & Goldman, 1993) reduce automatic appetitive responses to alcohol cues (Wiers et al., in press)? Similarly, do explicit strategies that link self-control-related goals to higher-order identities or important values, such as different forms of motivational

counseling (Cox & Klinger, 2004) change the way in which subsequent goal-related information is processed (Palfai, 2004). Better understanding of how features of automaticity are influenced by explicit intervention strategies will have important implications for the development of addiction treatments.

Controlled and Automatic Processes Interactions in Self-Regulation

A final issue to address in the development of interventions is the interaction between controlled and automatic processes. Although individual differences in automatic and conscious self-regulation skills account for unique variance in self-regulatory success (Diefendorff et al., 1998), at a functional level automatic and controlled processes that support self-regulation are tightly interconnected (Metcalfe & Mischel, 1999; Wegner & Bargh, 1998). In some circumstances, automatic and controlled processes may work at cross-purposes leading to less effective control (Wegner, 1994). A number of studies have shown that efforts to consciously suppress thoughts, feelings, and behaviors may lead to an increase in the very information that one is attempting to control (Wegner, 1994). As discussed above, Wegner (1994) suggests that the act of suppression initiates a conscious operating process that exerts self-control (i.e., eliminates information from awareness) and an automatic monitoring process that seeks out violations of the self-regulatory goal (e.g., information about the forbidden target). Thus, while the individual is intentionally attempting to eliminate certain target thoughts or feelings from awareness (e.g., the urge to drink), automatic monitoring processes may actually activate target-related representations in memory. Efforts of heavy social drinkers to suppress urges to drink when exposed to their favorite alcoholic beverage, for example, have been shown to increase the accessibility of alcohol-related expectancies in memory (Palfai et al., 1997). Such findings suggest that certain efforts to control responses may be successful at the level of awareness, but may actually lead to greater activation of systems that mediate addictive behavior.

Although these ironic effects are important in their own right, the implications of such findings are broader. Namely, conscious coping strategies may differentially influence automatic processes associated with addiction-related processing. This would suggest that optimal approaches to self-control would be those that are able to integrate automatic and controlled processes that support the self-control goal. This speaks to the importance of determining how conscious self-control strategies influence both "hot" and "cool" systems (Metcalfe & Mischel, 1999) within contexts when determining strategy effectiveness.

SUMMARY

In sum, research has identified a number of automatic processes associated with self-regulation that include (1) the automatic activation and utilization of goal-representations (Bargh & Ferguson, 2000), (2) the monitoring of goal-related and standard-related information (Lord & Levy, 1994), (3) the activation of goal-related means (Kruglanski et al., 2002), and (4) the inhibition of goal-irrelevant information (Diefendorff et al., 1998; Shah et al., 2002). These processes are central to the attainment of self-control goals such as efforts to change addictive behaviors. Clarifying the role of these automatic processes in self-regulation provides an expanded perspective on how the self-control of addictive behaviors may be facilitated. Future research on methods to increase the automaticity of self-regulation has important implications for the advancement of addictions treatment.

REFERENCES

Aarts, H., & Dijksterhuis, A. (2000). Habits as knowledge structures: Automaticity in goal directed behavior. *Journal of Personality and Social Psychology, 78,* 53–63.

Aarts, H., Dijksterhuis, A., & DeVries, P. (2001). On the psychology of drinking: Being thirsty and perceptually ready. *British Journal of Psychology, 92,* 631–642.

Abraham, C., Sheeran, P., & Johnston, M. (1998). From health beliefs to self-regulation: Theoretical advances in the psychology of action control. *Psychology & Health, 13,* 569–591.

Bagozzi, R. P., & Edwards, E. A. (1998). Goal setting and goal pursuit in the regulation of body weight. *Psychology & Health, 13,* 702–740.

Baker, T. B., Morse, E., & Sherman, J. E. (1987). The motivation to use drugs: A psychobiological analysis of urges. In C. Rivers (Ed.), *The Nebraska symposium on motivation: Alcohol use and abuse* (pp. 257–323). Lincoln: University of Nebraska Press.

Baker, T. B., Piper, M. E., McCarthy, D. E., Majeskie, M. R., & Fiore, M. C. (2004). Addiction motivation reformulated: An affective processing model of negative reinforcement. *Psychological Review, 111,* 33–51.

Bargh, J. A. (1982). Attention and automaticity in the processing of self-relevant information. *Journal of Personality and Social Psychology, 43,* 425–436.

Bargh, J. A. (1994). The four horsemen of automaticity: Awareness, intention, efficiency, and control in social cognition. In R. S. Wyer & T. K. Srull (Eds.), *Handbook of social cognition* (Vol. 1). Hillsdale, NJ: Lawrence Erlbaum.

Bargh, J. A., & Chartrand, T. L. (1999). The unbearable automaticity of being. *American Psychologist, 54,* 462–479.

Bargh, J. A., & Ferguson, M. J. (2000). Beyond behaviorism: On the automaticity of higher mental processes. *Psychological Bulletin,* 925–945.

Bargh, J. A., & Gollwitzer, P. M. (1994). Environmental control of goal-directed action: Automatic and strategic contingencies between situations and behavior. In W. D. Spaulding (Ed.), *Nebraska symposium on motivation* (Vol. 41). Lincoln: University of Nebraska Press.

Bargh, J. A., Gollwitzer, P. M., Lee-Chai, A., Barndollar, K., & Trotschel, R. (2001). The automated will: Nonconscious activation and pursuit of behavioral goals. *Journal of Personality and Social Psychology, 81,* 1014–1027.

Bargh, J. A., & Pratto, F. (1986). Individual construct accessibility and perceptual selection. *Journal of Experimental Social Psychology, 22,* 293–311.

Baumeister, R. F., & Heatherton, T. F. (1996). Self-regulation failure: An overview. *Psychological Inquiry, 7,* 1–15.

Brown, J. M. (1998). Self-regulation of addictive behaviors. In W. R. Miller & N. Heather (Eds.), *Treating addictive behaviors* (pp. 61–74). New York: Plenum.

Carver, C. S., & Scheier, M. F. (1998). *On the self-regulation of behavior.* Cambridge, UK: Cambridge University Press.

Cinciripini, P. M., Lapitsky, L., Seay, S., Wallfisch, A., Kitchens, K., & Van Vunakis, H. (1995). The effects of smoking schedules on cessation outcome: Can we improve on common methods of gradual and abrupt nicotine withdrawal? *Journal of Consulting and Clinical Psychology, 63,* 388–399.

Cox, W. M., & Klinger, E. (2004). *Handbook of motivational counseling: Concepts, approaches and assessment.* Chichester, UK: Wiley.

Dagenbach, D., & Carr, T. H. (1994). *Inhibitory processes in attention, memory, and language.* San Diego, CA: Academic Press.

Darkes, J., & Goldman, M. S. (1993). Expectancy challenge and drinking reduction: Experimental evidence for a mediational process. *Journal of Consulting and Clinical Psychology, 61,* 344–353.

Diefendorff, J. M., Lord, R. G., Hepburn, E.T., Quickle, J. S., Hall, R. J., & Sanders, R. E. (1998). Perceived self-regulation and individual differences in selective attention. *Journal of Experimental Psychology: Applied, 4,* 228–247.

Drobes, D. J., Meier, E. A., & Tiffany, S. T. (1994). Assessment of the effects of urges and negative affect on smoker's coping skills. *Behavior Research and Therapy, 32,* 165–174.

Fishbach, A., Friedman, R. S., & Kruglanski, A. W. (2003). Leading us not into temptation: Momentary allurements elicit overriding goal activation. *Journal of Personality and Social Psychology, 84,* 296–309.

Fitzsimons, G. M., & Bargh, J. A. (2004). Automatic self-regulation. In R. F. Baumeister & K. D. Vohs (Eds.), *Handbook of self-regulation: Research, theory and applications* (pp. 492–508). New York: Guilford.

Gollwitzer, P. M. (1999). How can good intentions become effective behavior change strategies. *American Psychologist, 54,* 493–503.

Gollwitzer, P. M., & Moskowitz, G. B. (1996). Goal effects on action and cognition. In E. T. Higgins & A. W. Kruglanski (Eds.), *Social psychology: Handbook of basic principles.* New York: Guilford.

Gollwitzer, P. M., & Oettingen, G. (1998). The emergence and implementation of health goals. *Psychology & Health, 13,* 687–715.

Greene, K., & Palfai, T. P. (2004, November). Implementation intentions and smoking. Paper presented at the annual meeting for the Association for the Advancement of Behavior Therapy, New Orleans, LA.

Kanfer, R. (1986). Implications of a self-regulatory model of therapy for treatment of addictive behaviors. In W. R. Miller & N. Heather (Eds.), *Treating addictive behaviors: Processes of change.* New York: Plenum.

Kanfer, R. (1996). Self-regulatory and other non-ability determinants of skill acquisition. In P. M. Gollwitzer & J. A. Bargh (Eds.), *The psychology of action: Linking cognition and motivation to behavior* (pp. 404–423). New York: Guilford.

Karoly, P. (1993). Mechanisms of self-regulation: A systems view. *Annual Review of Psychology, 44,* 23–52.

Karoly, P. (1999). A goal-systems self-regulatory perspective on personality, psychopathology, and change. *Review of General Psychology, 3,* 264–291.

Klinger, E., & Cox, W. M. (2004). Motivation and the theory of current concerns. In W. M. Cox & E. Klinger (Eds.), *Handbook of motivational counseling: Concepts, approaches and assessment.* Chichester, UK: Wiley.

Kruglanski, A. W. (1996). Goals as knowledge structures. In P. M. Gollwitzer & J. A. Bargh (Eds.), *The psychology of action: Linking cognition and motivation to behavior* (pp. 599–618). New York: Guilford.

Kruglanski, A. W., Shah, J. Y., Fishbach, A., Friedman, R., Chun, W. Y., & Sleeth-Kepper, D. (2002). A theory of goal systems. In M. Zanna (Ed.), *Advances in experimental social psychology* (Vol. 34). New York: Academic Press.

Kuhl, J. (1985). Volitional mediators of cognition-behavior consistency: Self-regulatory processes and action versus state orientation. In J. Kuhl & J. Beckman (Eds.), *Action control: From cognition to behavior* (pp. 101–128). New York: Springer-Verlag.

Kuhl, J., & Fuhrmann, A. (1998). Decomposing self-regulation and self-control: The volitional components checklist. In J. Heckhausen & C. Dweck (Eds.), *Life span perspectives on motivation and control* (pp. 15–49). Mahwah, NJ: Lawrence Erlbaum.

Kuhl, J., & Goshke, T. (1994). A theory of action control: Mental subsystems, modes of control, and volitional conflict-resolution strategies. In J. Kuhl & J. Beckmann (Eds.), *Volition and personality: Action versus state orientation* (pp. 93–124). Seattle, WA: Hogrefe & Huber.

Lord, R. G., & Levy, P. E. (1994). Moving from cognition to action: A control theory perspective. *Applied Psychology: An International Review, 43,* 335–398.

Metcalf, J., & Mischel, W. (1999). A hot/cool-system analysis of delay of gratification: Dynamics of willpower. *Psychological Review, 106,* 3–19.

Miller, W. R., & Brown, J. M. (1991). Self-regulation as a conceptual basis for the prevention and treatment of addictive behaviors. In N. Heather, W. R. Miller, & J. Greeley (Eds.), *Self-control and the addictive behaviors* (pp. 3–79). Sydney, Australia: Maxwell Macmillan.

Mischel, W., Cantor, N., & Feldman, S. (1996). Principles of self-regulation: The nature of willpower and self-control. In E. T. Higgins & A. Kruglanski (Eds.), *Social psychology: Handbook of basic principles* (pp. 329–360). New York: Guilford.

Monti, P. M., Rohsenow, D. J., Rubonis, A. V., Niaura, R. S., Sirota, A. D., Colby, S. M., et al. (1993). Cue exposure with coping skills treatment for male alcoholics: A preliminary investigation. *Journal of Consulting and Clinical Psychology, 61,* 1011–1019.

Moskowitz, G. B. (2001). Preconscious control and compensatory cognition. In G. B. Moskowitz (Ed.), *Cognitive social psychology: The Princeton symposium on the legacy and future of social cognition* (pp. 333–358). Mahwah, NJ: Lawrence Erlbaum.

Moskowitz, G. B. (2002). Preconscious effects of temporary goals. *Journal of Experimental Social Psychology, 38,* 397–404.

Moskowitz, G. B., Gollwitzer, P. M., Wasel, W., & Schaal, B. (1999). Preconscious control of stereotype activation through chronic egalitarian goals. *Journal of Personality and Social Psychology, 77,* 167–184.

Muraven, M., & Baumeister, R. F. (2000). Self-regulation and depletion of limited resources: Does self-control resemble a muscle? *Psychological Bulletin, 126,* 247–259.

Newman, J. P. (1998). Psychopathic behavior: An information processing perspective. In D. J. Cooke, R. D. Hare, & A. Forth (Eds.), *Psychopathy: Theory, research, and implications for society* (pp. 81–104). Dordrecht, The Netherlands: Kluwer.

Nigg, J. (2000). On inhibition/disinhibition in developmental psychopathology: Views from cognitive and personality psychology and a working inhibition taxonomy. *Psychological Bulletin, 126,* 220–246.

Palfai, T. P. (2004). Automatic processes and self-regulation: Implications for alcohol interventions. *Cognitive and Behavioral Practice, 11,* 190–201.

Palfai, T. P., Monti, P. M., Colby, S. M., & Rohsenow, D. J. (1997). Effects of suppressing the urge to drink on the accessibility of alcohol outcome expectancies. *Behaviour Research and Therapy, 35,* 59–65.

Powers, W. T. (1973). *Behavior: The control of perception.* Chicago: Aldine.

Rachlin, H. (2000). *The science of self-control.* Cambridge, MA: Harvard University Press.

Rothman, A. (2000). Toward a theory-based analysis of behavioral maintenance. *Health Psychology, 19*(Suppl. 1), 64–69.

Shah, J. Y., Friedman, R. S., Kruglanski, A. W. (2002). Forgetting all else: On the antecedents and consequences of goal shielding. *Journal of Personality and Social Psychology, 83,* 1261–1280.

Shah, J. Y., & Kruglanski, A. W. (2000). Aspects of goal networks: Implications for self regulation. In M. Boekaeris, P. R. Pintrich, & M. Zeidner (Eds.), *Handbook of self-regulation* (pp. 86–110). San Diego, CA: Academic Press.

Shiffrin, R. M., & Dumais, S. T. (1982). The development of automatism. In J. R. Anderson (Ed.), *Cognitive skills and their acquisition* (pp. 111–140). Hillsdale, NJ: Lawrence Erlbaum.

Shiffrin, R. M., & Schneider, W. (1977). Controlled and automatic human information processing: II. Perceptual learning, automatic attending, and a general theory. *Psychological Review, 84,* 127–190.

Tiffany, S. T. (1990). A cognitive model of drug urges and drug use behavior: Role of automatic and non-automatic processes. *Psychological Review, 97,* 147–168.

Vallacher, R. R., & Wegner, D. M. (1987). What do people think they're doing? Action identification and human behavior. *Psychological Review, 94,* 3–15.

Verplanken, B., & Faes, S. (1999). Good intentions, bad habits, and effects of forming implementation intentions on healthy eating. *European Journal of Social Psychology, 29,* 591–604.

Vohs, K. D., & Baumeister, R. F. (2004). Understanding self-regulation: An introduction. In R. F. Baumeister & K. D. Vohs (Eds.), *Handbook of self regulation: Research, theory and applications* (pp. 1–9). New York: Guilford.

Wegner, D. M. (1994). Ironic processes in mental control. *Psychological Review, 101,* 34–52.

Wegner, D. M., & Bargh, J. (1998). Control and automaticity in social life. In D. T. Gilbert, S. T. Fiske, & G. Lindzey (Eds.), *Handbook of social psychology* (4th ed., pp. 446–496). Boston: McGraw-Hill.

Wegner, D. M., & Erber, R. (1992). The hyperaccessibility of suppressed thoughts. *Journal of Personality and Social Psychology, 63,* 903–912.

Wiers, R. W., Van de Luitgaarden, J., Van den Wildenberg, E., & Smulders, F. T. Y. (in press). Challenging implicit and explicit alcohol-related cognitions in young heavy drinkers. *Addiction.*

Yates, J. (1985). The content of awareness is a model of the world. *Psychological Review,* 249–284.

CHAPTER 27

Relevance of Research on Experimental Psychopathology to Substance Misuse

PETER J. DE JONG, MEREL KINDT, AND ANNE ROEFS

Abstract: In the domain of the emotional disorders, many research efforts have focused on the role of implicit cognition. Findings from these studies have provided important clues with respect to the role of implicit cognitions in the persistence of psychopathological complaints as well as to the returns of complaints after treatment. In this chapter, we take the findings of this line of research as the starting point and explore how it relates to theories in the areas of addiction. We mainly focus on attentional processes in an attempt to provide some clues in answering the main question of this chapter, which is: Do implicit drug-related cognitions have causal effects on craving and substance misuse?

INTRODUCTION

An important impetus behind the increasing research in studies in the areas of cognition in psychopathology has been the rise of cognitive models implying that emotional disorders critically depend on the existence of maladaptive cognitive structures in memory (e.g., Beck et al., 1985). These so-called schemata are assumed to automatically influence all stages of individuals' information processing. Since relevant cognitions may not be accessible through introspection, empirical research testing the validity of these types of models predominantly relied on indirect performance-based measures of cognitive processes that are assumed to be functionally related to the underlying maladaptive schemata (Mathews & MacLeod, 1985).

One of the most studied phenomena in this respect is the involuntary tendency of anxiety patients to prioritize the processing of information that is relevant to their current concerns (often referred to as "attentional bias"). Recent models of addictive behaviors imply similar processes to be involved in substance use and misuse (Franken, 2003). In the last decade a rapidly growing number of studies appeared in the area of substance use and misuse focusing on "attentional" bias for drug-relevant stimuli (see also Bruce & Jones, Chapter 10; Field et al., Chapter 11). The basic assumption of the information processing models of psychopathology and addiction is the idea that prioritizing threatening (in anxiety) or appetitive (e.g., in substance misuse) information contributes to the intensity of the problems. That is, these types of processing biases are not simply a symptom of addictive/emotional disorders, but are assumed to play a vital role in their causation and maintenance (Williams et al., 1997). More specifically, in emotional disorders it is assumed that there is a reciprocal relationship between emotional distress (e.g., fear) and a failure to inhibit the allocation of attentional resources toward threatening information (MacLeod et al., 2002; Mathews & MacLeod, 1994). Similarly, in addiction, current approaches assume that there is a reciprocal relationship between craving and "attentional bias" (Franken, 2003). In line with this view, it has even been argued that the development of an attentional bias for drug stimuli may be the core process underlying compulsive drug use and craving (Lubman et al., 2000).

A first prerequisite of these information processing models is that patients suffering from particular disorders are characterized by a disorder-specific bias in attention allocation. Following this, most initial research efforts have focused on demonstrating an attentional bias for concern-relevant stimuli (e.g., spiders for individuals with spider phobia; high caloric food in disinhibited dieters). A subsequent series of quasi-experimental studies focused on delineating the factors that are vital to reliably elicit (or inflate) processing biases. By directly or indirectly manipulating the motivational state in unselected, analogue, and clinical samples, it was tested whether indeed activating (or removing) particular current concerns or motivational states elicited (or reduced) functionally related processing biases. A related series of studies tested the influence of context cues and/or environmental settings on the strength of attentional biases.

Only very few recent studies have begun to test the most critical assumption, namely that processing bias has a causal influence on the generation of complaints. In these studies, it has been investigated whether inducing a bias results in more distress in a subsequent stressful task. Relatedly, some recent studies took the opposite perspective and explored whether techniques to experimentally reduce the attentional bias in anxiety patients is also effective in reducing patients' complaints. In the remainder of this chapter, we discuss the results, promises, and potential implications of these various types of studies for the understanding and treatment of addictive behaviors.

IS SELECTIVE PROCESSING BIAS A GENERAL CHARACTERISTIC?

One of the most popular paradigms to investigate selective processing priority is the so-called modified Stroop test. In the computerized version, participants are shown a series of words or pictures on the screen that are presented in various colors. It is their task to name the color of the words (or the color of the pictures, or the color of the background on which the pictures are presented) as quickly as possible. The contents of some of the words (or pictures) that are presented relate to the relevant clinical disorder (e.g., "beer" in the context of alcohol abuse). In the original color Stroop there is a dimensional overlap between the task-irrelevant feature (the meaning of the word, e.g., green) and the required response (naming the color of the ink in which the word is printed) (MacLeod, 1991). The so-called modified Stroop, however, is structurally different from the original color Stroop in that there is no such overlap between the task-irrelevant (distracting) meaning of the word (e.g., beer) and the name of the color. Hence, what is usually called the emotional or modified Stroop test is in fact no Stroop test at all (cf. De Houwer, 2003). Following this, it seems more appropriate to refer to this task as the color-naming interference task. Although the precise source of heightened color-naming interference has not yet been identified

(Williams et al., 1996), it is a clear indicator of a cognitive-processing bias.

Color-Naming Interference Task (Formerly Known as Modified Stroop)

Clinical groups generally display heightened color-naming interference on trials displaying words related to their disorder. Accordingly, interference has been found for general threat words in generalized anxiety disorder (GAD; Mogg et al., 1995), spider-related words in spider phobia (Lavy et al., 1993), and food-related words in obesitas (Braet & Crombez, 2003). Similar results have been reported for pictorial stimuli in the context of spider phobia (Kindt & Brosschot, 1998) and bulimia nervosa (Stormark & Torkildsen, 2004). Taken together, the available evidence in the context of anxiety and eating disorders is in accordance with the idea that selective allocation of attentional resources is not restricted to threatening information but may be evident as well for attractive reward-related stimuli.

Adding to the idea that selective processing biases may also be a characteristic of approach-related motivational states, similar selective patterns of interference have been reported for alcohol-related words in alcoholics (Johnsen et al., 1994; Stormark et al., 1997), heroin cues in heroin-dependent inpatients (Franken, Kroon, Wiers, et al., 2000), smoke cues in smokers (Waters & Feyerabend, 2000), and gambling-related words in pathological poker machine players (McCusker & Gettings, 1997). All in all, it seems that selective processing biases are the result of preoccupations with motivational salient stimuli, which are difficult to ignore when confronted with.

Dot-Probe Task

Another paradigm that is often used to study attention allocation is the dot-probe paradigm. In the typical paradigm, participants are presented with pairs of words or pictures one of which is replaced by a dot. It is the participant's task to indicate as fast as possible the location of this dot. In some of the pairs one picture (or word) is related to the clinical concerns (e.g., glass of beer), and one is the neutral contrast (e.g., tool). The dot-probe paradigm capitalizes on the idea that when participants' attention is grabbed by the disorder-related stimulus, they are relatively fast on trials when the dot appears in the spatial vicinity of the disorder-related cue, and/or relatively slow when it appears in the spatial location of the control stimulus.

Similar to the results with color-naming interference tasks, results with the dot-probe test revealed heightened vigilance for general threat words in GAD (Mogg et al., 1995), and for food words in individuals scoring high on the Eating Disorder Inventory (EDI; Placanica et al., 2002). Similar results have been reported for visual stimuli. For example, social phobic individuals were found to display enhanced vigilance for angry faces relative to happy and neutral faces (Mogg, Philippot, et al., 2004) and women with bulimia nervosa for pictures of food items (see Dobson & Dozois, 2004).

In line with the idea that heightened vigilance for threatening information is related to an avoidance-related motivational state, a bias toward threatening information is typically only found for short (i.e., 500 ms) presentation times of the task-irrelevant pairs of stimuli, whereas the differential vigilance for angry faces in social phobics is absent when using longer presentation times (i.e., 1,250 ms; Mogg, Philippot, et al., 2004). Accordingly, significant avoidance for injury scenes was found at longer exposure duration (i.e., 1,500 ms) in participants with high levels of blood-injection-injury-fears, whereas a strong vigilance for these scenes was evident during the shorter (500 ms) presentations (Mogg, Bradley, et al., 2004). Similar results have been found using eye movement measurements during a visual search task (i.e., participants were instructed to detect a spider as fast as possible in complex naturalistic slides). Relative to controls, spider-phobic individuals not only detected spiders faster and fixated closer to spiders during initial search, they also fixated farther away from spiders following the detection of the spider (Pflugshaupt et al., 2005).

Unfortunately, within the existing literature there are thus far no studies in the context of eating disorders that used longer stimulus presentation times. So it remains to be seen whether the initial vigilance also shifts to avoidance in individuals suffering from eating disorders. An alternative and plausible hypothesis would be that the initial vigilance for "attractive" food stimuli would be sustained as would be predicted when selective attention for food stimuli is functionally related to an approach-related motivational state. Interestingly, this type of study has recently been done in the context of addictive behavior. Sustaining the idea that prioritizing drug-related information is indeed related to an approach-related motivational set, habitual smokers were found to display a maintenance of attention on smoking-related visual scenes when a longer (i.e., 2 s) stimulus duration was used (Mogg et al., 2003). A study measuring eye movements and gaze fixation during a similar dot probe test with a long stimulus presentation time (2 s), further confirmed the idea that addicted individuals are characterized by a biased maintenance of attention on smoking-related cues. Interestingly, this pattern was especially pronounced in participants who were experimentally deprived from nicotine (Field et al., 2004b), suggesting that nicotine deprivation promotes sustained attentional allocation to nicotine cues.

The majority of studies in the area of addiction, however, exclusively relied on the typical short (500 ms) stimulus presentation times, allowing only testing on the presence of initial vigilance. In general, these studies showed that substance misusers are characterized by heightened vigilance for drug-related stimuli. Accordingly, using a pictorial dot-probe test, Ehrman et al. (2002) revealed an attentional bias for smoke cues in heavy smokers, but not in individuals who never started smoking. Similarly, opiate-dependent individuals displayed a selective processing priority toward pictures of drug paraphernalia (Lubman et al., 2000), whereas heavy social drinkers were found to display vigilance for visually presented alcohol cues (Townshend & Duka, 2001). Corresponding to the alleged reciprocal relationship between initial vigilance and craving, correlations were found between individual's level of "craving" and differential attentional deployment in habitual smokers (Mogg et al., 2003), cocaine users (Franken, Kroon, & Hendriks, 2000), and recreational cannabis users (Field et al., 2004a). Because the level of craving (or the level of bias) in these studies was not experimentally manipulated, however, it remains to be seen whether these correlations have a causal (reciprocal) basis.

Findings with the Stroop and dot-probe tasks converge in several ways. Both tasks have identified specific biases in clinical groups but less consistent biases in nonclinical people. In addition, both tasks can be modeled in terms of processing along task-relevant and task-irrelevant pathways, with the effects arising because participants allocate attention to task-irrelevant pathways that convey threat or reward (Williams et al., 1996). Furthermore, both tasks are considered to tap relatively automatic processes that are difficult to control.

Spatial-Cueing Task

A third type of tasks that has been used to study attentional bias in anxiety, are spatial-cueing tasks (e.g., Derryberry & Reed, 1994, 2002). Most important, these tasks can differentiate between tendencies to shift attention toward particular stimuli versus difficulties in shifting away from these stimuli. This distinction is important as both forms of bias may have different implications for subsequent processes. Individuals who shift attention toward negative information may notice multiple threats but still process them rather superficially, resulting in only minor emotional distress. In contrast, those who have difficulty shifting away from threat may tend to lock onto the negative stimulus to process it deeply, resulting in stronger emotional responding (Derryberry & Reed, 1994). In a similar vein, both forms of attentional bias may differentially contribute to the generation of craving and substance misuse in addiction.

In the spatial-cueing tasks, participants are engaged in a motivated computer game in which they can gain or lose points depending on their speed in detecting simple circular targets. Before each target appears, a peripheral cue is presented that automatically orients attention to the positive location (where points can be gained if the response is fast enough) or the negative location (where points can be lost if the response is too slow). In half of the trials the target appears in the uncued location (invalid cue). Relatively fast responses on trials with a valid cue on the negative location are indicative of an attentional bias toward threat. Relatively slow responses on trials with an invalid cue on the negative location are indicative of a difficulty to disengage from threatening stimuli.

In keeping with the results from the other tasks, anxious participants showed a bias favoring threatening locations where points could be lost (Derryberry & Reed, 1994). Importantly, this bias only appeared when a cue on the negative location was followed by a target in the other (i.e., uncued) location. This finding questions the traditional view of the processes underlying the attentional bias phenomenon. That is, rather than facilitating attentional shifts toward threatening stimuli, it appears that anxiety delays the disengagement

of attention from threat. Such a view is compatible with both the Stroop and dot-probe results. Difficulty in shifting away from threatening information would slow down color-naming when the anxious individual has difficulty shifting from the irrelevant threatening meaning to the relevant color information. In line with the idea that interference effects in the dot-probe task are also due to delays in disengaging from threatening information, the bias in favoring threatening locations mostly arise from slow reactions to neutral locations rather than from fast responses to threat locations (Brosschot et al., 1999; Koster et al., 2004).

In the original setup, the cues did not predict the target's location and participants should not have been intentionally motivated to attend them. To test whether attentional biases also arise in situations that promote a more intentional use of attention deployment, the task has been adapted in a way that the peripheral cues actually predicted the target's location during the majority of trials. In such a modified task, anxious individuals still displayed a similar attentional bias, also when using relatively long time intervals between cue and target (500 ms), suggesting that apart from automatic processes also more voluntary attentional processes are involved in anxiety (Derryberry & Reed, 2002).

The authors are not aware of studies using this paradigm in addiction research. This paradigm, however, seems even more promising than the often-used color-interference or dot-probe tasks in disentangling the underlying mechanisms of compulsive drug use and craving. It allows differentiating between the tendency to shift attention toward attractive stimuli and individuals' difficulty to shift away from attractive reward-related information (i.e., the positive location). In addition, it can be modified in a way to evaluate the relative importance of automatic and more voluntary attentional processes in the area of addiction.

INFLUENCE OF EXPERIMENTALLY MANIPULATED CONTEXT AND/OR MOTIVATIONAL STATE

Deprivation

A series of studies employed quasi-experimental methods to directly or indirectly influence participants' motivational state in an attempt to investigate whether this would result in parallel changes in individuals' patterns of selective information processing. In what can be considered as a first rigorous exploration of this issue, Lavy and Van den Hout (1993) asked half of their participants to refrain from food for 24 hours before performing a color-naming interference task. As predicted, fasting resulted in a more positive evaluation of food stimuli, an increased urge to obtain food, and in a heightened color naming interference for appetitive (food) cues.

A subsequent study using the dot-probe task, further confirmed these basic findings, and showed that heightened visual attention toward food words was mainly found in participants in the fasting condition (Mogg et al., 1998). Furthermore, the strength of the bias was significantly correlated with hunger ratings and the estimated amount of food that could be eaten. This supports the hypothesis that such bias for appetitive cues is fueled by an approach-related motivational state. Together, it appears that "hunger" (and presumably also other drives and states) result in a difficulty to inhibit the allocation of resources to appetitive cues. This seemingly highly adaptive mechanism may become dysfunctional in restrained eaters who strongly try to regulate their food intake resulting in disinhibited eating patterns. The dysfunctional triggering of the vigilance for food cues may be further strengthened by the enhanced reward value of food after repeated periods of prolonged deprivation (cf. Brown et al., 1998).

A recent pictorial dot-probe study showed that fasting may not only induce a bias toward food in normal controls but may also change the focus of the habitually enhanced vigilance in analogue groups scoring high on the Eating Disorder Inventory (EDI; Placanica et al., 2002). More specifically, fasting resulted in an attentional shift from "healthy" low-caloric food items toward "unhealthy" high-caloric foods. This pattern of results may provide a clue for the apparent preference for high-caloric food in bulimia nervosa.

Together, these findings not only show that influencing motivational state results in predictable changes in attentional deployment, but also underline the importance of taking the motivational state during measurement procedures into consideration. Clearly, this type of process may also be involved in the context of addictions (see, e.g., Field et al., Chapter 11, for a discussion of the effects of nicotine deprivation on attentional bias).

Pre-Loads

Using a different approach to manipulate individuals' motivational state, Overduin and colleagues (1995) provided half of the participants with an "appetizer" (a bit of pudding) just before a color-interference task. As an index of individuals' motivational set they measured the amount of ice cream participants ate during a subsequent "taste test" that was carried out immediately following the interference task. Interestingly, compared to the "nonappetizer" control group, participants in the "appetizer" condition showed heightened color-naming interference during food-word trials. Although the appetite manipulation was not generally related to the amount of ice cream participants consumed, the level of color-naming interference did strongly correlate with participants' actual amount of ice cream intake. Hence, in support of the vigilance-approach hypothesis for appetitive cues, the processing priority of food words was not only inflated in the appetite condition but was also found to have predictive validity for subsequent food intake.

Using a similar strategy in the context of alcohol use, a group of social drinkers were sip-primed with alcohol immediately before starting a color-naming interference test including words referring to positive (reward/approach-related) alcohol outcomes and negative alcohol outcomes (Jones & Schulze, 2000). Similar to the results of Overduin et al. (1995), typically the alcohol-primed social drinkers displayed selective color-naming interference for positive alcohol words. Subsequent research presented a group of heavy and a group of light social drinkers with a "taste test" of either an alcoholic or a soft drink immediately prior to a color-naming interference test (Cox et al., 2003). In line with the pattern of previous findings, only heavy drinkers in the alcohol pre-load condition displayed relatively heightened color-naming interference for alcohol words compared to soft drink words. All in all, it appears that pre-loads of wanted/attractive consumables (e.g., food, drinks) can modify individuals' attention allocation. The crucial question that remains to be answered is whether this processing bias is causally related to craving, which in turn may support or disinhibit individuals' subsequent intake behaviors.

Treatment

Another way to test the influence of motivational saliency on attentional bias is to reduce its saliency via therapeutic interventions. The influence of treatment on attentional bias in addiction is still a largely unexplored area. Meanwhile, studies in the area of anxiety disorders and bulimia nervosa showed that when the motivational saliency of initially threatening (or attractive) stimuli is removed after successful treatment, individuals' attentional bias is likewise removed (e.g., Lavy, Van den Hout, & Arntz, 1993; Dobson & Dozois, 2004). It should be noted, however, that none of the apparently successful treatment studies included a no-treatment control group to test for mere test/retest effects. Meanwhile, the only study that did include such a no-treatment control group revealed that the reduction of color-naming interference for spider words in spider-phobic individuals was similar in the treatment and no-treatment control group (Thorpe & Salkovskis, 1997). Future studies including no-treatment control groups are necessary to more rigorously test whether reduction in attentional bias following treatment is indeed due to a reduction of the emotional saliency of disorder-relevant stimuli. In addition, it would be important for future studies to include follow-up assessments. From both a theoretical and a practical standpoint, it would be important to see whether a residual bias is predictive of the return of complaints (cf. de Jong et al., 1995). Unfortunately, thus far none of the studies on attentional bias tested the predictive power of residual attentional bias for relapse.

Context Cues

To test the influence of context cues on individuals' attentional bias, a series of studies experimentally manipulated the context cues during the measurement procedure. For example, Braet and Crombez (2003) presented obese and normal-weight control children with two different color-interference tests. One test used the traditional random version in which food words and control words are presented intermixed, whereas the other test used the so-called blocked format in which various categories of words are presented in separate blocks of trials. Although the mixed-presentation format is generally considered as the most stringent test of automatic attention allocation (e.g., less influence of post-attentional rumination; cf. Lavy & Van den Hout, 1993), the blocked version may be a better experimental analogue of the natural environment of obese children (or alcohol misusers, etc.). That is, in the natural environment of these children there is an abundance of food (and alcohol, etc.) cues. Thus, by mimicking the naturally abundant presence of food cues, the blocked format may be a more ecologically valid approach to detect the pathological attentional processes that are involved in these types of problematic behaviors.

As predicted, obese children showed stronger color-naming interference for food words than normal control children. Interestingly, this apparent hypersensitivity for food cues was considerably stronger in the blocked than in the mixed format. These findings are in line with the idea that the omnipresence of concern-related (e.g., food) cues may have a cumulative effect that hinders strategic attentional control. Eventually, the abundant presence of concern-related cues may lead to a breakdown when an individual is no longer able to expend sufficient extra effort to override the tendency for motivational salient stimuli to capture the individual's attention (cf. Mathews & MacLeod, 1994). Following this, in their natural environment, obese children may find themselves progressively unable to disengage their attention from food-related cues. In its turn, this may induce or enhance their craving for the forbidden food, with overeating as the eventual consequence. In line with this, a considerable correlation was found in the obese group between the level of color-naming interference and children being overweight. These findings are thought provoking and clearly point to the importance of studying the causal relationship between

(attenuated) "attentional control" and craving in the area of addiction.

Following a different strategy to create a more valid experimental analogue of the seducing natural environment of substance misusers, Cox and his colleagues exposed half of their participants to a color-naming interference task in a setting containing alcohol-related visual cues (i.e., participants were surrounded by alcohol posters). Keeping in line with the idea that the presence of motivation-relevant cues may elicit a tendency to allocate attention toward motivationally salient stimuli, heavy social drinkers only showed interference effects for alcohol-words in the alcohol poster condition but not in the control condition (Cox et al., 1999). It would be interesting to see how this type of manipulation affects alcohol-dependent individuals and how these enhancing effects may be influenced by successful interventions. To the extent that apparently successfully treated alcoholics are not able to divert their attention away from alcohol cues under potentiated conditions (e.g., blocked format, tested in negative mood state, or in a drinking-relevant environmental context), these individuals could be at risk for relapse.

ATTENTIONAL BIAS: CAUSAL AGENT OR EPIPHENOMENON?

As reviewed in the previous sections, there is evidence that anxiety and eating-disorder patients, as well as substance misusers, are characterized by selective processing biases, whereas these biases seem to be attenuated or even eliminated following treatment. Although this pattern of findings is consistent with (i.e., does not refute) the idea that attentional bias plays a critical role in the maintenance of psychopathological complaints, it is also consistent with the interpretation that attentional bias is a mere symptom of pathological anxiety (or addiction).

Following the motivational-cognitive model of emotional disorders, one of the most important questions regarding attentional bias is whether the bias precedes, and whether it contributes to, the development of complaints. In spite of its vital importance, only a small body of work has been undertaken to determine whether attentional bias has any influence on emotional dysfunction. In a first correlational approach, color-naming interference was assessed for supra- and subliminally presented general threat words in a group of women awaiting colposcopy ($N = 31$). A subgroup of these women ($n = 15$) later received a diagnosis of cervical pathology. It was found that the single best predictor of the seriousness of the elicited emotional distress in this subgroup was the level of color-naming interference on subliminal trials (MacLeod & Hagan, 1992). In other words, it appears that the subliminal interference effect represents an emotional vulnerability factor that is predictive of the level of experienced distress when faced with important stressors. Obviously, the women in this study experienced current situational stress of being in anticipation of a potentially threatening diagnosis during the assessment. To see whether the experience of current stress during assessment (which is likely to modulate attentional bias) is a necessary prerequisite for a predictive relationship to occur, a subsequent study was carried out in women who were not currently exposed to environmental stress. Yet, again, it was found that (subliminal) color-naming interference was the single best predictor of vulnerability to life stress (Van den Hout et al., 1995).

Using a conceptually similar approach, a group of nonanxious undergraduates ($N = 87$) with naturalistic variations in color-naming interference effects for panic-related threat stimuli were exposed to a biological-challenge task (brief inhalations of 20 percent carbon dioxide enriched air; Nay et al., 2004). Consistent with the idea that threat-biased attentional processing has a causal influence and reflects a premorbid anxiety vulnerability factor, color-naming interference effects for both subliminally and supraliminally presented panic words predicted emotional responding above and beyond self-reported anxiety sensitivity (ASI). It would be interesting to see whether an inflated premorbid attentional bias for reward rather than threat-related stimuli would set people at risk for substance misuse (cf. Franken, 2003).

Although thought provoking and clinically important, causality can still not be inferred from these prognostic studies. Yet, these findings did instigate several researchers to perform the next step to critically test whether processing bias is causally related to anxiety symptoms. Accordingly, MacLeod et al. (2002) experimentally induced an attentional bias using a modified dot-probe task and tested the impact of this manipulation on subsequent emotional vulnerability. They tested students with average anxiety levels. During a large number of training trials (576), half of the participants consistently moved toward negative stimuli (experimental condition: attentional bias induction) and half of the participants consistently moved away from the negative stimuli (control condition) in the modified dot-probe task. This manipulation successfully induced an attentional bias: In the experimental condition, participants were faster on (new) negative words than on (new) neutral words on test trials, and in the control condition the opposite was found. It is important to note that the training had no effect on mood during the training itself. After a stress task, however, the experimental group reported higher levels of distress than the control group (and again in a replication study in the same article). These results clearly support the idea that attentional bias can causally mediate emotional vulnerability, lending substance to the previously speculative suggestions concerning the proposed causal role of attentional bias (see also Mathews &

MacLeod, 2002, for additional evidence). Thus far, no attempts have been reported to induce a bias for appetitive stimuli to test the causal relationship between heightened (and/or prolonged) vigilance for substance cues and craving or misuse.

CHANGING DYSFUNCTIONAL ATTENTIONAL BIAS

The finding that a bias induction in nonanxious individuals can lower the threshold for evoking negative emotional reactions also points to an exciting therapeutic application. It suggests that a similar modified cognitive-experimental dot-probe task may also be used to reduce an already existent bias in anxiety patients, thereby reducing these patients' anxiety complaints. Indeed, research in a nonreferred sample of chronic worriers (40 percent met *DSM-IV* criteria for generalized anxiety disorder [GAD]), lent support to the idea that attentional retraining (AR) might be useful as a therapeutic tool (Vasey et al., 2002). At 5-day intervals, participants were exposed to five sessions of 30 minutes of AR using a modified dot-probe task. In the treatment condition, each session consisted of 216 trials in which probes followed neutral words on 204 trials. The placebo condition was identical to AR with the exception that probes followed neutral words on 50 percent of the trials and threat words on the remainder. The placebo condition did not affect individuals' bias for threat or their scores on the anxiety pathology questionnaires. Meanwhile, the treatment condition not only resulted in an attenuated threat bias, it also led to a considerable reduction of individuals' symptom scores. Adding to its clinical significance, these treatment effects compared favorably with the average effect for cognitive behavioral therapy for GAD in past-published studies.

In a similar vein, treatment-seeking socially phobic individuals ($N = 18$) completed eight sessions of either an attention training using a modified version of the dot-probe detection paradigm or a placebo condition (Amir et al., 2004). During the training sessions participants were presented with 160 trials depicting rejecting (disgusting) and neutral faces. In the experimental condition, the dot appeared in 80 percent of the trials on the location of the neutral face, whereas in the placebo condition it appeared in 50 percent of the trials on that location. The modification training was not only effective in changing biased attention in socially anxious individuals but also substantially reduced symptoms of social anxiety as assessed by an independent rater as well as by standardized self-report measures. This change was clinically significant and of similar size as reported for traditional cognitive behavioral interventions (see also Dandeneau & Baldwin, in press). Importantly, AR has promise as a new treatment tool in the context of complaints in which attentional bias is assumed to play a vital role (e.g., Wiers et al., 2004). Currently, we are eagerly waiting for the first AR studies to emerge in the context of addictive behaviors.

SUMMARY AND CONCLUSION

Several studies are presented that are relevant to the challenging hypothesis that processing biases for drug stimuli form the psychological nucleus of addiction (e.g., Lubman et al., 2000). Although several interesting studies appeared in the last years, most studies are still quasi-experimental. To test the viability of the current hypothesis, future research should focus on experimental designs in which processing biases are manipulated. The research area of addiction could profit from recent developments in anxiety research, in which experimental paradigms are developed to test the causal contribution of processing bias in the development and maintenance of complaints.

REFERENCES

Amir, N., Beard, C., Klumpp, H., Elias, J., Brady, R., & Hewett, J. (2004, September). *Modification of attentional bias in social phobia: Change in attention, generalizability across paradigms, and change in symptoms.* Paper presented at the 34th annual congress of the European Association for Behavioural and Cognitive Therapies, Manchester, UK.

Beck, A. T., Emery, G., & Greenberg, R. L. (1985). *Anxiety disorders and phobias: A cognitive perspective.* New York: Basic Books.

Braet, C., & Crombez, G. (2003). Cognitive interference due to food cues in childhood obesity. *Journal of Clinical Child and Adolescent Psychology, 32,* 32–39.

Brosschot, J. F., de Ruiter, C., & Kindt, M. (1999). Processing bias in anxious subjects and repressors, measured by emotional Stroop interference and attentional allocation. *Personality and Individual Differences, 26,* 777–793.

Brown, G., Jackson, A., & Stephens, D. N. (1998). Effects of repeated withdrawal from chronic ethanol on oral self-administration of ethanol on a progressive ratio schedule. *Behavioural Pharmacology, 9,* 149–161.

Cox, W. M., Brown, M. A., & Rowlands, L. J. (2003). The effects of alcohol cue exposure on non-dependent drinkers' attentional bias for alcohol-related stimuli. *Alcohol and Alcoholism, 38,* 45–49.

Cox, W. M., Yeates, G. N., & Regan, C. M. (1999). Effects of alcohol cues on cognitive processing in heavy and light drinkers. *Drug and Alcohol Dependence, 55,* 85–89.

Dandeneau, S. T., Baldwin, M. W. (in press). The inhibition of socially rejecting information among people with high versus low self-esteem: The role of attentional bias and the effects of bias reduction training. *Journal of Social & Clinical Psychology.*

De Houwer, J. (2003). A structural analysis of indirect measures of attitudes. In J. Musch & K. C. Klauer (Eds.), *The psychology of evaluation: Affective processes in cognition and emotion* (pp. 219–244). Mahwah, NJ: Lawrence Erlbaum.

de Jong, P. J., Van den Hout, M. A., & Merckelbach, H, (1995). Covariation bias and the return of fear. *Behaviour Research and Therapy, 33,* 211–213.

Derryberry, D., & Reed, M. A. (1994). Temperament and attention: Orienting toward and away from positive and negative signals. *Journal of Personality and Social Psychology, 66,* 1128–1139.

Derryberry, D., & Reed, M. A. (2002). Anxiety-related attentional biases and their regulation by attentional control. *Journal of Abnormal Psychology, 111,* 225–236.

Dobson, K. S., & Dozois, D. J. A. (2004). Attentional biases in eating disorders: A meta-analytic review of Stroop performance. *Clinical Psychology Review, 32,* 1001–1022.

Ehrman, R. N., Robbins, S. J., Bromwell, M. A., Lankford, M. E., Monterosso, J. R., & O'Brien, C. P. (2002). Comparing attentional bias to smoking cues in current smokers, former smokers, and non-smokers using a dot-probe task. *Drug and Alcohol Dependence, 67,* 185–191.

Field, M., Mogg, K., & Bradley, B. P. (2004a). Cognitive bias and drug craving in recreational cannabis users. *Drug and Alcohol Dependence, 74,* 105–111.

Field, M., Mogg, K., & Bradley, B. P. (2004b). Eye movements to smoking-related cues: Effects of nicotine deprivation. *Psychopharmacology, 173,* 116–123.

Franken, I. H. A. (2003). Drug craving and addiction: Integrating psychological and neuropsychopharmacological approaches. *Progress in Neuro-Psychopharmacology & Biological Psychiatry, 27,* 563–579.

Franken, I. H. A., Kroon, L. Y., & Hendriks, V. M. (2000). Influence of individual differences in craving and obsessive cocaine thoughts on attentional processes in cocaine abuse patients. *Addictive Behaviors, 25,* 99–102.

Franken, I. H. A., Kroon, L. Y., Wiers, R. W., & Jansen, A. (2000). Selective cognitive processing of drug cues in heroin dependence. *Journal of Psychopharmacology, 14,* 395–400.

Johnsen, B. H., Laberg, J., Cox, W., Vaksdal, A., & Hugdahl, K. (1994). Alcoholic subjects' attentional bias in processing of alcohol-related words. *Psychology of Addictive Behaviors, 8,* 111–115.

Jones, B. T., & Schulze, D. (2000). Alcohol-related words of positive affect are more accessible in social drinkers' memory than are other words when sip-primed by alcohol. *Addiction Research, 8,* 221–232.

Kindt, M., & Brosschot, J. F. (1998). Phobia-related cognitive bias for pictorial and linguistic stimuli. *Journal of Abnormal Psychology, 106,* 644–648.

Koster, E., Crombez, G., Verschuere, B., & De Houwer, J. (2004). Selective attention to threat in the dot probe paradigm: Differentiating vigilance and difficulty to disengage. *Behaviour Research and Therapy, 42,* 1183–1192.

Lavy, E., & Van den Hout, M. A. (1993). Attentional bias for appetitive cues: Effects of fasting in normal subjects. *Behavioural and Cognitive Psychotherapy, 21,* 297–310.

Lavy, E., Van den Hout, M. A., & Arntz, A. (1993). Attentional bias and spider phobia: Conceptual and clinical issues. *Behaviour Research and Therapy, 31,* 17–24.

Lubman, D. I., Peters, L. A., Mogg, K., Bradley, B. P., & Deakin, J. F. W. (2000). Attentional bias for drug cues in opiate dependence. *Psychological Medicine, 30,* 169–175.

MacLeod, C., & Hagan, R. (1992). Individual differences in the selective processing of threatening information, and emotional responses to a stressful life event. *Behaviour Research and Therapy, 30,* 151–161.

MacLeod, C., Rutherford, E., Campbell, L., Ebsworthy, G., & Holker, L. (2002). Selective attention and emotional vulnerability: Assessing the causal basis of their association through the experimental manipulation of attentional bias. *Journal of Abnormal Psychology, 111,* 107–123.

MacLeod, C. M. (1991). Half a century of research on the Stroop effect: An integrative review. *Psychological Bulletin, 109,* 163–203.

Mathews, A., & MacLeod, C. (1985). Selective processing of threat cues in anxiety states. *Behaviour Research and Therapy, 23,* 563–569.

Mathews, A., & MacLeod, C. (1994). Cognitive approaches to emotion and emotional disorders. *Annual Review of Psychology, 98,* 236–240.

Mathews, A., & MacLeod, C. (2002). Induced processing biases have causal effects on anxiety. *Cognition & Emotion, 16,* 331–354.

McCusker, C. G., & Gettings, B. (1997). Automaticity of cognitive biases in addictive behaviours: Further evidence with gamblers. *British Journal of Clinical Psychology, 36,* 543–554.

Mogg, K., Bradley, B. P., Field, M., & De Houwer, J. (2003). Eye movements to smoking-related pictures in smokers: Relationship between attentional biases and implicit and explicit measures of stimulus valence. *Addiction, 98,* 825–836.

Mogg, K., Bradley, B. P., Hyare, H., & Lee, S. (1998). Selective attention to food-related stimuli in hunger: Are attentional biases specific to emotional and psychopathological states, or are they also found in normal drive states? *Behaviour Research and Therapy, 36,* 227–237.

Mogg, K., Bradley, B. P., Miles, F., & Dixon, R. (2004). Time course of attentional bias for threat scenes: Testing the vigilance-avoidance hypothesis. *Cognition & Emotion, 18,* 689–700.

Mogg, K., Bradley, B. P., Millar, N., & White, J. A. (1995). Follow-up study of cognitive bias in generalized anxiety disorder. *Behaviour Research and Therapy, 33,* 927–935.

Nay, W. T., Thorpe, G. L., Roberson-Nay, R., Hecker, J. E., & Sigmon, S. T. (2004). Attentional bias to threat and emotional response to biological challenge. *Journal of Anxiety Disorders, 18,* 609–627.

Overduin, J., Jansen, A., & Louwerse, R. E. (1995). Stroop interference and food intake. *International Journal of Eating Disorders, 18,* 277–285.

Pflugshaupt, T., Mosimann, U. P., Von Wartburg, R., Schmitt, W., Nyffeler, T., Müri, R. M. (2005). Hypervigilance pattern in spider phobia. *Journal of Anxiety Disorders, 19,* 105–116.

Placanica, J. L., Faunce, G. J., & Job, R. F. S. (2002). The effect of fasting on attentional biases for food and body shape/weight words in high and low eating disorder inventory scorers. *International Journal of Eating Disorders, 32,* 79–90.

Stormark, K. M., Field, N. P., Hugdahl, K., & Horowitz, M. (1997). Selective processing of visual alcohol cues in abstinent alcoholics: An approach-avoidance conflict. *Addictive Behaviors, 22,* 509–519.

Stormark, K. M., & Torkildsen, O. (2004). Selective processing of linguistic and pictorial food stimuli in females with anorexia and bulimia nervosa. *Eating Behaviors, 5,* 27–33.

Thorpe, S., & Salkovskis, P. (1997). The effect of one-session treatment for spider phobia on attentional bias and beliefs. *British Journal of Clinical Psychology, 36,* 225–241.

Townshend, J. M., & Duka, T. (2001). Attentional bias associated with alcohol cues: Differences between heavy and occasional social drinkers. *Psychopharmacology, 15,* 67–74.

Van den Hout, M. A., Tenney, N., Huygens, K., Merckelbach, H., & Kindt, M. (1995). Responding to subliminal threat cues is related to trait anxiety and emotional vulnerability: A successful replication of MacLeod and Hagan (1992). *Behaviour Research and Therapy, 33,* 451–454.

Vasey, M. W., Hazen, R., & Schmidt, N. B. (2002, November). *Attentional retraining for chronic worry and generalized anxiety disorder (GAD).* Paper presented at the annual conference of the American Association of Behavioral Therapy, Reno, NV.

Waters, A. J., & Feyerabend, C. (2000). Determinants and effects of attentional bias in smokers. *Psychology of Addictive Behaviors, 14,* 111–120.

Wiers, R. W., de Jong, P. J., Havermans, R., & Jelicic, M. (2004). How to change implicit drug use-related cognitions in prevention: A transdisciplinary integration of findings from experimental psychopathology, social cognition, memory, and experimental learning psychology. *Substance Use & Misuse, 39,* 1625–1684.

Williams, J. M. G., Mathews, A., & MacLeod, C. (1996). The emotional Stroop task and psychopathology. *Psychological Bulletin, 120,* 3–25.

CHAPTER 28

Adolescent Changes in Implicit Cognitions and Prevention of Substance Abuse

Marvin D. Krank and Abby L. Goldstein

Abstract: This chapter explores the growth of implicit substance-use associations during early adolescence and their implications for the development of primary and secondary prevention programs. Increases in implicit measures of substance-use cognitions are highly correlated with, and prospectively predict, the initiation of youth alcohol and marijuana use. We propose that implicit memory measures may uniquely reveal decision-relevant indices of incentive motivation and behavioral choice. As such, implicit measures should be useful to (1) identify and target the stage of risk for substance-use initiation, (2) provide early sensitive measures of effective change from prevention programs, and (3) guide the development of new methods of persuasive messages that focus on behaviorally relevant cognitive changes.

Adolescence is a time of significant change, development, and risk. During the formative adolescent years, young people increasingly interact with the larger social world and acquire new cognitive representations that shape their current and future life choices. Curious adolescents explore their world, try new things, test limits, and take risks. Given the current prevalence and availability of both licit and illicit drugs, it is not surprising that this stage of novelty and exploration often involves the initiation of substance use (Johnston et al., 2004). Although substance use in adolescence typically involves experimentation, rather than problem use, adolescent substance use is associated with a host of consequences, including academic problems, risky sexual activity, and unsafe driving practices (Everett et al., 1999; National Institute of Alcohol Abuse and Alcoholism, 1997).

Recent evidence demonstrates that changes in cognitive representations, such as expectancies and memory associations, often predict and mediate changes in substance use. The research presented in this book illustrates how measures of implicit cognition provide a unique and powerful tool for assessing the cognitive changes that precede and accompany substance use. By identifying the cognitive structures and processes that underlie substance use, implicit cognition theory has the potential to inform the development of effective, theory-based prevention programs. The purpose of this chapter is to describe the application of implicit cognition to adolescent substance use and explore how models of implicit cognition may be used to develop effective and persuasive prevention programs that target the cognitive processes directly influencing adolescent substance use.

UNDERSTANDING ADOLESCENT SUBSTANCE USE

Generally, first substance use, including alcohol (especially intoxication), tobacco, marijuana, and other illicit drugs, occurs after age 12 and before age 24, with many transitions including initial experimentation and problem substance use occurring before age 18. These trends cross international borders and, although certain substances undergo cyclical changes in their overall prevalence and are characterized by changing trends in use (e.g., ecstasy, crystal methamphetamine; Johnston et al., 2004), the pattern of progression across the teen years remains remarkably steady. What is most evident and typical of studies across this age range is the remarkable growth of drug use across a range of measures and drugs.

Recently, researchers have focused on identifying individuals and situations with greater risk for substance use and abuse. Longitudinal examinations of substance use with latent growth curve modeling have resulted in the identification of subsets of users that differ in their substance use progression and substance-related problems. For example, Flory et al. (2004) classified adolescents into distinct subgroups based on their use (or nonuse) of alcohol and marijuana. For alcohol, early onset users had more dysfunctional outcomes (e.g., arrests,

alcohol abuse/dependence, marijuana abuse/dependence) than either late onset users or nonusers, whereas for marijuana both early and late onset users had more dysfunctional outcomes than nonusers.

Other researchers have identified risk factors that are associated with the growth of substance use in adolescence. These risks include substance use by peers (e.g., Brook et al., 1999), aggression and delinquent behavior (e.g., Raskin-White et al., 2001), and family factors such as family substance use, lack of parental monitoring, and parent-child conflict (Wills & Yaeger, 2003). Individual differences in personality traits and comorbid psychiatric disorders also contribute to youth transitions in substance use (see Conrod & Stewart, in press). These risk factors and the stage of progression in substance use are important to the development of effective prevention and early intervention for youth substance use and suggest the need for tailored programs addressing differing motivations and stages of substance use (see Stewart et al., 2005).

A further differentiation of individual risk derives from Prochaska and DiClemente's (1983) transtheoretical model of change, which proposes that the acquisition and cessation of behaviors progresses along a series of stages: precontemplation, contemplation, preparation, action, and maintenance. This stage model of behavior change has implications for treatment. The treatment goal is to move individuals from a more harmful stage to a safer one. Similarly, the acquisition of substance-use behavior in adolescents can be characterized according to stages of progression where substance use progresses along a continuum from nonuse, through intention to use, experimentation, regular use, abuse, and dependence (cf. Dimeff et al., 1999). The addition of intention as a construct dichotomizes nonusers into two groups: those who intend to use drugs or alcohol in the foreseeable future and those who have no intention to use. The rationale for including intention is similar to the readiness construct in the transtheoretical model. Individuals who are openly considering future substance use are hypothesized to be in a different stage of risk than those who have given it no thought or have concluded that they will never use. In addition, our work with alcohol use (Krank et al., 2003) suggests that intentions can be reliably measured and that intentions to drink increase concomitantly with changes in alcohol-related cognitions. This stage model is useful to illustrate how implicit cognitions may be used to measure the stage of risk and help to tailor prevention efforts before any actual use has occurred.

It is within this multistage framework of youth substance use that we explore the contribution of implicit memory to the prevention of substance abuse.

IMPLICIT COGNITION AND SUBSTANCE-USE TRANSITIONS IN YOUTH

Cognitive measures associated with substance use are useful adjuncts to understanding and predicting transitions in adolescent substance use. Substance-use associations change both concurrently and in advance of actual substance-use transitions (Goldman et al., 1999; Krank et al., 2003, 2005; Stacy, 1997). These methods can be used in prevention in a number of ways. First, they add a measure of risk to target individuals or populations for particular types or intensities of intervention. In addition, cognitive methods provide sensitive measures of intervention efficacy, potentially differentiating those who are reached by the intervention from those who are not. Further, we argue here that implicit memory measures tap the associative structures of adolescent incentive motivation and provide a window into the processes of behavioral choice related to substance use.

These potential applications indicate that implicit cognitive approaches provide an innovative theoretical basis for substance-use interventions and point to new directions for program development and evaluation.

COGNITIVE CHANGES AND THE PREDICTION OF SUBSTANCE USE IN ADOLESCENTS

There have been a number of approaches to measuring cognitive changes that predict substance use. Our focus is on associative memories about substance use and alternative behaviors. The measures we use include both explicit outcome expectancies, implicit behavioral associates, and ambiguous word associations (see below for details). Using the expectancy paradigm, studies in adolescents have shown that alcohol-related associations are formed prior to drinking initiation (Christiansen et al., 1982) and that positive alcohol outcome expectancies prospectively predict consumption in adolescent drinkers (Christiansen et al., 1989). Goldman et al. (1999) argue that alcohol outcome expectancies (1) correlate with alcohol use, (2) predate actual drinking experience, (3) predict future drinking, (4) are modified by drinking experiences, and (5) mediate other antecedent influences. Implicit measures of substance-use associations also reveal a strong proximal relationship with substance use. Evidence from alcohol use in adolescents demonstrates that implicit measures of substance-use memory associations (1) correlate independently with alcohol use when demographic and other cognitive variables are controlled, (2) change before substance use begins, and (3) predict future drinking independently of demographic, personality, and other cognitive variables.

We have examined the relationship between cognitive associations and substance use in a cross-sectional sample of 1,724 students in grades 7 through 12 of a single school district in British Columbia, Canada. The data were collected from groups of students by survey in the spring of 1997. Drug- and alcohol-use patterns are similar to those described above for national and regional surveys of youth in this age range (Krank & Johnson, 1999). The study investigated the relationship between cognitive associations and alcohol and marijuana use. Participants were administered two implicit measures, behavioral associates and ambiguous word associations (from Stacy, 1997), for both alcohol and marijuana. These implicit tests were placed at the beginning of the survey to prevent contamination with subsequent questions about drinking and marijuana use. Behavioral associates were assessed by asking students to write down the first behavior or action that came to mind in response to a number of outcome phrases, such as *having fun, feeling good,* or *feeling dreamy.* The phrases were selected as high-frequency, self-generated outcomes for drinking alcohol or smoking marijuana based on previous research (Stacy et al., 1994). Open-ended responses were coded as alcohol or marijuana associates or both (see Stacy, 1997; Stacy et al., Chapter 6) and composite scores were calculated based on the sum of responses that mentioned alcohol or drinking behavior as well as using marijuana, respectively. In the ambiguous word-association task students were asked to write the first word that came to mind in response to a word with dual meanings, one of which was related to alcohol or marijuana. For example, the probe *draft* might elicit responses of *paper* or *beer.* Similarly, word probes, such as *pot* and *weed,* have multiple meanings, but some responses, such as *reefer, stoned,* or *smoke* are clearly marijuana-related in the context of these probes. Again, cumulative scores of the number of alcohol and marijuana interpretations of target probes were taken as the implicit measures of alcohol or marijuana associations.

These implicit measures correlate strongly with measures of alcohol and marijuana use, respectively. Table 28.1 shows the results of regression analyses using implicit memory measures and alcohol outcome expectancies to predict each of three measures of alcohol use and one measure of intention to use alcohol. The intention analysis was conducted only on nondrinkers. All regression analyses controlled for grade and gender. This study also assessed explicit positive- and negative-outcome expectancies for alcohol use with a standardized questionnaire (Leigh & Stacy, 1993). Each of the four regression analyses was highly significant. Alcohol-implicit memory measures predict drinking quantity, frequency of use in past 30 days, and recency of use after controlling for outcome expectancies, grade, and gender. As expected, the outcome expectancy measures also predicted alcohol use after controlling for grade and gender. The implicit-alcohol association measures, however, predicted variance in alcohol use independently of the explicit measure of alcohol outcome expectancies. Intention to drink in nondrinkers was predicted by homographs and positive-outcome expectancies; however, neither behavior associates nor negative-outcome expectancies predicted intention. In the case of behavior associates, this is because very few nonusers produced any alcohol responses to the outcome phrases. By contrast, the behavior associates were stronger predictors of level of alcohol use in those students who had begun to drink.

In this same study, these implicit measures also predict current marijuana use and future intention to use in nonusers. The behavioral associates and homographs measures of marijuana associations strongly correlated, $r = .351$, $p < .001$. Nevertheless, both homograph and behavioral associate measures contributed independently to the prediction of marijuana use (beta = .210, $t(1, 771) = 6.0$, $p < .001$; beta = 1.85, $t(1, 771) = 5.25$, $p < .001$, respectively) and intention to use

Table 28.1   Regression of Implicit Cognitive Measures of Alcohol Associations and Grade and Gender on Measures of Alcohol Use and Intention

	Quantity		Days in past 30		Recency		Intention	
	Beta/R	t	Beta/R	t	Beta/R	t	Beta/R	t
Model	.587*		.468*		.620*		.302*	
Behavior Associates	.113	5.10*	.118	4.90*	.071	3.31*	.042	.76
Homograph	.131	5.86*	.166	6.81*	.135	6.24*	.150	2.74*
Positive Exp.	.260	11.8*	.216	8.97*	.229	15.4*	.258	4.58*
Negative Exp.	-.249	-11.7*	-.215	-9.25*	-.308	-14.9*	-.027	-.48
Gender	-.095	-4.6*	.001	.025	.021	1.08	.051	.91
Grade	.194	9.20*	.009	.399	.146	7.15*	-.078	-1.42

NOTE: Behavioral Associate = number of alcohol-related behavior responses to outcome cue words fun, relaxed, happy, good time, forgetting problems, and powerful (range 0–6); Homograph = number of alcohol-related responses to ambiguous words with possible alcohol meaning: draft, mug, ice, cooler, shot, bottle (range 0–6); Positive Exp. = average score on positive expectancy items from Leigh and Stacy (1993; range 0–6); Negative Exp. = average score on negative expectancy items from Leigh and Stacy (1993; range 0–6).

*All models significant at p < .001; Quantity, days and recency models df = 6, 1,587; Intention model df = 6, 306; * significant at p < .001.

443

(beta = .462, $t(1, 1411) = 20.2$, $p < .001$; beta = .191, $t(1, 1411) = 8.3$, $p < .001$, respectively) controlling for gender and grade in the model. This pattern contrasts slightly with that found for alcohol in that marijuana behavior associates were produced in nonusers and did predict intention to use (Krank et al., 2003). For both marijuana and alcohol, higher implicit memory scores predicted increased intentions to use in the future among nonusers. These observations suggest that implicit measures of memory associations may be valuable in predicting an early transitional stage in substance use. Given the strong relationship between intentions and actual behavior (Ajzen, 1985), these findings provide added support for implicit cognitions as prospective predictors.

Even stronger evidence that confirms Stacy's (1997) findings that implicit measures of alcohol are useful prospective predictors of alcohol use comes from longitudinal data that we have collected from 1,303 adolescents. In that study, implicit alcohol associations predict drinking 12 months later using a number of drinking measures including the number of days drinking in the past 30, usual number of drinks, recency of last drinking episode, and recency of last time drunk. Strikingly, the initiation of drinking during the 12 months was also predicted by the homograph measure in adolescents who had not had any previous drinking history (Krank et al., 2003, 2005). This is the same pattern as is found in the intention measure for nonusers in Table 28.1.

IMPLICIT MEMORY AND SUBSTANCE USE

We turn now to consider the question of why implicit memory is so strongly predictive of substance use. Our contention is that implicit memory measures reflect the same memory associations that underlie incentive motivation and behavioral choice. Specifically, implicit memory methods tap into the situation-behavior-reinforcer associations that are central to incentive motivation and other reinforcement-based explanations of behavioral choice. Implicit methods are uniquely important to substance use because they open new windows to these "memories" of motivationally significant relationships.

Implicit Cognition, Incentive Motivation, and Behavioral Choice Theory

Recent theories of substance use and addiction are heavily influenced by representations of substance-use behaviors and their association with reinforcing outcomes. Although not explicitly cognitive, incentive motivation theories of substance use are based on anticipation or memory of positive or reinforcing consequences of a behavior (Robinson & Berridge, 1993; for a review, see Krank, 2003). Behavioral choice theory provides another associative learning theory of addictive behavior (Vuchinich & Tucker, 1996). According to behavioral choice theories, preference for substance use depends on both the reinforcing outcome associated with substance use and the potential reinforcing outcomes of other activities. Both incentive motivation and behavioral choice theories postulate that substance use is governed by learned associations between actions and outcomes. Whereas incentive theories of addiction focus on the uniquely powerful or qualitatively distinct reinforcement value of abused substances arising from their direct action in particular brain regions, behavioral choice theories emphasize preference for an activity within the context of other activities and the availability of reinforcing substitutes. The analytical approach is behavioral, but the theory assumes cognitive representations of behavior-outcome associations. It is worth noting here that incentive motivation and behavioral choice theories do not necessarily involve conscious or rational decision making. Implicit cognition methods may be particularly powerful tools for investigating the unconscious influences on behavior choice.

Contributions of Implicit Cognition to Associative Theories of Substance Use

Implicit memory methods provide new measures to assess associations between substance use and its anticipated outcomes that are reflective of incentive motivations and behavioral reinforcer associations underlying choice. Indeed, measuring behavior-outcome associations without explicit awareness may overcome resistance in the assessment process (Stacy, 1997). Implicit methods may also access memories that are inaccessible to awareness (see e.g., Ames et al., Chapter 23) and reveal unconscious influences on behavior (Greenwald & Banaji, 1995; Jacoby & Kelley, 1990). Implicit cognition may be particularly important in adolescence, a developmental stage marked by impulsivity, risk-taking, and novelty-seeking. Such behaviors are more easily influenced by unconscious processes and are related to levels of early substance use (Cooper et al., 2003). The relative lack of preplanning in adolescents underscores the importance of prevention programs that identify the implicit factors influencing impulsive substance use. Finally, implicit cognition advances our understanding of substance abuse by expanding the focus beyond response outcome associations to include situational, contextual, and social stimulus elements (Krank & Wall, Chapter 19; Krank et al., 2005). Thus, implicit measures capture a richer complex of associative elements, including outcomes, words, contexts, and affect. Prevention approaches can turn this wealth of subjective information into material for building persuasive messages to mitigate risk.

IMPLICIT COGNITION AND PREVENTION

A wide array of methods has been applied to the prevention and treatment of substance abuse in adolescents (Monti et al., 2001; Wagner & Waldron, 2001). Our goal here is not to review the prevention literature; rather we will explore the ways implicit memory research can enhance prevention programs to reach a greater percentage of at-risk teens with more effective and individually tailored methods. From the transitional stage model described earlier, the goal of prevention is the modification of individual substance-use trajectories either to (1) impede progression to increased or more harmful use, or (2) aid in the return to reduced or less harmful use. Such prevention strategies are effective only to the extent that they make contact with the individual and change the individual's future behavior. The cognitive approach to prevention further assumes that changing the appropriate underlying cognitions in an individual will result in positive behavioral change. For example, many adolescents overestimate levels of substance use in their peers and society at large (e.g., Sussman et al., 1988). Programs that challenge these mistaken beliefs are effective in reducing problem use (e.g., Marlatt et al., 1998).

Implicit memory research indicates new directions for prevention, including (1) early identification of and intervention for at-risk individuals or populations, (2) sensitive measures of intervention success, and (3) targeting relevant cognitive representations for change (see also Wiers et al., 2004). In addition, the implicit processing approach to adolescent interventions has some general implications for effective persuasion. Specifically, prevention is persuasive only to the extent that the message is processed, relevant, and retrieved at the right time. To be effective, prevention programs must change the cognitive processing of associations that influence behavioral choice at the times of most ssignificant risk.

Early Identification of Levels of Risk in Individuals or Populations

Implicit measures of substance-use associations are proximal predictor variables and thus can be sensitive indicators of an individual's stage and level of risk. Recent approaches to secondary prevention have shown the value of identifying high-risk groups or individuals for targeted substance-use interventions (Conrod & Stewart, in press; Stewart et al., 2005). Identifying at-risk individuals or groups allows tailoring prevention programs to match individual needs (Dimeff et al., 1999; for a recent review, see Sussman et al., 2004). Tailoring prevention programs for target groups involves matching the intervention with the severity of risk and aligning prevention methods with the antecedent conditions of substance use. From our earlier discussion, stage of initiation differentiates individual differences in adolescent substance-use risk. Youth differ in their past history of substance use, problems associated with use, and their future intentions to use. Moreover, cognitive changes predict these progressive stages of risk. Thus, implicit memory measures may be used to identify the stage of risk and aid in identifying individuals who will benefit from different prevention programs. Specifically, individuals who have already started drinking need a different approach than those who are merely contemplating drinking or those who have not even begun to consider the possibility. Implicit memory measures provide unobtrusive ways of differentiating youth who are in these various stages of risk. In addition, the nature of substance-use associations at these stages of risk should lead to

tailored prevention programs that selectively target the memory associations that need to change.

Measuring Change

Implicit substance-use associations are also useful in identifying who has successfully benefited from prevention programming. We have already argued that implicit alcohol associations predict nonusers who intend to use alcohol and prospectively predict patterns of drinking in both drinkers and nondrinkers. Increases in implicit alcohol associations along with positive outcome associations independently predict alcohol risk-taking behaviors in adolescents. This means that effective prevention should impede the growth of such associations. In individuals who are nonusers or infrequent users, it may be difficult to determine whether an intervention has successfully resulted in behavior change. Intentions and cognitions, both explicit and implicit, may be the most effective means for determining the effects of a prevention program in nonusers and experimenters. Future research using implicit memory measures may provide further validation for the effectiveness of prevention programs targeted at altering specific substance-related cognitions.

Targeting Specific Cognitive Changes in Prevention

Beyond the predictive utility of implicit measures of substance use, evidence reviewed earlier suggests that associations with substance use are causal mediators of substance use in adolescents (see also Goldman et al., 1999; Krank et al., 2003, 2005; Stacy, 1997). Modifying the processing of memory associations that place individuals at risk can have a protective effect. From the perspective of incentive motivation and behavioral choice theories, the development of prevention programs should benefit from methods that minimize the effects of positive associations with substance use. Methods that should be helpful include enhancing negative associations with substance use, preventing the learning of positive associations with substance use, and promoting learning of positive associations with nonsubstance-use behaviors that would compete with substance use. Such prevention programs would target anticipated and actual changes in substance-use cognitions that increase the risk of substance-use transitions. Implicit methods are useful not only in identifying risky cognitions, but also in identifying alternative associations that have protective effects.

Normative Behavioral Associations and Behavioral Choice

Behavioral choice theories and behavioral economics have recently been applied to health-related behaviors (see Bickel & Vuchinich, 2000) and substance use (Vuchinich & Tucker, 1988). Madden (2000) defines behavioral economics as the examination of factors that influence consumer behavior. Accordingly, the choice to use substances varies as a function of (1) direct constraints on access to substances, and (2) the availability of other reinforcers and constraints on access to them (Vuchinich & Tucker, 1988). In a recent sample of British Columbia students, 56.6 percent and 45.5 percent of youth reported that alcohol and marijuana, respectively, were either "easy" or "very easy" to obtain. Consequently, to produce change, other behaviors of equal or greater reinforcement value need to be easily available for selection. For example, increasing constraints on access to substances (e.g., price increases for legal substances or enforcement strategies) should be coupled with decreasing constraints on access to alternatives (e.g., funding for after-school programs). According to behavioral choice theory, these methods fit well with community or family-oriented prevention designed to provide alternative activities.

Implicit memory approaches may be used to enhance the development of effective applications of behavioral choice theories through a more complete exploration of the associations governing adolescent choice at various stages of substance-use initiation. The behavioral associate (described above) and situational associate (see Stacy et al., Chapter 6) tasks illustrate how implicit measures may be used to assess the range of behavioral options available to adolescents and identify those behaviors that, from a behavioral choice perspective, may be substitutes for substance use. In both tasks, the response field is open to nondrug alternatives. In fact, we have found that nondrug users give exclusively nondrug-related responses to outcome probes such as *have fun*. Similarly, situational probes, such as *Friday or Saturday night*, elicit drinking responses in drinkers, but alternative behaviors in nondrinkers. These associations may translate into choices youth make when navigating environments in which both substance use and alternative behaviors are available.

Identifying potential behavioral substitutes available to adolescents may inform the development of substance-abuse prevention programs. Specifically, instead of promoting abstinence through emphasizing the negative consequences of alcohol use, interventions may highlight alternatives to substance use and broaden youths' menu of choices. As Bigelow (2001) stated, "The most effective way to reduce and eliminate an undesirable behavior is to provide a competing attraction" (p. 302). In prevention approaches, these normative activities that compete with substance use should provide contrast to develop discrepancies for change. The idea is that these contrasts would motivate alternative, safer behaviors much the same way that normative levels of drinking motivate reduced drinking in heavy users. Direct encouragement and training in alternative behaviors is obviously the strongest approach.

Such alternative behavior training fits well in community-, school-, and family-based approaches. Cognitive approaches that encourage alternative behavioral associations with contexts or outcomes that are often linked to substance use should be developed in primary prevention. These cognitive methods are particularly suited for those not yet involved in substance use.

General Implications of Cognitive Approaches to Future Prevention Efforts

The focus of the foregoing analysis is the cognitive impact of messages youth receive and their relevance to behavioral choice and prevention. We turn now to the general implications of the cognitive perspective in prevention. Wiers and colleagues (2004) have presented a detailed analysis of how some principles of learning and memory impact prevention approaches. We present here just a couple of salient points from this perspective to emphasize that prevention messages to be effective must be encoded in a manner that makes them retrievable in the situational context where decisions about substance use are made (typically not when parents are around). The encoded message must be relevant and result in new learning that counteracts risky cognitions. Unfortunately, few programs pay attention to how the prevention message is processed and even fewer evaluate its impact on cognitions that influence behavioral choice. Prevention programs need to evaluate the changes in the substance-use associations that are known to precede changes in behavior. Our analysis suggests that behavioral associations that compete with substance use are critical for change. We need to measure not only risky behaviors and cognitions, but also positive associations and other desirable outcomes to validate early whether an intervention is effective.

Discrepancy and Surprise

Recent motivational enhancement approaches to therapy emphasize the importance of discrepancy in persuasive messages (Miller & Rollnick, 2002). Both traditional learning and computational cognitive theories give insight into why discrepancy is so important. The central feature of the influential Rescorla and Wagner (1972) theory of associative learning was the discrepancy hypothesis. Simply stated, the degree of new learning depends on the discrepancy between an expected and an actual outcome. Surprising events are processed more, resulting in more associative or interpretive encoding. New learning depends on surprise generated by the contrast between expected and actual events. A prevention message that is surprising or unexpected is more likely to result in the new learning that is essential for change.

Retrieval Factors

The contexts of substance-use associations should be incorporated into the prevention message because they are likely to be critical to memory retrieval and behavioral decision making (see Krank & Wall, Chapter 19, for a more complete discussion). For example, substance-use associations about self and others like "me" (peers, role models, and family) are likely to be more influential than those about others. When making decisions about whether "I" should do something, associations of self with situations and outcomes become relevant retrieval cues. The social context of substance-use associations suggests that the target audience should identify with the messenger. The messenger must be believable. A cognitive perspective argues that social context is important to the prevention message. From the present perspective, future research should examine how the messenger might interact with the message to produce cognitive changes that are most effective in protecting the individual against substance use. More generally, prevention programs should consider their impact on the accessibility of substance use and alternative associations in contexts where decisions will be made.

FUTURE DIRECTIONS IN PREVENTION RESEARCH

From our analysis of behavioral choice and implicit memory theories, a primary goal of cognitive prevention approaches should be to produce alternative behavioral associations that are both incompatible with and more accessible than cognitive changes that antedate substance-use transitions. Recently, both primary (Cruz & Dunn, 2003) and secondary (Dunn et al., 2000) prevention programs have begun to address cognitive associations (substance-use outcome expectancies) directly. These approaches are based on the expectancy challenge approach to problem drinking (Darkes & Goldman, 1998; for a critical overview, see Jones et al., 2001). In the expectancy challenge, drinkers are confronted with a placebo drinking experience and led to face the conclusion that many of the effects of drinking are based on expectancy and not alcohol. The premise of this approach is that the realization that their positive expectancies are false will reduce drinking. In recognition that placebo drinking would not be appropriate in prevention, cognitive expectancy challenge procedures were designed to modify memory configurations and strengthen associations between alcohol and negative affect (e.g., *slow, sleepy*) and physical (e.g., *sick, rude*) effects. The application of implicit memories for substance-use associations should take this kind of cognitive approach in new directions.

Brief Screening and Targeted Intervention

Cognitive approaches to substance-use prevention efforts need to target the stage of risk. From our perspective, there is little value in challenging associations that are not currently present. Thus, cognitive challenge or false expectation approaches would not be appropriate in nonusers. In those who have not used, but intend to use, cognitive challenges to the expected effects of substance use would be appropriate. These challenges, however, are likely to differ from those aimed at individuals who are already drinking and have some direct experience with the drug's effects. We propose a two-stage brief intervention process for school-based prevention derived from the BASICS (Brief Alcohol Screening and Intervention for College Students) approach to secondary prevention (Dimeff et al., 1999). The first phase of the program would assess the current stage of risk in target school populations (e.g., grades 7 through 9). In addition to tools assessing the current level of use and other risk factors, we would add implicit measures of substance-use associations, long-term goals, alternative behaviors, and future intentions. In the second phase of the program, individuals would be grouped according to the current level of use and future intentions to use. Behavioral associations, alternative behaviors, and long-term goals would be used to provide individual feedback and tailor the prevention messages to the specific group. Although secondary prevention typically uses individual interventions, Marlatt and his colleagues (1998) have shown that it can be effective for heterogeneous groups.

Cognitive Inoculation Training

One specific example of how targeted approaches could be applied is inoculation training. Nonusers in particular would benefit from programs designed to protect them from media and peer influences. During the teen years, youth are increasingly exposed to drug and alcohol references in popular culture and through their exposure to individuals in their immediate environments, including family and friends. Advertising, music, and movies depict substance use with greater frequency than real life and often in images that typically show positive outcomes and rarely show adverse outcomes (Grube, 1993; McIntosh et al., 1999). Media exposure to others using drugs and alcohol is a significant risk for substance use (Villani, 2001). Implicit memory measures may be useful in identifying the nature of the changes that result from social learning before actual substance use begins (e.g., messages in popular media; Fleming et al., 2004; Stacy et al., 2004). One effective campaign to reduce teen smoking involved portrayals of cigarette manufacturers as manipulators (Goldman & Glantz, 1998). From a cognitive perspective, this prevention approach succeeds by "inoculating" teens against the messages found in smoking advertisements and movies depicting smokers. The prevention message allows the young person to encode cigarette exposure in the popular media as deception. Protection against veiled and often not so veiled messages about the positive consequences of substance use may be useful in prevention venues that target nonusers, intenders, and experimenters. Such inoculation training would be directed at a critical portrayal of media sources of information about substance use including alcohol advertising.

CONCLUSION

The real war on drugs is the battle for the hearts and minds of our youth. Adolescence is a critical period for the initiation of substance use and, for some, represents the first stage in an increasingly problematic continuum of use. Cognitive representations of substance use change concurrently and in advance of substance-use transitions. Implicit memory methods allow for their measurement without resistance, which may be particularly important for adolescents, whose propensity for impulsivity and risk-taking implies unconscious or unplanned behavior. Moreover, such measures tell us about the structure of the associations that influence choice behavior. Thus, further understanding of adolescents' implicit cognitions concerning substance use may serve as an important theoretical basis for the evaluation and development of substance-abuse prevention programs. This focus on implicit cognition has the potential to take the prevention field into several new directions, including (1) early identification of at-risk individuals or populations for targeted interventions, (2) sensitive measures of intervention success, (3) identification of cognitive representations that should be targets for producing behavior change, and (4) greater understanding of the most persuasive methods for message delivery that produce new learning and will be most effective when decisions about substance use are made.

REFERENCES

Ajzen, I. (1985). From intentions to action: A theory of planned behavior. In J. Kuhl & J. Beckmann (Eds.), *Action-control: From cognition to behavior* (pp. 11–39). New York: Springer.

Bickel, W. K., & Vuchinich, R. E. (Eds.). (2000). *Reframing health behavior change with behavioral economics*. Mahwah, NJ: Lawrence Erlbaum.

Bigelow, G. E. (2001). An operant behavioral perspective on alcohol abuse and dependence. In N. Heather, T. J. Peters, & T. Stockwell (Eds.), *International handbook of alcohol dependence and problems* (pp. 299–315). New York: John Wiley.

Brook, J. S., Kessler, R. C., & Cohen, P. (1999). The onset of marijuana use from preadolescence and early adolescence to young adulthood. *Development and Psychopathology, 11,* 901–914.

Christiansen, B. A., Goldman, M. S., & Inn, A. (1982). The development of alcohol-related expectancies in adolescents: Separating pharmacological from social learning influences. *Journal of Consulting and Clinical Psychology, 50,* 336–344.

Christiansen, B. A., Roehling, P. V., Smith, G. T., & Goldman, M. S. (1989). Using alcohol expectancies to predict adolescent drinking behavior after one year. *Journal of Consulting and Clinical Psychology, 57,* 93–99.

Conrod, P. J., & Stewart, S. H. (in press). A critical look at dual-focused cognitive-behavioral treatments for comorbid substance use and psychiatric disorders: Strengths, limitations, and future directions. *Journal of Cognitive Psychotherapy.*

Cooper, M. L., Wood, P. K., Orcutt, H. K., & Albino, A. (2003). Personality and predisposition to engage in risky or problem behaviors during adolescence. *Journal of Personality and Social Psychology, 84,* 390–410.

Cruz, I. Y., & Dunn, M. E. (2003). Lowering risk for early alcohol use by challenging alcohol expectancies in elementary school children. *Journal of Consulting and Clinical Psychology, 71,* 493–503.

Darkes, J., & Goldman, M. S. (1998). Expectancy challenge and drinking reduction: Process and structure in the alcohol expectancy network. *Experimental & Clinical Psychopharmacology, 6,* 64–76.

Dimeff, L. A., Baer, J. S., Kivlahan, D .R., & Marlatt, G. A. (1999). *Brief Alcohol Screening and Intervention for College Students (BASICS). A harm reduction approach.* New York: Guilford.

Dunn, M. E., Lau, C. H., & Cruz, I. Y. (2000). Changes in activation of alcohol expectancies in memory in relation to changes in alcohol use after participation in an expectancy challenge program. *Experimental & Clinical Psychopharmacology, 8,* 566–575.

Everett, S. A., Lowry, R., Cohen, L. R., & Dellinger, A. M. (1999). Unsafe motor vehicle practices among substance-using college students. *Accident Analysis & Prevention, 31,* 667–673.

Fleming, K., Thorson, E., & Atkin, C. K. (2004). Alcohol advertising exposure and perceptions: Links with alcohol expectancies and intentions to drink or drinking in underaged youth and young adults. *Journal of Health Communication, 9*(1), 3–29.

Flory, K., Lynam, D., Milich, R., Leukefeld, C., & Clayton, R. (2004). Early adolescent through young adult alcohol and marijuana use trajectories: Early predictors, young adult outcomes, and predictive utility. *Development and Psychopathology, 16,* 193–213.

Goldman, L. K., & Glantz, S. A. (1998). Evaluation of antismoking advertising campaigns. *Journal of the American Medical Association, 279*(10), 772–777.

Goldman, M. S., Del Boca, F. K., & Darkes, J. (1999). Alcohol expectancy theory: The application of cognitive neuroscience. In H. Blane & K. Leonard (Eds.), *Psychological theories of drinking and alcoholism.* New York: Guilford.

Greenwald, A. G., & Banaji, M. R. (1995). Implicit social cognition: Attitudes, self-esteem, and stereotypes. *Psychological Review, 102,* 4–27.

Grube, J. W. (1993). Alcohol portrayals and alcohol advertising on television: Content and effects on children and adolescents. *Alcohol Health & Research World, 17*(1), 54–60.

Jacoby, L., & Kelley, C. (1990). An episodic view of motivation: Unconscious influences of memory. In E. T. Higgins & R. M. Sorrentino (Eds.), *Handbook of motivation and cognition: Foundations of social behavior* (Vol. 2, pp. 451–481). New York: Guilford.

Johnston, L. D., O'Malley, P. M., Bachman, J. G., & Schulenberg, J. E. (2004). *Monitoring the future national results on adolescent drug use: Overview of key findings, 2003* (NIH Publication No. 04-5506). Bethesda, MD: National Institute on Drug Abuse.

Jones, B. T., Corbin, W., & Fromme, K. (2001). A review of expectancy theory and alcohol consumption. *Addiction, 96,* 57–72.

Krank, M. D. (2003). Pavlovian conditioning with ethanol: Sign-tracking (autoshaping), conditioned incentive, and ethanol self-administration. *Alcoholism: Clinical and Experimental Research, 27*(10), 1592–1598.

Krank, M. D., & Johnson, T. (1999). Retrieval and implicit memory for alcohol associations. *Alcoholism: Clinical and Experimental Research, 23*(5). Paper presented at the annual meeting of the Research Society on Alcoholism, Santa Barbara, CA.

Krank, M. D., Wall, A. M., Lai, D., Wekerle, C., & Johnson, T. (2003). Implicit and explicit cognitions predict alcohol use, abuse and intentions in young adolescents. *Alcoholism: Clinical and Experimental Research, 27*(5). Paper presented at the annual meeting of the Research Society on Alcoholism, Fort Lauderdale, FL.

Krank, M. D., Wall, A. M., Stewart, S. H., Wiers, R. W., & Goldman, M. S. (2005). Context effects on alcohol cognitions. *Alcoholism: Clinical and Experimental Research, 29,* 196–206.

Leigh, B. C., & Stacy, A. W. (1993). Alcohol outcome expectancies: Scale construction and predictive utility in higher order confirmatory models. *Psychological Assessment, 5,* 216–229.

Madden, G. J. (2000). A behavioral economics primer. In W. K. Bickel & R. E. Vuchinich (Eds.), *Reframing health behavior change with behavioral economics* (pp. 3–26). Mahwah, NJ: Lawrence Erlbaum.

Marlatt, G. A., Baer, J. S., Kivlahan, D. R., Dimeff, L. A., Larimer, M. E., Quigley, L. A., et al. (1998). Screening and brief intervention for high-risk college student drinkers: Results from a 2-year follow-up assessment. *Journal of Consulting and Clinical Psychology, 66,* 604–615.

McIntosh, W. D., Smith, S. M., & Bazzini, D. G. (1999). Alcohol in the movies: Characteristics of drinkers and nondrinkers in films from 1940 to 1989. *Journal of Applied Social Psychology, 29*(6), 1191–1199.

Miller, W. R., & Rollnick, S. (2002). *Motivational interviewing: Preparing people for change* (2nd ed.). New York: Guilford.

Monti, P. M., Colby, S. M., & O'Leary, T. A. (2001). Adolescents, alcohol, and substance abuse: Reaching teens through brief intervention. New York: Guilford.

National Institute of Alcohol Abuse and Alcoholism. (1997). *Youth drinking: Risk factors and consequences* (Alcohol Alert No. 37). Bethesda, MD: Author.

Prochaska, J. O., & DiClemente, C. C. (1983). Stages and processes of self-change of smoking: Toward an integrative model of change. *Journal of Consulting and Clinical Psychology, 51,* 390–395.

Raskin-White, H., Xie, M., Thompson, W., Loeber, R., & Stouthamer-Loeber, M. (2001). Psychopathology as a predictor of adolescent drug use trajectories. *Psychology of Addictive Behaviors, 15*, 210–218.

Rescorla, R. A., & Wagner, A. R. (1972). A theory of Pavlovian conditioning: Variations in the effectiveness of reinforcement and nonreinforcement. In A. H. Black & W. F. Prokasy (Eds.), *Classical conditioning II: Current theory and research* (pp. 64–69). New York: Appleton-Century-Crofts.

Robinson, T. E., & Berridge, K. C. (1993). The neural basis of drug craving: An incentive-sensitization theory of addiction. *Brain Research Reviews, 18*, 247–291.

Stacy, A. W. (1997). Memory activation and expectancy as prospective predictors of alcohol and marijuana use. *Journal of Abnormal Psychology, 106,* 61–73.

Stacy, A. W., Leigh, B. C., & Weingardt, K. (1994). Memory accessibility and association of alcohol use and its positive outcomes. *Experimental & Clinical Psychopharmacology, 2*, 1–14.

Stacy, A. W., Pearce, S. G., Zogg, J. B., Unger, J., & Dent, C. W. (2004). A nonverbal test of naturalistic memory for alcohol commercials. *Psychology & Marketing, 21*(4), 295–322.

Stewart, S. H., Conrod, P. J., Marlatt, G. A., Comeau, M. N., Thush, C., & Krank, M. D. (2005). New development in prevention and early intervention for alcohol abuse in youth. *Alcoholism: Clinical and Experimental Research, 29*, 278–286.

Sussman, S., Dent, C. W., Mestel-Rauch, J., & Johnson, C. A. (1988). Adolescent nonsmokers, triers, and regular smokers' estimates of cigarette smoking prevalence: When do overestimations occur and by whom? *Journal of Applied Social Psychology, 18, 537–551.*

Sussman, S., Earleywine, M., Wills, T., Cody, C., Biglan, T., Dent, C. W., et al. (2004). The motivation, skills, and decision-making model of "drug abuse" prevention. *Substance Use & Misuse, 39*(10–12), 1971–2017.

Villani, S. (2001). Impact of media on children and adolescents: A 10-year review of the research. *Journal of the American Academy of Child & Adolescent Psychiatry, 40*, 392–401.

Vuchinich, R. E., & Tucker, J. A. (1988). Contributions from behavioral theories of choice to an analysis of alcohol abuse. *Journal of Abnormal Psychology, 97*, 181–195.

Vuchinich, R. E., & Tucker, J. A. (1996). The molar context of alcohol abuse. In L. Green & J. H. Kagel (Eds.), *Advances in behavioural economics: Vol. 3. Substance use and abuse* (pp. 133–162). Norwood, NJ: Ablex Publishing.

Wagner, E., & Waldron, H. B. (Eds.). (2001). *Innovations in adolescent substance abuse intervention.* Oxford, UK: Elsevier Science.

Wiers, R. W., de Jong, P. J., Havermans, R., & Jelicic, M. (2004). How to change implicit drug use-related cognitions in prevention: A transdisciplinary integration of findings from experimental psychopathology, social cognition, memory, and experimental psychology. *Substance Use & Misuse, 39*(10–12), 1625–1684.

Wills, T. A., & Yaeger, A. M. (2003). Family factors and adolescent substance use: Models and mechanisms. *Current Directions in Psychological Science, 12*(6), 222–226.

CHAPTER 29

Implementation Intentions: Can They Be Used to Prevent and Treat Addiction?

ANDREW PRESTWICH, MARK CONNER,
AND REBECCA J. LAWTON

Abstract: Forming an implementation intention involves an individual planning when, where, and how to perform a specific behavior. Evidence relevant to the mechanisms of this intervention and its application to addiction and other health behaviors is reviewed. Implementation intentions have rarely been applied to addiction but, it is argued, they could be employed to successfully link critical environmental cues to nonaddictive behavior or techniques to refuse the addictive substance. Furthermore, it is proposed that they could inhibit addiction-related cognitions, maintain self-regulatory resources, promote adherence to treatments, or deal effectively with internal factors, such as stress, which increase the risk of addictive behavior. The chapter ends by detailing eight issues relevant to using implementation intentions for the prevention or treatment of addiction.

OVERVIEW

This chapter describes implementation intentions, a strategy successfully used to change behavior. It explains what implementation intentions (Gollwitzer, 1993) are, why they are important, how they work, and discusses applications and issues relevant to the prevention and treatment of addiction.

WHAT ARE IMPLEMENTATION INTENTIONS?

Forming an implementation intention involves an individual deciding when, where,

and how they will perform a behavior. Whereas a goal intention possesses the structure "I intend to achieve Z" with Z relating to an outcome or behavior to which the individual commits to, implementation intentions take the form of an if-then plan that links a behavior or cognitive response to a good opportunity to act ("If situation X occurs, then I will perform behavior Y" or "If I see a cigarette in my house before I go to work then I will leave without smoking it") as a means to achieve a goal. Through implementation intentions, individuals commit themselves to act when faced with a certain situation (e.g., seeing a cigarette at home before work) in a particular manner (leaving the house and not smoking). In contrast, with a goal intention, people commit themselves to a desired end state (e.g., not smoking/being healthy).

WHY ARE IMPLEMENTATION INTENTIONS NECESSARY?

A number of models (e.g., Theory of Planned Behavior; Ajzen, 1985) have viewed intention, reflecting how hard people are willing to try, as *the* direct precursor of behavior. Research indicates, however, that intentions do not always strongly predict behavior (cf. Sheeran, 2002). Intending or being motivated to perform a particular behavior is not enough (cf. Heckhausen, 1991). Changing addictive behavior is no different. Addicts could be aware of the negative consequences of addiction and strive for abstinence but processes outside of conscious awareness could elicit addictive behavior (e.g., McCusker & Gettings, 1997) implying motivational interventions are insufficient to tackle addiction.

HOW DO IMPLEMENTATION INTENTIONS WORK?

Deciding in advance the context in which to act allows one to select an appropriate situation that prompts few competing goals. Choosing a specific context increases the accessibility of environmental cues that eases detection of critical opportunities to act even when busy with other tasks. Research by Dellarosa and Bourne (1984) shows that making decisions enhances the accessibility of decision-consistent information, thus providing a theoretical basis for this proposition. Numerous studies argue that implementation intentions change behavior through this heightened accessibility of environmental cues (e.g.,

Brandstätter et al., 2001; Gollwitzer & Brandstätter, 1997), but research by Aarts et al. (1999) provides the strongest evidence for this position.

Aarts et al. (1999) requested participants collect a food coupon and half of them form an implementation intention relating to its collection. Before having the opportunity to collect the coupon, the participants completed a lexical decision task. Using speed to detect five environment-related words concerned with the collection of the coupon on this task as an index of the accessibility of environmental cues, participants forming implementation intentions showed significantly quicker response latencies for these words and greater success in collecting the coupon. After controlling for latency, the effect of planning on goal completion was nonsignificant. This suggested that the beneficial effect of planning on goal completion was produced by the heightened accessibility of specific environmental cues. Beyond this heightened accessibility, once the opportunity to act is detected, implementation intentions automatize behavior within the preplanned context. Action initiation becomes immediate, efficient, and occurs outside conscious awareness thus acquiring the features of automaticity found in habit (Bargh, 1997).

These features of habit have been illustrated within several implementation intention studies. Evidence for immediacy and efficiency were displayed by the research pertaining to heightened accessibility of environmental cues (e.g., Brandstätter et al., 2001; Lengfelder & Gollwitzer, 2000), while Malzacher (1992, cited in Gollwitzer, 1999) showed that implementation intentions could elicit behavior without awareness of the environmental cue that triggers it. Having to respond to an insult from an experimenter by directly complaining to him or her in a seemingly unrelated experiment, an implementation intention group, but not a control (goal intention only) condition, read negative adjectives faster and positive words slower after the subliminal presentation of the experimenter's face compared to a neutral face. Situational cues specified in the implementation intention, therefore, elicit cognitive processes without conscious intent, which facilitates initiation of intended behavior.

In sum, implementation intentions change behavior by helping the identification of good opportunities to act by heightening the accessibility of environmental cues. These environmental features then cue behavior so that it occurs immediately, efficiently, and without conscious awareness.

APPLICATIONS: HEALTH BEHAVIOR

Implementation intentions increase the performance of important health behaviors such as exercise (e.g., Milne et al., 2002) and healthy eating (e.g., Armitage, 2004). The effects of implementation intentions on changing health behaviors are summarized in Figure 29.1. The figure presents 21 measures across 16 studies with a total sample size of $N = 2,149$. Effect size r indicates the magnitude of the difference between implementation intention and control conditions at follow-up (unless otherwise stated). Correlations were in the range $r = .07$ to $.57$ with a sample-weighted average of $r = .25$, a small to medium effect size (Cohen, 1992).

To ensure health benefits, people need to maintain healthy behaviors but unfortunately implementation intention intervention studies have typically assessed behavior change over a period of less than 1 month. Only two studies, one promoting cervical cancer screening uptake (Sheeran & Orbell, 2000) and another breast self-examinations (Prestwich et al., in press), have monitored implementation intention manipulation over more than two months and although

successful, the actions were infrequently performed behaviors. Although it has been argued that implementation intentions would maintain behavior change, as they possess habit-like features (Milne et al., 2002; Sheeran & Orbell, 1999), more evidence is required.

APPLICATIONS: PREVENTING ADDICTION

To prevent drug use, gambling, or other addictive behaviors, strategies must be able to promote actions that hinder the development of problematic behavior. Research has indicated the use of implementation intentions for health protective behaviors such as breast self-examinations (Orbell et al., 1997; Prestwich et al., in press), vitamin C compliance (Sheeran & Orbell, 1999), and cervical cancer screening (Sheeran & Orbell, 2000). Implementation intentions could quicken the detection of breast abnormalities or cervical cancer as a means to prevent the risk of incurable cancer and the strategy could be used in a similar fashion for addiction prevention.

Even if an individual possesses an intention to refrain from drug use, encountering drug cues may trigger urges that temporarily override the intention to remain abstinent and prompt relapse (cf. Robinson & Berridge, 2003). Deciding when and where the urges are likely to occur and planning how to stop oneself from entering these situations or how to get out of them could prove helpful.

Higgins and Conner (2003) predicted that implementation intentions, relating to when, where, and how to refuse the offer of a cigarette, could be used to prevent the uptake or relapse of smoking in children aged from 11 to 12. Weak statistical power inhibited the emergence of a significant effect, although there was a trend in the predicted direction. None of the 51 nonsmokers in the intervention group tried smoking during the

8 weeks of the study compared to 3 of the 53 nonsmokers in the control condition (0 percent vs. 6 percent). The zero uptake of cigarettes in the experimental condition hints at the potential of this planning strategy for preventing the performance of unhealthy, potentially addictive behaviors.

APPLICATIONS:
TREATING ADDICTION

Higgins and Conner (2003) also included smokers in their sample. Although the study might not say much about treating addiction as few of the sample were likely to be addicted (only 6 adolescents out of 162 reported smoking more than 1 cigarette per week), it still allowed a test of whether the intervention could be used to reduce drug intake. Sixty-four percent of the smokers in the experimental group reported smoking at follow-up compared to 68 percent in the control condition. This weaker effect (see Figure 29.1) suggests that implementation intentions could be more useful for the prevention of addiction, rather than reduction of drug intake.

Murgraff et al. (1996), however, showed implementation intentions can be used to significantly reduce the performance of unhealthy, drug-related behavior. In this study, undergraduates were given information regarding the safe limits of alcohol intake per drinking occasion and negative consequences of binge drinking and were asked to try to drink within these limits. In addition, participants in the implementation intention condition selected a response that they could use to refuse a drink (e.g., "No thanks, I have to get up early tomorrow.") and planned when and where they would use this chosen strategy. The experimental group showed a significant reduction in drinking behavior in relation to the control group over a period of 2 weeks. Although the study did not try to eliminate drinking and the

reported analyses, based on the whole sample that comprised both frequent and infrequent binge drinkers, made it unclear how effective the intervention was in treating addiction, the significantly reduced intake could serve as an important step in the elimination of addiction and relapse prevention. This focus on reduction, rather than abstinence, still allows the internal system to receive some reward and might explain why implementation intentions were successful within this research but not in Higgins and Conner's (2003) work, particularly as implementation intentions have been shown to be more effective when behavior is enjoyable (e.g., Koestner et al., 2002).

Tiffany's (1990) cognitive model of addiction proposed drug use is triggered by the cueing of automatized action plans. By identifying the situations in which addictive behaviors could or do occur, implementation intentions might be used to promote alternative action plans that are incompatible with the previous addictive behavior. Using statements to refuse a drug can be countered by peer pressure. Alternative plans that prompt opposing behavior (e.g., planning to eat gum to avoid or counteract cigarette cravings: "If I feel smoking urges then I will buy and chew gum from the local shop.") might increase reliability. The automatic activation of a (enjoyable) counter-behavior could reduce addiction.

Implementation intentions could treat addiction indirectly by promoting attendance at clinics or counseling/support groups or compliance to antidrug regimens. Sheeran and Orbell (2000) showed that 92 percent of women asked to form an implementation intention in relation to their attendance at a cervical cancer screening subsequently attended compared to 69 percent in the control, no intervention, condition (but see Michie et al., 2004). Sheeran and Orbell (1999) indicated implementation intentions significantly increased vitamin C compliance over a period of 3 weeks. These findings have

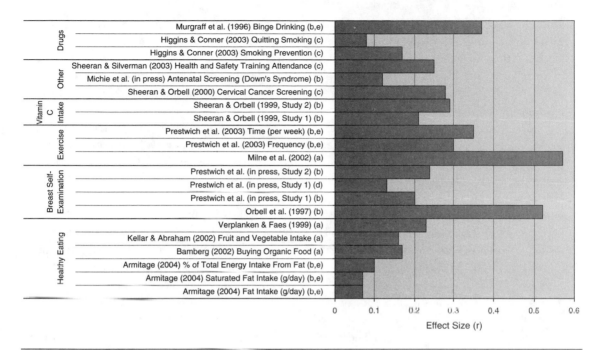

Figure 29.1 Effect sizes from implementation intention studies of health behaviors. (Intervention period: [a] = 1–7 days, [b] = 8 days–1 month, [c] = 1–3 months, [d] = 3–6 months. [e] Effect size reflects change from baseline to follow-up.)

implications for the treatment of addiction. A former addict on the verge of relapse forgetting to attend a support group or outpatient clinic could make the difference between them spiraling back into addiction or remaining abstinent.

STUDIES USING ADDICTS AND CLINICAL SAMPLES

Frontal regions of the brain are involved in decision making and judging the future consequences of one's actions (e.g., Bechara et al., 2000; Smith & Jonides, 1999). According to a review by Jentsch and Taylor (1999) long-term exposure to particular drugs reduces neural processing within these regions, meaning that addicts can display the same neuropsychological deficits shown by patients with frontal dysfunction. This dysfunction reduces cognitive inhibitory control and increases impulsivity, which can

encourage compulsive, addictive behavior and reflects a general lack of conscious control of action and poor decision making and judgment. Evidence that implementation intentions can be effective within frontal lobe patients suffering problems with action control (Lengfelder & Gollwitzer, 2000) is thus pertinent regarding the use of implementation intentions for the treatment of addicts. Furthermore, given the widespread use of student populations within implementation intention research, using clinical samples aids the generalization of conclusions concerning implementation intention-behavior relations.

Lengfelder and Gollwitzer (2000) used a dual-task procedure to measure two features of automatic action control—immediacy and efficiency in action initiation (Bargh, 1997). A Go/No-Go (secondary) task assessed immediacy by recording the speed of a button press in relation to a number, rather than a letter, appearing in a circle, while a tracking (primary) task, with easy and difficult levels, allowed the assessment of speed of response under low and high mental loads. Participants were brain-injured patients (with frontal lobe lesions or nonfrontal lobe lesions) and university students. All participants were asked to press the mouse button immediately when a number appeared in a circle and press it particularly quickly when the number 3 appeared. They were requested to use one of two strategies to accelerate their response to this number. Half formed an implementation intention ("If the number 3 appears, I will press the button particularly fast!"), while the other half familiarized themselves with the number 3 by filling in gaps on a sheet where the number should have appeared. The immediacy of implementation intentions was found as they speeded up critical button-press responses. There was also evidence that they seemed to reduce mental load and increase efficiency. First, implementation intentions improved tracking performance when a critical button-press was required during the difficult tracking. Second, practice effects emerged on noncritical trials on the secondary task within implementation intention, but not familiarization, conditions. This efficiency frees up cognitive capacities. By displaying these effects within frontal lobe patients, it appears that implementation intentions could be a useful self-regulatory strategy with automatic effects that could help organize the habitual performance of everyday activities within the people who need the most help—in this example, frontal lobe patients. In essence, however, anyone under high cognitive strain including addicts under withdrawal could benefit.

Brandstätter et al. (2001, Study 1) revealed implementation intentions are useful in promoting everyday activities within opiate addicts during withdrawal. They invited addicts during withdrawal and those no longer under withdrawal to write a short curriculum vitae (CV) before 5 p.m. Half of these participants were asked to specify when and where they would write the CV in addition to forming the goal intention to write it. The remaining half of the sample was requested to form the same goal intention but form an implementation intention irrelevant to the writing of the CV. Eighty percent of the addicts under withdrawal forming the relevant plan were successful compared to 40 percent of the participants no longer under withdrawal who formed such a plan. Of the participants forming an irrelevant plan, none wrote a CV, regardless of whether they were under withdrawal or not. The effects could not be attributed to increasing commitment to the task. The freeing up of resources, implied here and within Lengfelder and Gollwitzer's (2000) research, can be used for effective self-regulation in dealing with addiction-relevant problems. These issues include managing to adhere to antidrug regimens or attending support groups or clinics, or coping efficiently with factors that precipitate relapse, such as stress (cf. Goeders, 2004).

IMPLEMENTATION INTENTIONS, SELF-REGULATION, AND ADDICTION

Self-regulation controls one's own responses, including thoughts, emotions, impulses, and behavior. Failures of self-control contribute to personal and social problems, thus effective self-regulation is central to the avoidance of addiction (see Baumeister et al., 1994).

Conflicting goals often contribute to self-regulation failures. For example, addicts fail to stifle the desire for short-term, often pleasurable rewards derived from their source of addiction for long-term benefits. To obtain these long-term benefits, one must sustain high self-regulatory levels to resist temptation and ignore or avoid cues that trigger the addictive behavior.

Sustaining strong self-regulation is difficult as it is a limited resource that becomes depleted after use (e.g., Baumeister et al., 1998). Once self-regulatory capacity is emptied following an initial act of self-control, or "ego-depleted," an individual can become vulnerable to impulsive behaviors such as increased intake of addictive substances and poor decision making. Ego depletion could undermine the restraint displayed by addicts under withdrawal. For example, a study by Kahan et al. (2003) indicated ego-depleted individuals exhibited less dietary restraint than those individuals who avoided ego depletion.

Webb and Sheeran (2003) showed an implementation intention group demonstrated greater persistence on unsolvable puzzles than a control group after undergoing a Stroop task. The Stroop task was ego-depleting as it involved participants overriding a dominant, automatic response with voluntary control that could be likened to a smoker seeing a cigarette but overriding the automatic dominant response to smoke it. In a second experiment, ego-depleted individuals who formed implementation intentions performed as well as nondepleted controls on a Stroop task. As a strategy that prevents ego-depletion and offsets its negative effects (Webb & Sheeran, 2003), this is further evidence for the use of implementation intentions in preventing or treating addictive behaviors.

Koole and Van't Spijker (2000), using mediation analysis, found that implementation intentions speed up goal completion by reducing the number of interruptions incurred. This effect could emerge through selection of the most appropriate environment (i.e., one which holds the least distractions), or by cognitive inhibition of distracting stimuli (cf. Gollwitzer, 1999). Although implementation intentions, by themselves, do not aid the identification of contexts that elicit behavior, following help from a healthcare professional to identify these triggers, implementation intentions can be used to automatically elicit behavior that deals with precipitating risk factors or inhibit addictive cognitions (e.g., "When I feel stressed (tired, bored), I will perform yoga in my office."; "If I feel stressed, I won't think about drinking."). This is important because activating addiction-related cognitions in memory increases the risk of addictive behaviors implicitly by affecting the interpretation of stimuli and accessibility in memory of certain addictive behavioral options (e.g., Jones & Schulze, 2000).

Ironic effects increase thoughts about an object when one actively tries to suppress such cognition under high cognitive load (e.g., Wegner, 1994) and thus could threaten the effectiveness of implementation intentions for the suppression of addiction-related cognitions. Asking people not to think about drugs could heighten the problem as they could become more likely to think about drugs, particularly if they are under high cognitive strain. Nevertheless, implementation intentions can block habitual cognitive and emotional (i.e., not just behavioral) responses without causing ironic effects. Gollwitzer, Schaal, et al. (1999, cited in Gollwitzer, 1999) showed that implementation intentions (e.g., "When I see an old person, I tell myself: Don't stereotype!") can be used to suppress the automatic activation of stereotypical beliefs assessed across a range of measures of implicit cognition.

In essence, planning is effective in that consideration of many situations and instrumental behaviors can be made. This allows immediate goal pursuit when good opportunities to act in a way that prevents performance of their addictive behavior appear fleetingly in the relevant situation. Since planning occurs in advance, when encountering the situation few cognitive resources should be required, so few in fact, that action initiation may be automatic. This automatization of goal pursuit could promote anti-addictive cognitions and behavior, suppress addiction-related cognitions and protect the individual from other threats to their continued addiction such as ego-depletion, distractions, bad habits, and competing goals.

IMPLEMENTATION INTENTIONS AND ADDICTION: ISSUES

(1) Can Implementation Intentions Lead to Objective Changes in Health Behavior?

Although most implementation intention studies have used self-report measures, meta-analytic evidence shows greater effects with self-report ($N = 13$, $r = .35$) rather than objective ($N = 10$, $r = .26$) measures (Sheeran, 2001). Most studies that have employed objective criteria measured actual behavior once (e.g., writing a report, Gollwitzer & Brandstätter, 1997; collecting a coupon, Aarts et al., 1999). A small number of studies, however, have presented more indirect, but objective, evidence for significant changes in behavior that should be enacted frequently for health benefits to emerge (e.g., fitness changes to assess exercise, Prestwich et al., 2003; pill counts for vitamin C compliance, Sheeran & Orbell, 1999). Nevertheless, there is still a need for more studies to incorporate objective measures within long-term interventions to substantiate claims that implementation intention can change health behavior including the prevention and treatment of addiction.

(2) Can Implementation Intentions Change Complex Behavior?

Simple behaviors could be defined as those that involve a single action rather than complex behaviors that involve a chain of actions. Using this definition, addiction to drugs, which comprise drug-seeking and drug-taking behavior, can be classified as complex. Attendance for a health-related screening could be classified as complex behavior because it involves both arranging and attending the appointment, as would, for example, recycling (e.g., saving bottles and taking them to the bottle bank), eating healthily (e.g., buying healthy foods and eating them before they lose their freshness), or reducing binge drinking (e.g., taking a small amount of money on a night out, leaving a cash card at home, refusing drinks, and going home). The success of implementation intentions for these complex behaviors suggests that they can be used appropriately here (e.g., Rise et al., 2003; Sheeran & Orbell, 2000). Studies that have compared the effectiveness of implementation intentions for easy versus more complex/difficult tasks, however, have yielded mixed results (see Dewitte et al., 2003; Dholakia & Bagozzi, 2003; Gollwitzer & Brandstätter, 1997; Koestner et al., 2002) and implementation intentions have not been effective for all complex behaviors (e.g., Michie et al., 2004). Such research suggests that for really difficult behaviors, including addiction, implementation intentions may require additional interventions or strategies to be effective. Indeed, Verplanken and Faes (1999) have argued implementation intentions that specify *how* to perform a behavior become particularly important for complex behaviors that may be acted on in a variety of ways.

(3) Under Which Circumstances Are Implementation Intentions Most Likely to Work?

When Intentions Are Strong

There is now substantial evidence suggesting implementation intentions are most effective when intentions are strong. For example, Orbell et al. (1997) showed that 100 percent of women intending to perform breast self-examinations (BSE) and forming an implementation intention relating to its performance underwent a BSE over the following month, compared to 53 percent with equivalent intentions in the control group. These rates were higher than those obtained for those not holding strong intentions to perform BSE (64 percent in the implementation intention group vs. 14 percent of those in the control condition). In addition, Prestwich et al. (2003) reported stronger effects of a joint motivational-implementation intention intervention than an implementation intention intervention without a motivational manipulation in relation to exercise frequency and fitness improvements over four weeks. Lack of implementation intention effects when failure and arguably de-motivation had been previously encountered, provides further evidence for the need for strong motivation (Dholakia & Bagozzi, 2003).

For behavior change, including addiction, implementation intentions should be paired with a motivational intervention to maximize their effectiveness. Alternatively, those people who do not want to quit cigarettes, alcohol, heroin, shopping, gambling, or any other addiction will not benefit from implementation intention intervention. First, the individual must want to quit and then implementation intention manipulations can be used to plan how to quit.

When Goals Are Intrinsically Motivated

Self-concordant goals reflect personal interests and values while non-concordant goals are pursued for controlled reasons such as social pressure or financial gain. People may decide to quit drugs for extrinsic reasons such as to obtain praise from others, stop people nagging or to avoid jail, or for more intrinsic reasons: liking oneself more, to stop health damage, or to feel control in one's life

(Downey et al., 2001). Non-concordant goals are associated with less persistence and are less likely to lead to goal success than concordant goals (e.g., Sheldon & Elliot, 1998). The reasons behind quitting drugs are more intrinsic than extrinsic, and high intrinsic motivation relative to extrinsic motivation is strongly associated with successful abstinence (e.g., Curry et al., 1990; Downey et al., 2001) and as implementation intentions have been shown to be more effective for self-concordant or intrinsically motivated goals than those that are non-concordant or extrinsically motivated (Dholakia & Bagozzi, 2003; Koestner et al., 2002) they could prove a helpful strategy to tackle addiction.

(4) Collaborative Implementation Intentions

A variation of implementation intentions, collaborative implementation intentions (Prestwich et al., in press) involves an individual deciding, with another person, the context in which they will perform a behavior together. In their collaborative planning study, Prestwich et al. (in press) requested that all participants read an instruction sheet relating to how to perform a BSE and completed a motivational intervention derived from Protection Motivation Theory (Rogers, 1983) to increase their intentions to perform the exam in the next month. Participants were assigned to one of four conditions based on a 2 (involve partner or not) × 2 (form an implementation intention or not) factorial design to create collaborative implementation intention, implementation intention, partner involvement-no implementation intention, and no partner involvement-no implementation intention groups. Deciding to involve a partner, rather than perform it alone, increased the likelihood of BSE (90 percent vs. 48 percent), as did implementation intention formation versus nonformation (74 percent vs. 51 percent). There was no significant partner by group interaction although the collaborative implementation intention condition was 100 percent successful. Partner involvement increased ratings of perceived BSE enjoyment, which can increase implementation intention success (e.g., Koestner et al., 2002), while collaborative implementation intentions reduced forgetfulness.

Further, collaboration may make the planning particularly sound and thus more successful (Gollwitzer & Kinney, 1989, p. 532). Active involvement of a supportive other has been shown to be helpful in addiction treatment programs. For example, Carlson et al. (2002) showed that prospective quitters of cigarettes who brought a support person to a support-group session on at least one occasion showed higher cessation rates at 12-month follow-up than those who did not. Evidence such as this implies that a collaborative variant of implementation intentions could be useful for the treatment of addiction.

(5) Internal Cues

Implementation intentions are largely based on external cues that become accessible and likely to directly trigger behavior (e.g., Aarts & Dijksterhuis, 2000; Aarts et al., 1999). These cues may not be useful when removed or changed. For example, an implementation intention such as "I will go for a run around Hyde Park when my housemate arrives home from work." would not be effective if the housemate does not arrive home. An implementation intention based on internal cues ("I will go for a run around Hyde Park when I feel hungry.") may be more reliable in promoting behavior. Recently, Milne et al. (2003) showed that an implementation intention based on an internal cue was equally effective as one based on an external cue for the reduction of perceived stress.

In relation to drugs, plans could incorporate internal ("If I feel like smoking, then I will eat gum." or "If I feel stressed, then I will eat gum.") and external cues ("If I see a cigarette, then I will eat gum."). Which form is most effective remains to be tested but evidence that addiction is strongly associated with stress, depression, and anxiety (cf. Goeders, 2004) points to the potential, unique effectiveness of implementation intentions based on internal cues.

(6) Can Implementation Intentions Break Habits?

To overcome habits, the automatic effects of implementation intentions must be strong enough to overcome the automaticity associated with competing habits. Although habits and implementation intentions have been argued to hold the same characteristics (e.g., Aarts & Dijksterhuis, 2000) because addiction is manifest with repetitive, excessive, compulsive, and habitual behavioral patterns and automatic cognitive biases, it is hard to imagine that the automaticity generated through one mental act is sufficient to overcome the automaticity associated with habits.

Gollwitzer (1998), however, indicated that implementation intentions protect ongoing goal pursuit from competing habits. Supplementing a goal with an implementation intention prevents antagonistic habits, activated unconsciously via priming procedures, from derailing goal-striving. Higgins and Conner (2003) showed that using implementation intentions to change habitual, addictive behavior is difficult with nonsignificant effects in relation to smoking though this study suffered from a floor effect as very few adolescents took up (or gave up) smoking during the intervention period. The successful application of implementation intentions for the reduction of binge drinking by Murgraff et al. (1996) provides greater promise, although the intervention did not abolish binge drinking. Further, as such plans heighten the accessibility of environmental cues they could be used to divert attention to nonaddiction-related cues as a means to break attentional bias, a key feature in drug dependence, craving, and relapse (Townshend & Duka, 2001).

(7) *Immediate Costs Versus Long-Term Gains*

Attempting to break an addiction is associated with immediate, perhaps unpleasant, costs with long-term gains and such behaviors including exercise and BSE may be expected to benefit less from implementation intentions. Gollwitzer (1999) cites a number of studies that suggest this is not the case (e.g., Milne et al., 2002, exercise; Verplanken & Faes, 1999, healthy eating). These behaviors, however, also provide immediate benefits as well as costs. For example, exercise improves mood (Steinberg et al., 1998) and BSE may provide relief from worry. Not performing addictive behavior may be associated with even fewer immediate benefits. To deal with the physiological rewards of the addictive substance, one could form an implementation intention that instigates similarly rewarding actions in the contexts that trigger the addiction. Alternatively, one could use a plan that generates negative feelings associated with performing the addictive behavior when there is risk of addictive behavior (e.g., "If I see a cigarette, then I will get angry." or "If I think about alcohol, then I will think about the hangover.").

(8) *Can Implementation Intentions Maintain Behavior Change?*

Based on the postulation that they have habit-like qualities, implementation intentions have been argued to maintain their effectiveness (Milne et al., 2002; Sheeran & Orbell, 1999). Previous implementation

intention research, however, has ignored the problems associated with the maintenance of behavior over an extended period of time (months, years) and fails to address whether implementation intentions deal with or override them. Sheeran's (2001) meta-analysis provided statistical evidence for these concerns as it implied that the effectiveness of implementation intentions decreased over time and, apart from the study by Prestwich et al. (in press) that introduced collaborative implementation intentions, no study has attempted to improve their sustainability as a behavior-change intervention. This issue is important; treating addiction needs to maintain change and prevent relapse. Reasons for changing the addictive behavior should be intrinsic; strong intentions to stay sober need to be maintained and setbacks need to be handled. Implementation intentions would need to be combined with additional strategies to meet these criteria and maximize the likelihood of successful, implementation intention influenced, treatment.

SUMMARY

Implementation intentions involve individuals planning the context in which they will perform a behavior. Research has shown them to be an effective health intervention by automatically eliciting goal-directed behavior. After identifying the contexts that elicit the addiction or its precipitating factors, perhaps with the help of a healthcare professional, plans could be formed that automatically link the situation to nonaddictive behavior or techniques to refuse the addictive substance. They could be used to inhibit addiction-related cognitions and promote adherence to antidrug treatments and counseling. In addition, they are an efficient strategy that helps to maintain self-regulation, an important defense against addiction. Implementation intentions are certainly not a panacea. There have been few long-term interventions that have used objective measures and they tend to require strong, preferably intrinsic, motivation to maximize their effects. Evidence suggests, however, that they are effective in health behavior change even when it is complex and presents immediate costs against long-term benefits. There are promising variants that propose the use of internal cues or the joint involvement of another person in planning and action. Theoretically, implementation intentions could prove a helpful self-regulatory tool for the treatment and prevention of addiction. Further research is needed to put these theoretical ideas to the test.

REFERENCES

Aarts, H., & Dijksterhuis, A. (2000). Habits as knowledge structures: Automaticity in goal-directed behavior. *Journal of Personality and Social Psychology, 78,* 53–63.

Aarts, H., Dijksterhuis, A., & Midden, C. (1999). To plan or not to plan? Goal achievement or interrupting the performance of mundane behaviors. *European Journal of Social Psychology, 29,* 971–979.

Ajzen, I. (1985). From intentions to actions: A theory of planned behavior. In J. Kuhl & J. Beckmann (Eds.), *Action-control: From cognition to behavior* (pp. 11–39). Heidelberg, Germany: Springer.

Armitage, C. J. (2004). Evidence that implementation intentions reduce dietary fat intake: A randomized trial. *Health Psychology, 23,* 319–323.

Bamberg, S. (2002). Effects of implementation intentions on the actual performance of new environmentally friendly behaviors: Results of two field experiments. *Journal of Environmental Psychology, 22,* 399–411.

Bargh, J. A. (1997). The automaticity of everyday life. In R. S. Wyer, Jr. (Ed.), *The automaticity of everyday life: Advances in social cognition* (Vol. 10, pp. 1–61). Mahwah, NJ: Lawrence Erlbaum.

Baumeister, R. F., Bratslavsky, E., Muraven, M., & Tice, D. M. (1998). Ego depletion: Is the active self a limited resource? *Journal of Personality and Social Psychology, 74,* 1252–1265.

Baumeister, R. F., Heatherton, T. F., & Tice, D. M. (1994). *Losing control: How and why people fail at self-regulation.* San Diego, CA: Academic Press.

Bechara, A., Damasio, H., & Damasio, A. R. (2000). Emotion, decision making and the orbitofrontal cortex. *Cerebral Cortex, 10,* 295–307.

Brandstätter, V., Lengfelder, A., & Gollwitzer, P. M. (2001). Implementation intentions and efficient action initiation. *Journal of Personality and Social Psychology, 81,* 946–960.

Carlson, L. E., Goodey, E., Bennett, M. H., Taenzer, P., & Koopmans, J. (2002). The addition of social support to a community-based large-group behavioral smoking cessation intervention: Improved cessation rates and gender differences. *Addictive Behaviors, 27,* 547–559.

Cohen, J. (1992). A power primer. *Psychological Bulletin, 112,* 155–159.

Curry, S., Wagner, E. H., & Grothaus, L. C. (1990). Intrinsic and extrinsic motivation for smoking cessation. *Journal of Consulting and Clinical Psychology, 58,* 310–316.

Dellarosa, D., & Bourne, L. E. (1984). Decisions and memory: Differential retrievability of consistent and contradictory evidence. *Journal of Verbal Learning and Verbal Behavior, 23,* 669–682.

Dewitte, S., Verguts, T., & Lens, W. (2003). Implementation intentions do not enhance all types of goals: The moderating role of goal difficulty. *Current Psychology: Development, Learning, Personality, Social, Planned Behavior, 22,* 73–89.

Dholakia, U. M., & Bagozzi, R. P. (2003). As time goes by: How goal and implementation intentions influence enactment of short-fuse behaviors. *Journal of Applied Social Psychology, 33,* 889–922.

Downey, L., Rosengren, D. B., & Donovan, D. M. (2001). Sources of motivation for abstinence. *Addictive Behaviors, 26,* 79–89.

Goeders, N. E. (2004). Stress, motivation and drug addiction. *Current Directions in Psychological Science, 13,* 33.

Gollwitzer, P. M. (1993). Goal achievement: The role of intentions. In W. Stroebe & M. Hewstone (Eds.), *European Review of Social Psychology, 4,* 141–185. Chichester, UK: Wiley.

Gollwitzer, P. M. (1998). *Implicit and explicit processes in goal pursuit.* Paper presented at the symposium "Implicit vs. Explicit Processes" at the annual meeting of the Society of Experimental Social Psychology, Atlanta, GA.

Gollwitzer, P. M. (1999). Implementation intentions: Strong effects of simple plans. *American Psychologist, 54,* 493–503.

Gollwitzer, P. M., & Brandstätter, V. (1997). Implementation intentions and effective goal pursuit. *Journal of Personality and Social Psychology, 73,* 186–199.

Gollwitzer, P. M., & Kinney, R. F. (1989). Effects of deliberative and implemental mind-sets on illusion of control. *Journal of Personality and Social Psychology, 56,* 531–542.

Heckhausen, H. (1991). *Motivation and action.* New York: Springer-Verlag.

Higgins, A., & Conner, M. T. (2003). Understanding adolescent smoking: The role of the Theory of Planned Behavior and implementation intentions. *Psychology, Health & Medicine, 8,* 173–186.

Jentsch, J. D., & Taylor, J. R. (1999). Impulsivity resulting from frontostriatal dysfunction in drug abuse. Implications for the control over behavior by reward-related stimuli. *Psychopharmacology, 146,* 373–390.

Jones, B. T., & Schulze, D. (2000). Alcohol-related words of positive affect are more accessible in social drinkers' memory than are other words when sip-primed by alcohol. *Addiction Research, 8,* 221–232.

Kahan, D., Polivy, J., & Herman, C. P. (2003). Conformity and dietary disinhibition: A test of the ego-strength model of self-regulation. *International Journal of Eating Disorders, 33,* 165–171.

Kellar, I., & Abraham, C. (2002). *A brief research-based intervention promotes fruit and vegetable consumption.* Paper presented at the European Health Psychology Society Annual Conference 2002, Lisbon, Portugal.

Koestner, R., Lekes, N., Powers, T. A., & Chicoine, E. (2002). Attaining personal goals: Self-concordance plus implementation intentions equals success. *Journal of Personality and Social Psychology, 83,* 231–244.

Koole, S., & Van't Spijker, M. (2000). Overcoming the planning fallacy through willpower: Effects of implementation intentions on actual and predicted task-completion times. *European Journal of Social Psychology, 30,* 873–888.

Lengfelder, A., & Gollwitzer, P. M. (2000). Reflective and reflexive action control in frontal lobe patients. *Neuropsychology, 15,* 80–100.

McCusker, C. G., & Gettings, B. (1997). Automaticity of cognitive biases in addictive behaviors: Further evidence with gamblers, *British Journal of Clinical Psychology, 36,* 543–554.

Michie, S., Dormandy, E., & Marteau, T. M. (2004). Increasing screening uptake amongst those intending to be screened: The use of action plans. *Patient Education and Counseling, 55,* 218–222.

Milne, S., Gollwitzer, P. M., & Sheeran, P. (2003, September). *Using implementation intentions to control stress: Can we use internal cues to control behavior?* Paper presented at the annual conference of the Division of Health Psychology, Staffordshire, UK.

Milne, S., Orbell, S., & Sheeran, P. (2002). Combining motivational and volitional interventions to promote exercise participation: Protection motivation theory and implementation intentions. *British Journal of Health Psychology, 7,* 163–184.

Murgraff, V., White, D., & Phillips, K. (1996). Moderating binge drinking: It is possible to change behavior if you plan it in advance. *Alcohol and Alcoholism, 31,* 577–582.

Orbell, S., Hodgkins, S., & Sheeran, P. (1997). Implementation intentions and the theory of planned behavior. *Personality and Social Psychology Bulletin, 23,* 945–954.

Prestwich, A. J., Conner, M. T., Lawton, R. J., Bailey, W., Litman, J., & Molyneaux, V. (in press). Individual and collaborative implementation intentions and the promotion of breast self-examination. *Psychology & Health.*

Prestwich, A. J., Lawton, R. J., & Conner, M. T. (2003). The use of implementation intentions and the decision balance sheet in promoting exercise behavior. *Psychology & Health, 18,* 707–721.

Rise, J., Thompson, M., & Verplanken, B. (2003). Measuring implementation intentions in the context of the theory of planned behavior. *Scandinavian Journal of Psychology, 44,* 87–95.

Robinson, T. E., & Berridge, K. C. (2003). Addiction. *Annual Review of Psychology, 54,* 25–53.

Rogers, R. W. (1983). Cognition and physiological processes in fear appeals and attitude change: A revised theory of protection motivation. In J. T Cacioppo & R. E. Petty (Eds.), *Social psychophysiology: A source book* (pp 153–176). New York: Guilford.

Sheeran, P. (2001, March). *Meta-analysis of the effectiveness of implementation intentions in promoting behavior.* Paper presented at the centenary annual conference of the British Psychological Society, Glasgow, Scotland.

Sheeran, P. (2002). Intention-behavior relations: A conceptual and empirical review. In W. Stroebe & M. Hewstone (Eds.), *European Review of Social Psychology* (Vol. 12, pp. 1–30). Chichester, UK: Wiley.

Sheeran, P., & Orbell, S. (1999). Implementation intentions and repeated behavior: Augmenting the predictive validity of the theory of planned behavior. *European Journal of Social Psychology, 37,* 231–250.

Sheeran, P., & Orbell, S. (2000). Using implementation intentions to increase attendance for cervical cancer screening. *Health Psychology, 19,* 283–289.

Sheeran, P., & Silverman, M. (2003). Evaluation of three interventions to promote workplace health and safety: Evidence for the utility of implementation intentions. *Social Science & Medicine, 56,* 2153–2163.

Sheldon, K. M., & Elliot, A. J. (1998). Not all personal goals are personal: Comparing autonomous and controlled reasons as predictors of effort and attainment. *Personality and Social Psychology Bulletin, 24,* 546–557.

Smith, E. E., & Jonides, J. (1999). Storage and executive processes in the frontal lobes. *Science, 283,* 1657–1661.

Steinberg, H., Sykes, E. A., Nicholls, B., Ramlakhan, N., Moss, T., LeBoutillier, N., et al. (1998). Weekly exercise consistently reinstates positive mood. *European Psychologist, 3,* 271–280.

Tiffany, S. T. (1990). A cognitive model of drug urges and drug-use behavior: Role of automatic and nonautomatic processes. *Psychological Review, 97,* 147–168.

Townshend, J. M., & Duka, T. (2001). Attentional bias associated with alcohol cues: Differences between heavy and occasional social drinkers. *Psychopharmacology, 157,* 67–74.

Verplanken, B., & Faes, S. (1999). Good intentions, bad habits, and effects of forming implementation intentions on healthy eating. *European Journal of Social Psychology, 29,* 591–604.

Webb, T. L., & Sheeran, P. (2003). Can implementation intentions help to overcome ego-depletion? *Journal of Experimental Social Psychology, 39,* 279–286.

Wegner, D. M. (1994). Ironic processes of mental control. *Psychological Review, 101,* 34–52.

Section VII

COMMENTARIES AND GENERAL DISCUSSION

CHAPTER 30

Toward a Cognitive Theory of Substance Use and Dependence

Kenneth J. Sher

COMMENT ON THE *HANDBOOK OF IMPLICIT COGNITION AND ADDICTION*

Wiers and Stacy have done the field of addiction studies a major service by assembling this series of papers providing both a broad overview and in-depth analysis of the role of implicit cognition in addictive behavior. Indeed, I think the title of the book does a disservice to both the editors and the authors because, as it becomes readily apparent, the volume address the more general issue of cognition and addictive behavior because an analysis of "implicit" cognition requires consideration of more "explicit" cognition as illustrated by the discussion of dual-system approaches to cognition. One could take this observation further and suggest that because the study of addiction is so broad as to encompass a range of behaviors from initial experimentation and experience to profound physiological dependence, that the volume addresses the broader issue of cognition in goal-directed behavior and how it changes as a function of pharmacological experience (in the case of substance use and substance use disorders) and other behaviors (such as

normal gambling and pathological gambling) where there is a clear disjunction between compulsive reward seeking and the harm that such behavior causes.

To many readers of this volume, especially those like me who have not closely followed recent development in basic cognitive psychology and social cognition, new opportunities for conceptualizing various aspects of addictive are afforded by many of the analyses presented here. I've come to this perspective reluctantly and with some skepticism. I've been aware of a number of studies of implicit cognition starting in the later 1980s and was never sure exactly what it was buying us. Indeed, I recall discussions with co-editor and author, Alan Stacy, more than 15 years ago about experiments he was planning with Barbara Leigh where they planned to extend some of Russ Fazio's research on attitude accessibility to examine similar processes related to alcohol attitudes and expectancies. I had always found the rationale for studying "accessibility" compelling as it was clear from my own research that inquiring about an attitude or expectancy using so-called explicit measures would elicit an answer from a participant even is he or she never entertained the attitude object prior to reading the question. Using behavioral measures (i.e., reaction times or response latencies), we could learn something beyond what people were willing to tell us. . . especially those who were basically clueless as to the answer. However, over time (and, admittedly as a fairly ignorant observer) my interest in this research started to wane a bit. It wasn't that the research wasn't exceptionally clever (it often was) or appeared to provide unique sources of variance not provided by other measures (if often did), but there was not sufficient grounding of the findings in a more comprehensive model of cognition or mind. As such, I think many casual readers of this literature found the work interesting but somewhat tangential to their interests and not especially likely to deepen their understanding of addictive phenomena.

Additionally, I often found the discussion of what implicit measures represent to be inadequate. All too often authors would seem to tacitly assume there was something about "implicit measures" that measured something important but it wasn't often clear about whether this was an implicit measure of the same construct that could be measured explicitly but just subject to different experimental demands, or whether some related but entirely different phenomena was being measured. The conceptual vagueness that I often found in reading some of the early papers is well captured in De Houwer's (Chapter 2) overview of the lack of clarity in the literature and the conflating of various characteristics attributed to implicit cognition including automaticity, lack of awareness, capacity-free (as opposed to limited channel capacity processes), controllability, and directness (i.e., obtrusiveness) of measurement and the lack of precision in distinguishing aspects of the measurement procedure versus the constructs they are presumed to measure. Most psychologists are more interested in the processes tapped by various so-called implicit tasks and having them organized into coherent models with other processes that they coordinate and interact with. As described in the chapters addressing dual process models and neuroscience perspectives on cognition, this is precisely where the field is going. From this perspective, a broad consideration of processes that interact, vary in their controllability, automaticity, and bandwidth permits a more integrative synthesis that hold promises for understanding how the various "parts of the elephant" fit together.

Another satisfying aspect of the volume is that tasks not typically subsumed under the rubric of "implicit," but clearly are relevant, are considered. That is, discussions of implicit cognition are often restricted to data from tasks such as the Stroop, Word Association Tasks, the Implicit Attitude Test, and various types of priming paradigms with measures derived from behavioral data (e.g., response latencies, accuracy, and errors). However, some of the chapters in the volume address various kinds of psychophysiological approaches that use autonomic, skeletal (e.g., startle), and CNS electrophysiological and functional neuroimaging approaches. If there is something missing in the scope of approaches described, it is the general failure of existing researchers interested in implicit cognition to exploit facial actions and other automatic (and controlled) indices of emotion (but see Mucha, Pauli, & Weyers, Chapter 14, and Waters & Sayette, Chapter 21, for brief discussions of facial EMG data). This would help to further expand the discussion and, again, foster the integration of behavioral and biological explanations, while adding unobtrusive, online assessments of implicit processing to the arsenal of researchers interested in studying substance use motivation.

Of course, as noted in multiple chapters in the volume, the distinction between processes that could be, for sake of discussion, implicit or explicit (or impulsive or reflective; or system 1 or system 2) have a long tradition in both experimental psychology (e.g., Ebbinghaus's memory "savings"; Freud's primary and secondary process) and, as noted by Stacy, Ames, & Grenard (Chapter 6), word association approaches go back to times long before there was a science of psychology. Jung's classic work on word associations in schizophrenia has a long-lasting legacy in the area of experimental psychopathology where scientists continue to use a variety of cognitive tasks coupled with neuroimaging approaches to discover the nature and cause of information processing deficits in schizophrenia and other psychotic conditions.

However, what is truly intriguing in this volume is that the types of analyses presented in this volume can address long-standing problems of interest to clinicians interested in addictive behavior but that have received minimal attention from researchers. Bechara, Noel, and Crone (Chapter 15) address this in their analysis of "will power." The so-called conative (i.e., volitional or willful) aspects of behavior or "conation" seemed to have receded from the theories of psychologists over the past 100 years as modern cognitive and motivational psychologists keep stripping away the tasks ascribed to a central executive. (I suspect that some motivational theorists, especially those interested in self-determination and intrinsic motivation would disagree; however, to date, their influence in addiction studies and psychopathology has been limited.) However, the common-sense notion of will power is something that clinicians and patients find intuitively appealing but lay conceptions seem not to be particularly useful. Again, a dual system approach that examines the relative balance of implicit and explicit (or automatic and controlled) processes appears to produce a useful reframing that permits

more insightful analysis and could potentially yield more effective treatment approaches. Perhaps even more intriguing is the extent that central clinical concepts such as denial can be addressed. I am not aware of anywhere in the field of addiction studies where the "clinical wisdom" and scientific focus and explanation are further apart. Traditional psychodynamic perspectives (still the leading framework for understanding denial in the clinical literature) have failed to generate much in the way of testable hypotheses. Neurological approaches, generalizing from deficits seen in patients suffering from neurological disease or injury, focus on those brain areas that are often compromised in patients suffering from anosognosia (i.e., lack of awareness of their illness). The so-called transtheoretical model of behavior change simply describes a group of individuals who are "precontemplative"; implying that their lack of awareness of their problems is unmotivated although any reasonable description of individuals who are severely dependent strongly suggests that for many, this is anything but the case. Evans and Coventry's (Chapter 3) analysis of gambling suggests that when overwhelmed by overly strong automatic processes, higher-level control processes are rendered somewhat helpless and that the inferences the individual makes can reflect confabulation or faulty reconstructions of his or her experience. (I suspect a similar argument could be made in other conditions such as paranoia.) Thus, my sense is the promise of a better understanding of implicit processes will yield testable theoretical propositions that will permit us to recast certain clinical phenomena in a more helpful way.

There are several issues I would hope that research on implicit cognition in addiction will address in the coming years. I will briefly highlight these because I think they are both basic issues in the area of addictions and that I believe the study of implicit cognition can inform these areas.

(1) How do changes in implicit processes track the development and course of dependence? Increasing epidemiological evidence suggests that with alcohol and drug dependence, there is a rapid increase in late adolescence and a subsequent decrease during the third decade of life. The overwhelming majority of individuals who "mature out" or "naturally recover" from their dependence do so without formal treatment. Are implicit processes responsible for any of this or are the basic role incompatibilities of parent, spouse, and worker the clear majority cause. For those who fail to "mature out," is it that implicit addiction-related processes are stronger for them than for their peers who settle down?

(2) The assessment of dependence relies primarily upon self-reported symptoms. Can implicit assessment techniques be used to assess, more thoroughly, dependence criteria? As an aside, in clinical medicine and psychiatry, there is a distinction between sign (which can be observed) and symptom (which can be reported). Can implicit measures be used to supplement symptom reporting with signs not readily accessible to the individual.

(3) Is there a psychometric structure to various indices of implicit cognition and explicit cognition? Psychometricians interested in characterizing the basic structure of cognitive abilities have long used techniques such as factor analyses to construct models of different abilities and traits. Although math modeling approaches to the structure of associations and other sophisticated statistical techniques are described in this volume, a more comprehensive assessment of implicit cognitive measures (and there temporal dynamics) would be useful for theory building and for exploiting potentially useful assessment approaches for applied problems.

(4) Can modern data collection techniques that are used "in the field" (e.g., Web-based data collection; palm-top computers) be exploited to collect more "implicit" measures of cognition that would supplement survey and intensive longitudinal study designs? Clearly, innovators like Nosek and colleagues have made important initial strides in this regard, but the ultimate reliability and validity of these types of measures, typically administered in highly controlled laboratory, remains an open question.

The above four questions are just a few of many that have promise in furthering an understanding of addiction and a brief commentary like this one fails to do justice to the numerous ideas, provocative data, and excitement that is conveyed in this volume's chapters. However, it is clear that insights gained from a broader view of cognitive processing than has typically been held by addiction researchers hold considerable promise for pushing our rapidly expanding knowledge base further.

CHAPTER 31

Automatic Processes in Addiction: A Commentary

KENT C. BERRIDGE AND TERRY E. ROBINSON

S ections 3 through 5 present a fascinating set of chapters on the many different psychological processes that may contribute to pathological drug-seeking behavior in addiction, with an emphasis on implicit automatic processes. We briefly address some highlights.

SPLITTING PSYCHOLOGY OF ADDICTION INTO ITS TRUE COMPONENTS

The idea that addiction may result from dysfunction that alters the balance among multiple different psychological processes, which normally occur simultaneously in encounter with rewards or predictive cues for them, is featured in several chapters. For example, whether an abstinent addict either relapses or continues to abstain at any given point in time may be the result of complex interactions among multiple cognitive and motivational components, all of which may be activated by the same reward-related event. Thus, it is important to know the identity of the real components, differences between

them, and the balance that controls behavior at any moment. Yin and Knowlton (Chapter 12) describe the differences between three major categories of psychological process that produce appetitive responses: cognitive act-outcome understanding, simpler S-R (stimulus-response) habits, and middle-level, Pavlovian-triggered appetitive motivational components, which can include attribution of incentive salience to reward-related conditioned stimuli and their neural representations. Yin and Knowlton (Chapter 12) discuss how these three mechanisms operate simultaneously in animals as well as people, and review evidence that they are mediated by different underlying neural systems. Franken et al. (Chapter 13) further survey human neuroimaging studies of reward-related processes, and note the importance of identifying brain activations triggered by reward stimuli that actually mediate reward. These must be distinguished from activation due to other simultaneously activated psychological processes, such as memory and attention. Such efforts will be critical to map psychological components of addiction onto their respective brain mechanisms.

THE ROLE OF S-R HABITS

Ames et al. (Chapter 23) note that the idea that the development of pathological stimulus-response habits contributes to addiction has been prominent ever since William James wrote about habits over a century ago (James, 1890), and there recently has been renewed interest in this idea (Berke, 2003; Cardinal & Everitt, 2004; Everitt et al., 2001; Hyman & Malenka, 2001). Cox et al. (Chapter 17) help unpack the potential role of habits and related implicit goals in addiction. As a methodological issue, Ames et al. (Chapter 23) also point out the need to discriminate automatic habits from controlled cognition. Although habits may contribute to addiction, there are clearly other psychological processes involved too, including motivational ones that can give compulsive force to the act of taking drugs (Robinson & Berridge, 2003).

AFFECTIVE PROCESSES: THE ROLE OF NEGATIVE REINFORCEMENT

One of the most longstanding motivational hypotheses of addiction is the negative-reinforcement idea that addicts take drugs mainly to escape negative affect states of drug withdrawal, or of preexisting life stresses and other unpleasant situations. Curtin et al. (Chapter 16) provide a thoughtful contemporary argument for the negative reinforcement idea here, suggesting that negative affect might be viewed as the most important factor in driving addiction. In their view, implicit mechanisms trigger craving by quickly activating mechanisms of negative affect, while slower cognitive control mechanisms lag behind. For some addicts in some situations, such negative reinforcement explanations are surely plausible. As Wiers et al. (Chapter 22) note in support, "coping drinkers," at least, often may drink to avoid negative affect. Birch et al. (Chapter 18), however, conclude that evidence for the notion that negative reinforcement in general is the primary mechanism for addictive drug-taking is at best inconsistent. Indeed, they point out some studies indicate quite the opposite: Events that cause positive affect may markedly increase craving.

APPETITIVE PROCESSES

For these and other reasons, Wiers et al. (Chapter 22) note that in recent years the dominant research focus has been on implicit processes of positive reinforcement and on positive appetitive reactions underlying addiction. Cox et al. (Chapter 17) point out that people sometimes drink especially when they hold positive expectations. Bechara et al. (Chapter 15) demonstrate that some drug addicts also overrespond to other positive rewards, such as money won in a gambling task. Bechara et al. (Chapter 15) suggest in particular that amygdala-triggered positive reactions, mediated by somatic marker mechanisms (Damasio, 1996), can generally cause exaggerated appetitive response to incentive cues in addicts, most particularly drugs but not necessarily always limited to them. Fascinatingly, these authors show that dopamine manipulations alter money-based gambling decisions most in ambiguous conditions, that is, when players without explicit understanding of the payoff rules must rely on implicit knowledge cues. Among such exaggerated somatic marker reactions, Bechara et al. suggest that the reaction of incentive-wanting may be mediated in part by somatic markers occurring in the supracollosal sector of the anterior cingulate cortex, whereas liking (the hedonic experience following consumption of a reward) may involve somatic markers located in the insula and somatosensory cortex.

Related to distinguishing wanting from liking in addicts, Wiers et al. (Chapter 22) show that heavy drinkers have higher arousal responses to alcohol-related items in an implicit association task, compared to light drinkers. But heavy drinkers still have equally negative valence as light drinkers toward alcohol items. Wiers et al. (Chapter 22) suggest that this dissociation between positive arousal and negative affective reaction might reflect greater "wanting" for alcohol without greater "liking" for alcohol in heavy drinkers, as predicted by the incentive-sensitization theory (Robinson & Berridge, 1993, 2003). In support of the idea that incentive salience might be automatically attributed to cause dissociated "wanting" and influence behavior in an implicit manner, other evidence indicates that unconscious "wanting" without insight into accompanying behavior can be produced in both addicts and ordinary undergraduate students (Fischman & Foltin, 1992; Robinson & Berridge, 1993; Winkielman et al., 2005).

Regarding factors that control the strength of positive reactions, Cox et al. (Chapter 17) note that the brain response of heavy drinkers to alcohol cues is actually magnified immediately after they ingest alcohol. It seems noteworthy that the priming-enhanced motivated reaction to alcohol cues occurs even though negative reinforcement withdrawal should be lowest just after a drink. Thus, alcohol on board actually magnifies brain motivation-related responses, rather than medicating them down. Alcohol priming of neural responses perhaps reflects pharmacological activation of brain mesolimbic systems, which in these heavy drinkers generate even stronger incentive salience or "wanting" when under the influence of alcohol. Synergistic potentiation of incentive mechanisms might thus act dangerously to catapult a drinker into sustained alcoholic relapse. This phenomenon may also be related to the reinstatement of drug self-administration produced by drug priming so well described in preclinical studies (McFarland et al., 2004; Shaham et al., 2003; Vezina, 2004).

PERCEPTUAL SALIENCE

The ability of drug-related stimuli to draw the eye and attract attention is a crucial feature of the incentive salience hypothesis of dopamine-related mesocorticolimbic function, and its potentiation in drug users is predicted by incentive-sensitization theory of addiction. This feature is beautifully highlighted in several chapters. The perceptual/motivational interaction is described by Bruce & Jones (Chapter 10) as "salient stimulus properties grabbing attention in a preconscious, automatized and involuntary way," revealed best in spatial visual tasks. Field et al. (Chapter 11) describe how initial orientation and duration of eye fixation measures of drug users looking at drug stimuli correlate with measures of drug craving. Similarly, Waters and Sayette (Chapter 21) describe how smokers pay exaggerated attention to smoking cues, compared to nonsmokers. They also raise the interesting possibility that smokers may be more apt to notice cigarettes or other people smoking when they themselves are attempting to quit than when still smoking. Conceivably deprivation might potentiate mesolimbic brain activation of incentive salience mechanisms in these individuals, raising incentive salience attribution to appropriate cues in a way that is similar to how natural hunger, thirst, sodium depletion, and other deprivation states selectively raise the incentive value of their own appropriate stimuli (Berridge, 2004; Toates, 1986). Enhanced attentional process in addiction may also involve alterations in brain cholinergic systems, which have been shown to exhibit sensitization effects (Arnold et al., 2003).

MODULATION OF REACTIVITY BY CONTEXT, DRIVE STATE, DRUG, AND OTHER ADDICTIONS

Basic appetitive reactions and other automatic processes can be modulated by a variety of factors. Krank and Wall (Chapter 19) show that context is especially powerful as a modulator of addiction processes. They note the famous example of Vietnam veterans who gave up drugs when they returned to postwar civilian life, and suggest that context acts in part to influence addiction by modulating memory processes. Mucha et al. (Chapter 14) describe how basic automatic reactions are also modulated by other factors, including motivational state or drug state. They suggest that basic acoustic startle reflexes, which are modulated by motivational state and drugs, can be used to study mechanisms that overlap with automatic responses involved in addiction. In an interesting extension of modulation of appetitive reactions in a way that suggests cross-talk among different addictions, Zack and Poulos (Chapter 24) show that gamblers/drinkers exhibit facilitated IAT reactions to alcohol-related words immediately after gambling wins. Also, they note amphetamine administration appears to prime gamblers' motivation to gamble, an appetitive facilitation involving mesolimbic activation that may share mechanisms similar to a drug's ability to prime incentive motivation to take more of the same drug. One wonders if these phenomena are related to the cross-sensitization between drugs revealed in animal studies, and to the modulation of sensitization induction and expression by associative context (Anagnostaras et al., 2002; De Vries & Shippenberg, 2002; Robinson & Berridge, 1993).

CONTROLLED COGNITION VERSUS AUTOMATIC APPETITIVE PROCESSES

The complex interaction between automatic appetitive processes versus cognitive control ("willpower") is highlighted in several chapters. Fillmore and Vogel-Sprott (Chapter 20) suggest that cognitive control is especially vulnerable to disruption if a person samples drugs. They show that alcohol specifically impairs cognitive control processes, while leaving automatic processes unaffected. Selective inhibition of controlled cognition needed to abstain thus leaves automatic appetitive mechanisms free to trigger further problematic responses. Bechara et al. (Chapter 15) point out further that damage to ventromedial prefrontal cortex may occur in at least some addicts, and may specifically impair willpower and create special vulnerability to relapse. Finally, in an intriguing and novel twist on the competition between automatic versus controlled processes, Palfai (Chapter 26) suggests it might be possible to harness some automatic reactions to help, instead of hinder, efforts to abstain. Palfai notes that dieters' automatic responses to subliminal diet-related primes can be modified by self-control, and suggests that future therapies might possibly make a self-control reaction itself automatic, using it to aid the cognitive decision to abstain.

Altogether, these chapters help to clarify the nature of the multiple psychological processes that may contribute to addiction, especially implicit or automatic processes. They also reveal specific interactions between basic automatic processes and higher-level regulatory controls. In sum, the authors of this collection of chapters show that recent research on automatic processes has borne valuable fruit, and usefully point the way to research topics for the future.

REFERENCES

Anagnostaras, S. G., Schallert, T., & Robinson, T. E. (2002). Memory processes governing amphetamine-induced psychomotor sensitization. *Neuropsychopharmacology, 26*(6), 703–715.

Arnold, H. M., Nelson, C. L., Sarter, M., & Bruno, J. P. (2003). Sensitization of cortical acetylcholine release by repeated administration of nicotine in rats. *Psychopharmacology* (Berlin), *165*(4), 346–358.

Berke, J. D. (2003). Learning and memory mechanisms involved in compulsive drug use and relapse. In J. Q. Wang (Ed.), *Drugs of abuse: Neurological reviews and protocols* (Vol. 79, pp. 75–101). Totowa, NJ: Humana Press.

Berridge, K. C. (2004). Motivation concepts in behavioral neuroscience. *Physiology and Behavior, 81*(2), 179–209.

Cardinal, R. N., & Everitt, B. J. (2004). Neural and psychological mechanisms underlying appetitive learning: Links to drug addiction. *Current Opinion in Neurobiology, 14*(2), 156–162.

Damasio, A. R. (1996). The somatic marker hypothesis and the possible functions of the prefrontal cortex. *Philosophical Transactions of the Royal Society of London: Series B. Biological Sciences, 351*(1346), 1413–1420.

De Vries, T. J., & Shippenberg, T. S. (2002). Neural systems underlying opiate addiction. *Journal of Neuroscience, 22*(9), 3321–3325.

Everitt, B. J., Dickinson, A., & Robbins, T. W. (2001). The neuropsychological basis of addictive behaviour. *Brain Research Reviews, 36*(2–3), 129–138.

Fischman, M. W., & Foltin, R. W. (1992). Self-administration of cocaine by humans: A laboratory perspective. In G. R. Bock & J. Whelan (Eds.), *Cocaine: Scientific and social dimensions* (Vol. 166, pp. 165–180). Chichester, UK: Wiley.

Hyman, S. E., & Malenka, R. C. (2001). Addiction and the brain: The neurobiology of compulsion and its persistence. *Nature Reviews Neuroscience, 2*(10), 695–703.

James, W. (1890). *Principles of psychology.* New York: Henry Holt.

McFarland, K., Davidge, S. B., Lapish, C. C., & Kalivas, P. W. (2004). Limbic and motor circuitry underlying footshock-induced reinstatement of cocaine-seeking behavior. *Journal of Neuroscience, 24*(7), 1551–1560.

Robinson, T. E., & Berridge, K. C. (1993). The neural basis of drug craving: An incentive-sensitization theory of addiction. *Brain Research Reviews, 18*(3), 247–291.

Robinson, T. E., & Berridge, K. C. (2003). Addiction. *Annual Review of Psychology, 54*(1), 25–53.

Shaham, Y., Shalev, U., Lu, L., de Wit, H., & Stewart, J. (2003). The reinstatement model of drug relapse: History, methodology and major findings. *Psychopharmacology, 168*(1–2), 3–20.

Toates, F. (1986). *Motivational systems.* Cambridge, UK: Cambridge University Press.

Vezina, P. (2004). Sensitization of midbrain dopamine neuron reactivity and the self-administration of psychomotor stimulant drugs. *Neuroscience & Biobehavioral Reviews, 27*(8), 827–839.

Winkielman, P., Berridge, K. C., & Wilbarger, J. L. (2005). Unconscious affective reactions to masked happy versus angry faces influence consumption behavior and judgments of value. *Personality and Social Psychology Bulletin, 31*(1), 121–135.

CHAPTER 32

Addiction: Integrating Learning Perspectives and Implicit Cognition

DIRK HERMANS AND DINSKA VAN GUCHT

When I (Dirk Hermans) was a student of psychology—like many others probably—I was fascinated by studies that demonstrated "unconscious" influences on human behavior. These included work by cognitive psychologists on the impact of "nonattended" information, experiments from social psychology that showed that we have only limited introspection concerning the dynamics of our actions, and phenomena like blindsight, implicit memory, masked priming, and unconscious learning. In hindsight, these studies were probably so salient and appealing because they contrasted with a preexisting and prescientific perception of humans as logical and rational beings. These findings opened the possibility that at least some of our thoughts and actions are driven by processes that are concealed by the layer of rationality. The fact that it was empirical work that fueled these ideas, rather than theories from wise people, I experienced as most persuasive.

About two decades later, my view on this matter has changed a lot. I am no longer convinced that some of our actions and thoughts are ruled by "unconscious" processes. Actually, I believe that *most* (or even *all*) of them are. The study of automatic information processing and associative learning has sharpened the belief that the basis of actions resides largely outside of consciousness. At times, when in a deterministic mood and when immersed in metacognitions about human behavior, I tend to view humans as complex biological robots that are behaviorally shaped by the contingencies of life and the classical and operant learning principles that operate on these—fine-tuned automatons that interact with their environment in a rather flexible way as a result of fast-acting automatic information processing. This pondering usually ends with thoughts like "*But why then do we feel that we are consciously controlling our lives?*" And in a sense this is precisely where one of the crucial questions remains: It is not the existence or function of the "unconscious" (e.g., in terms of automatic processes) that has to be explained. It is "consciousness" that needs explanation. Why do we have consciousness? Do we need it? What is its function? It would take us too far to go into this debate here. Moreover, some of the most distinguished psychologists and philosophers have devoted highly readable monographs to this very topic (e.g., Dennett, 1991; Wegner, 2002; Wilson, 2002; see also Norretranders, 1998).

Nevertheless, whatever importance one likes to attribute to nonconscious/automatic processes, it will not be difficult to think of examples of situations where behavior is influenced by factors that are outside conscious control (e.g., Bargh & Chartrand, 1999). This is particularly evident within the context of psychopathology. Clinical fear is a prototypical example, addiction another. Faced with a multitude of negative consequences (physical, relational, financial, etc.) many addicts try to forcefully stop the damaging behavioral chain, often, however, without enduring success. Entering addiction-related contexts sometimes instigates acute craving or makes old behavioral action sets more probable; addiction-related stimuli activate meanings that were once associated with them and elicit approach tendencies that are difficult to resist. Attention, memory, and reasoning can be colored or distorted in ways that make resumption of the addictive behaviors more likely. These and other factors can hinder the execution of explicit and honest behavioral goals (e.g., stay sober). In fact, most often it is this clash between explicit personal goals and the actual (negative) behavioral outcome that is the basis for seeking professional help.

One of the merits of research in the broader domain of experimental psychopathology is that it has identified a number of cognitive and behavioral processes that are responsible for the origin and maintenance of psychological problems (e.g., Harvey et al., 2004; Williams et al., 1997). One of the characteristics that is shared by most of these mechanisms is that they run to completion in a rather implicit way.

Although a lot of this research originated in the context of anxiety and depression, there exists now a more than substantial body of evidence in the domain of addictions. Hence, it was timely to collect all this empirical work in one volume on implicit cognition and addiction. As the totality of about 30 separate contributions suggests, this has been a growing and fruitful field of research.

From the perspective that was sketched at the outset of this chapter, one of the major messages of this book is that the psychological mechanisms that are central to addiction are often automatic and occur outside the individual's introspection. This is of great consequence, as a lot of clinical work with addicts is strongly inspired by views that hinge on the importance of "willpower." Even widely accepted clinical theories like Prochaska and colleagues' "Stages of Change Model" (Prochaska & DiClemente, 1983; Prochaska et al., 1992) have a rather exclusive focus on the *intentional* decision making of the individual.

Yet, contrary to my private metacognitions concerning psychological determinism and human automatons, the significance of implicit processes is placed here within theoretically sound and empirically validated frameworks. Examples are dual-process models like the System 1/System 2 theories described by Evans and Coventry (Chapter 3) or the Reflective-Impulsive Model described by Deutsch and Strack (Chapter 4). These models weigh the impact of more automatic and more deliberate processes for addictive behavior. They describe how these two levels of processing interact, and when and how they influence addictive behavior.

The book is also rich in the description of implicit/indirect measures, including word-association paradigms (Stacy et al., Chapter 6), priming methodology (Houben et al., Chapter 7) and other reaction-time procedures (Bruce & Jones, Chapter 10; de Jong et al., Chapter 27; Fadardi et al., Chapter 9;

Wiers et al., Chapter 22). Without doubt, this wealth of new research methodology will further our views on addiction. The degree to which this endeavor will be successful, however, will depend on a number of factors. First, at a theoretical level, there is a need for a better understanding of what exactly is measured by each of these indirect procedures. Second, at a more practical level, the potential of indirect measures will depend on (1) the extent to which the relatively weak psychometric qualities of these tasks can be enhanced (e.g., reliability) and (2) the extent to which (and under what circumstances) these tasks will prove to be better predictors of addictive behavior (e.g., lapse, relapse) than classical paper and-pencil tests.

More generally, however, it is our conviction that the domain of addiction and implicit cognition would benefit from broadening its perspectives. A rather crude breakdown of the components of human cognition could be described as follows: (1) information is encoded by the organism, and is (2) stored in memory, where these representations remain dormant until (3) they are reactivated, and (4) influence/steer behavior. At present, the vast majority of studies on implicit cognition and addiction are devoted to the analysis of the cognitive representations of addiction-relevant information in addicts and controls (part "2") and the ways in which this information can be activated (part "3"). Less work has been devoted to the—probably complex—ways in which these representations steer addictive behavior (part "4"). Among others, this latter component includes the study of how and when the two layers of the dual-process models come into play, as well as the study of the predictive value of indirect measures for addictive behavior. And with respect to part "1," there has been surprisingly little attention to the processes that are involved in the encoding and storage of these "implicit cognitions" in addiction. Hence, our conviction that the

domain of addiction and implicit cognition would benefit from incorporating a "learning perspective" (for related arguments, see Hermans et al., 2003).

What would be the advantage of expanding toward a learning perspective? First of all, there are a number of identical research questions that develop quite separately in the domains of implicit cognition and the psychology of learning. Both would benefit from some cross-fertilization. Second, a number of recent insights from the domain of associative learning would be of interest for implicit cognition research. And finally, the integration would provide a more complete picture, with implications for clinical practice. Instead of reviewing these arguments in a more general manner, we will illustrate this line of reasoning with some examples.

No one will doubt that an individual's alcohol attitudes (explicit or implicit), outcome expectancies, and craving are based on learning experiences. Classical and operant conditioning can be seen as research paradigms "par excellence" by which people acquire new meanings and learn to interact with these meaningful stimuli or situations. Although there exists conditioning work in the context of addiction (see Curtin et al., Chapter 16; Krank & Wall, Chapter 19; Yin & Knowlton, Chapter 12), most of this is animal research and rather unrelated to the domain of implicit cognition. Particularly the study of *human* (classical) conditioning can be informative for those studying implicit cognition in addiction, because of a number of highly related research questions. For example, the translation of animal conditioning models to the understanding of human associative learning has opened the discussion of the relative importance of lower-level versus higher-level cognitive processes (e.g., De Houwer et al., in press; Lovibond, 2004; Öhman & Mineka, 2001). We believe that the "implicit cognition" debate concerning when and how lower- or higher-level cognitive processes influence (addictive) behavior should at least be informed by knowledge that is acquired in the context of the rather similar debate that is current in the human associative learning literature. At present, both domains proceed too much in isolation. Another example of a topic where cross-fertilization would be of interest is the study of context effects on the expression of (addictive) behavior.

In addition, a number of recent insights from the domain of associative learning are of relevance for the study of addiction and implicit cognition. For instance, animal as well as human studies have led to the conclusion that extinction does not entail "unlearning" (e.g., Rescorla, 1996). Rather, a new association is formed. Whether the "old" association (acquisition memory) or the new association (extinction memory) is active will (in part) depend on the context (Bouton, 2004). With respect to addiction, this implies that most treatments (e.g., abstinence, cue exposure) will not erase the old cognitive structures (part "2") that form the basis for craving, outcome expectancies, or drug/ alcohol attitudes. Confrontation with addiction-related conditioned stimuli might reactivate these old associations, particularly when encountered in contexts that had previously formed the background of addictive behaviors (see also Krank & Wall, Chapter 19). Indirect measures of the memory associations might be brought into play to assess this risk.

An interesting study that is rooted in experimental learning psychology and that relates the above-mentioned issues of "absence of unlearning" and context-dependency was published by Collins and Brandon (2002). These authors exposed 78 social drinkers to a series of visual-olfactory presentations of beer (i.e., without drinking; extinction training). One group of participants was subsequently tested for salivary responses and urge self-reports in the context where extinction training had taken place (same context group [SC]). A second group was tested in a different context (different context group [DC]). In line with expectations, the DC group showed significantly greater "renewal" of saliva and urge responses than the SC group. These findings demonstrate the context-dependency of extinguished alcohol cue reactivity (see also Crombag & Shaham, 2002). Interestingly, the authors included a third group that was also tested in a context that differed from the extinction context, but for this group a reminder cue was present (i.e., a stimulus that was also present in the extinction context). It was hypothesized that this cue might help to retrieve the extinction context and thereby reduce the renewal effect that was induced by the presentation of the alcohol cues outside the extinction context. This hypothesis was supported.

In sum, we believe that the study of addiction would benefit from a transdisciplinary integration between implicit cognition research and experimental learning psychology (see also Wiers et al., 2004). Insights into how (implicit) associations and cognitive structures develop and change (e.g., throughout treatment) will provide a more complete picture of human addictive behavior.

REFERENCES

Bargh, J. A., & Chartrand, T. L. (1999). The unbearable automaticity of being. *American Psychologist, 54,* 462–479.

Bouton, M. E. (2004). Context and behavioral processes in extinction. *Learning & Memory, 11,* 485–494.

Collins, B. N., & Brandon, T. H. (2002). Effects of extinction context and retrieval cues on alcohol cue reactivity among nonalcoholic drinkers. *Journal of Consulting and Clinical Psychology, 70,* 390–397.

Crombag, H. S., & Shaham, Y. (2002). Renewal of drug seeking by contextual cues after prolonged extinction in rats. *Behavioural Neuroscience, 116,* 169–173.

De Houwer, J., Vandorpe, S., & Beckers, T. (in press). On the role of controlled cognitive processes in human associative learning. In A. Wills (Ed.), *New directions in human associative learning.* Mahwah, NJ: Lawrence Erlbaum.

Dennett, D. C. (1991). *Consciousness explained.* Boston: Little, Brown.

Harvey, A. G., Watkins, E., Mansell, W., & Shafran, R. (2004). *Cognitive behavioural processes across psychological disorders: A trans-diagnostic approach to research and treatment.* Oxford, UK: Oxford University Press.

Hermans, D., Baeyens, F., & Eelen, P. (2003). On the acquisition and activation of evaluative information in memory: The study of evaluative learning and affective priming combined. In J. Musch & K. C. Klauer (Eds.), *The psychology of evaluation: Affective processes in cognition and emotion* (pp. 139–168). Mahwah, NJ: Lawrence Erlbaum.

Lovibond, P. F. (2004). Cognitive processes in extinction. *Learning & Memory, 11,* 495–500.

Norretranders, T. (1998). *The user illusion: Cutting consciousness down to size.* New York: Penguin.

Öhman, A., & Mineka, S. (2001). Fears, phobias, and preparedness: Toward an evolved module of fear and fear learning. *Psychological Review, 108,* 483–522.

Prochaska, J. O., & DiClemente, C. C. (1983). Stages and processes of self-change of smoking: Toward an integrative model of change. *Journal of Consulting and Clinical Psychology, 51,* 390–395.

Prochaska, J. O., DiClemente, C. C., & Norcross, J. C. (1992). In search of how people change: Applications to addictive behavior. *American Psychologist, 47,* 1102–1114.

Rescorla, R. A. (1996). Preservation of Pavlovian associations through extinction. *Quarterly Journal of Experimental Psychology, 49B,* 245–258.

Wegner, D. M. (2002). *The illusion of conscious will.* Cambridge, MA: MIT Press.

Wiers, R. W., de Jong, P. J., Havermans, R., & Jelicic, M. (2004). How to change implicit drug use-related cognitions in prevention: A transdisciplinary integration of findings from experimental psychopathology, social cognition, memory, and experimental learning psychology. *Substance Use & Misuse, 39,* 1625–1684.

Williams, J. M. G., Watts, F. N., MacLeod, C., & Mathews, A. (1997). *Cognitive psychology and emotional disorders* (2nd ed.). Chichester, UK: Wiley.

Wilson, T. D. (2002). *Strangers to ourselves: Discovering the adaptive unconscious.* Cambridge, MA: Harvard University Press.

CHAPTER 33

Being Mindful of Automaticity in Addiction: A Clinical Perspective

G. ALAN MARLATT AND BRIAN D. OSTAFIN

Clinical experience and research demonstrate that although interventions may initially benefit addictive behaviors, these effects typically do not last (Catalano et al., 1988). This lack of long-term improvement after an initial response characterizes treatment outcome for other disorders as well (Westen & Morrison, 2001). Utilizing implicit cognition in addiction theory and research may hold great promise for coming to a better understanding of both (1) the automatic processes that make addictive behaviors so difficult to change and (2) the treatment strategies that may alter those processes. The *Handbook on Implicit Cognition and Addiction* admirably consolidates the known research on these two points. We would like to use this commentary as an opportunity to elaborate on a clinical perspective of using implicit cognition theory and methods to model addiction.

Why do the majority of addicts who want to change have such a difficult time doing so? Two answers suggested by a number of the chapters are that automatic attentional biases and associative networks may conflict with explicit goals to inhibit use. This volume describes a range of implicit cognition tasks to measure these automatic processes. These tasks may provide important information about the likelihood both of young users developing substance-use disorders (and the need for preventive treatment; see Krank & Goldstein, Chapter 28) and of relapse for heavy users after an intervention (and the need for additional treatment; see Stacy et al., 2004; Waters et al., 2003). A corollary issue regards the treatment itself—that is, how to best effect changes so that automatic processes that facilitate addictive behavior do not prevail in those wishing to reduce or abstain.

AUTOMATICITY IN INITIAL USE: PREVENTING LAPSE

A point made in several chapters that we feel important to underscore is that to be successful, interventions may need to target more than one automatic process. This point may be illustrated with findings from an alcoholism intervention study by Marlatt (1979).

Results showed that by itself, aversion therapy demonstrated good short-term (3-month) but poor long-term (15-month) effects in alcoholics. These findings may be explained by basic learning research that indicates that although punishment may temporarily suppress a behavior, spontaneous recovery of that behavior is likely unless a new behavior (e.g., alternative coping response) can be added (Hilgard & Bower, 1966). In this vein, multifaceted intervention strategies may include (1) weakening automatic processes that facilitate substance use with components such as pharmacology (Bechara et al., Chapter 15; Cox et al., Chapter 17; Wiers et al., Chapter 22; Yin & Knowlton, Chapter 12), cue exposure (Ostafin & Palfai, Chapter 25; Palfai, Chapter 26; Wiers et al., Chapter 22; Zack & Poulos, Chapter 24), and attentional retraining (de Jong et al., Chapter 27; Field et al., Chapter 11); and (2) strengthening both automatic and controlled processes that inhibit substance use with components such as coping skills (Bechara et al., Chapter 15; Palfai, Chapter 26; Yin & Knowlton, Chapter 12), implementation intentions (Palfai, Chapter 26; Prestwich et al., Chapter 29), or creating nonsubstance incentives (Cox et al., Chapter 17).

The self-regulation of addictive behavior is often framed as a conflict between automatic appetitive processes and controlled inhibitory processes (Tiffany, 1990). It follows that because the effortful cognitive resources needed to utilize conscious (e.g., coping) strategies are limited (Muraven et al., 1998), successful self-regulation will often be disadvantaged. Several chapters suggest that this concern can be circumvented by using regulatory techniques that strategically utilize automatic processes. Although coping strategies can become automatic with extensive practice, other regulatory strategies may more inherently involve automatic processes. Thus, implementation intentions may be automatically activated in the presence of a cue (Palfai, Chapter 26; Prestwich et al., Chapter 29) and

developing nonsubstance-related incentives might weaken substance-reinforcement value associations (Cox et al., Chapter 17).

Recent research into mindfulness suggests it may be another way to circumvent obstacles inherent in an automatic facilitation versus effortful inhibition perspective of change. Mindfulness can be described as a metacognitive state of "awareness that emerges through paying attention on purpose, in the present moment, and nonjudgmentally to the unfolding of experience moment by moment" (Kabat-Zinn, 2003, p. 145). Although different meditative practices have been studied as clinical interventions for decades (see Marlatt & Kristeller, 1999), interest in mindfulness meditation has dramatically increased over the past 10 years. Mindfulness-based treatments have shown efficacy in reducing anxiety, depression relapse, ratings of chronic pain (Baer, 2003), and recent research in our lab indicates utility as a treatment for substance-use disorders (Bowen et al., 2005; Marlatt et al., 2004).

How mindfulness works is not well understood, though theoretical (see especially Bishop et al., 2004) and some empirical work suggest that it may alter the influence of automatic processes on psychopathology. Following other definitions of mindfulness (cf. Kabat-Zinn, 2003), Bishop et al. (2004) describe two components of mindfulness as consisting of increased attention to immediate (internal) experience and adoption of an attitude of openness and acceptance toward that experience. Each component may impact several automatic processes involved in substance use.

The first component of mindfulness is attention, which can be further divided into two skills. The first attentional skill consists of bringing greater awareness to physical sensations and body-feeling states. Baker et al. (2004) have suggested that substance users are often unaware of the internal cues of negative affect that elicit behavior directly leading toward the acquisition and consumption of substances. Thus, a user may almost unexpectedly find him- or herself lighting a cigarette or calling a dealer. Unnoticed internal cues may also elicit behavior that indirectly leads toward substance use through "apparently irrelevant decisions" in which a person may find him- or herself in a high-risk situation seemingly without warning (Marlatt & Gordon, 1985, p. 49). For example, a person who is trying to abstain from alcohol may take a shortcut past a favorite bar, a cue that may activate behavior (e.g., walking in, ordering a beer) that will directly lead to drinking. For deliberative, conscious processes to influence behavior so that unwanted substance use does not occur there needs to be an opportunity to do so (Fazio, 1990). That is, awareness of internal cues that activate substance-use behavior may create an opportunity for explicit goals and strategies to be utilized early on. Thus, a lack of internal awareness at the beginning of the sequence may delay the use of coping response such that the situation becomes like "closing the door after the horse has left the barn" (Kornfield, 1993, p. 279). Evidence that mindfulness is associated with increased awareness of internal experience (Brown & Ryan, 2003; Forte et al., 1987–1988) suggests that a mindful state would both reduce the likelihood of apparently irrelevant decisions resulting in high-risk situations and increase the opportunity to utilize coping skills early on. The latter idea could be examined by (1) teaching coping strategies to a sample who use substances for negative-reinforcement reasons and (2) creating a subtle negative affect induction (perhaps with subliminally presented stimuli; see studies discussed in Bargh & Chartrand, 1999) and assessing behaviors generated to negative reinforcement outcome stimuli with a continued association task (see Ames et al., Chapter 23). We would predict that greater awareness of incipient negative affect would be correlated with a greater number of nonsubstance-related coping responses.

The second attentional skill consists of sustaining attention on the object of one's current experience. Attentional biases to substance-use-related cues predict greater use (de Jong et al., Chapter 27; Field et al., Chapter 11). This may be because attention maintained on a substance cue continually reactivates affective and motor associations that facilitate use. Evidence that mindfulness is associated with increased ability to sustain attention (Davidson et al., 1976; Forte et al., 1987–1988) suggests that it would lead to reduced susceptibility to attentional intrusions of substance-related cues. We would predict that mindfulness would reduce attentional bias to substance-use cues and suggest this could be examined with methods such as the visual probe task (see Field et al., Chapter 11).

The second component of mindfulness is the orientation of an accepting attitude toward current experience. This involves "a conscious decision to abandon one's agenda to have a different experience and an active process of 'allowing' current thoughts, feelings, and sensations" (Bishop et al., 2004, p. 233). In many cases, simple attention to internal experience is not enough, as evidence suggests that awareness of internal state can increase the influence of affective representations on drinking behavior (Bartholow et el., 2000). An accepting attitude should lead to reductions in strategies to avoid unwanted aspects of one's experience. Experiential avoidance strategies such as thought suppression may facilitate substance use because suppression (e.g., of urges) can "ironically" make the content more accessible and likely to influence behavior (Palfai et al., 1997; Wegner & Smart, 1997). There is evidence indicating that reducing thought suppression mediates the effects of mindfulness training on substance use (Bowen et al., 2004). Decreases in thought suppression should also lead to reductions in chronic accessibility of substance-related information in users who are attempting to restrain. This could be examined with methods such as the lexical decision task. Ending the ironic effects of suppression could in turn change explicit representations of self as having more efficacy to handle high-risk situations, thus making a lapse less likely (Blume et al., 2003).

Additionally, an accepting attitude toward one's experience may provide insight into the nature of that experience as "passing events in the mind rather than as inherent aspects of the self or valid reflections on reality" (Bishop et al., 2004, p. 234). This relation toward one's experience has been called *metacognitive awareness* or *decentering* and has been found to be increased by mindfulness training and to predict less vulnerability to depressive relapse (Teasdale et al., 2002). We would predict that mindfulness would reduce identification of self with substance use. This could be examined with an implicit self-concept task (Rudman et al., 2001) assessing associations between self and substance-use concepts. Related, because an accepting, decentered perspective may weaken the experience of one's thoughts (e.g., "I have to get a drink.") as being valid, automatic thoughts should be less likely to be acted upon. We would predict that in users who want to restrain, the relation between implicit measures of substance-use attitudes and actual use would be moderated by mindfulness-based acceptance.

AUTOMATICITY IN CONTINUED USE: PREVENTING RELAPSE

This volume impressively details the automatic processes that may instigate substance use and the treatment strategies that may alter the processes so that use is less likely to occur. Although much work needs to be done to test these ideas, we think it will be valuable to also examine what happens after an initial lapse has occurred. That is, how is automaticity involved in whether a lapse exacerbates into a relapse and what treatment strategies may be useful to prevent this from happening? Initial use may affect a number of automatic processes that facilitate further use. It may be that the effects of the substance deplete the controlled-process resources available to inhibit automatic tendencies toward further use (see Fillmore & Vogel-Sprott, Chapter 20). Another way an initial lapse may facilitate continued use is by enhancing automatic appetitive processes. For example, compared to placebo, alcohol may enhance the accessibility of positive relative to negative outcome expectancies (Palfai & Ostafin, 2003), making continued consumption more likely.

In addition to tilting the balance from controlled inhibition of use to automatic facilitation of use, a lapse may also trigger automatic self-concepts (e.g., associations between self and low willpower concepts) that attribute the initial use to internal factors, leading to the experience of guilt. This may then lead to increased drinking to cope with the guilt as part of an abstinence violation effect (Marlatt & Gordon, 1985; Marlatt & Donovan, 2005). It is of note that substance users are not skilled at predicting what attributions they will make if they lapse after treatment (Curry et al., 1987). In addition to obtaining self-report, it may be useful to measure the automatic activation of self-internal attribution associations after imagining a lapse. This may allow better prediction of relapse and provide suggestions for cognitive restructuring during treatment. Besides cognitive restructuring and other explicit cognitive strategies to prevent relapse (Marlatt & Gordon, 1985), we would again suggest that mindfulness may lessen relapse likelihood by creating a decentered relation to negative affect and thoughts about self (see Breslin et al., 2002; Teasdale et al., 2002).

SUMMARY

Substance-use researchers not infrequently lament the slow transfer of theory and methods from basic science (Shiffman, 1993). The current volume represents fundamental research and theory that will likely spur innovative models of addictive behavior and approaches to treat it. In addition to the variety of treatment strategies mentioned, we would suggest that mindfulness-based interventions hold potential in substance-use treatment because they can influence a number of automatic processes that facilitate addictive behavior. In a review of the role of automatic processes in human behavior, Bargh and Chartrand (1999) borrowed from a Kundera (1984) novel for their title "The Unbearable Automaticity of Being." Although they concluded that the title belied the often-beneficial function of automaticity, we would keep the tenor of that title for the topic of automaticity in addiction. As mindfulness can create a decentered perspective on experience, allowing moments of pausing instead of reacting in the usual habitual manner, we would suggest another Kundera (1995) title to represent this treatment approach: "Slowness."

REFERENCES

Baer, R. A. (2003). Mindfulness training as a clinical intervention: A conceptual and empirical review. *Clinical Psychology: Science and Practice, 10*, 125–143.

Baker, T. B., Piper, M. E., McCarthy, D. E., Majeskie, M. R., & Fiore, M. C. (2004). Addiction motivation reformulated: An affective processing model of negative reinforcement. *Psychological Review, 111*, 33–51.

Bargh, J. A., & Chartrand, T. L. (1999). The unbearable automaticity of being. *American Psychologist, 54*, 462–479.

Bartholow, B. D., Sher, K. J., & Strathman, A. (2000). Moderation of the expectancy-alcohol use relation by private self-consciousness. Data from a longitudinal study. *Personality and Social Psychology Bulletin, 26*, 1409–1420.

Bishop, S. R., Lau, M., Shapiro, S., Carlson, L., Anderson, N. D., Carmody, J., et al. (2004). Mindfulness: A proposed operational definition. *Clinical Psychology: Science and Practice, 11*, 230–241.

Blume, A. W., Schmaling, K. B., & Marlatt, G. A. (2003). Predictors of change in binge drinking over a 3-month period. *Addictive Behaviors, 28*, 1007–1012.

Bowen, S., Dillworth, T. M., & Marlatt, G. A. (2004). Buddha and the bear: Relationships between meditation, thought suppression and substance use. Poster session presented at the annual conference of the American Psychological Association, Honolulu, HI.

Bowen, S., Witkiewitz, K., Dillworth, T. M., Chawla, N., Simpson, T. L., Ostafin, B. D., et al. (2005). *Mindfulness meditation and substance use in an incarcerated population.* Manuscript submitted for publication.

Breslin, F. C., Zack, M., & McMain, S. (2002). An information-processing analysis of mindfulness: Implications for relapse prevention in the treatment of substance abuse. *Clinical Psychology: Science and Practice, 9*, 275–299.

Brown, K. W., & Ryan, R. M. (2003). The benefits of being present: Mindfulness and its role in psychological well-being. *Journal of Personality and Social Psychology, 84*, 822–848.

Catalano, R., Howard, M., Hawkins, J., & Wells, E. (1988). Relapse in the addictions: Rates, determinants, and promising prevention strategies (1988 Surgeon General's Report on Health Consequences of Smoking). Washington, DC: Government Printing Office, Office of Smoking and Health.

Curry, S., Marlatt, G. A., & Gordon, J. R. (1987). Abstinence violation effect: Validation of an attributional construct with smoking cessation. *Journal of Consulting and Clinical Psychology, 55,* 145–149.

Davidson, R. J., Goleman, D. J., & Schwartz, G. E. (1976). Attentional and affective concomitants of meditation: A cross-sectional study. *Journal of Abnormal Psychology, 85,* 235–238.

Fazio, R. H. (1990). Multiple processes by which attitudes guide behavior: The MODE model as an integrative framework. In M. P. Zanna (Ed.), *Advances in experimental social psychology* (Vol. 23, pp. 75–109). New York: Academic Press.

Forte, M., Brown, D. P., & Dysart, M. (1987–1988). Differences in experience among mindfulness meditators. *Imagination, Cognition and Personality, 7,* 47–60.

Hilgard, E. R., & Bower, G. H. (1966). *Theories of learning* (3rd ed.). New York: Appleton-Century-Crofts.

Kabat-Zinn, J. (2003). Mindfulness-based interventions in context: Past, present, and future. *Clinical Psychology: Science and Practice, 10,* 144–156.

Kornfield, J. (1993). *A path with heart.* New York: Bantam.

Kundera, M. (1984). *The unbearable lightness of being.* New York: Harper & Row.

Kundera, M. (1995). *Slowness.* New York: HarperCollins.

Marlatt, G. A. (1979). A cognitive-behavioral model of the relapse process. In N. A. Krasnegor (Ed.), *Behavioral analysis and treatment of substance abuse* (Research Monograph 25, pp. 191–200). Washington, DC: National Institute of Drug Abuse Research.

Marlatt, G. A., & Donovan, D. (2005). *Relapse prevention: Maintenance strategies in the treatment of addictive behaviors* (2nd ed.). New York: Guilford.

Marlatt, G. A., & Gordon, J. R. (1985). *Relapse prevention: Maintenance strategies in the treatment of addictive behaviors.* New York: Guilford.

Marlatt, G. A., & Kristeller, J. (1999). Mindfulness and meditation. In W. R. Miller (Ed.), *Integrating spirituality in treatment: Resources for practitioners* (pp. 67–84). Washington, DC: APA Books.

Marlatt, G. A., Witkiewitz, K., Dillworth, T. M., Bowen, S., Parks, G. A., MacPherson, L. M., et. al. (2004). Vipassana meditation as a treatment for alcohol and drug use disorders. In S. C. Hayes, M. M. Linehan, & V. M. Follette (Eds.), *Mindfulness and acceptance: Expanding the cognitive-behavioral tradition* (pp. 261–287). New York: Guilford.

Muraven, M., Tice, D. M., & Baumeister, R. F. (1998). Self-control as limited resource: Regulatory depletion patterns. *Journal of Personality and Social Psychology, 74,* 774–789.

Palfai, T. P., Monti, P. M., Colby, S. M., & Rohsenow, D. J. (1997). Effects of suppressing the urge to drink on the accessibility of alcohol outcome expectancies. *Behaviour Research and Therapy, 35,* 59 65.

Palfai, T. P., & Ostafin, B. D. (2003). The influence of alcohol on the activation of outcome expectancies: The role of evaluative expectancy activation in drinking behavior. *Journal of Studies on Alcohol, 64,* 111–119.

Rudman, L. A., Greenwald, A. G., & McGhee, D. E. (2001). Implicit self-concept and evaluative implicit gender stereotypes: Self and ingroup share desirable traits. *Personality and Social Psychology Bulletin, 27,* 1164–1178.

Shiffman, S. (1993). Smoking cessation treatment: Any progress? *Journal of Consulting and Clinical Psychology, 61,* 718–722.

Stacy, A. W., Ames, S. L., & Leigh, B. C. (2004). An implicit cognition assessment approach to relapse, secondary prevention, and media effects. *Cognitive and Behavioral Practice, 11,* 139–149.

Teasdale, J. D., Moore, R. G., Hayhurst, H., Pope, M., Williams, S., & Segal, Z. V. (2002). Metacognitive awareness and prevention of relapse in depression: Empirical evidence. *Journal of Consulting and Clinical Psychology, 70,* 275–287.

Tiffany, S. T. (1990). A cognitive model of drug urges and drug-use behavior: Role of automatic and nonautomatic processes. *Psychological Review, 97,* 147–168.

Waters, A. J., Shiffman, S., Sayette, M. A., Paty, J. A., Gwaltney, C. G., & Balabanis, M. H. (2003). Attentional bias predicts outcome in smoking cessation. *Health Psychology, 22,* 378–387.

Wegner, D. M., & Smart, L. (1997). Deep cognitive activation: A new approach to the unconscious. *Journal of Consulting and Clinical Psychology, 65,* 984–995.

Westen, D., & Morrison, K. (2001). A multidimensional meta-analysis of treatments for depression, panic, and generalized anxiety disorder: An empirical examination of the status of empirically supported therapies. *Journal of Consulting and Clinical Psychology, 69,* 875–899.

CHAPTER 34

Common Themes and New Directions in Implicit Cognition and Addiction

ALAN W. STACY AND REINOUT W. WIERS

This book has presented many different perspectives on implicit cognitive processes in addiction. The diversity of measures, theories, and applications reflects the nature of a rapidly expanding, new area that has roots in different research areas and disciplines. Despite the variety, there are some important ways in which most of the chapters unite in their message and implications. In our view, one of the most important common messages is that an implicit cognition framework provides a new and useful way to conceptualize, understand, and prevent or treat addictions. Yet, these new ideas did not occur in a vacuum and have many historical roots. Another general theme is that paradigms established in basic research on cognition, affect, and underlying neural systems are shown to be quite applicable to an important, applied problem. As is common in the history of science, the application of new methods opens up many possibilities for new understanding, and possibly control, of a fundamental phenomenon. Another commonality across many chapters is optimism. Implicit cognition should not be viewed in terms of mysterious or untestable "dark forces" reminiscent of Freud's Id. Rather, implicit cognition can be scientifically studied using multiple converging methods and harnessed to help change behavior in a positive direction. Indeed, healthy and prosocial behaviors are probably governed largely by some of the same implicit processes that govern harmful behaviors.

More specific common themes emerge from the chapters. These include the importance of multiple systems, applications for intervention, triggering effects of broadly defined cues, contexts, or moods, and other points of convergence. Rather than reiterate major findings, we briefly highlight two of the specific themes below. Then, we summarize some of the challenges for the future.

AUTHOR'S NOTE: This chapter was supported in part by grants from the National Institute on Drug Abuse (DA16094) and from the National Science Foundation of The Netherlands (N.W.O.), VIDI grant 452.02.005.

SUPPORT FOR
MULTIPLE SYSTEMS
AND PROCESSES

The chapters have reviewed various classifications or distinctions relevant to implicit and explicit cognition. As is frequently the case, there is no clear consensus on the best use of all relevant terms. Many of the chapter authors agree, however, with the view that there are multiple systems of cognition and emotion relevant to addictions. In a set-theoretic approach, some investigators might consider implicit cognition the most all-inclusive term encompassing automatic processes, unconscious cognition, implicit memory, impulsive cognitive processes, Kahneman's (2003) "System 1," and so on. Others may prefer a different organization of terms (for discussion, see De Houwer, Chapter 2). Nevertheless, there is widespread evidence from diverse methods and multiple levels of analysis (neural to cognitive response) that these implicit processes play a fundamental role in behavior in general, and in addictive behaviors in particular. Even investigators who do not emphasize multiple *systems* (e.g., Krank & Goldstein, Chapter 28) still underscore the importance of addressing different *modes* of processing. In such a view, the transfer from encoding to retrieval situations, in terms of compatibility of cues and modes of processing, is the focus.

Different chapters presented multiple-system views at different levels of analysis and with different foci. Bechara et al. (Chapter 15) focused on the neural basis of two general systems, one supporting an impulsive system, the other supporting reflective judgments (including subsystems of impulse control and decision making). In a subgroup of addicts, the impulsive system can disrupt or completely "hijack" the reflective system. Curtin et al. (Chapter 16) focused on positive and negative reinforcement processes within an implicit system (analogous to Bechara et al.'s

impulsive system), and integrative, regulative, and monitoring functions within a cognitive control (explicit) system. Yin and Knowlton (Chapter 12) focused on the circuitry and behavioral implications of different neural systems supporting action-outcome (AO), stimulus-response (SR), and stimulus-outcome (SO) associations, noting that each system involves a set of circuits across multiple brain regions. Deutsch and Strack (Chapter 4) outlined a dual-process model of social cognition and behavior that can be linked in many ways to the neural substrates of impulsive/implicit and reflective/explicit systems outlined in other chapters and also to the neural basis of associations outlined by Yin and Knowlton. Evans and Coventry (Chapter 3) applied a general dual-process theory to gambling, providing evidence that a system analogous to the reflective system provides post hoc rationalizations for behavior caused by an implicit system. Fillmore and Vogel-Sprott (Chapter 20) showed that drug-use affects controlled processes much more than it does automatic or implicit processes, providing a different line of evidence supporting the view of multiple cognitive systems. McEvoy and Nelson (Chapter 5) reviewed evidence showing that memory responses are frequently influenced by both implicit and explicit processes; yet, these processes can be distinguished. The commentary by Berridge and Robinson (Chapter 31), as well as the primary chapters, outlined a number of ways in which multiple systems or processes delineated in the chapters may interact. An important topic in current neurobiological addiction research concerns cross-sensitization (see Berridge & Robinson, Chapter 31), and it is interesting to see that the first attempts are made to study this phenomenon in humans, using implicit cognition measures (Ostafin & Palfai, Chapter 25; Zack & Poulos, Chapter 24).

Support for multiple systems or processes does not imply that current measures are "pure" measures of only one process (De Houwer, Chapter 2). Indeed some current "implicit" measures have been shown to not only reflect automatic processes but the joint contribution of multiple qualitatively different processes (Conrey et al., in press). The possible influence of multiple systems/processes on assessment should be acknowledged, and evidence supporting a dominance of one system or process on assessment should be carefully weighed. Nevertheless, an earlier review (Ryan & Cohen, 2003) as well as chapters in this book have reported many *independent* lines of evidence supporting a distinction between multiple systems or processes. In a philosophy of science that underscores the importance of multiple operations (Cook & Campbell, 1979), convergence across truly independent methods of inquiry leads to confidence that the distinction is not the result of systematic method error and hence not a fiction of a particular research paradigm or discipline.

In summary, many chapters diverge in specific manifestations of multiple systems but they converge on several general conclusions regarding the distinction between systems:

1. Diverse neuroscientific and cognitive methods buttress the distinction using radically different assessments.

2. The distinction has clear implications for understanding a wide range of addictive or habit-forming behaviors, from drug use to gambling.

3. The distinction makes it difficult to rely solely on any single cognitive concept and instead suggests that multiple concepts are necessary for adequate explanation.

4. A multiple-system framework focuses scientific attention on the operation of (frequently) competing processes that may underlie the effectiveness (or failure) of interventions. This issue is addressed more fully below because it is one of the most common implications for intervention across chapters.

INTERVENTION APPLICATIONS

Most of the chapters that addressed interventions assumed the simultaneous operation of implicit and nonimplicit (explicit, executive, or control) systems or processes. These chapters reviewed or outlined procedures relevant to one or both classes of systems.

One common example suggests interventions to increase the effectiveness of nonimplicit systems. Systems involving explicit cognition, executive functions, or controlled processing can be harnessed in new ways to counteract implicit processes that may otherwise "hijack" good intentions or plans for change. Cox et al. (Chapter 17) outlined a comprehensive motivational therapy they refer to as Systematic Motivational Counseling. In part, this strategy attempts to influence the individual's motivation to change their behavior, focusing on the acquisition of other goals than substance use. Fillmore and Vogel-Sprott (Chapter 20) suggested it may be feasible to increase the effect of controlled processes on behavior even after a drug is consumed, potentially reducing the "free reign" of automatic or implicit processes. Birch et al. (Chapter 18) argued that participants in interventions should be trained to recognize mood triggers and resultant cognitive processes that foster drug abuse and that interventions should screen participants to identify their specific triggers. Such training may conceivably lead to a greater effect of controlled or executive processes on behavior, although effects on implicit processes also were suggested. Marlatt and Ostafin's commentary (Chapter 33) suggests a variety of additional ways in which "mindfulness" interventions can counter implicit processes, and the theory of Curtin et al. (Chapter 16) agrees that cognitive control processes are critical for countering drug-use motivation. Bechara et al. (Chapter 15) take a generally similar approach to control (or reflective) processes but focus on the addict's need for simultaneous relearning and corrective medication aimed at the system that shows a chemical imbalance—either one of the control (reflective) systems or the implicit (impulsive) system.

Several approaches, taken together, give strong indications that interventions can, and should, also address implicit systems. The general notion here is that interventions need to make automatic processes work in favor of intervention goals, not against those goals. Prestwich et al. (Chapter 29) review compelling findings showing that cues can come to automatically activate or elicit plans for behaviors (implementation intentions) that can serve as alternatives to a range of habits. A compatible approach from Palfai (Chapter 26) suggests that many if not all of the subprocesses of self-regulation have the *potential* to become automatized, becoming implicit processes. In a somewhat more general approach to the triggers of implicit processes, Ames et al. (Chapter 23) suggest that new associations in memory need to be a focus of interventions, to provide connections between the cues that normally precede risky behaviors and new, healthy skills, behavioral alternatives, goals, or other program elements. Work on mood by Birch and colleagues (Chapter 18), motivational state by Curtin and colleagues (Chapter 16), and context by Krank and Wall (Chapter 19) show that a wide range of affective and cognitive cues or triggers should be considered in such attempts. Such triggers could also be linked to cognitions about negative effects of addictive behaviors, which should have much more relevance to intervention effects if they become implicitly activated or at least more salient, as suggested by Wiers and colleagues (Chapter 22). If new associations are a focus of intervention, they must be assessed as potential mediators of program effects; chapters in this book suggest a variety of ways in which such associations can be measured (see Houben et al., Chapter 7; Stacy et al., Chapter 6).

Another approach to intervention in implicit systems focuses on attentional processes. Assessment of these processes to study prevention or treatment could lead to new insights about the origins of intervention effects. Most assessments of attentional biases in addictions have used varieties of modified Stroop and dot-probe tasks. In addition, several promising new tasks have been introduced, such as the "flicker paradigm" (see Bruce & Jones, Chapter 10; see also Waters & Sayette, Chapter 21, for an overview of tasks used in the area of smoking). Recent research has begun to focus on attentional subprocesses in addiction (initial orienting response vs. later disengagement; see Field et al., Chapter 11). This line of research also points to the importance of including other measures of brain functioning in attentional processes, such as eye movements (Field et al., Chapter 11), neuroimaging (Franken et al., Chapter 13), and psychophysiological measures (Mucha et al., Chapter 14). One interesting suggestion from recent studies in other areas of psychopathology is that an attentional retraining procedure may change an attentional bias, which could provide a direct way to influence the implicit cognitive system (see de Jong et al., Chapter 27; Fadardi et al., Chapter 9; and Field et al., Chapter 11). This is clearly an important new direction for intervention research. Indeed, initial results from different labs are promising (Wiers et al., submitted).

Although the issue of assessment inevitably emerges when considering new intervention possibilities, it is also relevant to understanding the effects of traditional interventions. Yet, the use of indirect assessment strategies or implicit cognition concepts to assess the influence of more traditional interventions has rarely been attempted. Exceptions include a study by Cox et al. (2002) on attentional bias as a predictor of treatment and a study by Wiers et al. (2005) that investigated effects of an expectancy challenge on implicit versus explicit alcohol cognitions. Further, to our knowledge no intervention study has yet included both measures of attentional bias and measures of implicit associations as potential mediators of program effects; use of both assessments together are rare in implicit cognition research even though the underlying concepts are theoretically related (e.g., Fadardi et al., Chapter 9).

Some chapters suggested how to integrate multiple systems in ways useful for intervention. One of several examples is the need to establish and consolidate more desirable alternatives to harmful habits (Cox et al., Chapter 17), probably through executive processes, in addition to forming new associations involving these alternatives, which may come to be triggered through an implicit system. A second example is the interplay between self-regulation or inhibitory processes and automatic processes (e.g., Bechara et al., Chapter 15; Curtin et al., Chapter 16), and the possibility of a transition from controlled to automatic processes in self-regulation (Palfai, Chapter 26). A transition in processing also needs to be addressed in the development of new associations of all types, whether between cues and goals or cues and other elements of an intervention. In addition, although they may bias cognition and channel behavior toward a certain direction, automatically activated associations acquired from an intervention may have much stronger effects if they involve goals that have motivational relevance to the individual, a point also relevant to Goldman et al.'s (Chapter 8) arguments. Indeed, motivation may be a cornerstone of successful treatment (Cox & Klinger, 2004; Miller & Rollnick, 2002) and prevention (Krank & Goldstein, Chapter 28; Sussman et al., 2004) programs,

which could in turn benefit from addressing associations in memory between motivational elements and a range of cues.

FUTURE CHALLENGES

The chapters in this book have suggested a number of clear, potentially fundamental directions for future research on basic processes as well as intervention. Although quite promising, this research area will continue to face challenges, many of which are common in other research areas. The challenges involve definitions, assessment, theory, and application.

Definitions

As De Houwer (Chapter 2) points out, there are definitional issues in this line of research. The title of this book focuses on implicit cognition only because it seemed to be the most descriptive, general term covering a diversity of approaches and disciplines, not because it was necessarily always the best term in any context. The editors agree with De Houwer that use of this and other terms in the domain needs to be accompanied by clear definitions.

The bottom line, perhaps, is that no single term is perfectly descriptive of the range of processes that do not originate from executive, control, or explicit cognitive processes. Whether a process is called implicit, automatic, unconscious, impulsive, non-declarative, procedural, or primed, any given research report needs to define what is meant in the context of that research. Readers of such reports should consider the full range of these types of processes, which include (1) those that may not involve any effects on consciousness or awareness, and (2) effects that originate in automatic/implicit forms of processing but get broadcast to conscious systems. Disposing of the latter process only in favor of the former may essentially throw out the baby with the bathwater, precluding study of one of the major phenomena.

Assessment

Assessment reliability, validity, and utility are fundamental to progress in this and other research areas on cognitive processes in addiction (see also Waters & Sayette, Chapter 21, and Sher's commentary, Chapter 30). To date, there are a number of promising assessment tools but no clear consensus on the best assessments. There is also little information about convergent validity among the various cognitive measures, that is, when the same research participants complete different measures. Existing multimethod support has usually come from discrete studies not the same study. Research that does not attempt multimethod support should at least provide documentation of reliability, and improving assessment should be a major goal in future research.

Despite the need for more assessment research, many indirect measures used in addiction research are identical or very similar to those well documented using diverse methods that uncover implicit processes in basic research. In several cases, the documentation is extensive. There are also instances, however, in which indirect measures used in addiction research are only slightly similar to previously validated indirect methods, may depart in fundamental ways from the spirit of indirect assessment, and also may have little or no direct support implicating implicit processes. When measures depart in any way from previously documented assessments of implicit processes, it should be the investigator's burden to delineate the difference and to study, or at least suggest, routes for validation. This suggestion does not imply that good indirect tests of implicit

processes cannot originate from addiction researchers but instead asks for attention to detail in documentation, as well as detail in the definition or sense of implicit process assessed.

Theory

There are a number of important areas of convergence in theory as outlined earlier in this chapter, but the development of theory is also faced with challenges. Although we, and many of the authors in this volume, view a multiple-systems theory as a useful way to address cognitive processes in addiction, some imply it is better to consider cognition as a unified entity akin to the general expectancy concept espoused by Goldman et al. (Chapter 8). Expectancies in research on problem behaviors were originally viewed in terms of quite explicit processes and if-then rules, as in applications of social learning and utility theories dating from the 1950s. In a different stream of research, Tolman (1932) and Bolles (1972) equated expectancies with a certain type of memory for predictive relations. Some scholars clearly fit this type of memory or relation under one specific neural system (see Berridge, 2001; Berridge & Robinson, Chapter 31; and Yin & Knowlton, Chapter 12), and a connectionist perspective could view Bolles and Tolman's expectancies as associations (acquired through an informational process) between behavior-outcome (R-S*) and cue-outcome (S-S*) elements (Stacy, 1995) rather than stored if-then rules. Yet, perhaps at a more global level of analysis expectancies can be defined as a general construct reflecting different anticipatory processes in the brain, as implied by Goldman and colleagues (Chapter 8; see also Krank & Wall, Chapter 19). Clearly the work on expectancies during the past two decades has generated valuable insights about cognitive processes in alcohol use and misuse in humans. As indicated by Goldman et al. (Chapter 8), "it is not the word *expectancy* that is of critical importance, but instead the recognition that the cognitive/information-processing system is in its essence a system shaped by evolutionary pressures to anticipate the future." For further theoretical development, it may prove useful to apply different names to the outcomes of different anticipatory and cognitive bias processes if these can be distinguished, even when at a more global level many of these different processes may be described as serving to anticipate the future (Berridge, 2001; Yin & Knowlton, Chapter 12).

Another theoretical challenge is understanding the development of implicit cognitions. This is an unsolved problem for basic research on memory, social cognition, and addiction. For example, although there are relevant laboratory studies in several literatures, no discipline can yet answer how associations in memory or attentional biases are established over time in humans outside of the lab. Applied to addiction, this question can be refined to ask how implicit cognition processes develop to influence behavior before and after substance use begins, and how these processes may change to either perpetuate or curtail the behavior.

A final example of a theoretical challenge is integration (also see commentary by Hermans & Van Gucht, Chapter 32). More specifically, research from multiple areas (neural circuits, learning, motivation, memory, attentional bias, social cognition, and experimental psychopathology) needs to become better integrated. As one example, research from each of these areas acknowledges the importance of connections or associations and triggering cues or circumstances, and this commonality could be more thoroughly applied toward a better integration relevant to addictive behaviors. In addition, some theories from basic research already attempt some integration, and these propositions should be addressed further in addiction research. For example, basic cognitive research has successfully integrated attention and memory concepts into single theories, either proposing that a fast-acting memory process provides codes that direct attention (Cowan, 1988) or by providing evidence that attention and memory responses originate from the same process assessed in different ways (Logan, 2002). Another example of a necessary integration is between cognitive and motivational research, whether studied at the neural or the behavior level. Much research in social cognition and experimental psychopathology provides evidence for cognitive or attentional biases that direct behavior and such evidence is often obtained without measuring motivational constructs. Cognitive and motivationally relevant variables need to be considered and measured together for a more complete understanding of their possibly parallel activation and effects on behavior. A recent example of the importance of assessing these constructs together comes from Winkielman et al. (2005). During a face-discrimination task (participants' task was to indicate gender), happy, neutral, or angry faces were presented subliminally (16 ms) before the neutral faces that were to be discriminated for gender. Priming with happy faces resulted in increased motivation to drink in the absence of changes in mood, in those participants who were thirsty. Interestingly, in participants who were not thirsty, the opposite happened (change in affect without effect on motivation to drink and drinking behavior). Hence, motivational state moderated the effects of implicit cognition on behavior and subjective mood.

Overall, the most thorough, and potentially useful, future integrations may require spanning the continuum from neural to behavioral levels of analysis and understanding the common ground in findings from different disciplines using diverse methods in both human and animal participants. Although some pioneering, integrative approaches to addiction certainly exist, as reflected in many of the chapters in this book, integration should become a much larger, multidisciplinary effort. Theory has not yet caught up to all of the available major findings from diverse, relevant disciplines.

Application

Many application potentials already have been addressed. These, however, pose a number of challenges. Most generally, implicit cognition research requires a more thorough translation of basic research findings into applicable, testable intervention procedures. One of many specific manifestations of this challenge is the translation of basic research on new associations into prevention or treatment interventions that target associations relevant to the intervention (Stacy et al., 2004). Another example is the need to translate (or reinterpret) existing intervention strategies in terms of implicit cognition processes, because some interventions already may be addressing these processes under a different name. If this translation is successful, then implicit cognition processes could be evaluated as potential mediators and predictors of program effects. Translations of basic research in many cases will require not only a thorough review and understanding of the relevant basic research literatures but also systematic program development (Sussman, 2001) and careful evaluation in collaboration with intervention specialists. Difficulties should not be surprising, because there are inevitable challenges with most any careful translation of basic research into intervention components. The hurdles must be addressed over time by a number of research programs to reach the full potential of this promising area.

FINAL THOUGHTS

Certain anonymous reviewers of the proposal for this book argued that something new is urgently needed in addiction research, both for theory and practice, and that this book would provide a much needed "new look" at the problem. Implicit cognition approaches and measures undoubtedly provide a different view of the processes that underlie addiction. The editors believe that the chapters in this book not only exemplify this "new look," but also illustrate a rare convergence of disciplines, levels of analysis, and independent methods. The diversity of multimethod support for multiple systems at dramatically different levels of analysis (e.g., neural to cognitive) may provide one of the most obvious advances over earlier cognitive research. This is important because most traditional research on cognitive predictors of addictive and other health behaviors has not provided multimethod support and often has relied on one class of techniques (e.g., explicit questions subjected to factor analysis), having rather minimal, or easily adjusted, criteria for falsifiability. Nevertheless, as with many assessments relevant to addiction, measures need to be better understood, improved, and in some cases better documented. Though this book provides a good sample of most of the available measures in this area, not all applicable measures and frameworks were represented and new assessments need to be explored.

Implicit cognition approaches have become an important stream of research in addiction and other areas of health behavior research. Undoubtedly, this research area provides new opportunities for advancing science and practice. The editors have enjoyed seeing many of the best scholars in the area come together in this single volume to learn from one another and share their best work. We hope their work will encourage others to join the effort.

REFERENCES

Berridge, K. C. (2001). Reward learning: Reinforcement, incentives, and expectations. In D. L. Medin (Ed.), *The psychology of learning and motivation: Advances in research and theory* (Vol. 40, pp. 223–278). San Diego, CA: Academic Press.

Bolles, R. C. (1975). *Theory of motivation* (2nd ed.). New York: Harper & Row.

Conrey, F. R., Sherman, J. W., Gawronski, B., Hugenberg, K., & Groom, C. J. (in press). Separating multiple processes in implicit social cognition: The quad model of implicit task performance. *Journal of Personality and Social Psychology*.

Cook, T., & Campbell, D. (1979). *Quasi-experimentation: Design and analysis issues for field settings*. Boston: Houghton Mifflin.

Cowan, N. (1988). Evolving conceptions of memory storage, selective attention, and their mutual constraints within the human information-processing system. *Psychological Bulletin, 104*(2), 163–191.

Cox, W. M., Hogan, L. M., Kristian, M. R., & Race, J. H. (2002). Alcohol attentional bias as predictor of alcohol abusers' treatment outcome. *Drug and Alcohol Dependence, 68*, 237–243.

Cox, W. M., & Klinger E. (Eds.). (2004). *Handbook of motivational counseling: Concepts, approaches, and assessment* (pp. 121–138). Chichester, UK: Wiley.

Kahneman, D. (2003). A perspective on judgment and choice: Mapping bounded rationality. *American Psychologist, 58*(9), 697–720.

Logan, G. D. (2002). An instance theory of attention and memory. *Psychological Review, 109*(2), 376–400.

Miller, W. R., & Rollnick, S. (2002). Motivational interviewing: Preparing people for change (2nd ed.). New York: Guilford.

Ryan, J. D., & Cohen, N. J. (2003). Evaluating the neuropsychological dissociation evidence for multiple memory systems. *Cognitive, Affective & Behavioral Neuroscience, 3*(3), 168–185.

Stacy, A. W. (1995). Memory association and ambiguous cues in models of alcohol and marijuana use. *Experimental & Clinical Psychopharmacology, 3*(2), 183–194.

Stacy, A. W., Ames, S. L., & Knowlton, B. J. (2004). Neurologically plausible distinctions in cognition relevant to drug use etiology and prevention. *Substance Use & Misuse, 39*, 1571–1623.

Sussman, S. (2001). *Handbook of program development in health behavior research and practice*. Thousand Oaks, CA: Sage.

Sussman, S., Earleywine, M., Wills, T., Cody, C., Biglan, T., Dent, C. W., et al. (2004). The motivation, skills, and decision-making model of "drug abuse" prevention. *Substance Use & Misuse, 39*, 1971–2016.

Tolman, E. C. (1932). *Purposive behavior in animals and men*. Oxford, UK: Appleton-Century.

Wiers, R. W., Cox, W. M., Field, M., Fadardi, J. S., Palfai, T. P., Schoenmakers, T., & Stacy, A. W. (submitted). The search for new ways to change implicit alcohol-related cognitions in heavy drinkers.

Wiers, R.W., Van de Luitgaarden, J., Van den Wildenberg, E., & Smulders, F. T. Y. (2005). Challenging implicit and explicit alcohol-related cognitions in young heavy drinkers. *Addiction, 100*, 806–819.

Winkielman, P., Berridge, K. C., & Wilbarger, J. L. (2005). Unconscious affective reactions to masked happy versus angry faces influence consumption behavior and judgments of value. *Personality and Social Psychology Bulletin, 31*, 121–135.

Name Index

Subject Index

About the Editors

Reinout W. Wiers is Research Associate Professor at Maastricht University, The Netherlands. He received his master's degree in psychonomics (experimental psychology and psychophysiology) at the University of Amsterdam (1992, with honors) and his PhD (with honors) in 1998 at the University of Amsterdam on cognitive and neuropsychological indicators of enhanced risk for alcoholism. He has published many articles in international journals on addiction research and in cognitive science. Wiers and colleagues were the first to apply the Implicit Association Test (IAT) to alcohol abuse and are currently focusing on theory, assessment, and practical applications of implicit drug-related cognitions with a grant from the Dutch National Science Foundation (N.W.O. VIDI grant). Stacy and Wiers are collaborating on an international project (N.W.O. Addiction and N.I.D.A.) on implicit cognition and prevention in high-risk youth.

Alan W. Stacy is currently the director of the USC Transdisciplinary Drug Abuse Prevention Research Center, funded by the National Institute on Drug Abuse. He is also an associate professor at the University of Southern California Department of Preventive Medicine. Stacy has published more than 80 peer-reviewed articles on addiction, focusing on cognitive models of drug use. He was one of the first investigators to apply implicit cognition approaches to the addiction area. His research on implicit cognition was recently acknowledged in the *10th Special Report to Congress on Alcohol and Health*.

About the Contributors

Susan L. Ames is a research associate at the Transdisciplinary Substance Abuse Prevention Research Center at the Institute for Health Promotion and Disease Prevention Research, Keck School of Medicine, University of Southern California. Her research emphasis is on the mediation of implicit processes and competing social, personality, and cultural constructs in the etiology and prevention of risk behaviors among at-risk youth and adults. Her research focuses on new assessments and prediction models of substance abuse as well as harm reduction strategies for addictive behaviors. Additional interests include neurobiological systems and brain structures associated with implicit processes and addictive behaviors.

Timothy B. Baker is a professor of psychology at the University of Wisconsin-Madison, and the director of research at the Center for Tobacco Research and Intervention in the University of Wisconsin Medical School. In addition, he is currently the editor of the *Journal of Abnormal Psychology*. Dr. Baker conducts research on the motivational mechanisms of addiction, and on psychosocial and pharmacologic treatments for addictive disorders, especially tobacco dependence.

Antoine Bechara is an associate professor of neurology at the University of Iowa Hospitals and Clinics. His research focuses on understanding the neural processes underlying how we make decisions and choices. He is known for his development of what became known as the Iowa Gambling Task (IGT), and for his studies of the decision-making capabilities of patients who have suffered injury to the ventromedial sector of their prefrontal cortex. His more recent research aims at integrating decision neuroscience with research in mental health, specifically substance addiction.

Kent C. Berridge is a professor in the Department of Psychology at the University of Michigan. His research interests span topics in affective neuroscience and hedonic psychology: emotion and motivation, brain systems for reward-liking and -wanting, neurobiology of pleasure, addiction, appetite, fear and stress and several other biopsychology topics, executive brain systems of action syntax, behavioral command systems, cognitive neuroscience, and animal neuroethology.

Cheryl D. Birch is a doctoral student in clinical psychology at Dalhousie University in Halifax, Nova Scotia, Canada. Her dissertation research, supervised by Dr. Sherry Stewart, concerns the impact of emotions and drinking motives on alcohol cognition and consumption behavior.

Jan Booij (MD, PhD) is a nuclear medicine physician and works as a staff member at the Department of Nuclear Medicine at the Academic Medical Center of the University of Amsterdam, The Netherlands. He is involved in preclinical as well as clinical research on neuroreceptor imaging with SPECT, with a special interest in disturbances of the central dopaminergic neurotransmission system in parkinsonism, schizophrenia, and addiction. In addition, he participates in large research projects on the possible neurotoxicity of ecstasy on the serotonergic system.

Brendan P. Bradley is a professor of clinical psychology research and a director of the Centre for the Study of Emotion and Motivation at the University of Southampton, United Kingdom. He previously held academic posts in the Department of Experimental Psychology, University of Cambridge, and the Institute of Psychiatry, London. He is joint editor of the *British Journal of Clinical Psychology* and consulting editor of *Emotion*. His research is primarily concerned with applying theoretical models and experimental methods from the fields of cognitive psychology and neuroscience to the study of addiction and emotional disorders, with a particular interest in anxiety and depression.

Gillian Bruce was awarded an MA with honors in psychology in 2001 from the University of Glasgow, Scotland. She subsequently completed an MSc in research methods in psychological science and currently holds an Economic and Social Research Council Postgraduate Studentship in the Psychology Department at the University of Glasgow. She is interested in the study of eye movements in relation to selective attention toward alcohol-related stimuli.

Mark Conner is a reader in applied social psychology at the Institute of Psychological Sciences, Leeds University, United Kingdom. His research interests include attitude-behavior models, and the social psychology of health behaviors. He has published widely in these areas.

Patricia J. Conrod is a clinical lecturer and "Action on Addiction" fellow at the National Addiction Centre, Institute of Psychiatry, King's College, London. Her research interests focus on biological and psychological approaches to personality in relation to the etiology of addictive behaviors, ranging from laboratory experimental studies to studies of targeted intervention and prevention.

Kate Coronges is a graduate research assistant at the Institute for Prevention Research at the University of Southern California. Her main research interest is in the interaction between social and cognitive domains. She is currently involved with projects applying social network analysis to theories of information processing.

Kenny Coventry is a reader in cognitive science at the University of Plymouth, United Kingdom. He has had a long-standing interest in why some gamblers lose control of their gambling behavior. In particular, he is interested in the role of decision making and its relationship with dissociation and arousal during the gambling process.

W. Miles Cox is professor of psychology of addictive behaviours, School of Psychology, University of Wales, Bangor, United Kingdom. He is the founding editor of *Psychology of Addictive Behaviors* (American Psychological Association [APA]) and past president of the APA Division on Addictions. His research and clinical activities focus on the interplay between drinkers' incentives in other life areas and their motivation to drink alcohol. A fellow in the American Psychological Association and a charter fellow in the American Psychological Society, Cox is the author of more than 100 publications, and the editor of four books.

Eveline A. Crone is an assistant professor of developmental psychology at Leiden University in The Netherlands. Her research focuses on neurocognitive development of control and self-regulation. She has developed child-friendly tasks based on the neuropsychological and cognitive literature (e.g., the Hungry Donkey Task, a child-version of the Iowa Gambling Task). To augment performance measures that are associated with self-regulation, she uses heart rate and skin conductance measures as indices of autonomic arousal, and neuroimaging techniques (fMRI) in children and adults.

John J. Curtin is an assistant professor in the Psychology Department at the University of Wisconsin-Madison. Dr. Curtin completed his undergraduate and graduate training at Johns Hopkins and Florida State Universities, respectively. He also completed a predoctoral clinical internship at Brown University. His research examines the contributions of affective and cognitive processes to alcohol and drug use, abuse, and dependence. His work draws heavily on current research in clinical psychology and cognitive and affective neuroscience.

Jack Darkes is a clinical psychologist and the associate director of the Alcohol and Substance Use Research Institute at the University of South Florida. He has published numerous articles and book chapters on the application of expectancy theory to substance use. His specific areas of interest are the mediational role of expectancies, the design and testing of expectancy theory–based strategies for behavior change, and the role of expectancy in postconsumption behavior. Dr. Darkes also serves as an assistant editor for the journal *Addiction* and on the editorial board of *Psychology of Addictive Behaviors*.

Jan De Houwer is professor of psychology at Ghent University in Belgium. Before that, he was a lecturer at the University of Southampton, United Kingdom, and obtained his PhD at the University of Leuven in Belgium. His main research interests are automatic affective processing and human associative learning, including the learning of preferences. One of his main contributions to research on automatic affective processing has been the development of the Extrinsic Affective Simon Task (EAST).

Peter J. de Jong is professor of experimental psychopathology at the University of Groningen, The Netherlands. The main focus of his research is on the role of automatic versus controlled cognitive processes in the origin and maintenance of various forms of psychopathology including anxiety disorders, eating disorders, and addiction.

Roland Deutsch is currently a postdoctoral researcher at the Ohio State University. In 2003, he received his PhD in social psychology from the University of Würzburg, Germany. His research is focused on evaluative learning, automatic evaluation, and the automatization of social-cognitive skills. In collaboration with Fritz Strack, he has developed a dual-system model of social cognition and behavior.

Jonathan St. B. T. Evans is professor of cognitive psychology at the University of Plymouth, United Kingdom. Since the early 1970s, he has conducted a major research program into thinking, reasoning, and decision making. He has over 150 scientific publications, which include numerous experimental studies of reasoning and judgment. He has made particular study of cognitive biases and established some of the major phenomena. He has also been one of the major authors contributing to the development of contemporary dual-process theories of thinking and reasoning.

Javad S. Fadardi is assistant professor of psychology at Ferdowsi University of Mashhad, Iran. His research interests are linked to motivational bases of implicit cognitive processes involved in various types of psychopathology and health behaviors. He completed his BA and MA studies in clinical and health psychology in Iran, and his PhD and postdoctoral studies in the United Kingdom. He is a member of the Iranian Psychological Association and has published several articles and books in both Persian and English.

Matt Field is a lecturer in psychology at the University of Liverpool, United Kingdom. He is a member of the British Association for Psychopharmacology and his research interests include cognitive and learning mechanisms in substance abuse and addiction. He obtained his DPhil from the University of Sussex in 2001 while under the supervision of Professor Theodora Duka, and he subsequently worked as a research fellow at the University of Southampton with Professors Karin Mogg and Brendan P. Bradley.

Mark T. Fillmore is an associate professor of psychology at the University of Kentucky. His research examines how acute drug effects on basic cognitive and behavioral processes play a role in the development of substance abuse and drug addiction. His work combines measures of cognitive functions with conventional assessments of drug-abuse liability in studies of individuals with and without histories of drug abuse. He has published extensively in the substance-abuse field and is an active member of several societies, including the American Psychological Association and the College on Problems of Drug Dependence.

Ingmar H. A. Franken is assistant professor at the Institute of Psychology of the Erasmus University, Rotterdam, The Netherlands. He trained as a clinical psychologist at Maastricht University. He completed his doctorate on cognitive and psychopharmacological mechanisms of drug craving at the Faculty of Medicine of the University of Amsterdam. His major research interest is the role of the reward system in psychopathology and personality. More specific topics include addiction, psychopharmacology and psychophysiology of reward, and reward-based decision making.

Mark S. Goldman is associate director of the National Institute on Alcohol Abuse and Alcoholism (NIAAA), and Distinguished Research Professor and director of the Alcohol and Substance Use Research Institute at University of South Florida (USF). He received his PhD in January 1972 from Rutgers University, and has been on the faculty at Wayne State University (1973–1985) and USF (since 1985). He is a Fellow of Divisions 3, 6, 12, 28, and 50, and a member of Division 40 of the American Psychological Association. In 1992, he received a MERIT Award from the NIAAA.

Abby L. Goldstein is currently an intern at the Brown University Clinical Psychology Training Consortium and is completing her PhD at York University in Toronto, Ontario, Canada. Ms. Goldstein's research interests include the cognitive and behavioral choice mechanisms underlying alcohol use and the development and evaluation of brief interventions for substance abuse and violence.

Jerry L. Grenard is a graduate research assistant at the Institute for Health Promotion and Disease Prevention Research at the University of Southern California. His specific interest is in memory associations and implicit cognition as applied to drug-abuse prevention among adolescents.

Dirk Hermans is a professor of psychology at the Center for the Psychology of Learning and Experimental Psychopathology, Department of Psychology, University of Leuven, Belgium. His research work focuses on associative and memory processes and their impact on the etiology and maintenance of emotional disorders (anxiety and depression).

Katrijn Houben is currently finishing her PhD at the University of Maastricht, The Netherlands, under the supervision of Dr. Reinout Wiers. The main focus of her project was investigating the role of implicit and explicit cognitions in the etiology and maintenance of addictive behaviors (primarily alcohol addiction). During this period, she mainly concentrated on the value of implicit techniques to assess alcohol-related cognitions. Her research interests include further development and validation of implicit measurement techniques that can be applied in addiction research and studying models of addiction etiology.

Barry T. Jones's undergraduate and postgraduate degrees were awarded by Durham and Edinburgh Universities in the United Kingdom. His early research was in the area of rat and monkey vision and his first faculty appointment was as lecturer in psychology at St. Andrews University in Scotland. He was subsequently given a personal chair in psychology at Glasgow University, also in Scotland, where he currently remains. After a midcareer shift in research interests to modeling clinical decision making in the mental health sector, he now researches the cognitions of the clients themselves— particularly in relation to alcohol, cannabis, and sleep problems.

Merel Kindt is professor of experimental clinical psychology at the University of Amsterdam, The Netherlands. Her research focuses on experimental models of anxiety disorders such as Posttraumatic Stress Disorder and Obsessive-Compulsive Disorder, information-processing and anxiety disorders, emotional memory, and mechanisms of change to reduce emotional disorders.

Eric Klinger is professor of psychology at the University of Minnesota, Morris and (adjunct) Minneapolis. His research activities focus on motivational processes, especially as these and emotional processes influence attention, recall, and the content of thoughts and dreams. He has contributed to basic theory of motivation and its extension to substance use, treatment of alcoholism, and depression. A fellow of the American Association for the Advancement of Science and of the American Psychological Association, and a charter fellow of the American

Psychological Society, Klinger is the author of more than 100 publications, including four books.

Barbara J. Knowlton received her BA in psychology in 1984 from Johns Hopkins University, where she was awarded the G. Stanley Hall prize. She received her PhD in neuroscience from Stanford University in 1990. In 1995, she was appointed assistant professor in the University of California, Los Angeles, Psychology Department and was promoted to associate professor with tenure in 2001. Since 2004, Her current research focuses on memory systems in the brain. Specific projects include functional neuroimaging studies of implicit, or unconscious, learning and neuroimaging studies of the encoding and retrieval of episodic memories.

Marvin D. Krank is dean of graduate studies and professor of psychology at the University of British Columbia Okanagan, Canada. Dr. Krank's research focuses on the role of learning and cognition in substance abuse. His past work includes studies of learning and drug tolerance, models of addiction, and adolescent substance-use initiation. With colleagues, including Anne-Marie Wall and Abby Goldstein, he recently completed data collection for the Project on Adolescent Trajectories and Health (PATH). PATH is a 3-year longitudinal study of the social and cognitive antecedents of adolescent risk-taking behaviors and their health consequences.

Rebecca J. Lawton is senior lecturer in health psychology at the Institute of Psychological Sciences, University of Leeds in the United Kingdom. Lawton is also a chartered health psychologist. Her research interests include understanding and predicting risky health and safety behaviors. She has published widely in this area in both mainstream and applied journals. She has also held grants funded by the Economic and Social Research Council, the National Health Service Regional, and the Department of Health.

G. Alan Marlatt is professor of psychology and director of the Addictive Behaviors Research Center at the University of Washington. He received his PhD in clinical psychology from Indiana University in 1968. After serving on the faculties of the University of British Columbia, Canada (1968–1969), and the University of Wisconsin (1969–1972), he joined the University of Washington faculty in the fall of 1972. His major focus in both research and clinical work is the field of addictive behaviors.

Danielle E. McCarthy is a clinical psychology PhD candidate working under the supervision of Timothy Baker, PhD, at the University of Wisconsin–Madison. She has been awarded pilot research grants to study the effects of nicotine dependence, nicotine abstinence, and stress on attention and to explore the feasibility of an intensive treatment for smokers adapted from exposure and response prevention treatments for anxiety. She also conducts research exploring smoking-cessation treatment mediation and nicotine-withdrawal dynamics at the University of Wisconsin Medical School Center for Tobacco Research and Intervention.

Cathy L. McEvoy is a professor of aging studies at the University of South Florida. Her research focuses on memory and aging, emphasizing how individuals use preexisting knowledge to augment age-related declines in memory for recently experienced information. Normal aging is marked by decrements in ability to recall recent experiences, while maintaining relatively stable knowledge and vocabulary, and Dr. McEvoy's research suggests that this stable knowledge becomes critical to remembering recent events as people age. Other research has focused on knowledge utilization in deaf and hearing-impaired adults.

Karin Mogg is a professor of psychology at the University of Southampton, United Kingdom, and a director of the Centre for the Study of Emotion and Motivation. Her main research interests concern cognitive processes in emotional disorders and addiction, and her work is largely supported by the Wellcome Trust. Recent awards and appointments include Wellcome Senior Research Fellow, editor of the *British Journal of Clinical Psychology*, and consulting editor for the *Journal of Abnormal Psychology*. Previously, she worked in the Department of Experimental Psychology, University of Cambridge, and also in London (Guy's and St. George's Hospitals) in both clinical and research settings.

Ronald Mucha is an addiction scientist living in Stuttgart, Germany, with research based in the Department of Psychology, University of Würzburg. Trained in physiological psychology and learning at the University of British Columbia and in behavioral pharmacology and addiction at the University of Toronto, he has conducted systematic research on drug dependence using experimental models ranging from isolated tissue out of the guinea pig, to rats in Skinner boxes, to schoolchildren learning to smoke. His numerous international publications reflect a specific interest in adaptation and learning produced by substances of abuse and how these modulate the risk of future drug consumption. He teaches courses on these topics at the University of Würzburg and at the Institute of Medical Psychology, University of Tübingen."

Douglas L. Nelson is a Distinguished Research Professor in the Department of Psychology at the University of South Florida. His research focuses on memory and cognition, with a specific emphasis on the influence of preexisting knowledge on the recall and recognition of recently experienced information. This work is formalized in a model of cued recall and recognition called PIER, for Processing Implicit and Explicit Representations. This model has been applied to understand the influences of substance abuse, aging, and deafness on memory.

Xavier Noel is currently a research assistant and clinical psychologist at the Clinic of Addictions of the Brugmann University hospital, Brussels, Belgium. He is trained in cognitive-behavior therapy and systemic therapy and he received his PhD in cognitive psychopathology from the University of Liège, Belgium. His research is focused on executive functioning deficits and cognitive biases that are involved in the development of dependence on alcohol, marijuana, tobacco, and the relapse. He is currently exploring the relationship between inhibition functions, attentional biases, and clinical impulsivity in individuals with alcoholism.

Brian D. Ostafin received his doctorate in clinical psychology from Boston University in 2004. He currently holds a postdoctoral fellowship in the Addictive Behaviors Research Center at the University of Washington Department of Psychology. His research interests revolve around the role of automatic affective processes in addictive behavior.

Tibor P. Palfai is an associate professor of psychology at Boston University who studies psychological mechanisms underlying health behavior change. His research is primarily on hazardous/harmful alcohol use among young adults. The goals of this work are to (1) clarify the influence of cognitive-motivational factors on alcohol-use patterns, (2) understand the effects of contextual cues on alcohol-related self-regulatory processes, and (3) construct intervention strategies to promote change in hazardous/harmful drinking.

Paul Pauli has been professor and chair of biological psychology, clinical psychology, and psychotherapy at the University of Würzburg, Germany, since 2001. Research

interests include anxiety disorders, affective disorders, somatoform disorders, and addiction as well as emotional influences on cognitive processes.

Megan E. Piper is a doctoral candidate in the clinical psychology program at the University of Wisconsin. She has been working for the University of Wisconsin's Center for Tobacco Research and Intervention since 1999. Piper's main research interests include defining, measuring, and understanding tobacco dependence; characterizing the affective components of tobacco dependence; and understanding gender differences in tobacco dependence. She completed her BA in chemistry at Carleton College, Minnesota, and her MA in clinical psychology at Miami University in Florida.

Constantine X. Poulos is a senior scientist in the Neuroscience Department at the Center for Addiction and Mental Health and professor of psychology at the University of Toronto, Ontario, Canada. His primary research interests are behavioral homeostasis and drug tolerance, addictions, memory processes, and impulsivity.

Andrew Prestwich is a senior research officer in the Department of Psychology at the University of Essex, United Kingdom. His research interests cover a diverse range of topics within social and health psychology and include implicit social cognition and health behavior promotion. Previously he worked in the Department of Experimental Psychology, University of Oxford, as departmental lecturer in social psychology. He completed his doctoral thesis on implementation intentions in September 2003.

Richard R. Reich, PhD, is the project coordinator of cognitive assessment at the Alcohol and Substance Use Research Institute (ASURI) and adjunct professor of psychology, University of South Florida. His research examines cognitive processes involved in alcohol expectancies. His current work investigates contextual factors resulting in alcohol-expectancy activation. He has presented his research at several departmental brown-bag and ASURI meetings. Dr. Reich has served as a reviewer for several journals in the alcohol field and he is a current member of the Research Society on Alcoholism.

Terry E. Robinson received his PhD from the University of Western Ontario, Canada, and in 1978 he moved to the University of Michigan, where he is now the Elliot S. Valenstein Collegiate Professor of Behavioral Neuroscience and professor of psychology. He is director of the National Institute on Drug Abuse Training Program in Neuroscience at Michigan, and editor-in-chief of the journal *Behavioural Brain Research*. Dr. Robinson is known internationally for his research concerning the behavioral and neurobiological consequences of repeated drug use, and the implications of these for addiction.

Anne Roefs is a postdoctoral research fellow at the Department of Experimental Psychology at Maastricht University, The Netherlands. Her research is in the field of applied cognitive psychology. For her PhD dissertation, her research concerned relatively automatic associations with food in obesity and eating disorders. In the next few years, her research will be about selective visual attention and body image.

Michael A. Sayette is professor of psychology at the University of Pittsburgh, with a secondary appointment as professor of psychiatry. His research examines cognitive, affective, and social processes in addiction, with an emphasis on tobacco and alcohol. His current work investigates (1) contextual factors affecting the experience of cigarette craving, (2) emotional factors influencing the prediction of future craving states and recall of past craving states, and (3) effects of alcohol on social bonding processes.

Dr. Sayette sits on several journal editorial boards and serves, or has served, as associate editor of the *Journal of Abnormal Psychology* and *Psychology of Addictive Behaviors*.

Kenneth J. Sher is Curators' Professor in the Department of Psychological Sciences at the University of Missouri–Columbia, where he directs the Alcohol Research Training Program and has been conducting research in the etiology and consequences of alcohol dependence for more than 25 years. He currently holds a MERIT award from the National Institute on Alcohol Abuse and Alcoholism (NIAAA) and is a member of NIAAA's National Advisory Council. He is a former associate editor of the *Journal of Abnormal Psychology* and *Psychological Bulletin* and a past president of the Society for a Science of Clinical Psychology.

Fren T. Y. Smulders is assistant professor at the Department of Experimental Psychology, Faculty of Psychology, at the University of Maastricht, The Netherlands. He obtained his PhD at the University of Amsterdam in 1993 with a dissertation on the effects of aging on information-processing stages and event-related brain potentials. Present research interests include attention and information processing and their modulation by emotion and personality.

Sherry H. Stewart is professor of psychology, psychiatry, and community health and epidemiology at Dalhousie University in Halifax, Nova Scotia, Canada. She is currently coordinator of the doctoral training program in clinical psychology at Dalhousie. She has published more than 100 journal articles, several book chapters, and one book. She holds a prestigious Investigator Award from the Canadian Institutes of Health Research to support her research on different pathways to substance abuse and comorbid mental health problems.

Fritz Strack is professor of psychology at the University of Würzburg, Germany. His research interests are in the domains of social judgment, cognition, and emotion. Together with Roland Deutsch he has received the Society for Personality and Social Psychology Theoretical Innovation Prize for their joint article "Reflective and Impulsive Determinants of Social Behavior." He is a former editor of the *European Journal of Social Psychology* and holds honorary memberships in several learned societies.

Wim van den Brink is a professor of psychiatry and addiction at the Academic Medical Center at the University of Amsterdam, The Netherlands, and director of the Amsterdam Institute for Addiction Research. In the last decade, his clinical epidemiological interests have been complemented with biological research regarding the underlying mechanisms of addiction and addiction treatment effectiveness. Since 1986, he has been involved in more than 300 scientific publications and more than 30 book chapters.

Dinska Van Gucht is a PhD student, funded by the Geoconcertcerde Onderzoeks Actie (GOA) that is based on the collaboration of two research groups in the Department of Psychology, University of Leuven, Belgium; the Center for the Psychology of Learning and Experimental Psychopathology; and the Research Group for Stress, Health and Well-Being. The project she is working on focuses on Pavlovian conditioning and more specifically on extinction and the return of conditioned responses. She is particularly interested in these processes with regard to health-related behaviors, for instance, smoking.

Muriel Vogel-Sprott is Distinguished Professor Emerita and adjunct research professor in the Department of Psychology, University of Waterloo, Ontario, Canada. Her research focuses broadly on factors that alter the behavioral and cognitive impact of alcohol and other drugs. Her studies examine the effects of environmental consequences of drug-induced behavioral impairment and ensuing learned expectancies that foster tolerance, as well as factors that alter the intensity of drug effects on particular cognitive processes governing behavior. Her publications include a book on behavioral tolerance to alcohol and its implications for addiction, as well as numerous book chapters, research papers, and monographs.

Anne-Marie Wall is an associate professor in the Department of Psychology at York University, Ontario, Canada. Her research focuses on substance use and abuse and its overlap with various forms of violence and health-compromising behaviors. Ongoing projects are directed at understanding familial, environmental, societal, and cognitive determinants of addictive behaviors and co-occurring maladaptive behavioral patterns.

Andrew J. Waters is an assistant professor in the Department of Behavioral Science at the University of Texas M. D. Anderson Cancer Center. His research examines cognitive processes in smoking initiation and smoking cessation. Dr. Waters conducts laboratory studies that examine the clinical utility of computerized cognitive tasks administered in smoking-cessation studies. He also conducts studies using handheld computers in an Ecological Momentary Assessment setting, and studies that investigate genetic associations with cognitive measures.

Peter Weyers has served as a research associate in the Department of Psychology, University of Würzburg, Germany, since 1989. His research interests include emotional facial expressions, addiction, stress and coping, and Attention Deficit Hyperactivity Disorder.

Henry H. Yin is currently a postdoctoral fellow at the Laboratory for Integrative

Neuroscience, National Institute of Alcohol Abuse and Addiction. He received his PhD in cognitive neuroscience from the University of California, Los Angeles. His work in graduate school focused on the role of the striatum in the acquisition and performance of goal-directed actions, and he is currently conducting research on the pharmacological modulation of synaptic transmission and plasticity in the striatum.

Martin Zack is a scientist in the Neuroscience Department at the Centre for Addiction and Mental Health and assistant professor of pharmacology at the University of Toronto, Ontario, Canada. His research focuses on pharmacological modulation of addiction-related semantic memory networks. Most of his work deals with problem gambling and problem drinking. The goal of this research is to advance the development of medications for these and other addictive disorders by examining how specific neurochemical probes influence cognitive processes related to addictive motivation.

Corien Zijlstra is a PhD student in the Department of Nuclear Medicine at the Academic Medical Center of Amsterdam. In December 2002, she graduated in neuropsychology (MSc) from Maastricht University, The Netherlands. Currently she is working on her thesis *Dopamine and Opiate Craving in the Human Brain: An Imaging Approach*. In this study, both SPECT and fMRI (3T) are used to relate instant and chronic drug-craving to the d_2 receptor density and activity, and brain activity in general.